T0127856

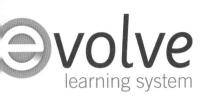

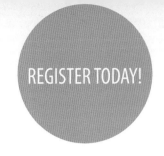

REGISTER TODAY!

To access the free Evolve Resources, visit:

http://evolve.elsevier.com/Sahrmann/extremities/

Evolve Student Learning Resources for Sahrmann: Movement System Impairment Syndromes of the Extremities, Cervical and Thoracic Spines *offers the following features:*

- **Additional Resources:** Printable versions of the appendices

- **References:** End of chapter references linked to Medline

- **Video:** Video simulations to supplement the chapters

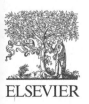

ELSEVIER

MOVEMENT SYSTEM IMPAIRMENT SYNDROMES
of the Extremities, Cervical and Thoracic Spines

Shirley Sahrmann and Associates

Shirley A. Sahrmann, PT, PhD, FAPTA
Professor, Physical Therapy, Neurology, Cell Biology & Physiology
Program in Physical Therapy
Washington University School of Medicine
St. Louis, Missouri

ELSEVIER
MOSBY

3251 Riverport Lane
St. Louis, Missouri 63043

MOVEMENT SYSTEM IMPAIRMENT SYNDROMES OF
THE EXTREMITIES, CERVICAL AND THORACIC SPINES
Copyright © 2011 by Mosby, Inc., an affiliate of Elsevier Inc.

ISBN: 978-0-323-05342-6

No part of this publication may be reproduced or transmitted in any form or by any means, electronic or mechanical, including photocopying, recording, or any information storage and retrieval system, without permission in writing from the publisher. Details on how to seek permission, further information about the Publisher's permissions policies and our arrangements with organizations such as the Copyright Clearance Center and the Copyright Licensing Agency, can be found at our website: www.elsevier.com/permissions.

This book and the individual contributions contained in it are protected under copyright by the Publisher (other than as may be noted herein).

Notices

Knowledge and best practice in this field are constantly changing. As new research and experience broaden our understanding, changes in research methods, professional practices, or medical treatment may become necessary.

Practitioners and researchers must always rely on their own experience and knowledge in evaluating and using any information, methods, compounds, or experiments described herein. In using such information or methods they should be mindful of their own safety and the safety of others, including parties for whom they have a professional responsibility.

With respect to any drug or pharmaceutical products identified, readers are advised to check the most current information provided (i) on procedures featured or (ii) by the manufacturer of each product to be administered, to verify the recommended dose or formula, the method and duration of administration, and contraindications. It is the responsibility of practitioners, relying on their own experience and knowledge of their patients, to make diagnoses, to determine dosages and the best treatment for each individual patient, and to take all appropriate safety precautions.

To the fullest extent of the law, neither the Publisher nor the authors, contributors, or editors, assume any liability for any injury and/or damage to persons or property as a matter of products liability, negligence or otherwise, or from any use or operation of any methods, products, instructions, or ideas contained in the material herein.

Library of Congress Cataloging-in-Publication Data
Movement system impairment syndromes of the extremities, cervical, and thoracic spines / [edited by] Shirley A. Sahrmann.
     p. ; cm.
  Includes bibliographical references and index.
  ISBN 978-0-323-05342-6 (hardcover : alk. paper)
  1. Movement disorders—Physical therapy.   2. Cervical vertebrae—Diseases—Physical therapy.   3. Thoracic vertebrae—Diseases—Physical therapy.   4. Extremities (Anatomy)—Diseases—Physical therapy.   I. Sahrmann, Shirley.
  [DNLM: 1. Movement Disorders.   2. Cervical Vertebrae–physiopathology.   3. Extremities—physiopathology.   4. Thoracic Vertebrae—physiopathology.   WL 390]
  RC376.5.M694 2011
  616.8'3—dc22

                                                                                    2010040828

Vice President and Publisher: Linda Duncan
Executive Editor: Kathryn Falk
Senior Developmental Editor: Christie M. Hart
Publishing Services Manager: Julie Eddy
Senior Project Manager: Laura Loveall
Designer: Margaret Reid

Printed in India

Last digit is the print number: 9 8 7

Working together to grow
libraries in developing countries

www.elsevier.com | www.bookaid.org | www.sabre.org

ELSEVIER   BOOK AID International   Sabre Foundation

*This book is dedicated to members of my family, both living and deceased,
both two-legged and four-legged, whether related by blood or love,
who have made my life so secure, happy, fulfilled, and productive.
You have made what many consider a lifetime of work to be
instead an amazing lifelong journey of joy.*

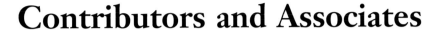# Contributors and Associates

Nancy Bloom, PT, DPT, MSOT
Assistant Professor
Program in Physical Therapy and Department of
    Orthopaedics
Washington University School of Medicine
St. Louis, Missouri

Cheryl Caldwell, PT, DPT, CHT
Assistant Professor
Program in Physical Therapy and Department of
    Orthopaedics
Washington University School of Medicine
St. Louis, Missouri

Suzy L. Cornbleet, PT, DPT
Assistant Professor
Program in Physical Therapy and Department of
    Orthopaedics
Washington University School of Medicine
St. Louis, Missouri

Mary K. Hastings, PT, DPT, ATC
Assistant Professor
Program in Physical Therapy and Department of
    Orthopaedics
Washington University School of Medicine
St. Louis, Missouri

Marcie Harris-Hayes, PT, DPT, MSCI, OCS
Assistant Professor
Program in Physical Therapy and Department of
    Orthopaedics
Washington University School of Medicine
St. Louis, Missouri

Gregory W. Holtzman, PT, DPT
Assistant Professor
Program in Physical Therapy and Department of
    Orthopaedics
Washington University School of Medicine
St. Louis, Missouri

Renee Ivens, PT, DPT
Assistant Professor
Program in Physical Therapy and Department of
    Orthopaedics
Washington University School of Medicine
St. Louis, Missouri

Lynnette Khoo-Summers, PT, DPT
Assistant Professor
Program in Physical Therapy and Department of
    Orthopaedics
Washington University School of Medicine
St. Louis, Missouri

Mary Kate McDonnell, PT, DPT, OCS
Associate Director of Residencies and Fellowships
Assistant Professor
Program in Physical Therapy and Department of
    Orthopaedics
Washington University School of Medicine
St. Louis, Missouri

Theresa Spitznagle, PT, DPT, WCS
Assistant Professor
Program in Physical Therapy and Obstetrics &
    Gynecology
Coordinator of Clinical Residency in Women's Health
Washington University School of Medicine
St. Louis, Missouri

Foreword

Recently, I was sharing my enthusiasm with a nonmedical friend about attending a research meeting with Dr. Shirley Sahrmann. I was trying to think of a way to describe the magnitude of her influence on the "world" of musculoskeletal medicine. The single thing I came up with was, "Her book has been published in seven different languages." My friend understood. I have been fortunate to work with and learn from an international rock star and her band, the Program in Physical Therapy at Washington University School of Medicine.

Movement is the activity that every patient with a musculoskeletal impairment wants to resume without pain and restriction. The assessment of movement has been at the core of my own training. However, early on, I recognized that there were several theories of thought without substantiation across the entire musculoskeletal system. It was obvious that to pursue the idea of reliably describing specific movement patterns in a clinical setting would take at least an entire career. Fortunately, Dr. Sahrmann has spent her career doing just that. *Movement System Impairment Syndromes of the Extremities, Cervical and Thoracic Spines* provides practitioners of musculoskeletal medicine with the theory and pictorials to describe movement impairments of the cervical and thoracic spine and extremities. This book extends the work of her preceding text, *Diagnosis and Treatment of Movement Impairment Syndromes*. Together the two books provide readers with a base of information to describe movement impairments across the entire musculoskeletal system.

A movement diagnosis is not a diagnosis that is uniformly established and then conveyed to the patient with a musculoskeletal disorder. With the advancement of technology and imaging, much attention is given to a structural injury or degenerative condition as the source of dysfunction and pain. Indeed, these advanced imaging techniques have promoted musculoskeletal evaluation and interventions. However, most are static images. To completely describe the patient with a musculoskeletal disorder, several observations should be summarized to determine the diagnosis. These include the clinical distribution and quality of symptoms, structural findings on imaging, and the movement observations. Certainly, the psychosocial setting in which all of these exist is important because the psychosocial attributes can affect any and all of these observations. In the setting of normal structural findings on imaging, the movement diagnosis is imperative. Unfortunately, this later diagnosis is not always clarified and instead the patient is told "there is nothing wrong" to "you're aging." As a result, movement retraining opportunities are missed, and the patient may go on to develop a chronic condition that could have been avoided.

Movement System Impairment Syndromes of the Extremities, Cervical and Thoracic Spines provides musculoskeletal healthcare practitioners a detailed method of examination to describe movement patterns and impairments in the clinical setting. Further, the spectrum of practitioners can benefit from reading and studying this work. Physical therapists that utilize the movement impairment system to diagnose and treat patients daily now have a detailed resource for examining and providing intervention for the cervical and thoracic spines and extremities. Other healthcare providers, (physicians, chiropractors, nurse practitioners, physician assistants, athletic trainers, and massage therapists) who provide musculoskeletal care can benefit from studying the movement impairment method of assessment. These latter practitioners may not have the same level of experience as physical therapists, but all have a unique background that can utilize this method of assessment in some way. The specificity of the description of the impairment leads to one of the key factors for intervention, specificity. Patients bring unique factors to even common impairments. As a result, a specific intervention is essential to maximize outcome. The movement impairment system of analysis provides that specificity.

Healthcare providers in musculoskeletal medicine have been waiting for *Movement System Impairment Syndromes of the Extremities, Cervical and Thoracic Spines*. The contents are worthy of the anticipated arrival.

Congratulations to Dr. Sahrmann and the faculty of Washington University School of Medicine Program in Physical Therapy. You have advanced musculoskeletal medicine one step further.

Heidi Prather, DO
Associate Professor
Chief of Section, Physical Medicine and Rehabilitation
Departments of Orthopaedic Surgery and Neurology
Washington University School of Medicine
St. Louis, Missouri

Preface

Alignment is the foundation for optimal movement and musculoskeletal health requires optimal movement to prevent or minimize painful movement syndromes.

The overall objectives of this book are the following:

1. Describe parts of the movement system and processes resulting in musculoskeletal pain syndromes.
2. Describe movement system syndromes.
3. Promote the importance of using diagnostic labels for movement system dysfunctions.
4. Create awareness that movement system syndromes are not single, isolated events but are part of a progressive condition affected by lifestyle that should be managed accordingly.
5. Describe the importance of assessing alignment, movement patterns of the painful region, and the effect of movements of other body segments on the painful region.
6. Promote the importance of monitoring the development and optimal function of the movement system throughout the lifespan.

Over the past 50 to 60 years, major transitions have occurred in knowledge, expectations, and attitudes regarding health. The transitions have been to (1) an acceptance of the critical importance of lifestyle, (2) an expectation that any pain and problem can be alleviated or fixed, and (3) an attitude that passive treatment may be as effective as active correction. Clearly, there is inconsistency between understanding that lifestyle is a major factor in health and the belief that any condition is not only amenable to passive treatment but is also effectively treated by medication. Because the transitions have taken place over many years, few people are aware of the extent of changes in lifestyle and expectations of medical care. The lack of awareness is consistent with the principle that everything is relative. People do not appreciate that our current lifestyle requires minimal physical activity or that we consume more and less healthier types of food than in years past. When I was growing up in the 1940s and 1950s, the prevailing belief was that whatever affected an individual's health was inevitable and uncontrollable. Heart attacks just happened. You developed high blood pressure or cancer.

Being overweight, or "pleasingly plump" as my Grandmother would say, might detract a bit from your appearance but not your health. In fact I am sure my Grandmother believed, "a little meat on your bones" made you healthier. Health insurance was just beginning to be provided by your employer, and the coverage did not include visits to the doctor's office. Thus you only went to the doctor if you were so sick you were unable to function. In fact, the insurance covered hospitalization but not office visits. When you consulted a physician, you hoped that he could diagnose the condition and provide some type of treatment. The feeling of inevitability of disease was consistent with the effects of the Great Depression and World War II. Both of these events created a feeling that many aspects of life were beyond your control, and thus the inevitability of medical problems was accepted. In addition, the cost of medical care served as another reason to limit visits to the physician, except if you had a serious problem. Clearly, the depth of knowledge of many systemic illnesses and the laboratory methods of identifying contributing or underlying factors was not known at that time.

From my perspective, the initial awareness of lifestyle as a factor in health was the identification of the relationship between smoking and lung cancer. When this fact was proclaimed by the Surgeon General in 1964,[1] it prompted additional investigations of the other numerous body systems affected by smoking. A real pioneer in recognizing and investigating the relationship between health and lifestyle, particularly the role of exercise, was John O. Holloszy, MD, at Washington University School of Medicine in St. Louis. His many studies[2-5] were a clear foundation for demonstrating that cardiovascular and metabolic conditions were related to insufficient exercise and dietary factors. Unfortunately, but as might be expected, humankind chose the path of least resistance. Medications were developed to treat the very conditions that Dr. Holloszy showed could be addressed by exercise and diet. But, instead of the medical community advocating active participation, the predictable path of passive consumption of medication was promoted and accepted. We have now reached a point where the numbers of overweight, obese, and inactive people and their associated medical problems have affected the economy of our country.

Why this long introduction to a book about musculoskeletal pain? I believe a parallel exists in what has happened to our metabolic and cardiovascular systems and what is happening to the musculoskeletal and/or movement system. Today, there is a great emphasis, although not followed by a majority of the population, on appropriate eating habits and adequate exercise. Again, in my younger days, if you asked the doctor about what food to eat or whether to take a vitamin pill, the attitude was not to worry because it really does not matter. Hardly a day goes by without an article being published about the importance of exercise in helping prevent or modify conditions ranging from diabetes and cancer to dementia.

But this all-important activity is not a common recommendation by physicians. Musculoskeletal pain is treated as if each episode is an isolated temporary inflammatory event rather than a progressive condition that is greatly influenced by lifestyle. Just as the prevailing behavior, if not belief, is that we can eat anything or as much as we want, there is a belief that we can sit or move in any way we want. Unfortunately, nothing could be farther from the truth. We get by with poor postural and movement habits for a while just like the consequences of smoking and hypertension take a while to cause health problems.

The sitting posture of children has only gotten worse since my initial comments 10 years ago in the first volume of this book. Sitting on the middle of the lumbar spine instead of sitting up straight with pressure on the ischial tuberosities is harmful to the spine and probably also the hip. Sitting and walking patterns are also affected by the social norm, as well as by clothing. I have learned from my younger patients that sitting up straight is "uncool." Pants that do not bend in the hips or shoes that interfere with a normal walking pattern all have an effect on the feet, knees, hips, and even the lower back. The bottom line is that there is a right and a wrong way to align the body and to move at individual joints, as well as among all the segments. Just because you can sit in the wrong way or move in less than optimal ways and there is no immediate effect does not mean that there will not be one eventually.

The public is unaware of the consequences of these poor choices. For the most part, the public believes that musculoskeletal pain just happens. Unfortunately, even many in the medical community are unaware that the onset and course of musculoskeletal pain can be modified. Providing the kind of guidance necessary to show individuals how to protect their musculoskeletal system requires a great deal of knowledge. Physical therapists should have that kind of knowledge. Consider the inconsistency in the importance that is placed on the alignment and health of the dental system compared to the importance placed on the musculoskeletal system. Many people use preventive and monitoring measures to optimize the appearance and health of their teeth, but the same measures are not used for the musculoskeletal system.

Certainly, a variety of exercise programs have become popular, and they often include "core" strengthening. Recognition of the importance of the trunk in providing a stable base for the function of the limb segments is good. What still needs to be appreciated is that just "strengthening" without regard for alignment and movement patterns is short-sighted. The public and health practitioners need to realize that alignment is the foundation for optimal movement and that musculoskeletal health requires optimal movement to prevent or at least minimize microtrauma that becomes macrotrauma and pain.

Awareness that movement system syndromes are a progressive rather than temporary condition requires a change in physical therapy practice. The immediate alleviation of symptoms does not address the underlying problem and should not be considered the completion of patient management. The physician does not just prescribe insulin for the patient with diabetes and cease his or her role with this resolution of the major sign of the disease. The physician examines the heart, kidneys, blood pressure, and lipid levels and orders numerous other laboratory tests to monitor how these systems are affected by the disease. The examination also includes assessing how physiological systems are affecting the diabetes. So, too, should the physical therapist examine all of the effects of alignment and posture, as well as movements of the limbs, on the region of the symptoms. In other words, all of the signs indicating that forces and movement patterns are contributing to the tissue trauma need to be addressed. Our knowledge of kinesiology and the interactions of all the segments of the body is what we bring to understanding musculoskeletal problems. We should not be satisfied by limiting our focus to what tissue is painful—which is the focus of the physician who lacks knowledge of kinesiology. Therapists should be asking, "Why did this tissue become painful?" and "What can be done to stop or slow the process?" Just as the physician continues to monitor the patient with diabetes so should the therapist continue to monitor the patient with musculoskeletal pain on a regular basis, similar to the yearly dental check-up.

Almost daily I am made aware that therapists are not recognized for their clinical decision-making abilities, as much as we tout our skill at this important process. We have not defined or described in a clear and cohesive way what decisions we make. We have not described the syndromes that we diagnose and treat. We have not used labels that can be recognized by the public and other health professionals. Those labels do not need to be the same as the physician uses. In fact, they cannot be when the physician's label requires tests that we cannot perform or order. Just as new pathologies of a physiological system are learned by the medical community so can the labels of movement system syndromes be learned by professionals who are not physical therapists. For example, 10 or even 5 years ago not many practitioners had heard of femoral acetabular impingement (FAI). Therapists are recognized for being able to guide exercise programs for patients after surgery or for strengthening programs that are considered rather generic. Even those indications for guidance by a therapist are in question. A leading orthopaedic surgeon told one of my patients that she did not need to go to physical therapy after shoulder joint replacement surgery. This patient had not been able to flex her shoulder above 90 degrees for 6 years before the surgery. Yet recovery of her ability to move and use her shoulder was considered relatively uncomplicated. At the other extreme, because physicians are not performing physical examinations, I frequently identify the actual sources of pain that have not been correctly diagnosed by the physician. A patient was referred for shoulder pain when the pain was originating from the cervical spine is just one of many examples. Physical therapists will have established their roles as diagnosticians and clinical decision-makers when physicians refer patients for diagnosis of the mechanical origin of a pain problem rather than for mere supervision of an exercise program or for symptom alleviation. The public and the healthcare system will be well served when the physician, having completed the diagnostic workup for a patient with thoracic area pain, cannot arrive at a diagnosis and refers the patient to physical therapy for a movement system diagnosis.

This book represents our current best effort at describing movement system syndromes of the cervical and thoracic spines and the extremities—syndromes that physical therapists should be able to recognize and manage. We have also provided very basic guidelines for acute conditions in which tissue protection is the emphasis. These syndromes are diagnoses that physical therapists should make. Our fervent hope is that these labels, among others, will be used and promoted to the public and to other healthcare practitioners.

Chapter 1 describes the kinesiopathological model and the proposed process in which repeated movements and sustained postures of daily activities can cause musculoskeletal pain problems.

Chapter 2 describes basic concepts of early stage tissue impairments. The management of conditions that begin with tissue protection, such as immediately after surgery or trauma, and progress to stage 2 and 3 for tissue strengthening for daily activities or if indicated for participation in sports is described.

Chapters 3 and 4 describe the movement system syndromes of the cervical and thoracic spines respectively. Each chapter provides the basic anatomy and kinesiology considered necessary to understand the normal performance of the relevant body area. The syndromes are described, and case examples are provided. Charts, traditionally known at the Washington University Program in Physical Therapy as "grids," are included as appendices to enable the therapist to have an overview of the key components of each diagnosis. Chapters 5, 6, 7, and 8 provide similar information for the hand, elbow, knee, ankle, and foot, respectively.

A video of the examination for each of the body regions described in this book is also included. Also, the exercises described in the first volume are relevant to many of the syndromes described in this book. The hand and elbow require special exercises, which are described in the appropriate chapter.

Shirley A. Sahrmann, PhD, PT, FAPTA

REFERENCES

1. The Reports of the Surgeon General: *Profiles in science: The 1964 report on smoking and health*, Bethesda, Md., 1964, National Library of Medicine.
2. Hurley BF, Hagberg JM, Goldberg AP, et al: Resistive training can reduce coronary risk factors without altering VO_2 max or percent body fat, *Med Sci Sports Exerc* 20(2):150-154, 1988.
3. Rogers MA, Yamamoto C, Hagberg JM, et al: The effect of 7 years of intense exercise training on patients with coronary artery disease, *J Am Coll Cardiol* 10(2):321-326, 1987.
4. Ehsani AA, Biello DR, Schultz J, et al: Improvement of left ventricular contractile function by exercise training in patients with coronary artery disease, *Circulation* 74(2):350-358, 1986.
5. Hagberg JM, Goldring D, Ehsani AA, et al: Effect of exercise training on the blood pressure and hemodynamic features of hypertensive adolescents, *Am J Cardiol* 52(7): 763-768, 1983.

Acknowledgments

Adequate expression of my deep gratitude to my colleagues who have not only participated in the development of information about movement system syndromes but who have also written the chapters in this book is not possible. As members of the faculty of the Program in Physical Therapy, Washington University School of Medicine in St. Louis, we have all been motivated and guided by the example set by the entire university for the pursuit of excellence. Specifically within the Program in Physical Therapy, our Program Director, Susie Deusinger, PT, PhD, FAPTA, has provided the vision, the ability, the resources, and the determination to ensure that the Program is one of the very best in the country and even the world. What I can never express adequately is how much I have learned from my colleagues at Washington University, how much I have enjoyed all of our interactions, and how much respect I have for their commitment to the profession and to hard work. In addition, they are also wonderful, caring people who have contributed so very much to my life. Many of us have worked together for over 20 to 30 years, and the newcomers joined us about 10 years ago. The group has the same enthusiasm and commitment today as when we first started on this pursuit of advancing the body of knowledge of physical therapy and the application to practice.

Those directly participating in the writing of this book were Nancy Bloom, PT, DPT, MSOT; Cheryl Caldwell, PT, DPT, CHT; Suzy Cornbleet, PT, DPT; Mary Hastings, PT, DPT, ATC; Marcie Harris-Hayes, PT, DPT, MSCI, OCS; Greg Holtzman, PT, DPT; Renee Ivens, PT, DPT; Lynnette Khoo-Summers, PT, DPT; Mary Kate McDonnell, PT, DPT, OCS; and Tracy Spitznagle, PT, DPT, WCS. Dr. Nancy Bloom deserves special comment because as a student, more years ago than we both want to acknowledge, she undertook the task of translating and transferring some rather rudimentary ideas. She converted what were mostly verbally expressed ideas and explanations into a written form that could then be developed, refined, and taught. Dr. Bloom has been a key contributor to the clarity, depth, and accuracy not only of the concepts and their application but also to the effectiveness with which they are taught. She has set a high standard for all of us to follow and from which we have learned and profited.

As acknowledged in the first volume of this book, Steven J. Rose, PT, PhD, FAPTA, was the first to recognize the importance of classification of clinical conditions and to point us in a direction of refining and describing the body of knowledge that constitutes the movement system. Steve knew that classification is the only way to truly achieve effective and efficient clinical practice and relevant research. As with all pursuits, support systems are the true keys to successful and outstanding outcomes. Barbara J. Norton, PhD, PT, FAPTA, has served in that role not just for me but for all of us at the Program in Physical Therapy. She has been a great friend, supporter, colleague, and most valued analyst (sometimes known as a critic). Dr. Norton has not only pulled me off many an intellectual limb but also has significantly contributed to the intellectual growth all of my colleagues. Barb has set high standards and shown us how to think clearly and critically. Linda Van Dillen, PT, PhD, has continued to carefully analyze both by laboratory and clinical research many of the basic concepts and their application to patients with low back pain. Linda has been able to think through the details and examine them in ways that reflect a depth of thought that most of us cannot even imagine. She has guided and elicited clinical studies and publications from most of us. Dr. Van Dillen is a truly outstanding mentor and the rigor of her research has produced results that are being recognized for their thoroughness and relevance.

What has been a major development since the publication of the first volume is the establishment of a faculty practice at the Program in Physical Therapy. The practice gives all of us an opportunity to interact as practitioners and further refine and test our ideas in the real life situation. How fortunate for the students in the Program in Physical Therapy when the specific faculty member who teaches the anatomy, kinesiology, clinical science, and diagnostic categories of a specific body region also sees patients with problems of the region of their specialty. This type of educational and practice organization has not only enhanced the education of the students but has also contributed to the further refinement of movement system syndromes. Because this book is the work of members of the faculty of the Program in Physical Therapy at Washington University School of Medicine in St. Louis, all profits will go to the Program to further the scholarship and research activities involved in movement system syndromes.

Several individuals have made important contributions to specific chapters of this book. Ann Kammien, PT, CHT, contributed to the development of the content and grids in Chapter 5 on the hand. She has also provided the photographs used in the chapter. Cindy Glaenzer, PT, CHT, proofread and provided valuable feedback for Chapter 5. Sara Culley, SPT, contributed to obtaining, organizing, and formatting the references for the chapters on the hand and the elbow. Michael Mueller, PT, PhD, FAPTA; Dave Sinacore, PT, PhD, FAPTA; and Jay Diamond, PT, made valuable contributions to the content of the chapter on the foot and ankle. These individuals have also been a major source of support for the work of Mary Hastings, PT, DPT, ACT, in particular.

Although the preparation of this volume of movement system impairment syndromes could not involve spirited discussion with Florence Kendall, her work did provide the foundational knowledge on which many of these concepts were developed. The terminology and some of the details regarding basic muscle biology may vary from concepts expressed by the Kendall's, nonetheless, the timeliness and the clarity of their insights is remarkable. Happily for me, I was able to take advantage of Florence's most valuable critic, her daughter and co-author, Betsy McCreary. Betsy was kind enough to review and add valuable comments to the first chapter of this book.

As with the first volume, my colleagues and I are indebted to the perseverance and invaluable assistance of our editor, Christie Hart. Christie truly made this book happen, and we are very indebted to her for keeping us on task. We regret all the distress we caused her during the process. We also appreciate all of those at Elsevier who have been instrumental in the preparation and completion of this book.

Contents

CHAPTER 1

Update of Concepts Underlying Movement System Syndromes

Shirley A. Sahrmann, Nancy Bloom

INTRODUCTION

Since 1980, the members of the physical therapy faculty at Washington University School of Medicine in St. Louis have been attempting to define, describe, and study the body of knowledge of physical therapy. A part of that pursuit has been the development of diagnostic categories or syndromes of conditions that are treated by physical therapists. Our efforts have resulted in the recognition that an important physiological system of the body is the *movement system* and that dysfunctions of this system can be classified into syndromes. These syndromes provide direction for diagnosis, treatment, and pursuing underlying kinesiopathology. The syndromes for orthopedic conditions causing musculoskeletal pain are (1) based on the movement directions or alignments that cause pain, (2) associated with movement impairments, and (3) improved by correction of the movement impairment that decreases or eliminates the symptoms. The systematic examination used to determine the diagnosis also identifies contributing factors. Based on clinical experience, research and analysis of the literature,[1-28] and organization of materials for academic teaching, key concepts of the movement system that contribute to the development of pain syndromes are proposed. Understanding the following key concepts and their application to patients with musculoskeletal pain will enable the practitioner to develop an appropriate movement system (MS) diagnosis and treatment program.

1. The majority of musculoskeletal pain syndromes both acute and chronic are the result of cumulative microtrauma from stress induced by repeated movements in a specific direction or from sustained alignments, usually in a nonideal position.
   - Musculoskeletal pain is the result of a progressive condition that is related to lifestyle and degenerative changes in tissues.
   - The transition from tissue microtrauma to macrotrauma is influenced by a variety of intrinsic (genetics, sex, and age) and extrinsic (amount and type of fitness, work activity) factors.
   - These repeated movements and sustained alignments occur during the performance of daily activities.

2. The site (joint region) that is moving or stressed in a specific direction is the site of pain generation.
3. The stress occurs most often during the initiation or earliest phase of the motion rather than at the end of the physiological motion.
4. Hypermobility, usually accessory motion hypermobility, is the cause of the pain. Therefore the offending motions are most often very subtle, and the more chronic the condition or the older the subject, the more subtle the motion.
5. The body follows the law of physics and takes the path of least resistance for motion, which contributes to the hypermobility.
6. The path of least resistance is affected by variation in the stiffness or relative flexibility of tissues attached to adjoining joints. Most activities involve movement across several contiguous joints that are arranged in series and one of these joints moves more *readily in a specific direction* than the other joints.
7. The predisposition of a joint to move *readily in a specific direction* contributes to the development of a movement pattern.
8. *Insufficient* muscle stiffness (because of greater relative flexibility) and increased resting muscle length are more problematic adaptations than specific muscle weakness and shortness.
9. The way everyday activities are performed is the critical issue. For efficiency, the body establishes a pattern of motion that reinforces the relative hypermobility and participation of specific joints, including the joint that moves the most readily in a specific direction. Hypermobility is reinforced and becomes habitual.
10. The relative participation of some muscle groups (disuse or overuse) is the result of movement patterns and biomechanical influences.
    - In the swayback posture, if the pelvis is tilted posteriorly and the hip is extended, the use of the gluteus maximus muscle is minimized.
    - The kyphotic posture without a posterior sway can reduce the participation of the abdominal muscles because they are not periodically working against gravity.

- In contrast, a kyphotic posture in the swayback position can be the result of abdominal muscle shortness or stiffness because the abdominals are the antigravity muscles of the trunk during standing.

11. Muscle performance is determined by the pattern of movement. Correction of faulty patterns is best achieved by training the correct pattern and not by isolated "strengthening" of a muscle.

12. The human body is highly capable of motor equivalency, which is the ability to realize the same motor outcome with different effectors. Over time, the repertoire of variability becomes limited. Stopping the offending motion at the joint that moves the most readily and redistributing the motion to other adjoining segments expands one's ability to vary patterns of motion.

13. The most important treatment is correcting the movement pattern that is causing the tissue to become painful or irritated rather than directing treatment to the affected tissue.

14. The critical issue is *how* an activity is performed not just performing the activity.
    - Proper movement strategy can optimize performance and minimize tissue injury. Faulty strategy can compromise performance and lead to tissue injury.

15. An exercise is not effective unless the exercise limits or corrects the movement at the painful joint and produces the desired appropriate movement at adjoining joints.
    - Redistributing the movement to appropriate joints is the goal.
    - The same exercise can be used for contrasting problems, depending on the instruction and performance (quadruped rocking to either increase or decrease lumbar flexion).

16. If a muscle contributes to the impaired motion of a painful joint, stretching the muscle will not stop the motion causing pain, but stopping the motion may stretch the muscle. If the tensor fascia lata-iliotibial band contributes to tibiofemoral rotation, stretching the band will not stop the impaired motion during the stretch or functional activities. If the tibiofemoral rotation is controlled and the hip joint does not medially rotate or abduct, the tensor fascia lata-iliotibial band can be stretched during walking.

17. Training movement patterns will induce appropriate muscular and biomechanical adaptations that will reinforce the development of optimal neuromuscular action.

18. All neuromuscular adaptations can *contribute to* and correct problems. Thus "indiscriminate" core strengthening exercises can become a cause of pain as readily as a lack of muscle strength can contribute to pain problems.

19. Every patient with musculoskeletal pain should have a MS diagnosis.

20. MS *syndromes* consist of multiple contributing factors or impairments that combine to produce the principal movement impairment that is the cause of the symptoms. The syndrome is named for this principal impairment.
    - The contributing factors are movement and neuromusculoskeletal adaptations.
    - A systematic examination is required to identify all of the contributing factors.

21. The examination must include tests and assessments of all regions of the body, including a determination of how all regions affect the movement of the painful joint because of the biomechanical interactions of the human body.

22. The movement system needs to be periodically examined, beginning in childhood and continuing into old age to (1) evaluate optimal tissue development, (2) ascertain the progression of degenerative changes, and (3) determine and guide exercises to maintain the health of the cardiovascular and metabolic systems.
    - Guiding exercise for appropriate use can prevent disuse, misuse, or overuse.

THE GENERAL PREMISE: MOVEMENT SYSTEM IMPAIRMENTS CAUSE PAIN SYNDROMES

Ten years have passed since publication of *Diagnosis and Treatment of Movement Impairment Syndromes*.[29] The purpose of the first book was to describe a generic model for organizing musculoskeletal pain conditions into syndromes that constitute diagnostic categories to direct treatment of the mechanical aspects of the problem. The belief is that correction or modification of factors altering the precision of motion (physiological motion but also as much as possible the accessory/arthrokinematic motion) alleviates or reduces the tissue irritation and thus the painful condition. The model also described the key contributing factors to the various diagnostic groups. A major premise of the model is that pain most often arises from tissues that are stressed by subtle impairments in movement or alignment and that key factors contribute to these particular impairments. One important factor is that the body, following the laws of physics, takes the path of least resistance for movement. The activities an individual performs require movements of multiple joints that are contiguous, in the same kinematic chain (i.e., in serial arrangement), and all of which have different flexibility characteristics. The result is that one joint of those that are anatomically arranged in series moves the most easily and most readily when an individual performs an activity. Our research supports the premise that the *ease and rapidity* with which a joint moves are more important factors in a movement pattern associated with pain than muscle shortness, soft tissue restrictions, or limited range of motion (ROM) of an adjoining joint.[6,8,15,16] These latter factors may have contributed to the initial development of the flexibility of the joint causing the pain, but once established, the offending motion has to be addressed primarily and the tissue adaptations, secondarily. Clearly, stretching muscles or soft tissues will *not* stop the offending motion. But when the offending motion is stopped or controlled, the appropriate tissues will be stretched.

The motion contributing to the stress occurs during the first few degrees of motion or with initiation of an activity. The primary impairment is believed to be an accessory rather than a physiological motion, which is consistent with the problem arising during the first few degrees of movement. Accessory motion hypermobility is an underlying characteristic of degenerative joint disease.[30-32] Lumbopelvic motion with lower extremity motions in patients with low back pain is an example of abnormal early onset joint motion. In the prone position, lumbopelvic rotation occurs earlier and to a greater extent during the first few degrees of knee flexion and hip rotation in patients with low back pain than in control subjects, and the pattern was specific to the MS category.[6,8,15,16] The predisposition of these joints to move readily contributes to the frequency of their movement and furthers the tendency for motion. Thus, a specific joint or joints of the lumbar spine, for example, develop a tendency or susceptibility to move readily in a specific direction (directional susceptibility to movement [DSM]) during all activities. In most joints, the accessory motion impairment is not clinically observable, thus the physiological motion associated with the pain is most often designated as the DSM.

Clarification of the meaning of *hypermobility* is essential. There are three possible meanings of hypermobility; the first is the joint ROM exceeds the ideal. The term can be applied to a physiological (osteokinematic) motion. For example, if the physiological motion of rotation between 2 cervical vertebrae is ideally 4 degrees or less, then 6 degrees of motion is hypermobility. Second, if the amount of accessory motion exceeds the normal. For example, translation between the cervical vertebrae, is 2 mm, then 3 mm of translation is hypermobility. Accessory motion hypermobility can occur even though the joint's physiological motion is less than normal. Third, the frequency of movement of a specific joint in a specific direction occurs more often than is considered ideal. If an individual has a habit of constantly moving the head and neck when talking, the cervical vertebrae that move the most readily will also be moving the most frequently. Also, excessive frequency of motion can occur in the presence of *cervical hypomobility*. In the cervical spine with degenerative disc disease and exostosis, motion at some joints may be markedly restricted but limited to a lesser extent at other joints. As the individual attempts to rotate the head and neck, although the ROM of every joint is less than normal, there will still be some joints that move more readily and will move more frequently than optimal. Accessory motion will probably occur the most readily and will be greater than normal, although the

physiological motion is less than normal. The attempt to achieve maximum voluntary motion with limited physiological motion will cause tissue stress and pain.

As might be suspected, when a joint moves more readily than other joints in the same kinetic chain, the repeated movements and prolonged postures associated with everyday activities can be the precipitating, as well as the perpetuating, factors of the joint's DSM. As a result, movement in the offending direction has been associated with pain and is often impaired (deviates from the kinesiological standard). When the movement is corrected, the symptoms decrease or are eliminated. Based on the premise that the diagnosis should direct treatment, the DSM is most often also the diagnosis. Correcting the pattern or stopping the movement in the painful direction is the focus of treatment because the symptoms are decreased or eliminated by this action.

For example, rotation of some cervical vertebrae can occur more readily than other vertebrae. Supporting the shoulders can alleviate the motion restriction of the cervical vertebrae caused by the tautness of the cervicoscapular muscles. When the shoulders are supported during rotation, the motion of those vertebral joints that are usually restricted is increased. Another example is found in some individuals who move more readily at the carpometacarpal (CMC) joint of the thumb than in the metacarpophalangeal (MP) joint because the MP is the stiffest of the two joints, and the neuromuscular recruitment pattern has adapted to this difference in the two joints. When the patient grasps an object, the movement of the thumb will occur more readily and be greater in range at the CMC joint than at the MP joint. As a result, because of the increased frequency of motion, there is a greater likelihood over the years of degenerative changes at the CMC joint.

What cannot be emphasized enough is that in some regions the movement impairments are often very subtle, and detection takes practice and involves tactile, as well as visual, cues. Cervical motion is a good example. One examination method is to have the therapist assess the pattern of cervical rotation by monitoring the movement with the hands. The patient sits in a chair with the forearms on armrests that are elevated enough to alleviate the downward pull on the neck from the weight of the upper extremities. The therapist, while standing behind the patient, lightly places the hands almost all the way around the posterolateral aspects of the cervical spine with the fingers on the jaw and thumbs at the base of the skull (Figure 1-1). The patient actively rotates the head and neck, as the therapist goes "along for the ride" to be able to detect the natural pattern of motion rather than just assessing ROM or controlling the motion. In patients with neck pain, a common pattern is a very rapid upper cervical motion with either slight side-flexion, or extension motion in the lower cervical area rather relatively precise rotation. Precise motion is envisioned as rotation around a rod running through the head and cervical spine. These patients may also complain of popping or clicking

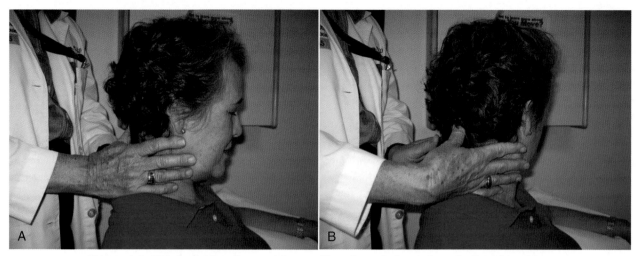

Figure 1-1. Hand position for assessing quality of cervical rotation. **A,** Initial position. **B,** Therapist initially follows the motion as the patient actively rotates the head and neck. If there is a movement fault, the therapist gently guides the motion to provide precision as the patient actively rotates the head.

during the motion. Most often the therapist also has to correct the starting alignment of the patient's head and neck before the patient initiates the motion. Then the patient is instructed to very *easily* turn the head and neck. When the patient exerts a minimal rather than a "natural" effort, the range will be the same, but the clicking and popping will cease or be minimal. The therapist also very easily guides the motion so that its pattern is more precise than the natural pattern. By minimizing the muscle contraction the muscles are not developing as much tension in either the rotational or the stabilizing direction, which decreases interjoint forces and the compression among the cervical vertebrae. The patient established a pattern of recruitment that was necessary to overcome the usual amount of tension required to rotate the head and neck because of the downward pull of the shoulders or some other perceived resistance. Although the load was reduced by supporting the arms, the active tension was not automatically adjusted. Often, once the patient "learns" to use less active tension and to perform the motion precisely, the new pattern can be used even without arm support.

As stated previously, the movement direction or alignment that most consistently causes or increases the patient's symptoms and that, when corrected, decreases or alleviates the symptoms is considered the diagnosis. Movements of the limbs also impose forces and motions on spinal segments, so the symptoms can also be elicited by limb movements. The complete description of all the impairments evident as signs or causing symptoms that contribute to the offending or principal movement impairment is the syndrome. As with other diagnoses used by medical practitioners, factors contributing to the diagnosis are delineated as part of the description of the syndrome. The formulation of a theory of the underlying mechanisms, as well as the specific syndromes and contributing factors, then becomes a basis for research.

This book attempts to clarify and develop consistency in explaining the concepts and the terminology used to describe MS syndromes. The conditions described in this book are characterized as problems of the MS because the emphasis has been on identifying the offending movement, alignment and role of contiguous joints, and general limb movements in the condition. The movement problem and many of the contributing factors are considered as impairments rather than pathological conditions, at least early in the development of the condition. *Impairment* is defined as any disorder in structure or function resulting from anatomical, physiological, or psychological abnormalities that interfere with normal activities.[33] In this book, impairments at the tissue level are described in stages that guide the progression from tissue protection to progressive and systematic stress. The staging addresses the changes in classification from tissue protection to a MS syndrome that can be determined once the patient's condition permits the performance of the necessary examination.

THE HUMAN MOVEMENT SYSTEM

The human movement system is a physiological system of the body that produces motion of the body or its component parts, or the functional interaction of the structures that contribute to the act of moving.[34] As depicted in Figure 1-2, the physiological actions of other body systems combine to compose the movement system, with biomechanics playing an important role as the interface among the skeletal, muscular, and nervous systems.

In an attempt to understand the development of musculoskeletal pain, the original kinesiopathological model has been expanded to provide a more complete although complex description of some of the contributing factors to MS syndromes (Figure 1-3). *Kinesiopathological* refers

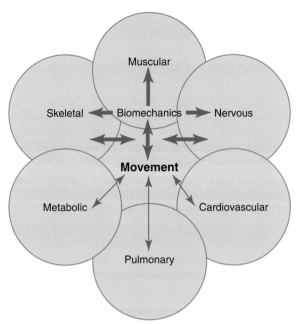

Figure 1-2. Schematic of the physiological systems that comprise the movement system and depiction of biomechanics as an important interface. The relative width of the arrows indicates amount of contribution. The arrows in both directions indicate that not only do these systems produce movement but that they are all also affected by movement.

to how movement that is excessive, imprecise, or insufficient contributes to the development of pathology. The complexity of the model stems from an attempt to provide a relatively complete description of the major factors and interactions that contribute to movement becoming imprecise, causing pain and pathological problems. In addition to providing theories for research, this model is particularly important for purposes of diagnosis and treatment of musculoskeletal problems. Based on kinesiology, no one segment or region of the system can be affected in isolation. A traditional approach to musculoskeletal conditions is to identify and treat the tissues considered to be the source of the pain or the pathoanatomical structures. *Most often, the painful tissues have been progressively subjected to microtrauma because of movement impairments or alterations in the precision of motion, and the end result is macrotrauma.* As stated by Adams and Dolan, "Skeletal tissues respond actively to their mechanical environment so that the end result of mechanical loading can vary between *adaptive remodeling and biological 'degeneration,'* depending on the precise circumstances."[35] Importantly, the adjoining body regions are most often a contributing factor to the movement impairment.

Although tissues of the body are known to be subjected to progressive degeneration from aging and microtrauma,

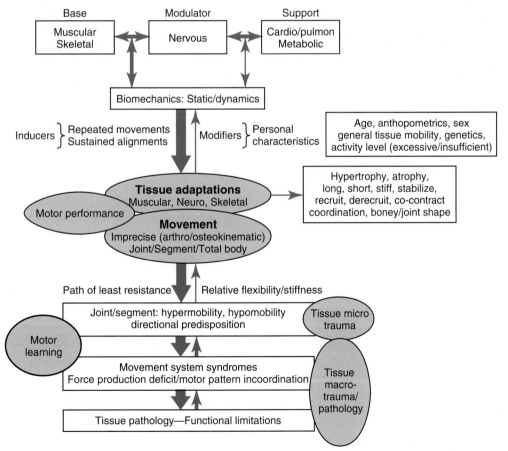

Figure 1-3. The kinesiopathological model of the human movement system depicting factors leading to the development of movement system (MS) syndromes.

the traditional approach to understanding the condition is not based on assessing the interactions of these two factors. Rather, treatment has been more consistent with a condition that (1) arises from an isolated trauma to one specific painful site and (2) can be immediately rectified by treatment focused on that site. The concepts proposed in this book are designed to have the practitioner consider all anatomical, physiological, and biomechanical interactions of the multiple body regions that contribute to the cause and that perpetuate the microtrauma and eventual macrotrauma of one specific region of the body. Research and clinical practice has demonstrated that alterations in motor control and muscle deficiencies underlie many of the biomechanical interaction contributing to the development of MS syndromes. We have subclassified the syndromes as motor pattern incoordination or force produce deficit problems. In some patients, both factors are present. The human movement system consists of highly interactive components, thus diagnosis and treatment must take this into consideration. Simply said, the movement of the hips and even the arms can cause and contribute to low back pain,[4,25] just as movements of the arms can contribute to neck pain and movement of the shoulder can contribute to hand problems. The alignment of the trunk contributes to back and neck pain, and the alignment of the pelvis and trunk affects the knee, as well as the foot. A comprehensive appreciation for these relationships and for the multiple tissue adaptations that become contributing factors is essential, and this model is an attempt to share the information that has been developed, with full appreciation that this is only a beginning, and to provide a useful foundation for future studies and clinical analysis.

ELEMENTS OF THE MODEL

The model, consisting of base, modulator, and support elements, describes the generalized contributions and functions characteristic of a dynamic system and the factors contributing to the development of musculoskeletal pain conditions.

Base Elements

The components of the base elements are the muscular and skeletal systems. These systems are considered the base elements because they consist of the tissues that provide the foundation and the structure of the system.

Modulator Element

The component of the modulator element is the nervous system. The term *modulator* is used to emphasize the regulator activity of the nervous system. Besides the role of modulating muscular activity, the nervous system also plays a role in the psychosocial aspects of musculoskeletal pain. Although psychosocial aspects are important regulators in the development of the condition, reaction to the condition, and participation in resolution of the condition, these aspects are beyond the intention and scope of this book.

Support Elements

The components of support elements are the cardiovascular, pulmonary, and metabolic systems. These systems do not contribute directly to movement, but as indicated by the term *support*, they provide the nutrients and substances required for maintaining the viability and health of those systems that do directly produce movement. The lack of physical activity or exercise causes pathological changes in the cardiovascular and metabolic systems and thus compromises the health of the individual. This book does not discuss or describe the type of exercise designed to optimize the components of the support elements, but the importance of the type of training required for optimizing endurance and cardiovascular and metabolic function is recognized. Often, individuals cannot initiate or continue with endurance exercise because of musculoskeletal pain. Therefore material about optimizing movement is considered essential to preventing or minimizing the development of musculoskeletal pain conditions that prevent participation in endurance exercise.

BIOMECHANICS

The model indicates that biomechanics is an interface between muscular and neurological activity. The pattern of muscular recruitment is highly influenced by relationships to gravity, as well as the force required to move the extremity and react to external forces. The design of the movement system also provides a variety of strategies to develop a moment about a joint. Many of those strategies are determined by biomechanics. For example, control of knee flexion in the standing position can be (1) the direct result of eccentric contraction of quadriceps muscle, or (2) an indirect result of contraction of the hamstrings acting as hip extensors as long as the foot is fixed. The demands on the force requirements from these muscles is either increased or decreased, depending on whether the line of gravity is anterior or posterior to the knee joint. If the line of gravity is anterior to the knee joint, the demand on muscle force is decreased. If the line of gravity is posterior to the knee joint, the demand on muscle force is increased. Gravitational forces also influence the shape of weight-bearing bones and joints (discussed in the "Tissue Adaptations of the Skeletal System" section). Specific examples of how the therapist needs to consider biomechanical factors are detailed in subsequent sections.

TISSUE ADAPTATIONS

The dynamic and biological characteristics of the components of the movement system enable tissues to adapt to the demands placed on them.[36] The specific tissue adaptations are normal biological responses to forms of stress but may contribute to deviations from principles of kinesiology. For example, alterations in muscle length, strength, and stiffness can affect the precision in joint motion. In combination, these adaptations can become problematic. The key adaptations of the skeletal, muscular, and nervous systems and how they contribute to the development of musculoskeletal pain are described in some detail in the appropriate section.

Inducers

The repeated movements and sustained alignments associated with everyday activities are the inducers of the tissue adaptations. When an individual undertakes a "training program," either for increasing muscle strength or improving cardiovascular endurance, there is an expectation that tissues will change. What is not readily appreciated is that every aspect of an individual's activities, whether passive or active, also induces changes in tissues. Although the physically active person will improve and increase the size of muscles and connective tissues, at the same time, the risk of injury also increases. Musculoskeletal pain problems and injuries of athletes mostly occur from noncontact stress. Golfers develop back, elbow, wrist, shoulder, and knee problems.[37] Tennis players also develop shoulder, elbow, and knee problems. Studies have been directed toward identifying the injuries associated with sports activities because of the frequency and costs.[38] The repetitive use of specific segments of the body combined with high and rapid force development can exceed tissue tolerance, resulting in microtrauma. Obviously, not all golfers, tennis players, or other athletes use the same movement patterns, and some of those patterns are more optimal than others. At the other extreme, even individuals who are inactive induce changes by the alignment and movements while sitting and during work activities. Alignments maintained for prolonged periods can induce changes in muscle length. Without activity, muscle and connective tissues are not stressed enough to provide optimal tissue health. Similarly, constantly leaning in one direction or rotating frequently to one side can also induce changes in muscles, joint alignment, and the precision of motion. A relatively frequent example is evident in women who have held babies on their hip, usually the left hip if they are right handed. The typical postural adaptation is for the trunk to shift to the right, slightly rotate to the right, and side flex to the left. Needless to say, the more prolonged the activity in hours per day, days per week, weeks per year, and for extended years, the more exaggerated the posture. Most often the patient is totally unaware of this adjustment. Importantly, even though the activity has ceased, the ideal alignment is not restored unless a specific effort is made to correct the posture. If a patient has decreased ROM of the knee joint, the treatment is to perform repeated movements to improve and increase the ROM. Improvement is achieved by changes in the tissues. When everyday activities involve repeated movements in a specific direction, the movement in that direction occurs more readily and easily because of the tissue changes. *Also, once a joint develops a tendency to move easily and readily in a direction, that movement will occur with all activities involving that joint and not just the one that induced the joint changes.* The therapist must obtain information about the activities (work, fitness, and leisure) that the individual performs on a regular basis.

Awareness of how an individual performs an activity is particularly important. After completing the examination and identifying the DSM, that information is used to assess whether the patient's activity involves the offending motion. For example, if the patient has neck pain that occurs with rotation and the evening activity is watching television, the viewing position often involves maintaining a rotated position because the chair does not face the TV. As explained in Chapter 3, a common factor in neck pain is that the patient is constantly moving the head and neck when communicating as part of body language. The therapist begins to gather pertinent information by observing preferred positions and body language, as well as from the history.

Modifiers

Although repeated movements and sustained alignments are proposed as inducers of tissue adaptations, there are modifiers that affect the adaptations. The modifiers are factors such as age, sex, height, weight, and genetic characteristics that include predisposition to osteoarthritis, benign general joint hypermobility, structural or anthropometric characteristics, and the amount and type of activity. A few generalizations about these modifiers can be useful in assessing their role in the development of movement impairments.

Age

In young individuals, tissues are more extensible and joints more flexible than in older individuals. Thus the offending motions are usually of greater ROM than the motions in an older patient. The health of the tissues is better in the younger individual than in the older individual because some degree of degeneration is already present with aging, although degenerative changes in the spine have been reported in individuals who are only 20 years of age.[39] In older individuals or those with a chronic condition, the movement impairments are usually more subtle so that the examination requires careful observation and usually slight corrections. The treatment using movement corrections and stabilizing exercises requires even greater precision in the older individual than in the younger patient. The way everyday activities are performed becomes even more critical in the older than in the younger individual. For example, a younger individual can sit leaning on one arm for prolonged periods without experiencing pain, but a short duration of leaning to one side can cause pain in an older individual. The prolonged alignments that have been used for years have usually induced tissue, bony, and structural changes in the aging such as the reduced height of intervertebral discs and changes in the facet joints. Other structural changes that can contribute to the pain syndrome are loss of the normal cervical curve and an acquired kyphosis or degenerative scoliosis.

Sex

Studies of patients with low back pain have demonstrated a difference in the pain-inducing movements and alignments between men and women.[11,17] The broader shoulders, higher center of gravity, and larger and stiffer muscles in men as compared to women also contribute to differences in tissue adaptation and movement patterns. The greater incidence of anterior cruciate ligament (ACL) injuries in women as compared to men is an example of variations in tissue adaptation that can be attributed to sex.[40,41] Recent studies demonstrate that women use more quadriceps activity during jumping than men and less hip extensor activity, creating different forces at the knee joint.[42,43]

Tissue Mobility

Of the genetic factors, benign joint hypermobility syndrome is one of the important problematic characteristics.[44] Individuals with hypermobility (Figure 1-4) seem to be more disposed to musculoskeletal pain problems than individuals with tissues that limit joint excursions; this occurs not only with the physiological motion but particularly in the accessory motions. Maintaining good alignment and precise motion is more difficult if the individual is hypermobile as compared to individuals with tissue stiffness. For example, individuals with tissue hypermobility tend to have depressed shoulders and the downward pull on the neck can contribute to the development of neck pain. These problems are particularly evident in women with large breasts whose bra straps exert a downward pull and who have held children in their arms for long periods of time over several years. These tissue adaptations do not reverse after cessation of the activity. Maintaining good alignment of the trunk and the knees is also difficult for the patient with joint hypermobility. In the presence of joint hypermobility, the individual with a supinated foot will tend to have knee hyperextension,

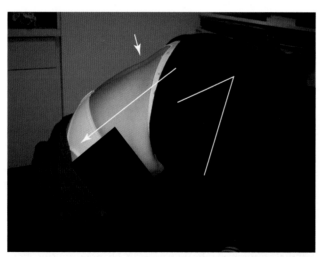

Figure 1-4. Forward bending with excessive hip flexion indicates generalized joint hypermobility. The lack of passive tension of the hip extensor muscles contributes to the failure to reverse the lumbar curve during forward bending. Low back pain is alleviated because of the unloading of the spine and the distraction of the trunk in this position. This condition makes maintaining good alignment and movement control difficult.

whereas another individual without a rigid foot will tend to develop a pronated foot. Therefore one of the important assessments during the examination is obtaining information about the general tissue and joint mobility and the effects on alignment and movement patterns. Treatment programs for these individuals are usually more challenging than for individuals with tissue stiffness because most often, specific exercises are not as useful as constant attention to alignments. The hypermobile individual will usually respond quickly to exercises to correct alignment, but equally as rapidly the original alignment will return, which is why these individuals must correct their alignment frequently during the day.

Anthropometrics

Body proportions are also a contributing factor in predisposing an individual to musculoskeletal problems. For example, a long trunk is usually associated with depressed shoulders and often neck pain. The reason is that the armrests on chairs are too low for an individual with a long trunk; therefore the shoulders are allowed to drop to support the forearms. The structure of the thorax is also a factor because the rib cage can be more barrel-shaped with a greater anterior-posterior dimension than a medial-lateral dimension. The barrel shape affects the position of the scapula and can contribute to shoulder joint problems. The carrying angle of the elbow is also related to the width of the pelvis. This aspect of assessment overlaps with the identification of structural variations.

Activity Level

The activity level can range from excessive, which tends to exacerbate the development of musculoskeletal pain problems, to insufficient activity. The consequence of insufficient activity is usually related to metabolic and cardiovascular problems, although musculoskeletal problems can also develop because of muscle weakness and poor support of the trunk. If the individual initiates an exercise program that is not carefully designed, injuries can develop more readily than if they had been previously active. The therapist needs to also factor into the examination whether the pain condition is from excessive activity that can be associated with problems from muscle hypertrophy and associated stiffness, as well as motor pattern incoordination, or from a lack of activity in which a systematic increase in physical activity and exercise to improve the force production deficit is necessary. In the former situation, part of the treatment may be to decrease the demands on specific muscles and increase the extensibility of those muscles.

Excessive activity in a young male. A competitive 36-year-old male cyclist developed neck pain because of the shortness and stiffness of the rectus abdominis muscle combined with the extended position of the cervical spine. The intense activity of the competitive cycling requires the abdominal muscles to contract about 60 times per second during the increased rate and dept of breathing. In addition, the abdominal muscles are stabilizing the pelvis, which is necessary to stabilize the attachments of the proximal hip muscles involved in the pedaling action. These actions of the abdominal muscles are occurring in a position in which the muscles are in a shortened length. This individual also is a stock broker who sits all day working on several computer screens. His head, neck, and thorax will be in the same position working on the computer and riding the bicycle. He also frequently rotates his head and neck to view the multiple computer screens. The hypertrophy of the abdominals in the shortened position depresses the chest and restricts the elevation of the rib cage. The depression and restriction to elevation of the rib cage creates a downward pull on the scaleni muscles that attach to the rib cage. Because these muscles flex and rotate the cervical spine, excessive tension on the attachments of the scaleni muscles would increase the resistance to neck extension and rotation. This patient needs to elongate the abdominal muscles and refrain from performing abdominal muscle exercises.

Excessive activity in a female with structural and genetic modifiers. A competitive 28-year-old female cyclist developed knee pain. She has a wide pelvis with prominent trochanters, femoral anteversion, and genu valgus. The characteristics of her hips are consistent with coxa vara that is associated with genu valgus. During forward bending, she has 100 degrees of hip flexion, which is indicative of general tissue hypermobility. When cycling, her femur is directed medially, while her tibia is laterally rotated. The cycling in the hip flexed position with the tibia in lateral rotation has resulted in shortness of the tensor fascia lata-iliotibial band (TFL-ITB). During the hip flexor length test, her tibia laterally rotates from the passive tension of the TFL-ITB as the hip is lowered to the fully extended position, and knee pain is experienced. The lateral rotation of the tibia is decreased if the hip is allowed to abduct during the length test. During a step up as well as during sit-to-stand and reverse, her knee is directed medially. If she actively contracts the hip lateral rotator muscles during these movements, the knee pain is reduced. The femoral anteversion and genu valgus has predisposed her to tibiofemoral rotation of the knee, which has become exaggerated by the intensity of her cycling. She needs to correct the tibiofemoral rotation during basic activities, and she can also stretch the TFL-ITB by using the 2-joint hip flexor test position and letting the hip abduction during the lowering to neutral from hip flexion. When lowering the leg, she needs to actively medially rotate her leg. Once she is in the neutral or hip extended position, she can adduct her hip but stop the motion if she has pain in the knee. If she sleeps on her side, she needs to sleep with a pillow between her knees and not allow her hip to be flexed and medially rotate while the tibia is laterally rotated.

Activity in an aged female with structural changes. A 68-year-old female who is recently retired decided to undertake a weight training program. She has lost 2 inches in height, and she has a marked thoracic kyphosis and a very prominent abdomen. She is doing lat pull downs on a weight training machine. She is sitting forward on the seat and trying to pull the bar down behind her head. She is also using an abdominal strengthening machine in which she sits and holds onto pads with her arms and rotates from one side to the other. She is beginning to develop thoracic pain and some pain in her legs. Observation indicates that as her shoulders flex to begin the lat pull down her rib cage elevates and her lumbar spine extends. Then, during the pull down phase of the motion, the thoracic spine flexes. When her shoulders are flexing, she is compensating for the thoracic kyphosis by extending her lumbar spine. The pull of the lattisimus dorsi muscle is also extending her lumbar spine. Because of insufficient strength in her latissimus dorsi muscle, she is flexing her thoracic spine instead of isolated shoulder extension. During the abdominal muscle exercises, she rotates at the apex of the thoracic flexion curve and extends her lumbar spine. This woman's pectoral muscles are stiffer than her abdominal muscles; therefore, when she eccentrically contracts her pectorals, they elevate the rib cage. Her thoracic pain is caused by the elevation of the rib cage during the lat pull down exercise, which is also contributing to the thoracic kyphosis. The abdominal machine is causing rotation of her rib cage at a specific segment that is predisposed to rotation because of the kyphosis. The increase in lumbar extension is causing her to develop symptoms in her legs from the narrowing of the intervertebral space associated with extension. She already has compromised spacing of the vertebrae as indicated by the loss of height. To correct the performance of these exercises, she needs to contract her abdominals as the bar is going up and not try to restrain the motion with her shoulder flexor muscles. She needs to sit against the back of the seat and pull the bar forward, and she needs to avoid both thoracic flexion and lumbar extension. She also needs to contract her abdominal muscles during the pull down phase. She should stop the trunk rotation exercise.

Tissue Adaptations of the Skeletal System

Although skeletal structures seem relatively fixed, bone is a dynamic tissue that is constantly being modified by the forces acting on it. For purposes of this material, the modifications of skeletal structure and alignment can be considered both dynamic and static. Dynamic conditions are correctable and sometimes easily modifiable, whereas the static conditions are relatively permanent or structural. The dynamic conditions are the postural malalignments associated with an acquired thoracic kyphosis, whereas the static or permanent kyphosis is present in individuals with Scheuermann's disease. The alignment of the thorax is a major factor in patients with neck pain. A thoracic kyphosis requires the individual to extend the head and neck. In younger individuals without changes in the cervical discs or vertebrae, the alignment will not

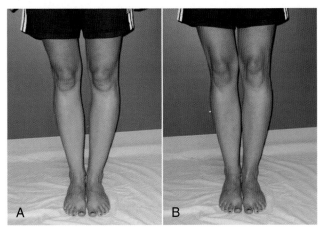

Figure 1-5. Genu varus and correction. **A,** Postural genu varus of the left knee from hip medial rotation and knee hyperextension. **B,** Correction of knee alignment by contracting hip lateral rotator muscles.

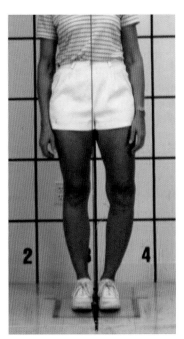

Figure 1-6. Structural genus varus of left knee. This degree of varus and the enlargement of the knee is indicative of degenerative joint disease.

be immediately pain inducing. In the older individual with degenerative joint changes in the cervical spine, the forced cervical extension from a thoracic kyphosis is usually pain inducing. The therapist must determine if the kyphosis is acquired or fixed in order to be able to develop a feasible and effective treatment program. Acquired rotation of the thoracic spine can be the result of sitting postures, throwing or even carrying a backpack, whereas a fixed scoliosis in a younger individual or a degenerative scoliosis in an older individual is permanent. In Chapter 4, the differences in postural and structural scoliosis are discussed. Similarly, as described in Chapter 7, there are acquired postural faults, such as standing with the knees in varus as the result of hip medial rotation and knee hyperextension, that can be corrected (Figure 1-5). In contrast, some individuals have a structural varus that is not correctable but needs to be monitored because of a predisposition to or the presence of degenerative knee joint disease (Figure 1-6).

Another consideration is the effect of prolonged forces on the shape of bones and joints. The changes that take place in the shape of long bones and in the joint when an individual has stood for many years in knee hyperextension is consistent with Wolff's Law.[45] Wolff (1836-1902) proposed that "changes in the form and function of bones, or changes in function alone, are followed by changes in the internal structure and shape of the bone in accordance with mathematical laws." During development, the bones will adopt a shape according to the forces imposed on them. In mature bone in which the general shape is established and no changes are made in the distribution of forces, the change is in the mass according to the mechanical demands. Prolonged standing with the knees in hyperextension results in sagittal plane varus (bowing) of the tibia and fibula, changes in the shape of the articular surface of the tibia, and changes in the alignment of the femur and the tibia (Figures 1-7 and 1-8). Changes in the shape and alignment of the joint also affect the characteristics of the ligaments and the distribution of

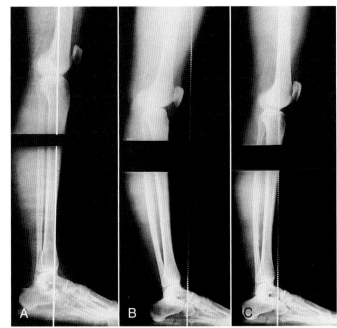

Figure 1-7. **A,** Normally aligned knee. **B,** Hyperextended knee. **C,** Hyperextended knee in the corrected position. The bowing of the tibia and fibula in the knee that has been maintained in hyperextension for years is consistent with the effects on bone expressed in Wolff's law. (From Kendall FP, McCreary EK, Provance PG: *Muscles: testing and function,* ed 4, Philadelphia, 1993, Lippincott Williams & Wilkins.)

forces on the articular cartilage, as well as alter the precision of joint motion. As noted in Figure 1-7, *B,* the position of the patella in the individual with hyperextended knees is lower than in the individual with well-aligned knees. Even in the corrected knee position (see Figure

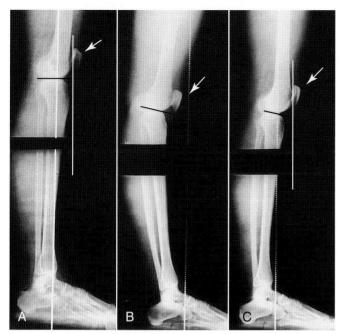

Figure 1-8. **A,** Normally aligned knee. **B,** Hyperextended knee. **C,** Hyperextended knee in the corrected position. In addition to the bowing of the tibia and fibula in the hyperextended knee, a number of other factors could predispose this knee to injury. The articular surface of the tibia is not horizontal, the femur is forward of the tibia, stressing the cruciate ligaments, and the patella sets low, reflecting minimal use of quadriceps. (From Kendall FP, McCreary EK, Provance PG: *Muscles: testing and function,* ed 4, Philadelphia, 1993, Lippincott Williams & Wilkins.)

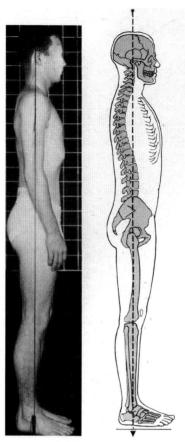

Figure 1-9. Ideal alignment. Optimal distribution of forces on bones and joints and the length and balanced stiffness of muscles and supporting structures. Also, with this type of alignment, when the individual leans forward slightly, the posterior muscles become active. When the individual leans backward, the anterior musculature becomes active. Thus ideal alignment aides the balanced participation of musculature. (From Kendall FP, McCreary EK, Provance PG: *Muscles: testing and function,* ed 4, Philadelphia, 1993, Lippincott Williams & Wilkins.)

1-7, *C*), the patella still sits inferiorly. Such positioning is consistent with the reduced use of the quadriceps because of the knee remaining in the locked position as compared to the frequent intermittent use of the quadriceps to prevent knee flexion that occurs in individuals with well-aligned knees (see Figure 1-7, *A*).

A major consideration is how skeletal alignment, both acquired and structural, affects the demands on muscle participation. Individuals with good alignment where the line of gravity is only *slightly* behind (hip) or in front (knee) of the joint center when standing are constantly altering the participation of the anterior and posterior musculature as the line of gravity oscillates from posterior-to-anterior relationships to the joint (Figure 1-9). The same principle applies to the trunk: If the trunk is swayed forward, the back extensors and hip extensor muscles become active (Figure 1-10, *A*). If the trunk sways backward, the abdominal and hip flexor muscles become active (Figure 1-10, *B*). The initial observations of a patient with pain problems should be an assessment of the alignment and the participation of musculature based on the relationship to the line of gravity. Awareness of the structural and muscular consequences of postural faults reinforces the belief that beginning in childhood, all individuals should be monitored on a yearly basis to assess acquired skeletal malalignment and monitor structural variations. Based on the results of the

examination, the therapist can recommend corrective postural training and exercise programs.

Tissue Adaptations of the Nervous System

Obviously, the contributions of the nervous system to movement are essential and have been the subject of many books, but what is only recently becoming widely accepted is that motor control plays a key role in musculoskeletal pain. Currently, there are two general theories about changes in movement in patients with musculoskeletal pain. One theory is that pain causes the change in movement patterns and alters motor control.[46] The other theory is that changes in movement patterns cause the problems that result in pain.[29] Certainly an acute and intense onset of pain can affect the patient's alignment and movement patterns. But the major question is, "What precipitated the pain episode?" As suggested by the model, the repeated movements and sustained postures of daily activities induce the changes in tissues and movement patterns that cause the pain problems. Therefore the pathological changes are secondary to the altered movement pattern

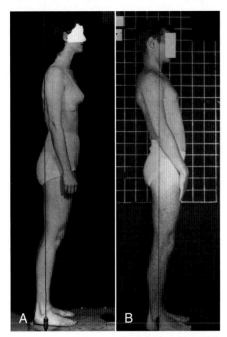

Figure 1-10. Two variations in the relationship of the trunk to the line of gravity. **A,** In the forward-leaning individual with the line of gravity posterior to the trunk, the back extensor muscles are active. **B,** In the backward-leaning individual with the line of gravity anterior to the trunk, the abdominal muscles are active. (From Kendall FP, McCreary EK, Provance PG: *Muscles: testing and function*, ed 4, Philadelphia, 1993, Lippincott Williams & Wilkins.)

and motor control and not primary. Both concepts require that treatment emphasize correction of the movement patterns and the altered motor control. If altered movement patterns cause the problem, then guidelines for prevention are possible. If the pain causes the problem, then the precipitating factors may not be easy to identify. Clinical experience with correcting movement patterns and alleviating symptoms supports the belief that the altered movement patterns are the key factor in causing pain and that correcting the movements and the contributing factors is the most effective long-term treatment.

A prevailing characteristic of the human body is to reduce the degrees of freedom when establishing a movement pattern, thereby achieving a degree of efficiency and minimizing energy expenditure. Movement patterns become established as they are repeated, and the pattern is reinforced by changes in both the nervous and muscular systems. Different stages are involved in motor learning.[47] The initial stage is *motor performance*, in which conscious effort is required to learn a new skill. With practice, the skill no longer requires conscious effort but becomes relatively automatic, performed efficiently and with skill. The final state is termed *motor learning*. Every activity that an individual performs involves this process. A classic example is learning to ride a bicycle: You learn to pedal to propel the bicycle, but at the same time, you learn how to balance and keep your center of gravity appropriately within the base of support provided by the bicycle. Mainly

subconsciously, you are learning the relationship between speed and body adjustments to manage the line of gravity. After practice with conscious effort to master the requirements for balance and pedaling, riding the bike then becomes automatic, and even after many years without cycling, the skill is quickly restored. Another aspect to consider is that even though the pedaling seems simple and straightforward, not everyone uses the same strategy. Studies have shown variations in muscle patterns during cycling, depending on skill and other activity.[48-50] One can also suspect that there are variations in how much hip extensor muscle versus knee extensor muscle activity is used, whether one lower extremity exerts more force than the other. If there are toe clips, how much force used by the hip and knee flexors versus the extensors can vary. Similarly, even though many studies of normal gait have provided the characteristic movement of the center of gravity, the joint angles, and the muscle recruitment patterns, gait is still highly individual, which is how we are able to recognize someone at a distance by the gait pattern, long before we can see the face.

When considering the factors contributing to musculoskeletal pain problems, the patterns of recruitment and derecruitment are primary. The belief is that the patterns are established by the requirement of the activity, personal characteristics, and intensity of use.

Case example. The patient is a 32-year-old right-handed construction worker with pain in the left scapular area between the vertebral border of the scapula and the thoracic spine (Figure 1-11, *A*). During left shoulder flexion and the return from flexion, the patient had marked winging and anterior tilt of the scapula, which was markedly abducted and internally rotated in the rest position (Figure 1-11, *B* and *C*). Both manual and electrophysiological testing did not indicate any muscle weakness or denervation of the serratus anterior muscle. The abducted position of the scapula is also not consistent with serratus anterior muscle weakness. Typically, with serratus anterior muscle weakness, the scapular rest position is adduction.

Key finding. Careful observation of the shoulder motion indicated that the patient was moving the scapula and humerus in a 1:1 ratio both during active shoulder flexion and the return from flexion.

Diagnosis. Scapular winging—motor pattern incoordination.

Treatment. The patient was instructed to face the wall with his elbow flexed and the little finger side of his hand against the wall and to easily slide his hand up the wall to flex his shoulder. On the return, the therapist lightly supported the inferior angle of the scapula and instructed the patient to let his elbow drop to return to the starting position. The purpose of the instruction was to have the patient relax the scapulohumeral muscles more rapidly than he was relaxing the serratus anterior muscle. After approximately 20 repetitions, the patient was able to let his shoulder extend without scapular

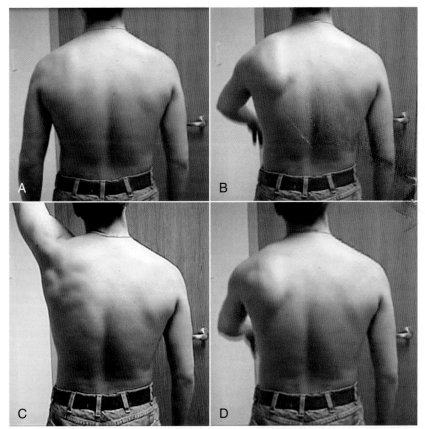

Figure 1-11. A right-handed construction worker with pain for 2 years in the left scapular area. All diagnostic studies were negative. **A,** Abduction, anterior tilt, and internal rotation of the left scapula. **B,** Shoulder flexion causes almost immediate scapular anterior tilt, abduction, and internal rotation, causing the scapula to appear to wing. **C,** The patient has almost full range of motion (ROM) of shoulder flexion without scapular winging, which is inconsistent with severe weakness of the serratus anterior muscle. **D,** During the return from shoulder flexion, the scapula abducts, tilts anteriorly and internally rotates, the same faults evident during flexion.

winging or tilt. The explanation of this motor control–induced problem is that as a right-handed laborer, the primary activity of his left hand was to hold things or objects in place for hammering or sawing. Thus he trained his left upper extremity musculature to maintain a constant long duration co-contraction of the glenohumeral musculature. Finally, his pattern was to lower the arm by allowing the scapula to downwardly rotate, while still maintaining the same glenohumeral alignment, rather than changing the glenohumeral joint position. In other words, he elongated the serratus anterior muscle more rapidly than the scapulohumeral muscles. The pattern became established and was generalized to all other activities involving his left shoulder motion. Undoubtedly, the fact that he was right handed and did not perform a wide repertoire of movements or skills with his left arm contributed to the problem. After training him to change the recruitment and derecruitment patterns, he was able to change the movement patterns affecting his scapula and eliminate his pain problem. When the patient returned for the third time 2 months later, his scapula was no longer winging (Figure 1-12).

The challenge for the therapist is to identify the movement strategy and if the pattern is painful or inconsistent with the kinesiology of the movement, then to retrain the patient. A prevailing belief is that as long as the body is able to move in a certain way, the movement is acceptable and not necessarily potentially harmful. Such a belief is no more accurate than a belief that an individual can eat any type of food and without limit. Similarly, those of us involved in exercise, learn with experience that developing the appropriate program for an individual is not easy if you are aware of all the things that need to be considered.

Case example. A patient has knee pain related to a learned pattern of lower extremity movement. This example of a learned motor pattern that can affect the knee and foot is one of allowing the knees to come together (adduct and medially rotate) when going from sit-to-stand and reverse (Figure 1-13, *A*). This type of pattern was considered "lady-like" and used by those with proper training. Also, women were taught to sit and hold their knees together. When performed frequently and for long periods of time, the result was decreased

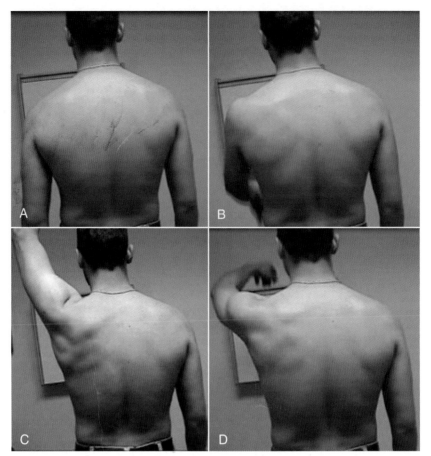

Figure 1-12. **A,** Two months later, third physical therapy visit. The scapula alignment is still impaired, but the vertebral border is not as prominent and the humerus is not as abducted or internally rotated, suggesting improvement in the scapular alignment. **B,** During shoulder flexion, the scapula no longer tilts anterior or internally rotates, thus not appearing to wing. **C,** Shoulder flexion range of motion is increased. **D,** During the return from shoulder flexion, the scapula is not tilting anteriorly or rotating internally, thus not appearing to wing.

performance of the hip abductor and lateral rotator muscles. Also, the hip adductors became over recruited.

Diagnosis. Tibiofemoral rotation: motor pattern incoordination with force production deficit. The consequence at the knee was tibiofemoral rotation and often the foot became pronated.

Treatment. The patient was instructed to practice sit-to-stand and reverse with knees apart (Figure 1-13, *B*), as well as sidelying hip lateral rotation from hip and knee in a flexed position and hip abduction. Side stepping was also recommended.

Learned gait patterns that are characterized by decreased push-off or knee hyperextension are also examples of normal adaptations using motor control mechanisms that result in imprecise movements and are reinforced by muscular and supporting tissue adaptations. In these instances, pain does not have to initiate the motor control adaptation. but the motor control adaptation can lead to the development of pain.

In summary, motor control can be considered a major contributing factor to the development of movement patterns that cause musculoskeletal pain syndromes. *The critical factor is not what you do as much as how you do it.*

Many of us can downhill snow ski, but only a few of us will ever reach a competitive level, much less the Olympic level. The way the nervous system and the responding musculoskeletal system control the performance is the issue, not the participation in skiing. The same mechanisms apply to movement patterns and musculoskeletal pain conditions.

As depicted in the model (see Figure 1-3), these patterns start as motor performance, which is the first stage in motor learning. With continued practice or repetitions, performance becomes motor learning and thus the pattern is considered relatively permanent. At that point, cognitive effort and retraining is necessary to alter the pattern. The therapist needs to recognize that the patient's reference for movement is the continuation of basic patterns that have been used for years. There is no internal sensing system that tells us when performance is optimal (we do what is familiar and not what is right). If a patient's habitual posture is one of a thoracic kyphosis with a forward head, correcting that alignment requires recognition of the fault and conscious practice of the correct alignment. Because the patient does not know what is right but only what is familiar, correction is

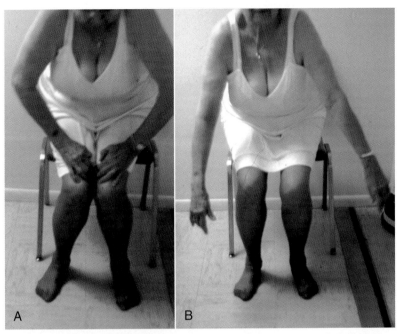

Figure 1-13. Learned movement pattern and correction with instruction. **A,** During sit-to-stand, the patient demonstrates her learned pattern of putting her knees together by hip adduction and internal rotation, as well as using her hands as an additional support. **B,** Able to come to standing while keeping her hips and knees in correct alignment and without support from her hands.

difficult. In addition, the patient needs to be instructed in the appropriate strategy for correcting the alignment fault and movement pattern. Most individuals correct a kyphosis by increasing lumbar extension. They should decrease the thoracic kyphosis by increasing the use of the thoracic back extensor muscles. The primary indicator of problems with performance is the development of pain. Recognition of the role of motor control and musculoskeletal adaptations in mechanical pain strongly suggests that passive treatment can only be viewed as temporary and palliative, rather than a means of (1) alleviating the contributing factors, (2) delaying recurrence, and (3) slowing the progression of the condition. The patient should be informed that changing motor patterns is at least a 4- to 6-week process, depending on the frequency and constancy of the correction. Inter-estingly, that is about the same time required for muscular hypertrophy. The changes in both systems help achieve and reinforce the eventual correction.

Tissue Adaptations of the Muscular System

The adaptations of muscle are changes in (1) length, both increased and decreased; (2) tension development capacity, hypertrophy, and atrophy; and (3) stiffness, the resistance to passive elongation. Traditionally, physical therapy and athletic communities have been concerned about the development of short muscles that need to be stretched. The manifestations of what is often attributed to muscle shortness is twofold. One example is the decreased ROM of a joint (e.g., lack of 80 degrees of hip flexion with the knee extended during the straight-leg raise). The decreased hip flexion is attributed to shortness of the hamstring muscles. The second manifestation is flexion of the lumbar spine resulting from posterior pelvic tilt when the hamstrings are stretched, either during the straight-leg raise or during knee extension when sitting (Figure 1-14). The effect on the lumbar spine is believed to be caused by the lack of sufficient hamstring muscle length. The standard treatment is to stretch the hamstring muscles to eliminate the effect on the pelvis and lumbar spine. Yet, shortness of the hamstring muscles is not a sufficient explanation for the pelvic tilt and the lumbar flexion. Why is the explanation not sufficient, and what are the implications for treatment? If the complete explanation was that the hamstrings are too short, then how are other findings explained? For example, in other patients, when their hamstring muscles are stretched, the pelvis does not tilt and the lumbar spine does not flex but rather the knee does not fully extend. An explanation lies in the relative stiffness of the tissues affecting the lumbar spine as compared to the stiffness of the hamstring muscles.

Relative Stiffness/Flexibility

Based on clinical testing of the muscle lengths of many patients over the past 50 years, the number of individuals with actual muscle shortness is far fewer than the number of individuals who have a "relative stiffness or flexibility" problem. Muscle stiffness is defined as the change in tension per unit change in length.[51] Stiffness refers to the resistance present during the passive elongation of muscle and connective tissue. The stiffness is a normal property of muscle and is the passive tension of a muscle when stretched. The combination of active and passive tension is also referred to as *stiffness.* But, in the current

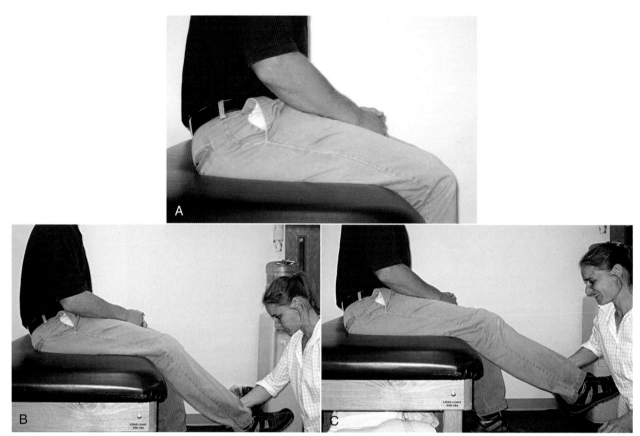

Figure 1-14. A, Patient's hip joint angle is almost 90 degrees with his knees flexed. **B,** With passive knee extension to only 45 degrees, his pelvis tilts posteriorly, and his lumbar spine flexes. The position of the pelvis and lumbar spine indicates that the hamstring muscles are stiffer than the supporting tissues of the lumbar spine. The alignment change occurred before the end of the excursion of the hamstring muscles. **C,** When the hip joint angle is maintained at 90 degrees, the knee cannot be fully extended. The hamstring muscles are short.

discussion and incumbent in this theory, the term *stiffness* is restricted to the passive property of muscle. When a muscle is being elongated and there is movement at the proximal attachment of the muscle, the best explanation is that the tissues stabilizing the joint are not stiff enough relative to the stiffness of the muscle being stretched. Consider the following scenario. Hamstring length is assessed with the patient sitting in a chair with the hip flexed to 80 degree and the knee extended (Figure 1-14). First, when the therapist passively extends the knee, the resistance that is felt is the passive stiffness of the hamstring muscles. If, as the knee is passively extended from 90 degrees of flexion to 45 degrees, the pelvis posteriorly tilts and the lumbar spine flexes, this motion is not an indication of hamstring muscle length. This behavior is an indication of the relative flexibility of the lumbar spine versus the hamstring muscles. If the back extensor muscles attaching to the pelvis and spine are as stiff or stiffer than the hamstring muscles, the pelvis would not tilt and the knee could not be extended (see Figure 1-14, *C*). The range of knee extension would be determined by the length of the hamstrings. Often, in the individual whose pelvis posteriorly tilts and the lumbar spine flexes as the

knee is being passively extended, if the pelvis and the lumbar spine are stabilized at 80 degrees of hip flexion, the knee *can be fully extended* to 0 degrees of flexion (see Figure 1-15). The concept is that the hamstrings and the tissues (muscles and ligaments) of the lumbar spine are springs in series. When the passive tension of the spring being stretched (hamstrings) is greater than the passive tension of the spring in series (lumbar spine tissues), there will be motion at the intervening joint (Figure 1-16). Reasonably, the earlier the movement at this joint the greater the indication of the lack of "stiffness or stability" of the joint. In other words, if the hamstrings are passively stretched and the knee is within 20 degrees of full extension before the pelvis tilts and the lumbar spine flexes, the spine is fairly stiff or stable. If the pelvis begins to tilt posteriorly and the lumbar spine flexes after only 20 degrees of passive knee extension, the spine is very flexible. What the therapist should note is the resistance that is associated with the passive knee extension, as well as the timing of the associated movement. If the patient is actively contracting the hip flexor muscles preventing posterior pelvic tilt posteriorly the motion of the pelvis and lumbar spine would be prevented.

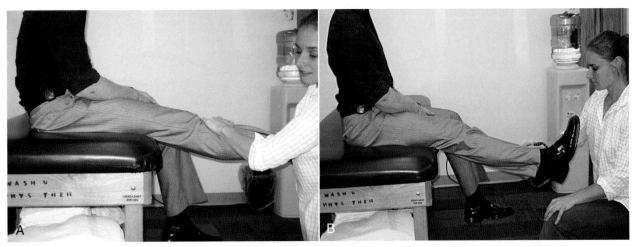

Figure 1-15. **A,** The patient's pelvis is tilted posteriorly, and his lumbar spine is flexed when his knee is passively fully extended. The position of the pelvis and spine can be the result of relative flexibility, which indicates that the hamstrings are stiffer than the supporting tissues of the lumbar spine but not that the hamstring muscles are short. **B,** The patient's hip joint angle is 90 degrees, and no motion of the pelvis or lumbar spine occurs when the knee is fully extended passively. The hamstring muscles would not be considered short.

The mechanism of the relative stiffness/flexibility problem is multifold. For example, as the intervertebral discs lose their height, the attached ligaments become slack rather than remain taut, which changes the passive tension about the joint. Another factor is the passive tension (stiffness) of the hamstring musculotendinous unit versus the passive tension of the back extensor musculotendinous unit. A major source of the passive tension (stiffness) in muscle fibers is an intracellular contractile protein called *titin*.[52,53] Titin is the largest connective tissue protein in the body and provides the passive tension for both striated and cardiac muscle (Figure 1-17). Titin attaches the myosin filament to the Z-line of the sarcomere and there are 6 titin proteins for every myosin filament. Therefore, muscle hypertrophy that increases the number of sarcomeres in parallel and consequently the amount of myosin will also increase the passive tension or stiffness of the muscle. A study examining the passive stiffness of the elbow flexors demonstrated a very high correlation between muscle volume and passive stiffness[54] (Figure 1-18).

A reasonable implication is that one of the important roles of muscle hypertrophy is the effect on passive tension. Realizing that an intrinsic property of the human body is the minimization of energy expenditure when inactive or even when active, the role of passive tension becomes particularly important. Passive tension is a primary contributing factor to alignment, often stability, and even the timing and effectiveness of the mechanical event connected with muscle contraction. Therefore the therapist should note the detected amount of tension as the muscle is passively stretched. This information is indicative of the tension across a joint and can be a source of the stabilizing force across a joint, the compression of the joint, and the resistance to the antagonistic muscle

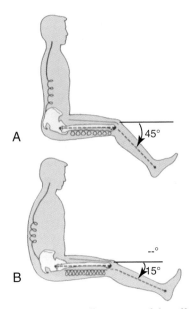

Figure 1-16. Diagrammatic illustration of the effect of relative stiffness of the back extensor muscles and the hamstring muscles. **A,** The back extensor muscles are stiffer than the hamstring muscles, so the knee does not extend. **B,** The back extensor muscles are less stiff than the hamstrings, therefore the pelvis posteriorly tilts and the lumbar spine flexes as the knee extends.

when it contracts. For example, if the patient is sitting and there is marked resistance as the knee is passively extended, then the quadriceps are working against that resistance during active knee extension. Also, if there is a lot of resistance from the hamstrings and that is combined with the tension generated by the quadriceps, then the compressive forces into the joint are going to be greater than if the hamstrings are not stiff. The *passive tension* provided by muscle plays an important role in joint stability, alignment, and in some situations contributes to pain. Thus an

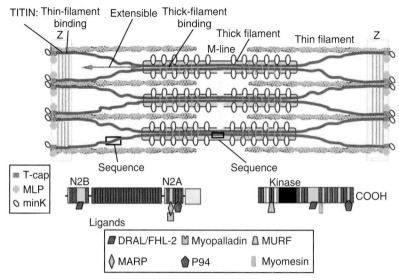

Figure 1-17. Schematic of the sarcomere illustrating the attachments of titin. (From Granzier HL, Labeit S: The giant protein titin: a major player in myocardial mechanics, signaling, and disease, *Circ Res* 94:284-295, 2004.)

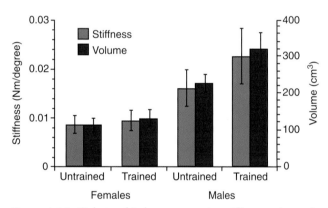

Figure 1-18. Relationship between passive stiffness and muscle volume. There is a high correlation between muscle size and passive stiffness, therefore the greater the hypertrophy of a muscle the greater the resistance to passive elongation. (From Chleboun GS, Howell JN Conatser RR, et al: The relationship between elbow flexor volume and angular stiffness at the elbow, *Clin Biomech* 12(6):383-392, 1997.)

individual's postural alignment is indicative of the passive tension and the length of trunk and opposing muscles. In Figure 1-19, *A*, the preferred, most energy-efficient posture is a swayback alignment with a thoracic kyphosis and forward shoulders. The patient also appears to be in a slight anterior pelvic tilt. Clearly, the rectus abdominis is stiffer than the thoracic back extensors as indicated by the kyphosis. The swayback alignment means that the upper body is behind the line of gravity so that the rectus abdominis is the antigravity lumbar muscle and thus is active. By swaying back, the back extensor muscles are not active and therefore not contributing to the anterior pelvic tilt. The anterior pelvic tilt also suggests that the passive tension from the hip flexors is greater than the tension generated by the rectus abdominis and external oblique abdominal muscles to posterior tilting of the pelvis (see Figure 1-19, *A).* When the subject corrects her

alignment, the strong effort required to lift her chest and decrease the thoracic kyphosis is evident (see Figure 1-19, *B).* This corrected alignment is not energy efficient because of the strong contraction required by the thoracic back extensors, particularly against the stiffness of the rectus abdominis muscle. What an amazing design is incorporated in a system that rewards you when you are at rest for the work you do actively. In other words, performing appropriate abdominal exercises not only "strengthens" the abdominal muscles so that they generate increased active tension, but these muscles also provide control and stability of the trunk when not contracting because of the passive tension or stiffness. But, as illustrated by this example, the stiffness can also contribute to alignment impairments. Consider the alignment of the pelvis. If the hip flexor muscles (e.g., rectus femoris and iliacus muscles) are hypertrophied, the passive tension will pull the pelvis into an anterior tilt (Figure 1-20). To achieve optimal alignment, the rectus abdominis and the external oblique muscles must have a similar, if not a greater, degree of passive tension to maintain the neutral or optimal alignment of pelvic tilt. This situation becomes more complex when considering the contribution of the lumbar back extensor muscles that also anterior tilt the pelvis anteriorly. If the pelvis is tilted anteriorly, the passive tension at the necessary length of the abdominal muscles does not offset the pull of the rectus femoris, the other hip flexors, and the back extensors. But, clearly, such muscle dynamics are not the only possibilities, and further examples are useful.

The alignment of a thoracic kyphosis can develop from a variety of factors. In some cases, the *abdominal muscle strength (and associated passive tension) can be contributing* to the kyphosis while in other cases, the *abdominal muscles are weak* because of the kyphosis.

An individual participates in fitness activities, such as cycling, or has performed numerous sit-up exercises, the

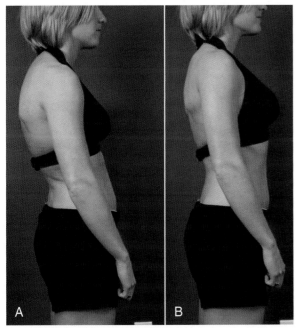

Figure 1-19. Implications of standing alignment and passive stiffness. **A,** Natural standing alignment with minimum energy expenditure. The swayed back trunk with the thoracic kyphosis indicates the thoracic back extensor muscles are not as stiff as the rectus abdominis muscle. The swayback minimizes the activity of the lumbar back extensor muscles, thereby not contributing to anterior tilt of the pelvis that is associated with action of these muscles. The anterior pelvic tilt indicates that the hip flexors are stiffer than the abdominal muscles that do not generate counter-balancing passive tension at the correct length to maintain ideal pelvic alignment. **B,** Active contraction of thoracic back extensor muscles improves her thoracic alignment. The emphasis of her treatment program is to improve the participation of the external oblique abdominal muscle more than the rectus abdominis to achieve correct pelvic tilt without increasing the thoracic kyphosis. The permanent correction requires enough change in the *passive tension and length* of the abdominal and thoracic back extensor muscles to "hold" the correct alignment *passively* and not actively.

abdominals will be stiff and/or short (see Figure 1-19). The exercise or activity has resulted in abdominal muscles that are stiffer than the thoracic back extensors. Thus the abdominal muscles are contributing to the kyphosis. Therefore the back extensor muscles may be pulled into the elongated position and have to work against the passive tension of the abdominals. Thus to correct the alignment, the thoracic back extensor muscles in this individual have to become stronger than the abdominals and have to generate enough tension passively at a shorter length than the muscle currently demonstrates.

A variation occurs when the trunk is swayed back so that the abdominals are the antigravity muscle of the trunk. This is a frequent posture of men who have performed many sit-up exercises (Figure 1-21). This individual is swayed back enough that his abdominal muscles are holding the trunk against gravity. The demands on his abdominal muscles are exaggerated because his shoulders are broad and in line with his trunk. The hypertrophy of the abdominal muscles and the associated passive stiffness means that the thoracic back extensor muscles have to generate more tension to correct the kyphosis than if the abdominal muscles were not stiff. In this swayback position, the back extensor muscles are not required to support his trunk and, thus, are usually atrophied. As evident from his posterior pelvic tilt and flat lumbar spine, neither the back extensors, nor the hip flexors are generating sufficient passive tension to counterbalance the tension of the abdominal muscles and correct the alignment of the thoracic and lumbar spine as well as the pelvis and hip joint. This passive tension of a muscle is NOT "inhibited" by any type of nervous system mechanism. This passive tension is a function of the intrinsic connective tissue proteins of muscle. Also noteworthy is that in these situations the antagonist to the thoracic back extension, the rectus abdominis muscle, becomes a source of resistance. This situation is one in

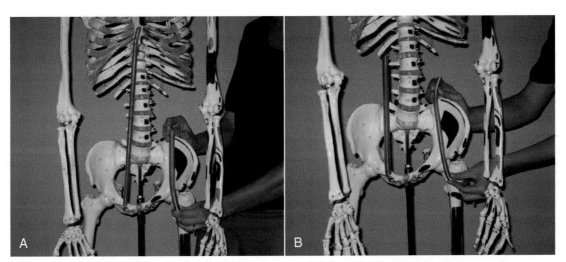

Figure 1-20. Springs depicting the passive tension of the abdominal and hip flexor muscles. The passive tension (stiffness) of muscles exerts an almost constant pull on its attachments. **A,** When the least stiff spring is the abdominal muscles, the stiffer spring of the hip flexors will pull the pelvis into an anterior pelvic tilt. **B,** When abdominal muscles are stiffer than the hip flexor muscles, the pelvis will be maintained in the correct alignment.

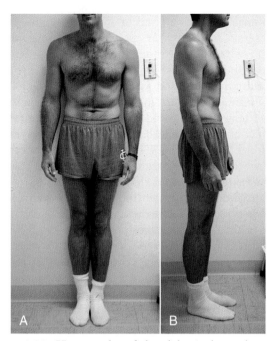

Figure 1-21. Hypertrophy of the abdominal muscles maintained by being the antigravity muscles of the trunk. **A,** Anterior view indicating the muscle definition of the abdominal muscles. **B,** The side view demonstrating that the head and shoulders are swayed back so that the line of gravity is anterior to the trunk. The patient also worked with his arms in front of him causing even more posterior sway of the trunk.

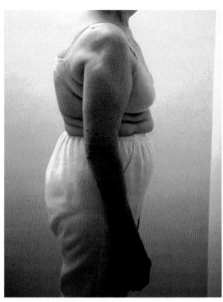

Figure 1-22. Thoracic kyphosis associated with excessive length of the thoracic paraspinal muscles and with laxity of the abdominal muscles.

which the body is acting as a resistance machine. The stiffness of the abdominal muscles is resistance to the thoracic back extensor muscles. Correction of this situation requires that the patient stands with his back against the wall to correct the sway back alignment. He should try to actively extend his back as he flexes his shoulders. During the day, he should frequently lean forward while trying to keep his back straight to increase the use of his back extensor muscles and the gluteus maximus muscles. He has to be careful when lifting weights, because he will automatically sway back and use his abdominal muscles to stabilize his trunk.

A third situation is one in which the individual has allowed the trunk to remain flexed out of habit, and the thoracic back extensors have lengthened and do not have the passive tension at the right length to keep the thoracic spine correctly aligned (Figure 1-22). In this individual, the abdominal muscles are weak without a great deal of passive tension (stiffness). Correction of the kyphosis requires frequent and sustained contraction of the thoracic extensor muscles until the length and the passive tension of the muscles is sufficient to maintain the correct alignment of the thoracic spine.

A high degree of muscular passive tension can also influence the effectiveness of an active muscle force. Consider the situation of the abdominal muscles in two individuals with very different muscle conditions. In one individual, the abdominal muscles, attaching to the ribcage and the pelvis, are notably hypertrophied so that

the individual has a flat abdomen and obvious muscle definition (see Figure 1-21). These abdominal muscles will be exerting tension on the pelvis and the rib cage. The second individual has notable distension of the abdomen and an obvious lack of muscle definition (Figure 1-23). If the first individual elicits a minimal contraction of his abdominal muscles, there is immediate delivery of tension to the rib cage and pelvis and the tension will be effective because of the hypertrophy. In the second individual with the distended abdomen and poor muscle definition, contraction of the abdominal muscles requires a great effort and the development of tension would be relatively slow because of the slack that has to be taken up to have an effect on the rib cage and pelvis. The eventual delivery of tension would be relatively small because of the lack of sarcomeres in parallel in the muscle cells. The timing of electromyographic (EMG) activity might be similar in both individuals, but the rate and the effectiveness of force development would be very different.

Assessment of the contributing factors to the patient's condition is essential to develop an effective treatment program. Consider the variations in the three individuals described as having different contributing factors to their thoracic kyphosis (see Figures 1-19, 1-21, and 1-22). These individuals may consider abdominal muscle exercises as an important part of their fitness program, but in some cases, such exercises would not be an impediment, but in other cases, they would be. In the first example (see Figure 1-19), the patient should perform exercises that emphasize the external oblique muscles, particularly the action of a posterior pelvic tilt. The patient should flatten the back against a wall and then try to extend the thoracic spine and try to hold the position for as long as possible. The forward shoulder posture helped minimize

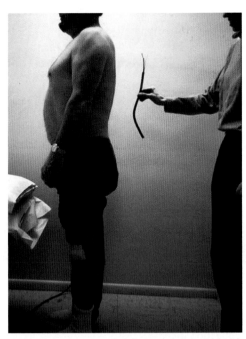

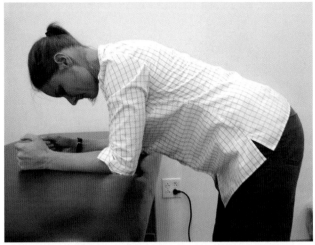

Figure 1-24. The modified quadruped position can be used to decrease the thoracic kyphosis and help elongate the trunk. The patient is instructed to allow the upper back to relax, letting the chest drop toward the table. The patient can then rock backward, which provides a slight stretch of the trunk.

Figure 1-23. Prominence of abdomen consistent with diminished abdominal muscle stiffness and a diastasis of the linea alba above the umbilicus. Contraction of abdominal muscles with this condition will have a minimal effect on the alignment of the pelvis and rib cage.

the demands on her abdominals to hold her trunk against gravity. Using hand weights, performing shoulder flexion to 90 degrees in the corrected position would also hypertrophy the thoracic back extensor muscles, helping to induce the changes in passive stiffness that is needed to achieve the change in the alignment. When performing shoulder flexion, she has to posteriorly tilt and externally rotate her scapula to correct the alignment. Contraction of the serratus anterior muscle and the trapezius to maintain the scapular position will increase the passive stiffness of the muscle, which is necessary to correct scapular and shoulder girdle position.

In the second individual (see Figure 1-21) with the swayback posture with the abdominal muscles functioning as an antigravity muscle, correcting the swayback is extremely important. As mentioned, this individual should perform exercises that emphasize thoracic and lumbar back extensor muscle activity and even hip flexion exercises to correct the posterior pelvic tilt. The individual should frequently stand with the back against the wall and practice aligning the shoulders and the hips. This individual could also practice external oblique abdominal exercises but should avoid any type of trunk curls. The abdominal muscles would be an even greater source of resistance to the thoracic back extensors than in the first individual. Both of these individuals should practice standing straight and taking deep breaths, particularly after exercising such as riding a bike. Lateral thoracic and not lumbar side flexion would also be beneficial to stretch the abdominal muscles. The final

individual (see Figure 1-22) with the assumed thoracic kyphosis needs to practice the correct thoracic alignment but does not have the resistance of the abdominal muscles. Abdominal exercises for the external oblique abdominal muscles in particular could be performed. She should not do any trunk-curls, which would add to the kyphosis, and because she is probably at risk for osteopenia. The program should emphasize frequent performance rather than a lot of repetitions at one time. If the individual has a lumbar lordosis, then abdominal muscle exercises, again particularly for the external oblique muscles, would be important. These exercises emphasize posterior pelvic tilt and not thoracic flexion movements. The patient has to try to elongate her trunk while performing exercises. Two exercises that are useful for elongating the trunk are shown in Figures 1-24 and 1-25.

These may be subtle variations, but such detail adds to the effectiveness and the efficiency of the treatment. Obviously, correction of the thoracic kyphosis requires contraction of the thoracic back extensor muscles sufficiently to achieve the optimal spinal alignment. Then the back extensor muscles have to hypertrophy enough that they can maintain the thoracic spine in the correct alignment with passive and not active tension.

Too often such a patient is given back extension exercises without ensuring that the thoracic spine is extending and instead the patient is extending the lumbar spine. Instead, the most effective exercise would be for the patient to stand with the back against the wall and lift the chest while trying to perform a posterior pelvic tilt with the external oblique abdominal muscles and then perform bilateral shoulder flexion. Once the patient has the correct thoracic alignment, lifting light weights while standing in the optimal alignment can be added to the program. The purpose is to hypertrophy the thoracic back extensors

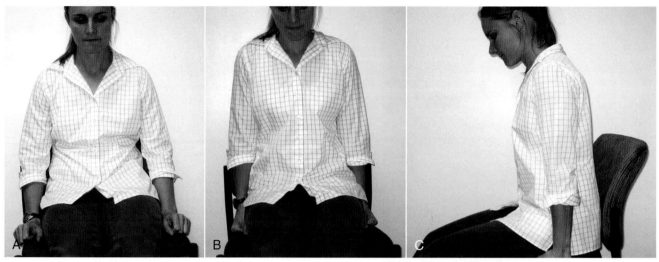

Figure 1-25. A, Patient sitting slumped with a thoracic kyphosis. **B,** Pushing up in the chair to elongate the trunk. She is not lifting her buttocks off of the chair, but she is just elongating the trunk by pushing into the seat of the chair and locking her elbows. The patient then tries to contract all of her trunk muscles to maintain the trunk alignment, and then she lifts her hands off the seat of the chair. **C,** Side view of the trunk elongation exercise.

with the goal of the musculature developing enough passive stiffness at the right length so that the posture is maintained without active effort. All three individuals should also do the quadruped exercise that allows the thoracic spine to flatten. In the same position, performing shoulder flexion while maintaining the corrected alignment contracts the thoracic back extensor muscles at the correct length.

In ideal alignment, there is optimal muscle participation that is not present when alignment is impaired as in the previous examples (see Figure 1-9). If an individual has ideal alignment in the standing position, when leaning forward slightly, the back extensors are activated because they are the antigravity muscle. When this individual leans backward slightly, the abdominal muscles are activated because they are the antigravity muscles. This type of oscillation in muscle participation contributes to balanced use of both anterior and posterior trunk muscles rather than almost constant use of one group of muscles.

In summary, muscle stiffness is an extremely valuable property of muscle that enables the body to be supported with minimal energy expenditure. The foregoing examples demonstrated the importance of optimal passive tension of muscles attaching to either side of a joint. Good alignment is indicative of balanced passive tension of muscles attaching to a joint or skeletal segment, such as the thorax or pelvis. The passive tension, which also has a high correlation to active tension, is the key to the alignment and stabilizing properties of the joint. As in all things, stiffness can become excessive or insufficient. The relative stiffness/flexibility properties are often the contributing factor to (1) alignment impairments, (2) one joint moving more readily than an adjoining joint, and (3) inadequate stabilization or inappropriate movement during the passive elongation of a muscle.

Case example. A young woman with right thoracic pain played volleyball and soccer. She illustrated another variation of the role of relative stiffness. For both soccer and volleyball, she had developed a great deal of trunk rotation to the right and very limited rotation to the left. As a right-handed individual, she used her right hand for spiking, which she performed frequently causing hypertrophy of her right pectoral muscles.

Key finding. In the supine position, when her right shoulder was passively or actively flexed, the right side of her ribcage elevated. When her left shoulder was passively or actively flexed, the left side of her ribcage did not elevate. The explanation is that the abdominal muscles attaching to the right side of her ribcage were elongated, allowing the excessive trunk rotation, therefore the passive tension from the pectoral muscles that are stretched with shoulder flexion elevated her ribcage because the passive tension from the abdominals was not sufficient.

Diagnosis. Thoracic rotation motor pattern incoordination. The asymmetrical effect on the ribcage was contributing to the rotation of the thoracic spine and her thoracic pain.

These examples also indicate how excessive or asymmetrical passive tension from muscles, such as the abdominals, can contribute to pain problems. Another example is how passive tension of the abdominal muscles can contribute to neck pain and limited ROM (see Chapter 3). Because the scalene muscles attach to the ribcage, if the rectus abdominis and the external oblique muscles are stiff and/or short, they pull down on the ribcage and the attachment of the scaleni muscles. Passively elevating of the ribcage in these patients, enables them to increase the rotation of the cervical spine, as well as alleviate their neck pain (Figure 1-26). One of the methods used to assess the

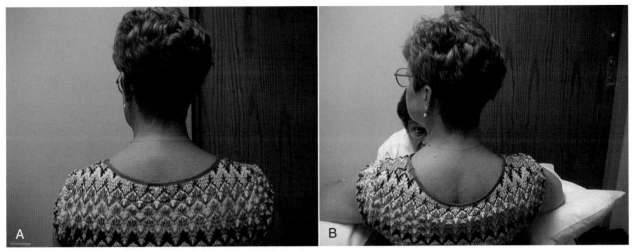

Figure 1-26. Stiffness of the scaleni muscles limiting rotation of head and cervical spine. Patient with severe headaches and neck pain with short and stiff abdominal muscles. **A,** Maximum head and neck rotation. **B,** Increased rotation of head and neck when arms are supported and the rib cage is passively elevated.

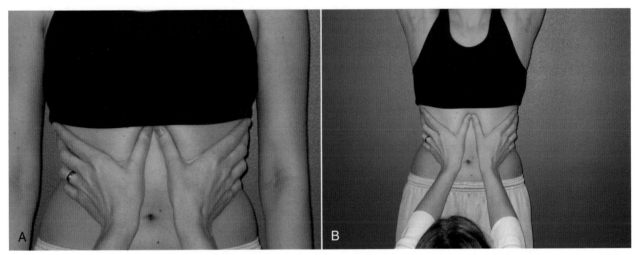

Figure 1-27. Assessing the infrasternal angle as an indication of abdominal muscle resting length. **A,** Narrow infrasternal angle associated with stiffness and/or shortness of the external oblique abdominal muscles. **B,** If the external oblique abdominal muscles are short, the change in diameter of the rib cage during maximum inhalation is less than 2 inches.

abdominal muscle extensibility is to measure the change in the circumference of the ribcage between maximum exhalation to maximum inhalation. The ideal change is 3 in or 7 cm. As the individual ages, the excursion decreases, but a change of 2 in or less in a young individual is not optimal. The same assessment of the change in the diameter of the ribcage is made during bilateral shoulder flexion, which stretches the abdominals. If the excursion is markedly limited, again the abdominal muscles are considered too short or stiff. If the infrasternal angle is less than 70 degrees, this could be another indicator of short or excessively stiff abdominals, particularly the external oblique muscles (Figure 1-27).

Muscle Length Adaptations

Increased length. Another muscle adaptation that clinically seems to be more common than loss of muscle length is increased resting muscle length. Possibly, small changes in muscle length are changes in passive resting tension, while greater increases in muscle length are associated with addition of sarcomeres in series in the muscle fibers. Although evidence for increased sarcomeres in series in adult human muscle is very limited,[55] such adaptations have been demonstrated in animals as the result of both passive immobilization[56] (Table 1-1 and Figure 1-28) and active use in a lengthened position.[57] A recent review paper suggests that short-term muscle lengthening is associated with changes in sensation, the subject's response to the discomfort of muscle stretching.[51] The effects from long-term muscle lengthening have not been studied,[51] but based on clinical observations, some muscle behaviors are best explained by such muscle length adaptations. The implications are important for both resting alignment and active motions. For example, individuals

TABLE **1-1**

Muscle Belly Length, Sarcomere Number, and Sarcomere Length Measurements of Young and Adult Muscles Immobilized in the Lengthened and Shortened Positions*

	Muscle Belly Length (mm)		Sarcomere Number		Sarcomere Length (μm)	
	Experimental	**Control**	**Experimental**	**Control**	**Experimental**	**Control**
ADULT						
Lengthened	[10·6 ± 0·16	10·8 ± 0·24]	2560 ± 36	2215 ± 14	2·43 ± 0·049	3·13 ± 0·021
Shortened	[6·3 ± 0·12	6·1 ± 0·17]	1824 ± 28	2283 ± 18	2·08 ± 0·050	1·41 ± 0·018
YOUNG						
Lengthened	5·3 ± 0·25	7·0 ± 0·15	1281 ± 31	1739 ± 24	2·64 ± 0·124	3·10 ± 0·093
Shortened	4·3 ± 0·17	5·7 ± 0·16	1005 ± 19	1826 ± 20	2·40 ± 0·072	1·62 ± 0·081

*In each case, muscles from five animals were used. Data in brackets are not significantly different from each other (P > 0.1).
(From Williams PE, Goldspink G: Changes in sarcomere length and physiological properties in mobilized muscles, *J Anat* 127:458-459, 1978.)

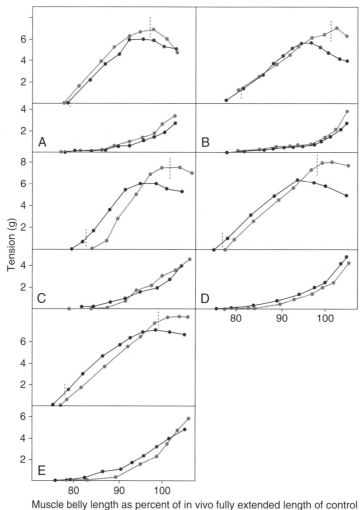

Muscle belly length as percent of in vivo fully extended length of control

Figure 1-28. Active and passive length-tension curves of mice muscles that have been immobilized in a lengthened position for 3 weeks and compared to control muscles. Note the curves of the lengthened muscles are shifted to the right. *Red line*, Control muscle; *blue line*, experimental-lengthened muscle. (From Williams PE, Goldspink G: Changes in sarcomere length and physiological properties in immobilized muscles, *J Anat* 127:459-468, 1978.)

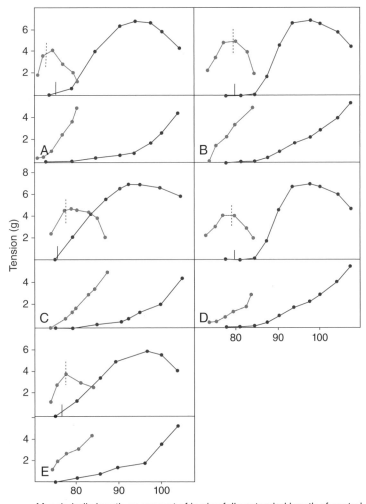

Figure 1-29. Active and passive length-tension curves of mice muscles that have been immobilized in a shortened position for 3 weeks and compared to control muscles. Note the curve of the shortened muscle is shifted to the left. *Red line,* Control muscle; *blue line,* experimental-shortened muscle. (From Williams PE, Goldspink G: Changes in sarcomere length and physiological properties in immobilized muscles, *J Anat* 127:459-468, 1978.)

whose shoulders are depressed not only are increasing the stress on their neck, but they are also changing the resting alignment of their shoulder at the sternoclavicular joint and at the glenohumeral joint. If the shoulders are very depressed, there has to be an associated change in the length of the upper trapezius and the serratus anterior muscles. This change in length of the muscles not only affects the resting alignment of the shoulders but also affects the characteristics of the movement of the shoulder joint because of the shift in the length-tension curve to the right. Thus the development of appropriate tension to upwardly rotate and elevate the scapula will not be possible if the underlying condition is an increase in the number of sarcomeres in series.

Decreased length. As shown by experiments in animals,[56] the development of true muscle shortness is associated with loss of sarcomeres in series in muscle fibers. Animal studies have shown that muscles maintained in a shortened position or at a short resting length

for as little as 3 weeks will lose sarcomeres in series and prevent the full excursion of the joint to which it is attached[56] (Figure 1-29). A typical example is the lack of 80 degrees of hip flexion with the knee extended that is considered an indication of "short" hamstrings. There is a lack of clarity in clinical practice about the various mechanisms involved in muscle shortness and tissues affected by stretch or the need to stretch. Possibly because "muscle stretching" is such a long-standing part of practice that, in spite of the efforts of various investigators to clarify the process,[58,59] confusion exists about methods to be used. A reasonable way to consider the appropriate intervention for variations in hamstring length is as follows. For example, if the decreased ROM of hip flexion with the knee extended is only 10 to 15 degrees and can be regained by stretching for a few minutes, the alteration can best be explained by the creep or viscoelastic properties of muscle. Repetitions of the stretch produce a temporary change in the resting length of the muscle, conveying the impression that the muscle is "longer" or "stretched." But this is a temporary state, and the muscle will return to its original resting length over a period of minutes, partially depending upon the duration of the stretching. In contrast, if the hamstring muscles are limiting the motion of the joint by 30 to 40 degrees, then the most likely explanation is that the muscle fibers have lost sarcomeres in series and the treatment has to be stretching of long duration (for example, 30 minutes or more, several times a day for many days) and as sustained as possible. Stretching should not be forceful because a reasonable explanation for this condition is that the muscle has lost sarcomeres in series and that requires protein synthesis and not just a change in the conformation of the proteins in the muscle cells.

Although muscles can become shortened by loss of sarcomeres in series, this is not the most common problem contributing to musculoskeletal pain. The most common problem is the relative stiffness of muscles attaching to the joint. If an individual stands with the pelvis in an anterior pelvic tilt, the therapist should not assume that the hip flexors are short. Rather, a likely explanation is that the passive stiffness of the hip flexors, anteriorly tilting the pelvis, is greater than the passive stiffness of the rectus abdominis and the external oblique muscles, posteriorly tilting the pelvis, at the length necessary to maintain the pelvis in the optimal position. The back extensor muscles could also be contributing to the anterior tilt of the pelvis, further increasing the demands on the passive tension of the abdominal muscles. These concepts are discussed in the section on relative flexibility/stiffness.

Accurate assessment of the contributing factors is important to the development of the treatment program. If the problem is a relative stiffness problem, then stretching the hip flexors is *not* going to change the pelvic alignment. Rather, the external oblique and rectus abdominis muscles must be able to generate the necessary *passive tension* at the right length, which requires hypertrophying the abdominal muscles so that the amount of titin increases. But the exercises must be performed in such a way as to optimize the hypertrophy with the abdominal muscles at the right length. The actively performed exercises must produce the desired change in length and passive tension, which means that performing exercises, such as leg raises or leg lowering in the supine position, may be counter productive because they are also a hip flexor muscle exercise and performed with the hip flexors in a shortened position. This would be problematic in individuals with large and heavy thighs or long lower extremities. Thus the stiffness of the hip flexors at a short length may be increasing more rapidly than the desired changes in the abdominal muscles.

Muscle Performance

The term *muscle performance* is preferred as compared to *muscle weakness* to place an emphasis on whether all factors influencing the muscle's participation are performing optimally. Performance includes timing, length,

passive tension, and the ability to generate active tension and endurance. Assessment of muscle strength provides information about muscle performance, and the results of the test can provide at least four possible determinations about the muscle. These test results indicate how a muscle is being used, characteristics of the adaptations, and insights into the movement patterns. The inference is that all factors that determine recruitment and use patterns are not optimal. The implication is that strengthening the muscle will not adequately address the problem because the "weakness" is the *result* not the cause. This rationale, of course, does not apply to conditions in which there is denervation, disease, or direct trauma to the muscle. Manual muscle testing (MMT) can be used to discern whether the muscle is (1) weak because of atrophy and the lack of sarcomeres in parallel and thus unable to develop adequate active tension; (2) strained because of being subjected to forces that have torn or disrupted the Z-lines of the sarcomeres and unable to develop adequate active tension; (3) too long, having added sarcomeres in series, and the muscle does not develop the appropriate tension throughout the ROM (Figure 1-30), or (4) normal.

Determination of these four possibilities is based on the following test findings. The MMT methods used are those that apply pressure with the 1-joint muscle at its shortest length, as developed by Kendall et al.[60] For example, when testing the lower trapezius muscle, the shoulder is placed in about 145 degrees of abduction with the glenohumeral joint laterally rotated and the scapula upwardly rotated. The therapist applies pressure to the forearm as the patient attempts to hold the position. If the patient is able to hold the test position when the therapist applies maximum pressure, the muscle is graded *strong/normal* or 5/5. If

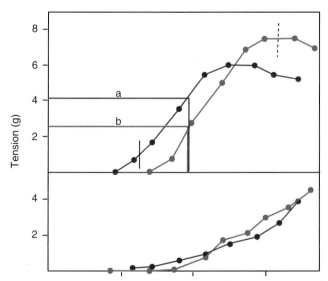

Figure 1-30. Illustration of the effect on the active tension of lengthened muscle. If the control muscle and the lengthened muscle are tested in the same position *(line a)*, the tension is less for the lengthened muscle than for the control *(line b)*. (Data adapted from Williams PE, Goldspink G: Changes in sarcomere length and physiological properties in immobilized muscles, *J Anat* 127:459-468, 1978.)

when the therapist applies pressure, the patient is not able to hold the position and the arm and scapula are unable to tolerate the pressure throughout the range, the muscle is considered *weak* and the grade can range from 3+ to 4+, depending on the amount of pressure the therapist applies that causes the arm to move. If the therapist applies pressure and the patient is unable to hold at the initial test position, but after a few degrees of motion of the arm and scapula, the patient is able to resist the continued pressure, the muscle is considered *long* but not weak. The final possible test finding is that if the patient has tenderness in the muscle belly of the muscle to palpation, then strain is suspected. If during testing, when the therapist applies pressure, the patient complains of pain and the muscle tests weak because the shoulder position cannot be held throughout the range as pressure is applied by the therapist, and the muscle is considered *weak because of muscle strain*. Clearly, these conditions require different interventions. The strained muscle must not be subjected to continued stress so healing can take place. The weak muscle must be strengthened by an appropriately designed progressive resistance exercise program. The long muscle must be used in shortened ranges, and the load decreased enough to allow the part to which it attaches to be moved through its optimal ROM.

The following examples are given to clarify and illustrate these possible muscle performance conditions and relate them to other tissue conditions and adaptations. Although this book does not discuss MS syndromes of the shoulder girdle, for syndromes of the neck, elbow, and the hand, part of the treatment involves optimizing shoulder girdle function. The performance of the serratus anterior muscle is used as the example.

Case example 1. A 40-year-old woman has not been physically active, but her appearance is important to her so she has tried to stand up straight and hold her shoulders back to have good posture. She has developed neck pain and some discomfort on the top of her shoulder that occurs when she performs tasks that involve reaching overhead. She is 5 ft 5 inches tall and weighs 140 lbs.

Physical examination. The examination indicates that the vertebral border of her scapula at the spine of scapula is 2 inches away from her thoracic spine. Therefore, her scapula is in adduction (retraction), which means the resting position of the serratus anterior muscle is longer than the optimal length. When she performs shoulder flexion, her scapula only upwardly rotates 40 degrees, instead of the optimal 50 to 55 degrees, and the inferior angle of the scapula barely reached the side of her thorax rather than reaching the midaxillary line. Her shoulder flexion was 175 degrees. MMT of the serratus anterior demonstrates that she could not hold the test position and that her arm gave through the range as the therapist applied pressure. Based on the pressure the therapist applied, the muscle was determined to be weak and graded 4−/5.

Key findings. The patient's scapula was not moving correctly because the upward rotation was only 40 degrees, not the appropriate 50 to 55 degrees, but she was flexing her shoulder almost 175 degrees. Therefore, as compensation for the decreased scapular upward rotation and abduction, the glenohumeral flexion was greater than 120 degrees. The serratus anterior muscle tested weak. No resistance was noted during assisted scapular motion. Correction of the scapular motion eliminated the pain in the shoulder.

Diagnosis. Scapular downward rotation syndrome with force production deficit.

Treatment. The patient was given two main exercises for this condition. First, she was instructed to perform shoulder flexion by facing the wall, with her elbow flexed and then sliding the little finger side of her hand up the wall as she flexed her shoulder and extended her elbow. When the patient initially performed this exercise, her scapula did not move through the optimal ROM, and she commented on the discomfort at the top of her shoulder. The therapist then assisted the scapular motion as the patient performed the shoulder flexion so that there was optimal scapular upward rotation and abduction. The therapist *did not note any resistance* as she assisted the scapular motion. The therapist continued to assist the patient with the exercise, providing verbal, as well as manual cues, so that the patient was able to produce the correct scapular motion during the shoulder flexion. The important point is that the patient was *not* given serratus anterior muscle strengthening exercises, such as the push-up plus, but was given an exercise that required the optimal motion of the scapula. *Improving the "strength" of a muscle does not automatically mean or ensure that the scapula will move correctly.* To be sure the end result is that the scapula moves correctly, the therapist must see the scapula move correctly as the patient performs the motion. There is no magic in an exercise unless the exercise is producing the desired result at the time of performance. For the second exercise, the patient is in the quadruped position to ensure activity of the serratus anterior muscle, which supports the thorax through its attachment to the scapula as the weight is placed on the upper extremity. The patient's initial position was one of scapular adduction and slight winging. She was instructed to rock backward, decreasing the loading on her shoulder girdle and allowing her scapulae to abduct and upwardly rotate. The therapist provided some assistance in guiding the scapula into the correct position. The patient then rocked forward to the starting position while maintaining the abducted position of the scapula and controlling the winging. She stopped coming forward at the point she could not control the scapula. Again, the major point is that the serratus anterior muscle is forced to develop tension, but the correct control of the scapular motion is the criterion for being an acceptable exercise. The exercises will progress as the patient is able to demonstrate the proper movement of the scapula and does not have pain. The goal is to improve the support of the scapula by the serratus anterior muscle so that the downward pull from the cervicoscapular muscles is reduced, thus reducing stress on the neck.

Case example 2. The second case is a 28-year-old male who performs a regular program of resistive exercises and plays tennis at least twice a week. He also has neck pain that increases when he plays tennis. He is 5 ft 11 inches tall and weighs 185 lbs. He has a very muscular build with marked hypertrophy of his shoulder girdle muscles.

Physical examination. In the standing position, his shoulders are depressed and his scapula are adducted, with the vertebral border of the spine of the scapula 2½ inches from his thoracic spine. The muscle definition of the rhomboids is particularly obvious. On completion of shoulder flexion, the scapula was upwardly rotated 45 degrees (55 degrees is normal) and the inferior angle reached the posterolateral border of the thorax, not the midaxillary line, yet shoulder flexion was 175 degrees. MMT of the serratus anterior muscle indicated that the patient could not maintain the initial test position when the therapist applied pressure, but after a 15-degree change in the shoulder angle because of scapular downward rotation, he was able to maintain the position against maximum pressure. The test performance indicated that the serratus anterior muscle was long but not weak. When the patient was asked to perform the exercise of shoulder flexion by sliding the little finger side of his hand up the wall, the therapist had to assist the movement of the scapula. The therapist noted that there was *marked resistance to the assistance given to the scapula* in the direction of upward rotation and abduction.

Key findings. The interpretation is that the serratus anterior was too long to move the scapula through the optimal range and the resistance to the motion was from the stiffness of the hypertrophied rhomboid muscles. The serratus anterior muscle had to generate enough tension to overcome the passive resistance of the rhomboids, as well as shorten enough to move the scapula through the optimal range.

Diagnosis. Scapular downward rotation—motor pattern incoordination. In this situation, the assistance of the therapist in moving the scapula also helped improve the extensibility of the rhomboid muscles.

Treatment. The patient was encouraged to frequently perform shoulder flexion with a major emphasis on abducting and upwardly rotating the scapula. He was also advised to avoid any tendency to "hold" his shoulders back and to cease any type of scapular adduction exercises. The patient also performed the quadruped exercise with the major emphasis on abducting and upwardly rotating the scapula.

Another consideration is how these tissue adaptations contribute to the stress on the cervical spine. First, the hypertrophy of the shoulder girdle musculature increases the weight of the upper extremities and the support by the cervicoscapular muscles adds to the compressive forces on the cervical spine. The passive stiffness of these muscles can also restrict the ease of cervical rotation. Second, when the patient uses his arms, particularly during the overhead motion that requires scapular upward rotation and abduction, the passive stiffness of the levator scapulae muscle could exert a rotational, as well as a compressive, force as it is being stretched during the scapular motion. Also, the passive resistance from the stiffness of the rhomboids requires the upper trapezius to develop greater tension than if there were minimal resistance to scapular upward rotation and elevation. The increased demands on the upper trapezius muscle can further add to the compressive force on the cervical spine. If the patient has neck pain during shoulder flexion, support of the scapula by the therapist during the shoulder motion can decrease or even eliminate the symptoms, which supports the hypothesis about the contributing factors. Improving the participation of the serratus anterior muscle and decreasing the stiffness of the rhomboid muscles would reduce the stress on the cervical spine. These examples illustrate the influences of the intersegmental demands and explain why the therapist needs to consider multiple influences on the painful joint during the examination when developing the treatment program.

In summary, in both patients, the movement impairment of the scapula was similar, but the underlying contributing factors were markedly different, requiring a different emphasis in the treatment program. In both conditions, the primary emphasis has to be on ensuring that the scapula moves correctly. In the first patient, a major contributing factor was the actual weakness, or inability to develop sufficient contractile tension, as well as the increased length of the serratus anterior muscle. In the second patient, the serratus anterior muscle was not weak but was long and had to develop enough tension to overcome the resistance from the rhomboid muscles. In both of these cases, the shoulder flexion was 180 degrees, which means that glenohumeral motion occurred more readily and was a site of compensation for the deficient scapular motion. Because the scapular motion was insufficient to achieve the 180 degrees of shoulder flexion, the glenohumeral motion exceeded the standard of 120 degrees. Improving scapular motion will decrease the stress on the glenohumeral joint structures by stopping the excessive excursion. These scenarios both address movement imprecision and the body's tendency to the path of least resistance. Additional discussion of tissue adaptations is provided in the first volume of this book, *Diagnosis and Treatment of Movement Impairment Syndromes.*

Imprecise Movement

The end result of the tissue adaptations, whether skeletal, muscular, and neurological, is that movement is altered and no longer precise. As stated frequently, our hypothesis is that alteration in the accessory or arthrokinematic motion is probably the most common and most important contributing factor. Excessive physiological or osteokinematic motion has to be associated with altered accessory motion. As discussed in the previous case examples, the lack of scapular motion resulted in excessive glenohumeral

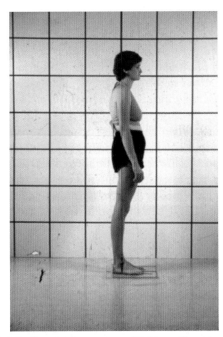

Figure 1-31. Swayback posture with line of gravity posterior to hip joint, decreasing the hip extensor moment. Associated with poor definition of the gluteal muscles.

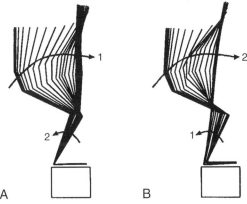

Figure 1-32. Motion analysis display of two strategies controlling the knee motion during stepping up on a footstool. **A,** Strategy in which the body is moved toward the knee that emphasizes control by the knee extensor muscles. **B,** Strategy in which the knee is pulled toward the body that emphasizes control by the hip extensor muscles. (From Sahrmann SA: *Diagnosis and treatment of movement impairment syndromes*, St Louis, 2002, Mosby; courtesy Amy Bastian, PhD, PT.)

motion. This also means excessive accessory motion of either or both superior glide or anterior glide. Assessment of accessory motion impairments is indeed difficult, and most often the fault is implied when pain is present during the performance of a physiological motion. Often, gentle assistance by the therapist to control movement precision as the patient performs the motion can confirm that the slight alteration in motion is the cause of the pain. The therapist guiding the pattern of rotation of the head and cervical spine can be used to assess whether the movement fault is the problem (see Chapter 3). Similarly, as discussed in Chapter 7, having the patient correcting the tibiofemoral rotation can alleviate the pain during knee extension in weight bearing. Although the focus is on the painful joint, it is very important to consider the pattern of movement and control evident in all of the other joints of the limb, as well as the alignment of the entire body. The therapist needs to assess the precision of motion of the painful joint, the entire limb segment, and the whole body. An example is a young patient with knee pain who stands in a swayback posture with knees hyperextended, hip extended, and shoulders posterior to the hip joint. There is poor definition of the gluteal muscles (Figure 1-31). During single-leg standing, the painful knee hyperextends and medially rotates. When going up steps, there is tibiofemoral rotation and the patient brings the knee back to meet the body rather than the body up to the knee (Figure 1-32). The patient also leans forward in an exaggerated manner when going up the steps. One reasonable explanation is that the patient is placing an abnormal amount of stress on the anterior knee joint, which may be changing the articular surface of the tibia over time. The cruciate ligaments will

be subjected to inappropriate stress.[7] The weight line of the body will be anterior to the knee joint, which decreases the demands on the quadriceps. The poor definition of the gluteal muscles suggests that the hamstrings are the dominate muscle (see Figure 1-32). The deep lateral rotator muscles of the hip are also likely to be poorly developed. During the step up, the femur is rotating medially because the lateral rotation is not controlled by the gluteal muscles or the deep lateral rotators. In fact, the medial hamstrings could be contributing to excessive medial rotation. The observation that the patient brings the knee back to meet the body is consistent with use of the hip extensors for knee control rather than the quadriceps. Leaning forward with the trunk can also reduce the demands on the quadriceps. Thus, control of the knee joint is affected not only by the precision of motion at the knee joint itself but also by control of the entire segment and of the entire body. Every tissue adaptation that alters alignment has the potential of affecting the precision of joint motion. As mentioned previously, one of the challenges for the therapist is to differentiate structural variations in alignment from acquired changes in alignment. The therapist must also perform a detailed assessment of muscular and motor control performance. Patients need to understand that their alignment and movement patterns are based on what is familiar and not what is optimal or right. The body does not have an internal referencing system that gives immediate feedback about optimal versus nonoptimal alignment or movement. A major responsibility of the therapist is to identify the impairments in muscle performance and movement patterns and provide the instruction in both exercise and movement correction during activities.

A recent radio program featured a physician who specializes in foot problems, a podiatrist, and a fitness expert who also specializes in running. They all seemed to agree that walking was automatic, all people walked in the same way, and there was not much to change. They did seem to believe that running was different and that some instruction in how to run would be useful. Clearly, they have not made the observation of recognizing someone by how they walked without seeing the face. The variations in gait are many, from lack of push-off to excessive push-off, from excessive hip adduction and lumbopelvic rotation to trunk lateral sway. The wear pattern on shoes is a good indicator of variations in walking and even the impressions in the top of the shoes. Some individuals extend their toes so much that the impression of the toes is very evident in the top of the shoe. One patient has deep gouges on the inside of the heel part of his shoes because his hips adduct so much during the swing phase that he hits the contralateral shoe on swing phase, not a little but a lot. Another indication of variation in muscle strategies during walking is the callous distribution. Some individuals, even long distance runners, do not have any notable callouses, but other individuals have very thick callouses. These individuals push the feet into the supporting surface, creating shear in their shoes, whereas people without callouses generate much of their swing phase with proximal muscles. They do not have to control the movement of their line of gravity with their feet but by the control of their trunk. All of these variations reflect alterations in the precision of motion. The task is to ascertain how alterations are affecting the painful joint and not get lost in the variations merely because they exist.

Path of Least Resistance

The movements of the joints of the body follow the rules of physics and take the path of least resistance. Forced to select the most important and useful observation pertaining to musculoskeletal pain, this concept is the clear choice. The symptoms in the majority of patients, particularly the nonacute patients, are reduced or eliminated when the painful area is stabilized and not allowed to move. Undoubtedly that accounts for the current popularity of "stabilizing" exercises or "core" exercises. The other most common factor that can be present at the same time is compression or loading of the joint. In fact, identifying whether compression is part of the problem is extremely important because abdominal muscle exercises can add to the compression. Because movements involve the participation of multiple joints, many of them in series, the joint that moves the most readily is the one that has the least resistance. One of the key controlling factors of the path of least resistance is the relative stiffness or flexibility of the tissues attaching to a joint. A few examples illustrate how generally this rule applies to a variety of situations. One example is found in individuals that have cardiac bypass surgery in which the thorax is opened. After the surgery, the scar tissue and stiffness of the chest is so great that patients become abdominal breathers. The abdomen becomes distended because they are no longer able to expand the ribcage during inhalation. Another example is the development of changes in the vertebrae

above and below after spinal fusion, known as *adjacent segment disease.*[61] One explanation is that the movement of the adjoining vertebral segments is increased because of the lack of motion at the fused joint. Other factors, such as the variations in joint degeneration, also influence the path of least resistance. For example, during cervical rotation, if degenerative changes are greater in the lower cervical joints than the upper cervical joints, then the movement will occur more readily in the upper cervical region than the lower. Because movement occurs along the path of least resistance, which means that the joint that moves the most readily in a specific direction, is subjected to a greater frequency of motion. When the frequency becomes excessive by changing the extensibility of the tissues and there is an associated alteration in the precision of the joint motion, the result is microtrauma. The vicious cycle of the readiness of the joint to move furthering the frequency of motion eventually causes microtrauma that becomes macrotrauma. With increased frequency of motion, there will be associated changes in flexibility and extensibility of the supporting tissues and a resulting change in the precision of the joint motion. The tissue trauma associated with repeated motion has been well documented.[39,62,63] A very useful guideline when determining the diagnosis and developing the treatment program is to presume that pain is arising from the site that is moving and the movement is occurring at this site because it is the path of least resistance. In addition, not only does the path of least resistance determine the site but also the direction of the offending motion.

Joint Mobility

The adaptations of the skeletal, nervous, and muscular systems are normal biological responses to repeated movements and sustained alignments. Over time, however, they can combine to cause alterations in the precision of motion. As discussed in the previous sections, the modifiers or variations in individuals explain why not all people develop pain problems or at least not as readily as other people. The primary means of preventing, as well as correcting, the cause of mechanically induced pain is to maintain precise movement of the joint. As depicted in the model, the problematic outcome of the tissue adaptations is the development of a relative stiffness or flexibility condition that becomes exaggerated because the body takes the path of least resistance for movement. The result of this cascade of events is that a joint develops hypermobility. Hypothetically, the hypermobility is an accessory or arthrokinematic motion rather than physiological or orthrokinematic motion. One of the consequences of imprecise movement is the development of points of high contact stress because of inadequate distribution of forces within the joint. For example, disc degeneration can begin as young as 20 years of age and is a process of structural failure.[39] The disc damage is attributed to compression, bending, and torsion.[35,62] Once the disc undergoes structural change, the loading is altered and the joint begins to become unstable because the length and tension of supporting structures is altered. If motion is imprecise, the trauma to tissue is further increased. The changes in the spine begin with hypermobility that progresses, and the final phase is hypomobility.[35] At this stage, the degenerative process has affected the joint to such an extent that motion has become limited and there are numerous tissue changes, including loss of cartilage and the development of exostosis. Although most studies have been of the degenerative process of the spine, a similar process has to apply to all joints. The most effective form of treatment will correct or minimize the hypermobility. This supports the rationale for "stabilization or core" exercises, but generic stabilization exercises are not sufficient. The components necessary for an effective program are identifying the offending movement direction and the contributing factors and retraining the patient to move the affected segment correctly, redistributing the movement, and using the appropriate timing.

This major emphasis on joint hypermobility does not mean that some painful conditions do not involve a form of a sustained malalignment or a stress into a malaligned position. Such conditions can respond to an abrupt and possibly forceful form of treatment. But the questions that remain, even if there is immediate relief of pain, are (1) what caused the condition to develop in the first place, (2) does it mean that the painful tissues are now fully restored to an optimal state, (3) what will prevent the condition from arising again, (4) does the patient understand the condition, and (5) is the patient aware of the contributing factors and how to avoid a repeat episode? Has the patient been given an active strategy to address the condition or is the patient dependent on passive intervention? In our experience, even conditions that respond to a form of manipulation can also be addressed by active treatment during the acute episode, and certainly, active treatment is required for long-term management. Furthermore, as reported in the literature, the resolution of acute pain is not as costly as the resolution or prevention of chronic pain.[64] Chronic pain problems are most often the ones associated with forms of tissue degeneration and strategies to prevent, slow, or minimize tissue trauma and degeneration have to be of particular importance. Because there is a discernible pattern to the resulting pain problem, the condition can be classified as a specific syndrome. The syndrome would be named for the movement direction or the sustained alignment that (1) most consistently causes symptoms; (2) is imprecise; and (3) when corrected, decreases or eliminates the symptoms.

SUMMARY

This book describes the MS syndromes of the cervical and thoracic spines, the elbow, hand, knee, and foot. The most complete picture as possible of the contributing factors, the tests used in the examination, and the treatment program is presented. Treatment consists of specific exercises, as well as instruction in changing movement patterns to correct the problems of relative stiffness or flexibility. As noted in the model, a further delineation in the syndromes is undertaken by attempting to identify whether the important contributing factors are from motor control, resulting in motor pattern incoordination, or from muscle weakness or force production deficit. The individual with hypertrophied muscles who uses muscles in patterns causing problems is at one extreme, and the individual who has generalized weakness or marked weakness of key muscles is the other extreme. Many patients fall somewhere on the continuum between these two extremes. The value of sublabeling is to help the practitioner and the patient understand that treatment is not just a function of strengthening muscles but also retraining. In fact, excessive muscle strength can be a contributing factor to movement impairments. One of the most challenging aspects of guiding an individual's exercise program is designing one that promotes optimal tissue health and prevents tissue injury because improper exercise can also contribute to problems.

In the future, the syndromes described in this book and its predecessor will most likely be modified by research, as well as by careful clinical analysis. As with pathological conditions of other systems of the body, advances in treatment and insights into causes depend on classification or delineations of subclassifications or diagnostic groups. This pattern exists for all pathophysiological and kinesiopathological conditions. The goal is to provide adequate information to enable others to participate in the process of using and clarifying MS syndromes. If the hypothesis on the "causes" of musculoskeletal pain syndromes has merit and preventive examinations are instituted, the impact on costs associated with these conditions should be significantly reduced. If, after an initial episode of pain, the patient seeks or is referred for an examination to identify impaired alignments, movement patterns, and muscle performance, the cost savings could be substantial. Of course, this supposes that patients will follow the recommendations. Clearly, as health care costs continue to escalate, emphasis on prevention and personal responsibility for healthful living is going to increase. As the consequences of insufficient exercise and excessive eating are shown to contribute to disease development, individuals are going to have to assume responsibility for their health. Individuals, as well as practitioners, will learn that these problems are not the inevitable outcome of aging and activity and that the progression of these disorders can be modified. The medical practitioner is now fully aware of how lifestyle is a major contributor to the development of cardiovascular and metabolic disorders. Musculoskeletal pain syndromes are also lifestyle disorders. Research currently underway will provide insights into the accuracy of that belief.

As depicted in the model, the consequence of the cascade of events is the development of a musculoskeletal pain syndrome or more accurately, a MS syndrome. Therapists must develop a specific diagnosis of these conditions. Our hypothesis is that these syndromes describe the cause of the problem as compared to the source, the pathoanatomical structure, that is painful. *The source of pain is the consequence of impaired motion.*

Clearly, other practitioners and the public will not appreciate the expertise of physical therapists in identifying syndromes unless terminology is used that encapsulates the condition. Terminology to describe the patterns represented by these syndromes needs to be accepted to communicate among ourselves and to the public. Just as other practitioners used diagnostic manuals describing the syndromes of the body system for which they have responsibility, so, too, physical therapists must have diagnostic manuals describing MS syndromes.

In addition to insights gained from ongoing analysis of the model and all of its components, trends in health care that were beginning to emerge 10 years ago are becoming clear. The impact of these trends on physical therapy is also becoming evident. Several factors suggest that physical therapy must undergo a paradigm change. The change is from a practitioner providing episodic care after acute injury to a practitioner providing preventive, as well as restorative, care on a yearly basis throughout life. The content of this book and the first volume provides information that (1) identifies the key factors contributing to the development of musculoskeletal pain and (2) can be used for the yearly examination and a patient-centered program. The factors supporting the importance of having a practitioner with expertise in the movement system are (1) that musculoskeletal pain is part of the degenerative process characteristic of the human biological system and is affected by lifestyle; (2) structural variations that can predispose an individual to pain problems, depending on the sports or fitness activity that they select; (3) the continuing evidence that exercise is the most potent agent for maintaining and restoring health; and (4) the rapidly rising cost of health care.

The monitoring of the movement system should consist of an examination of muscle performance, alignment, movement patterns, general conditioning, and the appropriateness of exercise programs and sports adaptations. As already stated, exercise is critical to the maintenance of health, and optimal exercise requires optimal development of the MS of the human body. The physical therapist's expertise should be in assessment and program development for prevention and diagnosis of MS dysfunctions when they occur. Individuals should have a yearly (or at the least every 2 years) examination of their movement systems, and such examinations should begin early in life and continue throughout life. The expertise that is required is knowledge of 1) structural variations that affect the appropriateness of specific activities and sports, 2) musculoskeletal development, and 3) the condition of the cardiovascular system. Clearly, all individuals must participate in exercise and activity that will optimize their health. To be able to sustain their activity level injury, prevention is a necessity and the physical therapist is ideally prepared for this role.

This type of practice can be considered analogous to the role of the dentist who monitors, recommends, and treats the dental system from early childhood through old age. This role of the physical therapist in guiding, monitoring, diagnosing, and treating the human movement system is increasingly important as the practice of medicine continues to change. The majority of physicians lack knowledge of the mechanical aspects of musculoskeletal disorders, as well as the examination skills, to detect a wide variety of relatively minor musculoskeletal conditions. Rather, a physician's expertise is needed primarily to identify severe disorders of other systems, such as the cardiac or nervous system, as well as potential neoplasms. Physicians are relying more and more on chemical and radiological assessments and not just on the physical examination. A practitioner who is skilled in a movement examination can help differentiate between the radiological findings suggesting the site of pain-generating tissue and the clinical examination suggesting a different site. For example, a skilled clinical movement examination can help differentiate whether pain in the shoulder area is coming from the cervical spine or the shoulder joint. Similarly, pain in the hip region can arise from the lumbar spine, the hip joint, or both. Radiological changes in both regions may be present or even misleading, and a thorough movement examination can be the method of identifying not only the actual pain generating site but also the mechanical interaction of these joints that is often contributing to the tissue injury. For example, if the hip joint does not extend easily during walking, then rotation will be imposed on the pelvis and the lumbar spine, contributing to tissue microtrauma and eventually macrotrauma. The pain in the hip region can be from early degenerative hip joint changes or from lumbar spine motion or from both. Radiological assessments to determine the site causing the pain, particularly in an aged population with multiple sites of degeneration can be misleading and a skilled MS examination can be particularly useful.

Tissue impairment diagnoses as they pertain to the different regions of the body are described in some detail in this book and how some of these diagnoses are associated with MS syndromes. The practice pattern used is one in which patients are not typically seen for frequent treatments. Rather, the treatment plan places the emphasis for remediation on the patient. In other words, the therapist completes a standard examination, determines a diagnosis, explains the diagnosis to the patient, and plans and teaches the patient a very specific exercise program, but the patient is given the responsibility of correcting the problem. The exercises address the needed tissue and movement corrections, and the therapist reviews and instructs the patient in the necessary modification of the way basic, sports, and fitness activities are performed. The instruction by the therapist includes several methods by which the patient can alleviate the symptoms. These include changes in movement or alignment or even types of supports such as pillows or armrests when sitting. Our experience is that such methods not only empower the patient but help reduce the anxiety that accompanies pain. This type of practice is compatible with the model of a yearly visit for preventive purposes. Of course, if a problem develops then the therapist is in a good position to offer an efficient and effective program because the patient is already known to the therapist. The contents of this book and its predecessor should serve as a guide to understanding MS syndromes, determining a diagnosis, and developing a treatment program. There will be changes as research and clinical experience provide additional information, but this information should provide a useful basis for current patient care, as well as future analysis.

REFERENCES

1. Scholtes SA, Norton BJ, Lang CE, et al: The effect of within-session instruction on lumbopelvic motion during a lower limb movement in people with and people without low back pain, *Man Ther* 15:496-501, 2010.
2. Harris-Hayes M, Holtzman GW, Earley JA, et al: Development and preliminary reliability testing of an assessment of patient independence in performing a treatment program: standardized scenarios, *J Rehabil Med* 42(3):221-227, 2010.
3. Harris-Hayes M, Sahrmann SA, Van Dillen LR: Relationship between the hip and low back pain in athletes who participate in rotation-related sports, *J Sport Rehabil* (1):60-75, 2009.
4. Van Dillen LR, Maluf KS, Sahrmann SA: Further examination of modifying patient-preferred movement and alignment strategies in patients with low back pain during symptomatic tests, *Man Ther* 14(1):52-60, 2009.
5. Harris-Hayes M, Van Dillen LR: The inter-tester reliability of physical therapists classifying low back pain problems based on the movement system impairment classification system, *PMR* 1(2):117-126, 2009.
6. Scholtes SA, Gombatto SP, Van Dillen LR: Differences in lumbopelvic motion between people with and people without low back pain during two lower limb movement tests, *Clin Biomech* (Bristol, Avon) 24(1):7-12, 2009.
7. Andrade GT, Azevedo DC, De Assis Lorentz I, et al: Influence of scapular position on cervical rotation range of motion, *J Orthop Sports Phys Ther* 38(11):668-673, 2008.
8. Gombatto SP, Norton BJ, Scholtes SA, et al: Differences in symmetry of lumbar region passive tissue characteristics between people with and people without low back pain, *Clin Biomech* (Bristol, Avon) 23(8):986-995, 2008.
9. Van Dillen LR, Bloom NJ, Gombatto SP, et al: Hip rotation range of motion in people with and without low back pain who participate in rotation-related sports, *Phys Ther Sport* 9(2):72-81, 2008.
10. Gombatto SP, Klaesner JW, Norton BJ, et al: Validity and reliability of a system to measure passive tissue characteristics of the lumbar region during trunk lateral bending in people with and people without low back pain, *J Rehabil Res Dev* 45(9):1415-1429, 2008.
11. Scholtes SA, Van Dillen LR: Gender-related differences in prevalence of lumbopelvic region movement impairments in people with low back pain, *J Orthop Sports Phys Ther* 37(12):744-753, 2007.
12. Harris-Hayes M, Wendl PM, Sahrmann SA, et al: Does stabilization of the tibiofemoral joint affect passive prone hip rotation range of motion measures in unimpaired individuals? A preliminary report, *Physiother Theory Pract* 23(6):315-323, 2007.
13. Van Dillen LR, McDonnell MK, Susco TM, et al: The immediate effect of passive scapular elevation on symptoms with active neck rotation in patients with neck pain, *Clin J Pain* 23(8):641-647, 2007.
14. Caldwell C, Sahrmann S, Van Dillen L: Use of a movement system impairment diagnosis for physical therapy in the management of a patient with shoulder pain, *J Orthop Sports Phys Ther* 37(9):551-563, 2007.
15. Gombatto SP, Collins DR, Sahrmann SA, et al: Patterns of lumbar region movement during trunk lateral bending in 2 subgroups of people with low back pain, *Phys Ther* 87(4):441-454, 2007.
16. Van Dillen LR, Gombatto SP, Collins DR, et al: Symmetry of timing of hip and lumbopelvic rotation motion in 2 different subgroups of people with low back pain, *Arch Phys Med Rehabil* 88(3):351-360, 2007.
17. Gombatto SP, Collins DR, Sahrmann SA, et al: Gender differences in pattern of hip and lumbopelvic rotation in people with low back pain, *Clin Biomech* (Bristol, Avon) 21(3):263-271, 2006.
18. Van Dillen LR, Sahrmann SA, Caldwell CA, et al: Trunk rotation-related impairments in people with low back pain who participated in 2 different types of leisure activities: a secondary analysis, *J Orthop Sports Phys Ther* 36(2):58-71, 2006.
19. Harris-Hayes M, Van Dillen LR, Sahrmann SA: Classification, treatment and outcomes of a patient with lumbar extension syndrome, *Physiother Theory Pract* 21(3):181-196, 2005.
20. Van Dillen LR, Sahrmann SA, Wagner JM: Classification, intervention, and outcomes for a person with lumbar rotation with flexion syndrome, *Phys Ther* 85(4):336-351, 2005.
21. McDonnell MK, Sahrmann SA, Van Dillen L: A specific exercise program and modification of postural alignment for treatment of cervicogenic headache: a case report, *J Orthop Sports Phys Ther* 35(1):3-15, 2005.
22. Van Dillen LR, Sahrmann SA, Norton BJ, et al: The effect of modifying patient-preferred spinal movement and alignment during symptom testing in patients with low back pain: a preliminary report, *Arch Phys Med Rehabil* 84(3):313-322, 2003.
23. Van Dillen LR, Sahrmann SA, Norton BJ, et al: Movement system impairment-based categories for low back pain: stage 1 validation, *J Orthop Sports Phys Ther* 33(3):126-142, 2003
24. Hollman JH, Deusinger RH, Van Dillen LR, et al: Knee joint movements in subjects without knee pathology and subjects with injured anterior cruciate ligaments, *Phys Ther* 82(10):960-972, 2002.
25. Van Dillen LR, Sahrmann SA, Norton BJ, et al: Effect of active limb movements on symptoms in patients with low back pain, *J Orthop Sports Phys Ther* 31(8):402-413; discussion 414-418, 2001.
26. Maluf KS, Sahrmann SA, Van Dillen LR: Use of a classification system to guide nonsurgical management of a

patient with chronic low back pain, *Phys Ther* 80(11):1097-1111, 2000.

27. Van Dillen LR, McDonnell MK, Fleming DA, et al: Effect of knee and hip position on hip extension range of motion in individuals with and without low back pain, *J Orthop Sports Phys Ther* 30(6):307-316, 2000.

28. Van Dillen LR, Sahrmann SA, Norton BJ, et al: Reliability of physical examination items used for classification of patients with low back pain, *Phys Ther* 78(9):979-988, 1998.

29. Sahrmann S: *Diagnosis and treatment of movement impairment syndromes*, St Louis, 2002, Mosby.

30. Lukoschek M, Boyd RD, Schaffler MB, et al: Comparison of joint degeneration models. Surgical instability and repetitive impulsive loading, *Acta Orthop Scand* 57(4):349-353, 1986.

31. Guilak F, Fermor B, Keefe FJ, et al: The role of biomechanics and inflammation in cartilage injury and repair, *Clin Orthop Relat Res* (423):17-26, 2004.

32. Lota JC, Ulrich JA: Innervation, inflammation, and hypermobility may characterize pathologic disc degeneration: review of animal model data, *J Bone Joint Surg Am* 88:76-82, 2006.

33. *Mosby's medical dictionary*, ed 8, St Louis, 2009, Mosby.

34. *Stedman's dictionary*, ed 28, Philadelphia, 2005, Lippincott Williams & Wilkins.

35. Adams MA, Dolan P: Recent advances in lumbar spinal mechanics and their clinical significance, *Clin Biomech* 10(1):3-19, 1995.

36. Mueller MJ, Maluf KS: Tissue adaptation to physical stress: a proposed "physical stress theory" to guide physical therapist practice, education, and research, *Phys Ther* 82:383-403, 2002.

37. Gosheger G, Liem D, Ludwig K, et al: Injuries and overuse syndromes in golf, *Am J Sports Med* 31(3):438-443, 2003.

38. Conn JM, Annest JL, Gilchrist J: Sports and recreation related injury episodes in the US population, 1997-99, *Inj Prev* 9(2):117-123, 2003.

39. Adams M, Bogduk N, Burton K, et al: *The biomechanics of back pain*, 2 ed, 2006, Churchill Livingstone.

40. Brophy R, Silvers HJ, Gonzales T, et al: Gender influences: the role of leg dominance in ACL injury among soccer players, *Br J Sports Med* 44:694-697, 2010.

41. Prodromos CC, Han Y, Rogowski J, et al: A meta-analysis of the incidence of anterior cruciate ligament tears as a function of gender, sport, and a knee injury-reduction regimen, *Arthroscopy* 23(12):1320-1325, 2007.

42. Sigward SM, Powers CM: The influence of gender on knee kinematics, kinetics and muscle activation patterns during side-step cutting, *Clin Biomech* (Bristol, Avon) 21(1):41-48. 2006.

43. Pollard CD, Sigward SM, Powers CM: Limited hip and knee flexion during landing is associated with increased frontal plane knee motion and moments, *Clin Biomech* (Bristol, Avon) 25(2):142-146, 2010.

44. Remvig L, Jensen DV, Ward RC: Epidemiology of general joint hypermobility and basis for the proposed criteria for benign joint hypermobility syndrome: review of the literature, *J Rheumatol* 34:804–809, 2007.

45. Taylor RT: A discussion of Wolff's law, *J Bone Joint Surg Am* S1-S15:221-231, 1902.

46. Sterling M, Jull G, Wright A: The effect of musculoskeletal pain on motor activity and control, *J Pain* 2(3):135-145, 2001.

47. Halsband U, Lange RK: Motor learning in man: a review of functional and clinical studies, *J Physiol* (Paris) 99:414-424, 2006.

48. Wakeling JM, Horn T: Neuromechanics of muscle synergies during cycling, *J Neurophysiol* 101:843-854, 2009.

49. Chapman AR, Vicenzino B, Blanch P, et al: Leg muscle recruitment during cycling is less developed in triathletes than cyclists despite matched cycling training loads, *Ex Brain Res* 3:503-518, 2007.

50. Chapman A, Vicenzino B, Blanch P, et al: Do differences in muscle recruitment between novice and elite cyclist reflect different movement patterns or less skilled muscle recruitment? *J Sci Med Sport* 12;1:31-34, 2009.

51. Weppler CH, Magnusson SP: Increasing muscle extensibility: a matter of increasing length or modifying sensation? *Phys Ther* 90:438–449, 2010.

52. Wang K, McCarter R, Wright J, et al: Regulation of skeletal muscle stiffness and elasticity by titin isoforms: a test of the segmental extension model of resting tension, *Biophysics* 88:7101-7105, 1991.

53. Labeit S, Kolmerer B: Titins: giant proteins in charge of muscle ultrastructure and elasticity, *Science* 270:293-296, 1995.

54. Chleboun GS, Howell JN, Conatser RR, et al: The relationship between elbow flexor volume and angular stiffness at the elbow, *Clin Biomech* 12:6;383, 1997.

55 Boakes JL, Foran J, Ward SR, et al: Case reports: muscle adaptation by serial sarcomere addition 1 year after femoral lengthening, *Clin Orthop Rel Res* 456:250-253, 2007.

56. Williams P, Goldspink G: Changes in sarcomere length and physiological properties in immobilized muscle, *J Anat* 127:459-468, 1978.

57. Lynn R, Talbot JA, Morgan DL: Differences in rat skeletal muscles after incline and decline running, *J Appl Physiol* 85:98, 1998.

58. Gajdosik RL: Passive extensibility of skeletal muscle: review of the literature with clinical implications, *Clin Biomech* 16:87, 2001.

59. Lieber RL: Muscle structure and function, and plasticity. *The physiological basis of rehabiltation*, ed 3, Philadelphia, 2010, Lippincott Williams & Wilkins.

60. Kendall FP, McCreary EK, Provance PG, et al: *Muscles testing and function with posture and pain*, ed 5, Baltimore, 2005, Lippincott Williams & Wilkins.

61. Kaito T, Hosono N, Mukai Y, et al: Induction of early degeneration of the adjacent segment after posterior lumbar interbody fusion by excessive distraction of lumbar disc space, *J Neurosurg Spine* 12;6:671, 2010.

62. McGill S: *Ultimate back fitness and performance*, ed 2, Waterloo, Ontario, 2004, Wabuno Publishers, Backfitpro Inc.

63. Marras WS: The case for cumulative trauma in low back disorders, *Spine J* 3:177, 2003.

64. Becker A: Chronic low back pain associated with high health care costs, *Spine* 35(18):1714, 2010.

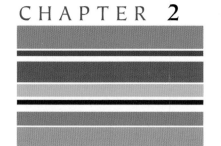

CHAPTER 2

Staging System
for Rehabilitation

Gregory W. Holtzman, Marcie Harris-Hayes

INTRODUCTION

Sustained postures and repeated movements are often found to be the cause of a musculoskeletal pain problem, and such impairments are well addressed by a thorough examination of the movement system and subsequent treatment. The physical therapist also needs to consider the actual pathoanatomical tissue that is injured or painful; this is otherwise known as the *source* of symptoms.

In some cases, such as postoperative conditions or acute injury, the source of symptoms becomes particularly relevant because thorough assessment of movement or posture is not possible as the result of specific restrictions or precautions, severe pain, or other constitutional symptoms. For example, a patient that presents to physical therapy after rotator cuff repair will likely have precautions on active range of motion (AROM). Given these restrictions, a full movement examination could not be performed. However, a limited problem-centered examination could be used to obtain information on the integrity or health of the tissues involved, as well as functional limitations.

Regardless of whether a thorough movement examination can be performed, the therapist needs to recognize what tissues are potentially affected by the injury, surgery, or musculoskeletal pain problem. Because biological tissue responds to physical stress in known and predictable ways, identifying the source of symptoms and the phase of healing enables the physical therapist to establish a prognosis for treatment and to develop an effective intervention plan.

The staging system for rehabilitation was developed to describe the involvement of biological tissue associated with a musculoskeletal pain problem in the presence or absence of specific movement impairments (Figure 2-1). This staging system serves to clarify the level of injury or phase of healing of each tissue involved and can be used with both the established movement system diagnoses or with the physician's diagnosis of the physiological or anatomical system that is pathological and for which he or she has responsibility.

This chapter explains in detail a staging system of tissue impairment used to describe the source of symptoms. First, the physical stress theory (PST) is described, as well as how this general framework can be used to understand the mechanism of injury to a specific tissue. Second, we briefly review how specific biological tissues respond to the application or removal of physical stress and how each could affect the healing process. Third, detailed information is provided on each stage of rehabilitation and an algorithm explains the movement system evaluation process, with special attention given to the source of symptoms. Finally, case studies illustrate the evaluation process and the use of staging of biological tissue to help guide evaluation and treatment.

MECHANISM OF INJURY: THE PHYSICAL STRESS THEORY

Physical stress is defined biomechanically as the force applied to a given area of biological tissue. This definition is true for all mechanical systems, including the human body. Based on substantive research across multiple disciplines, biological tissue, such as muscle,[1-8] bone,[9-13] or ligament,[14-16] clearly responds to such physical stress in predictable ways. Biological tissues may respond favorably (i.e., hypertrophy of muscle) or may respond negatively (i.e., atrophy of muscle, potentially leading to impairment or injury). A thorough discussion of specific tissue impairments related to physical stress is beyond the scope of this book; however, consideration of a theoretical construct that can guide the practicing therapist in staging specific tissue impairments and providing subsequent, appropriate intervention is useful. The PST, which was defined by Mueller and Maluf,[17] provides such a framework.

A basic tenet of the PST is that biological tissue can adapt or become more tolerant of stress when specific stresses are applied at or above a certain level. However,

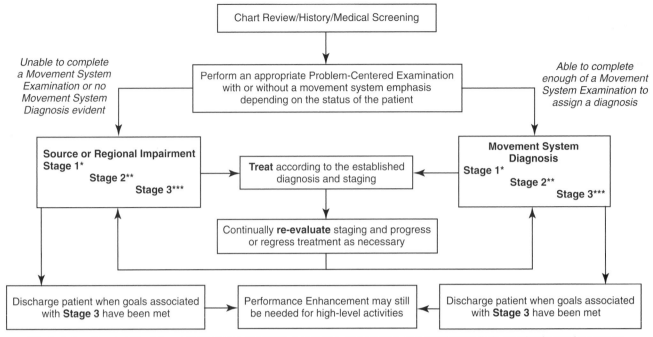

Stage 1: Low threshold for injury, or high tissue irritability. Symptoms, precautions, and restrictions limit examination and treatment. Levels of stress to affected tissues should be minimal.

**Stage 2: Moderate threshold for injury.* Precautions and restrictions may still be in place, but treatment should begin to emphasize progression of appropriate physical stress to targeted tissues.

***Stage 3: High threshold for injury,* or low tissue irritability. Treatment should emphasize tissue adaptation and hypertrophy. Generally, precautions have been lifted. Focus on return to work and higher level sport activities.

Figure 2-1. General diagrammatic representation of the diagnostic process. According to the physical stress theory, the stages used within the flow chart can generally be defined by stress restriction/progression. Staging should continually be evaluated.

for each type of biological tissue, there is also a threshold of adaptation, above which tissue injury or death may occur. Understanding this continuum is important for describing the mechanism of injury and for developing treatment strategies for rehabilitation.

The mechanism of injury to a specific biological tissue depends on (1) the intensity of physical stress applied to the tissue, (2) the duration that the stress is applied, and (3) the specific characteristics of the tissue.[17] The easiest example to understand is the injury that occurs as a result of a trauma. In this case, a high amount of physical stress is applied in a relatively short period of time (i.e., motor vehicle accident or fall). The tissue damage in this example is often readily apparent, and significant protection of the tissue might be required for proper healing and recovery of function. Tissue injury can also occur when a moderate amount of stress is applied over a moderate duration, as is the case with repetitive motion injuries. Often these injuries are associated with less than optimal movement patterns as well. Finally, a low amount of physical stress applied to a specific biological tissue over a prolonged period of time can also lead to tissue injury. Thus sustained postural malalignment could result in tissue degeneration and subsequent injury.

Injury to biological tissue, whether sudden (i.e., trauma), progressive (i.e., degeneration), or controlled (i.e., surgery), results in a more narrow window for adaptation relative to healthy tissue. In other words, lower amounts of physical stress are required for tissue injury and re-injury can occur much more quickly. Therefore, to allow for healing, injured biological tissue must often be protected from physical stress. As healing occurs with time, the biological tissue becomes more receptive to different types of physical stress. Eventually, additional physical stress is required by the injured tissue to fully adapt and to improve stress tolerance. By increasing the overall strength of an injured tissue, the likelihood of re-injury is decreased.

Thus a physical therapist should be able to generally evaluate the state of biological tissue after injury and determine whether that tissue should be protected or whether physical stress should be applied to promote tissue adaptation and recovery. The physical therapist should also consider physiological, movement and alignment, extrinsic (i.e., assistive devices, orthotics, etc.), and psychosocial factors when making this decision. Ultimately, the basic concepts of stress restriction and stress progression in response to tissue injury provide the foundation for the stages for rehabilitation presented in this

TABLE **2-1**
Variables Used to Determine Stage for Rehabilitation

Variable	Stage 1	Stage 2	Stage 3
Time since injury	Recent	—	Remote
Symptoms	↑Severity	—	↓Severity
	↑Irritability		↓Irritability
Outcome scores	Low-level function	Medium-level function	High-level function
	↑Disability		↓Disability
Functional mobility	↓Use of segment in function	Segment used in function, not optimal	↑Optimal use of segment in function

chapter and are used to develop appropriate examination and treatment strategies.

STAGES FOR REHABILITATION

An understanding of the basic mechanisms of tissue injury, subsequent healing and recovery processes, and the predictable manner in which biological tissue responds to stress has sparked the development of a staging system that should be used with any movement system syndrome.[18] To be clear, staging in the biomedical field is not unique. Staging systems are used for a wide variety of pathological conditions and describe wound healing,[19] musculotendinous injuries,[20-22] rotator cuff tears,[23] fracture severity,[24] and low back pain.[25] Most of the staging systems documented in the literature are specific to a type of biological tissue or a specific region of the body and help to describe the severity of the tissue injury. However, no formal staging system exists that can be used to specifically guide the physical therapist through the rehabilitation process, regardless of the body region affected. The stages for rehabilitation were developed to describe the general rehabilitation continuum of tissue healing from the initial injury to full recovery.

Specifically, three stages (Stage 1, Stage 2, or Stage 3) have been identified, and they illustrate the amount of protection required for an injured biological tissue or the amount of physical stress that can be applied to a tissue that is healing. Essentially, these stages describe the threshold for injury for the biological tissue involved. Tissues in the first stage have a low threshold for injury, whereas tissue in the third stage has a high threshold for injury.

The threshold for injury is specific to the biological tissue involved, but the stages are generally more comprehensive in that they are not limited by loosely defined time constraints as is the terminology of acute, subacute, and chronic. Rather, the stages used in this system incorporate moderating factors such as physiological co-morbidities, functional activity performance, precautions and restrictions to movement, psychosocial status, and pain. Thus this staging system provides a framework for the rehabilitation of an individual with a tissue injury, rather than just the tissue itself. As such, the stages for rehabilitation should be used to characterize the source of symptoms for all movement system syndromes, as well as for physician's diagnoses with undiagnosed or unidentifiable tissue impairments such as an ankle sprain.

Because there is no specific timeframe that defines each of the stages used in this system, there is no clear demarcation between each of the stages. However, Table 2-1 illustrates four key variables that are useful to consider when determining the proper stage: time since injury, symptoms, outcome scores, and functional mobility. Each of these variables provides a general framework for determining the stage for rehabilitation; however, all potential data obtained in the history and examination need to be considered when making a final decision regarding staging. In the next section, each stage is described in detail, including how you determine progression or regression from one stage to another.

Stages: Definition and Assessment

Stage 1 describes a state of *low threshold for injury*, or high tissue irritability and/or vulnerability. Generally, symptoms, precautions, and restrictions limit the thoroughness of the examination and the intensity of the subsequent treatment. Individuals at Stage 1 often are postsurgical or have had an acute injury or trauma. Thus performing a complete examination might be limited because of pain or physician's orders. Levels of stress to the affected tissues should be minimal, and the emphasis of treatment is on the protection of the injured tissue. Stage 2 describes a state of *moderate threshold for injury*. Normally, a complete movement system examination can be performed. Often, patients in this stage do not have precautions or restrictions, but their functional mobility is limited because of pain or other symptoms. For patients presenting to physical therapy postoperatively or after an acute injury, precautions and restrictions may still be in effect. In either case, treatment should begin to emphasize appropriate physical stress to targeted tissues. Stage 3 describes a state of *high threshold for injury*, or low tissue irritability and/or vulnerability. Generally, all precautions and restrictions have been lifted at this stage and an objective examination may include assessment of high level sport or work activities. For this stage, treatment should emphasize the gradual addition of physical stress to promote tissue adaptation or hypertrophy to restore an optimal level of function.

Table 2-2 provides a summary of key tests and assessments that are used to stage patients appropriately. For each stage, the potential findings for specific examination components are described. As noted previously, there is often no clear demarcation between each of the stages with regards to examination findings. Therefore the purpose of Table 2-2 is to provide a basic description of what might be evident for each of the stages during the examination process. The examination items will not be discussed in detail because that would be beyond the scope and objective of this text. In the next section, however, we discuss in detail specific treatment guidelines for each of the stages. Understanding intervention strategies for each of the stages should enable the reader to more fully grasp the staging system and to appropriately progress patients during treatment.

TREATMENT GUIDELINES FOR STAGES FOR REHABILITATION

With any patient, regardless of the stage at which he is initially diagnosed, the emphasis of treatment should be to restore range of motion (ROM) and strength of the involved segment, as well as the overall function of the individual without adding excessive stresses to the injured tissues. Specific movement impairments should also be addressed during rehabilitation to ensure optimal recovery and to promote proper performance of functional activities to prevent the recurrence of a specific injury or pain problem. General treatment guidelines are given for each stage and related to several key components of a rehabilitation program.

Precautions and Restrictions

Patients that present in Stage 1 may have had an acute injury or a recent surgery and often have restrictions or precautions in regard to movement or weight bearing that have been issued by the referring physician. Such orders serve to protect the injured tissue and to facilitate the recovery process. During the examination, the patient's understanding of these precautions or restrictions needs to be assessed, and the patient's ability to adhere to them needs to be determined. Precautions and restrictions should be strictly followed during the examination, and treatment options may be initially limited. Subsequent communication with the referring physician is important to progress the patient within an appropriate timeframe.

Patients that present in Stage 2 may or may not have physician-imposed precautions or restrictions still in place. Often, the progression to Stage 2 from Stage 1 is marked by a change in the degree of precautions or restrictions. For example, a postoperative patient might be progressed from non–weight-bearing status to 25 percent weight-bearing. In other cases, ROM restrictions may be progressed. Regardless of the restrictions or precautions ordered by the physician, patients in Stage 2 should be able to tolerate a certain amount of physical stress at the target tissues.

Patients that present in Stage 3 generally have no precautions or restrictions that would limit the progression of physical therapy. However, some individuals may enter Stage 3 with precautions or restrictions that will be in place for an extended period of time. Communication with the physician is important if any ongoing precautions or restrictions should be adhered to by the patient. If not, intervention can be progressed to gradually increase the amount of physical stress imposed on the involved tissues to increase the tolerance of the tissues.

Pain

Any pain complaint requires clarification of the location, quality, and intensity of the symptoms. This clarification enables the therapist to more accurately assess the actual source of pain and to develop an appropriate treatment plan that can then be progressed according to pain severity.

When treating an individual with pain, the therapist should consider the results of the assessment process to develop a staging diagnosis, as well as whether the patient presented to therapy after a surgical procedure or initiated therapy because of a pain problem or an acute injury. For the patient in Stage 1 who has had a recent surgery, some pain will likely be associated with exercises within the first 2 weeks of the postoperative period. Gradually over the next few weeks after surgery, pain associated with the exercise should lessen.

Pain can be used as a guide to the rehabilitation process. Sharp, stabbing pain should be avoided. Mild aching is expected after exercises but should be tolerable for the patient. This postexercise discomfort should decrease within 1 to 2 hours of the rehabilitation. Complaints of increasing pain, pain that is not decreasing with treatment, or burning pain are all indicators that the treatment is too aggressive or that there is a disruption in the usual course of healing. Coordinating the use of analgesics with exercise sessions may be beneficial. Splinting, bracing, and/or assistive devices may be used during this period to protect the injured tissue.

In contrast to the postsurgical patient, Stage 1 individuals with an acute injury or a pain problem should not reproduce their pain with exercise. Modalities, such as ice or electrical stimulation, and external support, such as taping or bracing, may be helpful to decrease pain.[26-29] The patient may also require the use of an assistive device during the early phases of healing.

The specific tissue pain present during Stage 1 should be significantly decreased for patients that present in Stages 2 or 3. However, as the treatment for the patient is progressed, he or she may report increased pain or discomfort with higher level exercises, fitness activities

TABLE 2-2
General Key Tests and Assessments for Staging

Stage 1	Stage 2	Stage 3
• Low threshold for injury or high tissue irritability. • Symptoms/precautions/restriction limit examination and treatment. • Levels of stress to affected tissues should be minimal.	• Moderate threshold for injury. • Precautions/restrictions may still be in place, but treatment should begin to emphasize progression of appropriate physical stress to targeted tissues.	• High threshold for injury or low tissue irritability. • Treatment should emphasize tissue adaptation/hypertrophy. Generally, precautions have been lifted. • Focus on return to work/higher level sport activities. • Emphasis of treatment is placed on gradually increasing stress to the tissues to restore to optimal level of function.
PRECAUTIONS • Check physician's orders and protocols. Assess patient's ability to adhere to precautions. • No resisted testing according to precautions. • Assess immobilization requirements.	• Check physician's orders and protocols for changes in precautions. Assess patient's ability to adhere to precautions. • Precautions and/or restrictions may be lessened.	• Check physician's orders and protocols for changes in precautions. Assess patient's ability to adhere to precautions. • Precautions likely to be lifted. • Resisted testing as allowed by precautions.
SYSTEMIC SIGNS/SYMPTOMS • Vital signs: Monitor with position changes. Heart rate may be increased secondary to pain. • Constitutional symptoms: Assess for signs of infection, including temperature changes.	• Vital signs: Monitor response to progression of activity.	• Vital signs: Monitor response to increasing levels of activity/exercise. • May have reduced tolerance of aerobic activities.
PAIN • Assess location and intensity of pain at rest and with movement. • Assess regimen of analgesics. • Pain may be severe at this stage (6-10/10).	• Assess location and intensity of pain at rest and with movement. • Pain management should be improving and intensity of pain should be less severe (3-6/10).	• Assess location and intensity of pain at rest and with movement. • Pain should be minimal at this stage (0-3/10).
NEUROLOGICAL STATUS • Establish baseline after all surgical procedures, particularly of the spine. • May report neurological symptoms secondary to injury or surgery, such as constant pain, numbness, and tingling, or motor loss, which may significantly limit functional activity performance.	• Monitor for change in status. • Activity tolerance is still limited, but neurological symtoms have improved enough to allow for progression of exercise and activity.	• Monitor for change in status. • Neurological symptoms should be intermittent at worst and manageable with correct movements and postures. Activity no longer limited by neurological symptoms.
FUNCTION • Assess patient's ability to perform functional activities while maintaining precautions and proper movement pattern. Education may need to be provided before assessment. • Significant limitations in functional abilities noted. May require external assistance for completion of activities.	• Assess patient's ability to perform functional activities as precautions change and movement patterns are more evident. • Patient able to perform most functional activities but is limited by symptoms.	• Assess patient's ability to participate in higher level activities. • Sport-specific activities. • Work-specific activities. • No limitations noted in the ability to perform required functional activities. Patient may be limited in the intensity or duration of functional activity performance.

Continued

TABLE **2-2**
General Key Tests and Assessments for Staging—cont'd

Stage 1	Stage 2	Stage 3
ALIGNMENT • Assess alignment and resting position. • Assess need for equipment. • Assessment may be limited secondary to precautions or restrictions.	• Assess alignment and resting position within the context of a movement system examination. • Poor alignment may be noted secondary to injury, surgery, or immobilization. Structural changes should be considered.	• Assess alignment and resting position within the context of a movement system examination. • Poor alignment may be noted secondary to injury, surgery, or immobilization. Structural changes should be considered.
APPEARANCE • Incision or portal may be present. Note the amount and type of drainage. • Note the location, mobility, and sensitivity of the scar if incision is healed. Initially, scar may be hypersensitive and restricted. • Assess for bruising and edema. Bruising and edema will likely be significant. • Note the location and amount of muscle atrophy. Common following immobilization.	• Incision or portal should be healed though some scabbing may still be present. • Scar should be less hypersensitive but may still be restricted with regard to mobility. • Bruising and edema present, but fluctuating. • Muscle atrophy still likely to be significant.	• Incision/portal should be well healed. • Scar should be soft and supple. • Edema, bruising, and atrophy may still be present, but no longer limiting function.
PALPATION • Perform when incision has healed. • May be acutely painful and diffuse.	• Should be able to palpate on and around incision site or area of injury. Pain may be more localized. May still have some hypersensitivity around incision.	• Incision/portal site should be mobile and supple. • Minimal pain (0-3/10) should be noted with palpation.
ROM • Assess involved joint and adjacent joints PROM and AROM (within precautions). • PROM and AROM likely to be limited and painful. Edema may contribute to loss of ROM.	• Assess involved joint and adjacent joints PROM and AROM (within precautions). • PROM and AROM may still be short of functional or normal ROM. Pain and tissue stiffness still limiting factors.	• Assess involved joint and adjacent joints PROM and AROM (within precautions). • AROM/PROM should be full or progressing as expected. Generally no ROM precautions.
MUSCLE PERFORMANCE (RECRUITMENT/STRENGTH) • Assess involved and surrounding musculature. • Resisted tests may be limited secondary to precautions and restrictions or pain. • Significant deficits in muscle performance likely noted in both involved and surrounding musculature, which limits functional activity performance.	• Consider movement impairments and assess involved and surrounding musculature as needed. • Deficits in muscle performance likely. Pain may still be present with testing. Muscle performance may limit the intensity and duration of functional activity performance.	• Consider movement impairments and assess involved and surrounding musculature as needed. • Muscle recruitment may still be deficient for higher-level sport or work activity. Deficits in muscle strength likely still noted.

AROM, Active range of motion; *PROM*, passive range of motion; *ROM*, range of motion.

such as walking or running, and return to the previous work or sport intensity. Thus the location of pain and discomfort should be closely monitored. Muscle soreness is expected, similar to the response of muscle to an overload stimulus (i.e., weight training). Usually, general muscle soreness should be allowed to resolve within 1 to 2 days before repeating a specific bout of activity. Pain described as stabbing should always be avoided.

Edema

Edema is quite common after surgery or an acute injury. Therefore the Stage 1 patient should be specifically educated in the use of edema control. Techniques that can safely be used during Stage 1 to control edema include the following:

- AROM
- Splinting to immobilize and rest the tissue
- Compressive garments or wraps
- Milking massage
- Ice or other modalities[30]
- Elevation

The patient should be encouraged to keep the extremity elevated as much as possible, particularly in the early phases (1 to 3 weeks). Application of ice after exercise is generally recommended. Ideally, a measurement of the edema should be taken at each visit to gauge progress. A sudden increase in edema may indicate that the rehabilitation program is too aggressive or that a possible infection has started. If an infection is suspected, the physician should be contacted immediately.

The time it takes for edema around the involved tissue to resolve is variable among patients and surgical procedures. Although edema should decrease significantly in the first 2 to 4 weeks after surgery or injury, some edema may persist for several months. Thus care should be taken to continually manage edema for individuals in Stages 2 and 3. As noted previously, techniques such as icing, elevation, and compression may be used successfully after exercise to minimize potential swelling with new or higher level activities. Additionally, Stages 2 and 3 patients might need to be instructed on how to moderate and progress their activity level. If activities and exercises are progressed appropriately, the edema should continue to decrease gradually with time.

Appearance

After surgery, the area around the incision or the involved joint should be closely monitored for a developing infection. An infection should be suspected if the involved area appears to be red, hot, and swollen. As noted previously, the physician should be consulted immediately if infection is suspected. An infection is most likely to occur during Stage 1 rehabilitation, but the patient should be monitored throughout the rehabilitation process.

Bruising after surgery or after a traumatic injury is common, and the patient should be monitored continually for any changes suggesting bruising. Again, an increase in bruising during the rehabilitation process may indicate an infection or additional injury.

Consideration should also be given to changes in hair growth, perspiration, or color because such symptoms may indicate some disturbance to the sympathetic nervous function, especially if in combination with the complaint of excessive pain.

During Stages 2 and 3, the incision should be well healed. Although bruising may still be present, it should be diminishing. As with Stage 1, signs of increased bruising or changes to the incision site are indicators of an adverse response to exercise or activity and the patient should be immediately referred to the physician.

Scar

Although scarring is a normal process of healing, it must be managed well during the rehabilitation process, particularly for the patient in Stage 1. Exercise, massage, compression, silicone gel sheets, and vibration are commonly used for scar management, although the use of silicone gel is best supported by the evidence.[31,32]

The gradual application of stress to the scar or incision site helps the scar remodel to allow the necessary gliding between tissue structures. A dry incision that has been closed and reopens as the result of the stresses applied with scar massage indicates that the scar massage is too aggressive. Additionally, a hypersensitive scar will require some level of desensitization.

A scar may continue to remodel for up to 2 years. Although they are probably most effective early in the healing process, scar management techniques may be effective until the scar matures. Therefore patients in Stages 2 and 3 may also benefit from education on scar management.

Range of Motion

ROM is often an important component of treatment for the patient in Stage 1. Depending on the type of injury, the patient may have ROM precautions or restrictions per the physician's orders to protect the healing tissues. If so, splinting or bracing is commonly used to adhere to the ROM precautions while allowing for the initiation of exercise as soon after surgery as possible.

Early initiation of ROM exercises is important to prevent muscle contracture or loss of flexibility as a result of immobilization.[33,34] In the early stages of rehabilitation, the patient should perform ROM exercises multiple times a day, and all exercises should be performed within pain tolerance. The uninvolved joints should also be exercised to prevent the development of restricted ROM at those joints. Decreasing pain and edema and improving ROM are typical indicators that the exercises can safely be progressed.

The typical exercise progression begins with gentle passive ROM and progresses gradually to active-assisted ROM (AAROM) and AROM; however this may vary in cases of injury to muscle or tendon. If resistance is allowed, proprioceptive neuromuscular facilitation (PNF) techniques, such as contract-relax or hold-relax, can be used to achieve ROM goals. If these techniques are used in Stage 1, the applied resistance should be gentle.

When performing ROM exercises near a fracture site, special attention should be given to hand placement during the exercises to minimize the stresses placed on the healing fracture site.

For patients in Stages 2 and 3, ROM precautions or restrictions have generally been reduced or lifted altogether. ROM in each of the stages, particularly Stage 2, may still be limited. However, exercise to increase ROM should be progressed and made more aggressive to achieve normal or functional range if appropriate.

Finally, joint mobilization may be a useful technique for any of the stages to facilitate an increase in ROM.[34] However, the physician should be consulted before initiating joint mobilization after a fracture or a specific joint injury.

Strength or Muscle Performance

For patients in Stage 1, strengthening or resistance training often does not begin until after the initial phase of healing (4 to 6 weeks). Thus the emphasis of treatment for these patients is on education, immobilization, edema management, and gradual progression of ROM with the correct movement pattern. Occasionally, light resistance is applied during exercises to improve the recruitment pattern of a specific muscle or muscle group, but such exercises should not be used to overload and strengthen the involved muscles. Also, if light resistance exercises are used, they should not violate any precautions or restrictions set forth by the physician.

Approximately 4 to 6 weeks after the surgery or the injury, strengthening may be gradually incorporated into the intervention program. By this time, patients have general progressed into either Stage 2 or Stage 3. Progression to a resistive exercise program is based on the patient's ability to perform ROM with a good movement pattern and without a significant increase in symptoms. For patients in Stages 2 and 3, weights, elastic bands, or isokinetic equipment may be used to enhance muscle performance. Specific exercise protocols provided by physicians and physical therapists should be evaluated to ensure that all exercises are appropriate for the individual's situation. Electrical stimulation or biofeedback may also be used to increase muscle strength and to improve motor recruitment.[35-38]

Proprioception and Balance

Proprioception and balance[39] are important components of fitness that can be incorporated into a rehabilitation program to improve functional activity performance and to hasten the return to high-level work or sport activities. Consideration of weight-bearing and ROM precautions or restrictions must be made for the patient in Stage 1. Therefore the initiation of these types of activities during

Stage 1 might vary according to the body region involved, the surgical procedure performed, or the injury incurred.

During Stages 2 and 3, proprioception and balance activities should be prescribed gradually to ensure proper postural control and patient safety. These exercises can be modified as necessary to incorporate any remaining precautions or restrictions. As the patient progresses into and through Stage 3, the balance and proprioceptive exercises prescribed by the therapist should be relevant to the sport, work, or functional activity that the patient needs to perform.

Cardiovascular Endurance

If not contraindicated by co-existing medical complications or specific precautions or restrictions, cardiovascular endurance activities should begin as soon as possible. During Stage 1, aerobic activities may need to be performed at a relatively low intensity and for a short duration. Thus these individuals may benefit from more frequent performance of cardiovascular exercises.[40] Interestingly, patients at any stage performing cardiovascular endurance exercises may have the added benefit of reduced pain and increased feelings of well-being.[40,41]

In Stages 2 and 3, the intensity, duration, and frequency of the exercise can be progressed as tolerated. For athletes, the cardiovascular exercises prescribed should be relevant to their sport or training regiment. For other patients interested in fitness, the cardiovascular exercise program should be tailored to prevent the potential onset of symptoms, to encourage correct movement patterns, and to promote optimal compliance.

Mobility

Early functional use of the injured segment should be encouraged while protecting the healing tissue. Educate the patient regarding precautions/restrictions, the use of the involved extremity during activities of daily living (ADLs), and the use of an appropriate assistive device as needed, including braces or splints. Compensatory techniques for mobility may be required during Stage 1 to protect the involved tissue and to promote optimal function. As precautions/restrictions allow, the patient should be instructed on the proper way to perform common functional mobility tasks using more normal, essential component-based strategies for movement. In addition, the assistive device used by the patient should be modified or eliminated according to the improvement in the patient's condition.

Work/School/Higher Level Activities

A patient in Stage 1 may be off work or restricted from regular activities during the immediate postoperative period or after an acute injury. When the patient is cleared to return to work or sport, he or she should be instructed in a gradual resumption of normal activities. The patient in Stage 1 who is required to return to work may benefit from instruction in specific modifications to the environment, or from imposed restrictions for light or limited duty. While at work, the patient should emphasize edema control and pain management. The goal is to prevent re-injury of the involved tissue.

A patient in Stage 2 may still have restrictions or limitations imposed for work or school activities. However, an effort should be made in therapy, if appropriate, to return the patient to his or her prior level of function at work or with a specific sports activity. Specifically, education about and practice of specific work or sport activities should be included in the intervention program. Edema and pain management should continue to be emphasized, in addition to the treatment of specific movement impairments related to deficits in muscle performance, joint mechanics, flexibility, or balance.

Finally, a patient in Stage 3 should be able to fully return to work or sport activities. In this stage, additional physical stress is applied during therapy to improve the ability of the patient to perform such higher level activities correctly for the necessary amount of time. Pain control and edema management may still be necessary, but the emphasis of treatment is on the optimal performance of the work or sport activity specific to the patient.

Sleep

Sleep is often disrupted in the immediate postoperative period or after an acute injury. During Stage 1, the patient should avoid sleep positioning that may encourage increased edema or possible contracture of the involved segment. For all stages, the patient should be educated on optimal sleep positions to reduce prolonged stress to the involved body regions. To fully correct a patient's sleep posture, regardless of stage, external supports, such as pillows or towels, may be used.

External Support

After surgery, the patient in Stage 1 may need to use a splint or a brace to protect the surgical site, depending on the specific surgical procedure or the type of injury sustained. During treatment, the therapist should ensure that the brace or splint fits the patient comfortably. The patient should also be educated in the timeline for wearing the brace. If the wearing time is not clear, the therapist should refer to the specific protocol prescribed by the physician or consult with the physician if no specific orders are provided.

A splint or brace might also be necessary for a patient who has sustained an acute injury. In addition, taping techniques may be used as an adjunct to treatment to help decrease symptoms and to control movement, depending on the underlying movement impairment.[42-45]

The recommendations concerning the need for splinting, bracing, or taping for prolonged periods are varied. Therefore communication among the physician, the patient, and the physical therapist is essential to determine the need for external support for the Stage 2 or Stage 3 patient.

Medications

During Stage 1, physical therapy could be timed with analgesic administration if possible, which should typically be 30 minutes after the administration of an oral medication. Communication with nurses and physicians is critical to ensure optimal pain relief for the patient. Otherwise, medications for patients in all stages should be reviewed to ensure that they are being taken appropriately. The therapist should be aware of any potential side effects of the medications that the patient is taking so that any problems that develop will be easily recognized and any impact on the treatment or the performance of daily functional activities can be minimized.

Modalities

For patients in all stages, modalities or physical agents can be used for pain relief, edema control, strengthening, and flexibility. For example, interferential current and sensory level transcutaneous electrical stimulation (TENS) has been shown to be helpful in decreasing pain and edema.[46-48] There is also some evidence to suggest that ultrasound can be used to enhance tissue healing[49-51] or to improve tissue extensibility through deep heating.[52] Finally, electrical stimulation is commonly used for muscle strengthening. Recent studies support the use of electrical stimulation to improve both motor recruitment and strength.[35-37] Regardless of the modality chosen, the therapist should determine if the patient is appropriate for a specific modality and check to ensure that there are no contraindications. Also, the therapist should be aware of specific precautions for each type of modality with regard to application. Ultimately, modalities can be a useful adjunct to treatment at any stage, but they should not be used alone.

Patient Education

Regardless of the stage for rehabilitation, patient education is an essential aspect of the treatment program. Therefore the following educational principles should be incorporated into the treatment of patients as appropriate. First, educate the patient regarding the structure and tissues involved in the injury, pain problem, or surgical procedure, as well as the approximate timeline for recovery and return to activity. Often, the patient will also need additional instructions regarding specific medical or surgical precautions ordered by the physician. Specifically, the patient should be instructed on how to maintain the prescribed precautions during various functional activities such as ambulation and transfers. If the patient has or obtains a brace or a splint, the patient should be educated on specific donning and doffing procedures, a schedule for use, and the appropriate care of the device. Finally, if appropriate, the patient should be educated regarding any specific movement impairment he or she might have and on how to move correctly throughout all daily activities and exercises.

TABLE 2-3
Examples of Naming Process*

Source/Physician's Diagnosis or Presenting Problem	Surgical Procedure Performed	Able to Determine MS Diagnosis	Unable to Determine MS Diagnosis or No MS Diagnosis Evident
Rotator cuff tear	Rotator cuff repair	Scapular downward rotation, s/p rotator cuff repair, Stage 3	Rotator cuff tear, s/p rotator cuff repair, Stage 1
Shoulder pain	None	Scapular downward rotation and humeral anterior glide, Stage 2	Shoulder impairment, Stage 1
Nonspecific low back pain	None	Lumbar rotation, Stage 2	Lumbar spine impairment, Stage 1
L4-L5 disc herniation	Lumbar fusion	Lumbar flexion, Stage 1	L4-L5 disc herniation, s/p lumbar fusion Stage 1
Acetabular labral tear	Labral repair	Femoral anterior glide, s/p labral repair, Stage 2	Labral tear, s/p labral repair, Stage 1
Hip osteoarthritis	Total hip arthroplasty	Femoral hypomobility, Stage 3	Hip osteoarthritis, s/p total hip arthroplasty, Stage 2
Knee pain	Arthroscopic knee surgery removal of loose bodies	Tibiofemoral rotation, s/p arthroscopic knee surgery for removal of loose bodies, Stage 2	Knee impairment, s/p arthroscopic knee surgery for removal of loose bodies, Stage 1
Ankle sprain	None	Supination (ankle/foot), Stage 2	Ankle sprain, Stage 3

MS, Movement system; s/p, status-post.
*Diagnostic labels used to describe the status of a patient's movement system after an examination using the diagnostic process described in Figure 2-2.

Changes in Status

For each stage, the therapist should carefully consider patient reports of increased pain or edema, decreased strength, or a significant change in ROM, especially if any of these occur in combination. The patient should be questioned about any precipitating factors related to the change in status (i.e., time of onset, daily activities performed before onset).

If the patient is postsurgical and the integrity of the surgery is in doubt, contact the physician promptly, particularly if there is fever and erythema observed at the incision site, which might indicate a potential infection.

In the next section, the diagnostic and treatment process is discussed with regard to the stages for rehabilitation. In doing so, we address how changes in patient status may affect the physical therapist's decision-making strategy and ultimately specific patient intervention.

THE DIAGNOSTIC PROCESS

When performing an evaluation of the movement system, the physical therapist should be able to recognize the potential source of symptoms or the biological tissues involved. More importantly, however, the therapist should attempt to determine the actual cause of the patient's symptoms by using a thorough examination of a patient's movement and posture. In doing so, a movement system diagnosis that can be used to develop a treatment plan and to progress the patient appropriately can be established.

Often, the cause of symptoms cannot be determined because of acuity or because a movement impairment simply does not exist. In either case, as shown in Table 2-3, the physical therapist should be able to establish a source or regional impairment diagnosis that can be used to treat the patient. Regardless of the diagnosis established, staging for rehabilitation should be an integral part of the diagnostic process for physical therapy. An understanding of this process should enable both the novice and expert physical therapist to implement a logical system for patient evaluation and re-evaluation to prescribe an optimal treatment program and to modify the intervention plan as needed.

Figure 2-2 illustrates the movement system evaluation process. This diagram presents a series of questions and steps that can be used to establish a diagnosis with a specific stage and illustrates the diagnostic process that more specifically demonstrates the use of staging. Rather than describe each step in detail, the following three cases demonstrate the decision-making processes used by expert clinicians to determine a movement system diagnosis and to stage the affected tissues. Figure 2-2 can be used to follow the decisions made for each case.

With any diagnosis that is established using the algorithm in Figure 2-2, it is important to continually re-evaluate the patient and modify the diagnosis, staging, or treatment as needed. At any time during a patient intervention, staging and the associated treatment can be progressed, regressed, or discontinued. In addition, the actual diagnosis may change if an impairment of the movement system develops. Thus the diagnostic process presented here should serve as a guide for the therapist to follow to establish an accurate diagnosis and an effective treatment plan, but the therapist must recognize the fluidity of this process to use it successfully.

CASE PRESENTATION
Anterior Cruciate Ligament Reconstruction
Symptoms and History

A 28-year-old female patient presents to an outpatient physical therapy clinic 2 days after an anterior cruciate ligament (ACL) reconstruction using a patellar tendon graft, in addition to a repair of the lateral meniscus. Surgical protocols following an ACL reconstruction vary across regions of the country and across physicians, but for the purposes of this case, the patient was weight bearing as tolerated for the first 6 weeks after the surgery with a hinged brace locked into full extension for all weight-bearing activities. The patient was using bilateral axillary crutches for ambulation. No ROM restrictions or precautions were ordered by the physician, but resisted testing of the involved quadriceps was contraindicated.

A history and medical screening using the movement system evaluation process to guide the initial visit is performed. The patient is medically stable and safe to treat, thus a working movement system or source diagnosis should be established. The working diagnosis is based on the information learned from the history, including the date of surgery; the results of standardized outcome measures to assess overall level of function, visual appraisal of the patient, and knowledge of specific precautions and restrictions. The working diagnosis helps guide the examination process to ensure that the appropriate tests are used and the patient is not subjected to re-injury. In this case, a working movement system diagnosis cannot be established. Rather, based on her presentation, a working diagnosis of a Stage 1 Knee Impairment would be more appropriate.

Key Tests and Signs

Precautions, restrictions, pain, and acuity limit the tests that can be used to assess for specific movement system impairments. Therefore, a limited problem-centered evaluation is performed that emphasized measurement of ROM and edema, assessment of functional activities such as gait and transfers, and visual observation of the incision site. Certainly, other tests and measures may be incorporated, but the therapist should recognize when certain movement tests should not or cannot be performed. For any test or measurement performed during the limited problem-centered evaluation, the therapist should note any observed movement faults that might be related to an underlying movement system diagnosis. For example, if the patient in this case were to demonstrate femoral adduction/medial rotation or tibial lateral rotation during the assessment of knee flexion ROM, the therapist considers a working movement system diagnosis of tibio-femoral rotation syndrome.

Diagnosis and Staging

Based on the results of the examination, the patient is given a diagnosis of ACL and lateral meniscal tear, s/p ACL reconstruction with lateral meniscal repair, Stage 1. By convention, neither symptoms nor a specific procedure should be used as the actual diagnosis. In this example, ACL and lateral meniscal tear is the actual diagnosis. This is the source diagnosis provided by the physician and is based on the tests the physician can perform or order. The inclusion of the surgical procedure (ACL reconstruction with lateral meniscal repair) and the stage for rehabilitation in the diagnosis provides additional information to describe the patient's status and to direct the development of a treatment program. Note that if no specific physician's or source diagnosis is provided, the physical therapist should name the diagnosis according to the region that is impaired. For example, if the patient had been seen prior to being diagnosed with the ACL tear, the diagnosis would be knee impairment, Stage 1. In the next two cases, we will review the diagnostic naming procedures.

Treatment

Once a diagnosis has been established, the physical therapist can initiate treatment. For this patient with a Stage 1 condition, the emphasis of treatment is on tissue protection. However, the therapist should always be aware of specific movement impairments that become evident during low-level exercise and activity. For this case, the actual treatment provided is not discussed because the primary objective here is to illustrate the diagnostic process. Once a patient has begun treatment, the therapist should continually re-evaluate the level of staging. In doing so, the physical therapist should consider patient progress, pain complaints, the status of precautions or restrictions, and patient tolerance of an examination with a movement system syndrome emphasis.

The patient progressed according to the expected timeframe for tissue healing, and after 6 weeks, when she was able to unlock her brace, she was able to be examined using a complete a problem-centered evaluation with a movement system syndrome emphasis.

Based on her complaints of pain and specific movement impairments, the patient is given a diagnosis of tibiofemoral rotation with secondary patellar lateral glide syndrome s/p ACL reconstruction and lateral meniscal repair, Stage 2 (see Chapter 7). The stage was determined based on considerations of her overall level of pain, the time since her surgery, the progress noted in ROM and functional activity performance, and the elimination of all restrictions.

Once the diagnosis is made, treatment is progressed to address the specific movement impairments and to increase the adaptive physical stress applied to the tissues that were initially weakened by both the injury and the

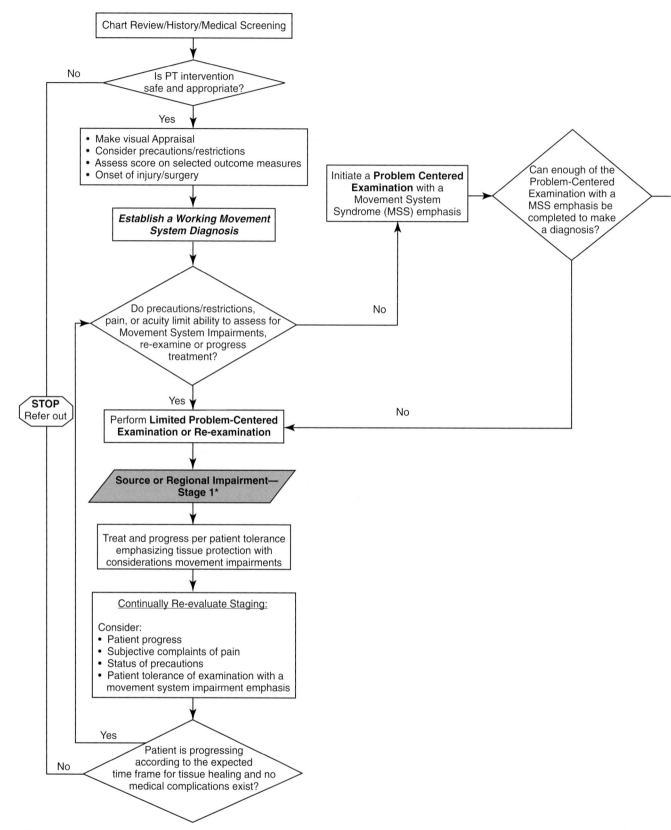

Chart Review/History/Medical Screening

Is PT intervention safe and appropriate? — No

Yes

- Make visual Appraisal
- Consider precautions/restrictions
- Assess score on selected outcome measures
- Onset of injury/surgery

Establish a Working Movement System Diagnosis

Initiate a **Problem Centered Examination** with a Movement System Syndrome (MSS) emphasis

Can enough of the Problem-Centered Examination with a MSS emphasis be completed to make a diagnosis?

Do precautions/restrictions, pain, or acuity limit ability to assess for Movement System Impairments, re-examine or progress treatment? — No

STOP Refer out

Yes

Perform **Limited Problem-Centered Examination or Re-examination**

No

Source or Regional Impairment— Stage 1*

Treat and progress per patient tolerance emphasizing tissue protection with considerations movement impairments

Continually Re-evaluate Staging:

Consider:
- Patient progress
- Subjective complaints of pain
- Status of precautions
- Patient tolerance of examination with a movement system impairment emphasis

Yes

Patient is progressing according to the expected time frame for tissue healing and no medical complications exist?

No

*Stage 1: Low threshold for injury, or high tissue irritability. Symptoms, precautions, and restrictions limit examination and treatment. Levels of stress to affected tissues should be minimal.

Figure 2-2. The movement system evaluation process. According to the physical stress theory, the stages used within the flow chart can generally be defined by stress restriction/progression. Staging should continually be evaluated. *PT,* Physical therapy.

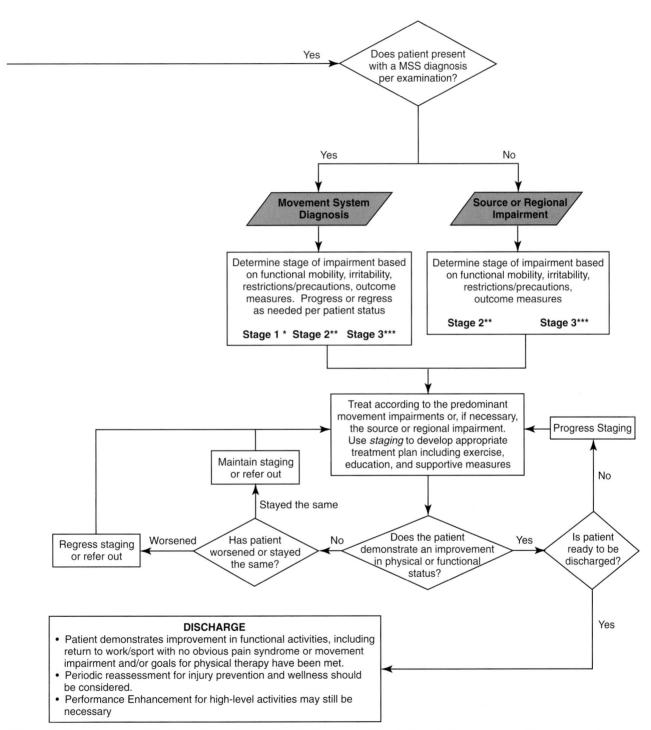

***Stage 2: Moderate threshold for injury.* Precautions and restrictions may still be in place, but treatment should begin to emphasize progression of appropriate physical stress to targeted tissues.

****Stage 3: High threshold for injury,* or low tissue irritability. Treatment should emphasize tissue adaptation and hypertrophy. Generally, precautions have been lifted. Focus on return to work and higher-level sport activities.

surgery. As expected, during a thorough re-examination 6 weeks later, the patient demonstrated continued improvement, reporting minimal pain and demonstrating normal ROM and adequate quadriceps performance. However, she was still not ready for discharge because she had not started to run. Therefore her staging was progressed to Stage 3, and her treatment was modified accordingly to include higher-level activities such as running and jumping.

Staging is somewhat unique to each individual. In this case, the patient was young and athletic with specific fitness and sports-related goals. Therefore, to ensure completion of these goals, treatment during Stage 3 was rather aggressive and discharge occurred when those goals were achieved. For other patients, the specific Stage 3 goals and subsequently, the intensity of treatment may differ based on such factors as age, medical co-morbidities, or prior level of function, but the completion of these goals is necessary for discharge.

Outcome

The patient achieved her goals for physical therapy, including running without pain and with no specific movement impairments, and was deemed ready for discharge.

CASE PRESENTATION
Chronic Lower Back Pain

Symptoms and History

A 42-year-old male presents to physical therapy with chronic lower back pain. The patient reports an insidious onset of pain 8 months ago that has gradually worsened. The patient's symptoms are localized to his right lower back with no radiating symptoms. The patient notes that on average his pain is about a 4/10 with an Oswestry score of 22%. Although he has some pain throughout the day, he continues to perform all of his daily activities, including his work responsibilities that are mostly sedentary. However, the patient has increased pain with running and with racquetball and is therefore no longer participating in these activities.

Key Tests and Signs

After a medical screening, including a brief review of systems, the determination is made that it is safe to proceed with evaluation and treatment. Based on the history provided, visual observation and the Oswestry score, a working diagnosis of lumbar rotation is established. The patient has no precautions, and his current symptoms will not limit the performance of the standard movement system examination.

Diagnosis and Staging

After a thorough movement system examination, the patient is diagnosed with lumbar rotation syndrome, Stage 2. The stage was determined by multiple factors discussed previously, including the time since the onset of pain, the relatively low pain level and Oswestry score, his functional activity performance, and his current limitations.

Treatment

Although this patient has a moderate level of tissue irritability, he should be able to accept some level of adaptive physical stress with treatment. Since a movement system diagnosis is established, treatment emphasizes the correction of specific movement faults or incorrect postures with exercise and education. Thus treatment is based on both the movement system diagnosis, as well as the stage for rehabilitation.

Outcome

As the patient improves and his tissue irritability decreases, he can be progressed to Stage 3 and then treated accordingly. Treatment for lumbar rotation syndrome, Stage 3 includes exercise and education to improve tolerance of higher level sport activities such as running and racquetball. Once the patient is able to return to these activities and manage his pain, he will be discharged.

CASE PRESENTATION
Moderate Ankle Sprain

Symptoms and History

A 16-year-old male basketball player presents to physical therapy after a moderate ankle sprain 6 months ago. During the history, the patient notes only moderate and infrequent pain in the lateral aspect of his ankle. His primary complaint is stiffness that is limiting his mobility during running and cutting activities. His score on the Foot and Ankle Ability Measure (FAAM) activities of daily living (ADLs) subscale is 92%, whereas his score on the FAAM sports subscale is only 72%. The physician provides a prescription for physical therapy to evaluate and treat ankle pain.

Key Tests and Signs

After a medical screening and a thorough history, the therapist determines that it would be safe to proceed with the evaluation to confirm a working diagnosis of ankle impairment. Because the patient has minimal pain and because the injury is not acute, the examination is not limited.

Diagnosis and Staging

According to the results of a thorough movement system examination, the patient does not present with any obvious or consistent movement impairments. For this reason, the patient is diagnosed with Ankle Impairment.

Again, staging for this patient is determined by the time since the initial injury, pain, functional activity level, and the functional outcome measure.

This patient is functioning at a high level and demonstrates a low level of tissue irritability, both of which are associated with Stage 3.

Treatment

The emphasis of treatment is on aggressive ROM techniques to decrease hypomobility and sports-specific training to optimize performance.

Although this patient was not initially diagnosed with a movement system diagnosis, it is still important to attend to the patient's movements and posture during functional activities and exercise to ensure that he does not develop any faulty movements during the rehabilitation process or with the return to sport after an injury.

CONCLUSION

As the previous case studies illustrate, the diagnostic process is both complex and continual. Consideration of the actual tissues involved in a specific musculoskeletal pain problem is essential for this process to occur appropriately without risk to the patient. Attending to the Stage for Rehabilitation allows the therapist to incorporate or exclude certain examination items, to emphasize specific educational principles, and to develop an appropriate treatment strategy. In addition, by understanding the state of the specific source of symptoms, you are more likely to positively affect the actual cause of symptoms. Throughout the remainder of this book, you will be introduced to many diagnoses related to movement system syndromes, otherwise referred to as the potential cause of symptoms. The Stages for Rehabilitation should be used with each of these diagnoses to successfully develop, modify, and progress a treatment program that is designed to ultimately optimize patient outcomes.

REFERENCES

1. Garrett WE: Muscle strain injuries, *Am J Sports Med* 24(Suppl 6):S2-S8, 1964.
2. Yarasheski KE, Pak-Loduca J, Hasten DT, et al: Resistance exercise training increases mixed muscle protein synthesis rate in frail women and men > 76 years old, *Am J Phys* 277:E118-E125, 1999.
3. Fitts RH, Riley DR, Widrick JJ: Physiology of a microgravity environment invited review: microgravity and skeletal muscle, *J Appl Physiol* 89:143-152, 2000.
4. Trappe S, Williamson D, Godard M, et al: Effect of resistance training on single muscle fiber contractile function in older men, *J Appl Physiol* 89:143-152, 2000.
5. Yu ZB, Gao F, Feng HZ, et al: Differential regulation of myofilament protein isoforms underlying the contractility changes in skeletal muscle unloading, *Am J Physiol Cell Physiol* 92(3):C1192-C1203, 2007.
6. Terzis G, Stattin B, Holmberg HC: Upper body training and the triceps brachii muscle of elite cross country skiers, *Scand J Med Sci Sports* 16(2):121-126, 2006.
7. Crameri RM, Cooper P, Sinclair PJ, et al: Effect of loading during electrical stimulation training in spinal cord injury, *Muscle Nerve* (1):104-111, 2004.
8. Starkey DB, Pollock ML, Ishida Y, et al: Effect of resistance training volume on strength and muscle thickness, *Med Sci Sports Exerc* 28(10):1311-1320, 1996.
9. Turner CH: Three rules for bone adaptation to mechanical stimuli, *Bone* 23:399-407, 1998.
10. Holick MF: Perspective on the impact of weightlessness on calcium and bone metabolism, *Bone* 22:105S-111S, 1998.
11. Notomi T, Lee SJ, Okimoto N, et al: Effects of resistance exercise training on mass, strength, and turnover of bone in growing rats, *Eur J Appl Physiol* 82:268-274, 2000.
12. Leblanc AD, Schneider VS, Evans HJ, et al: Bone mineral loss and recovery after 17 weeks of bed rest, *J Bone Miner Res* 8:843-850, 1990.
13. Schroeder ER, Wiswell RA, Jaque SV, et al: Eccentric muscle action increases site-specific osteogenic response, *Med Sci Sports Exerc* 31(9):1287-1292, 1999.
14. Wren TA, Beaupre GS, Carter DR: A model for loading-dependent growth, development, and adaption of tendons and ligaments, *J Biomech* 31:107-114, 1998.
15. Hayashi K: Biomechanical studies of the remodeling of knee joint tendons and ligaments, *J Biomech* 29:707-716, 1996.
16. Woo SL, Gomez MA, Akeson WH: Mechanical properties of tendons and ligaments. II. The relationships of immobilization and exercise on tissue remodeling, *Biorheology* 19(3):397-408, 1982.
17. Mueller MJ, Maluf KS: Tissue adaptations to physical stress: a proposed "Physical Stress Theory" to guide physical therapist practice, education, and research, *Phys Ther* 4:383-403, 2002.
18. Sahrmann SA: *Diagnosis and treatment of movement impairment syndromes*, St Louis, 2002, Mosby.
19. Pressure ulcers in adults: prediction and prevention, AHCPR Publication No. 92-0047, Rockville, MD, 1992, US Department of Health and Human Services (USDHHS).
20. Johnson KA, Strom DE: Tibialis posterior tendon dysfunction, *Clin Orthop* 239:196-206, 1989.
21. Pang HN, Teoh LC, Yam AK, et al: Factors affecting the prognosis of pyogenic flexor tenosynovitis, *J Bone Joint Surg Am* 89(8):1742-1748, 2007.
22. Burkhead WZ, Arcand MA, Zeman C, et al: The biceps tendon. In Rockwood C Jr, Matsen FA III, eds: *The shoulder*, ed 2, Philadelphia, 1998, Saunders.
23. Neer CS: Anterior acromioplasty for the chronic impingement syndrome in the shoulder: a preliminary report, *J Bone Joint Surg Am* 54:41-50, 1972.
24. Peterson HA: Physeal fractures. Part 3. Classification, *J Pediatr Orthop* 14(4):439-448, 1994.
25. Delitto A, Erhard RE, Bowling RW: A treatment-based classification approach to low back syndrome: identifying and staging patients for conservative treatment, *Phys Ther* 21:381-388, 1995.
26. Michlovitz SL: *Thermal agents in rehabilitation*, ed 3, Philadelphia, 1996, FA Davis.
27. Robinson AJ: Transcutaneous electrical nerve stimulation for the control of pain in musculoskeletal disorders, *J Orthop Sports Phys Ther* 24:208-226, 1996.

28. Johnson MI, Ashton CH, Thompson JW: An in-depth study of long-term users of transcutaneous electrical nerve stimulation, *Pain* 44:221-229, 1991.

29. Johnson MI, Tabasam G: An investigation into the analgesic effects of interferential currents and transcutaneous electrical nerve stimulation on experimentally induced ischemic pain in otherwise pain-free volunteers, *Phys Ther* 83:208-223, 2003.

30. Lessard L, Scudds R, Amendola A, et al: The efficacy of cryotherapy following arthroscopic knee surgery, *J Orthop Sports Phys Ther* 26:14-22, 1997.

31. Reish RG, Eriksson E: Scars: A review of emerging and currently available therapies, *Plast Reconstr Surg* 122:1068-1078, 2008.

32. Mustoe TA, Cooter RD, Gold MH, et al: International clinical recommendations on scar management, *Plastic Reconstr Surg* 110: 560-571, 2002.

33. Donatelli R, Owens-Burckhart H: Effects of immobilization on the extensibility of periarticular connective tissue, *J Orthop Sports Phys Ther* 3:67-72, 1981.

34. Kisner C, Colby LA: *Therapeutic exercise: foundations and techniques*, Philadelphia, 2007, FA Davis.

35. Delitto A, Rose SJ, Lehman RC, et al: Electrical stimulation versus voluntary exercise in strengthening the thigh musculature after anterior cruciate ligament surgery, *Phys Ther* 68:660-663, 1998.

36. Fitzgerald GK, Piva SR, Irrgang JJ: A modified neuromuscular electrical stimulation protocol for quadriceps strength training following anterior cruciate ligament reconstruction, *J Orthop Sports Phys Ther* 33:492-501, 2003.

37. Stevens JE, Mizner RL, Snyder-Mackler: Neuromuscular electrical stimulation for quadriceps muscle strengthening after bilateral total knee arthroplasty: a case series, *J Orthop Sports Phys Ther* 34:21-28, 2004.

38. Draper V: Electromyographic biofeedback and recovery of quadriceps femoris muscle function following anterior cruciate ligament reconstruction, *Phys Ther* 70:11-17, 1990.

39. Hewett TE, Paterno MV, Myer GD: Strategies for enhancing proprioception and neuromuscular control of the knee, *Clin Orthop* 1:76-94, 2002.

40. American College of Sports Medicine. *ACSM's guidelines for exercise testing and prescription*, Philadelphia, 2000, Lippincott Williams & Wilkins.

41. Suomi R, Collier D: Effects of arthritis exercise programs on functional fitness and perceived activities of daily living measures in older adults with arthritis, *Arch Phys Med Rehabil* 84:1589-1594, 2003.

42. Warden SJ, Hinman RS, Watson MA Jr, et al: Patellar taping and bracing for the treatment of chronic knee pain, *Arthritis Rheum* 59:73-83, 2008.

43. Selkowitz DM, Chaney C, Stuckey SJ, et al: The effects of scapular taping on the surface electromyographic signal amplitude of shoulder girdle muscles during upper extremity elevation in individuals with suspected shoulder impingement syndrome, *J Orthop Sports Phys Ther* 37:694-702, 2007.

44. Hyland MR, Webber-Gaffney A, Cohen L, et al: Randomized controlled trial of calcaneal taping, sham taping, and plantar fascia stretching for the short-term management of plantar heel pain, *J Orthop Sports Phys Ther* 36:364-371, 2006.

45. Crossley K, Bennell K, Greeen S, et al: Physical therapy for patellofemoral pain: a randomized, double-blinded, placebo-controlled trial, *Am J Sports Med* 30: 857-865, 2002.

46. Christie AD, Willoughby GL: The effect of interferential therapy on swelling following open reduction and internal fixation of ankle fractures, *Physiother Theory Pract* 6:3-7, 1990.

47. Johnson MI, Wilson H: The analgesic effects of different swing patterns of interferential currents on cold-induced pain, *Physiotherapy* 83:461-467. 1997.

48. Young SL, Woodbury MG, Fryday-Field K: Efficacy of interferential current stimulation alone for pain reduction in patients with osteoarthritis of the knee: a randomized placebo control clinical trial, *Phys Ther* 71:252, 1991.

49. Binder A, Hodge G, Greenwood M, et al: Is therapeutic ultrasound effective in treating soft tissue lesion? *Br Med J* 290:512-514, 1985.

50. Ebenbichler GR, Erdogmus CB, Resch KL, et al: Ultrasound therapy for calcific tendinitis of the shoulder, *N Engl J Med* 340:1533-1538, 1999.

51. Enwemeka CS: The effects of therapeutic ultrasound on tendon healing, *Am J Phys Med Rehabil* 6:283-287, 1989.

52. Wessling KC, DeVane DA, Hylton CR: Effects of static stretch versus static stretch and ultrasound combined on triceps surae muscle extensibility in healthy women, *Phys Ther* 67:674-679, 1987.

CHAPTER 3

Movement System Syndromes of the Cervical Spine

Mary Kate McDonnell

INTRODUCTION

The joints and all of the structures that move and support them are subjected to degenerative forces arising from repeated movements, prolonged postures, and simply through the process of aging. The cervical spine is particularly susceptible to degenerative changes because normal day-to-day activities require frequent movements of the head and cervical spine. The inevitable degeneration process leads to injury, altering the precision of movement that negatively impacts the rate and type of degeneration. In addition, many individuals perform excessive motions of their head and cervical spine as part of their body language or use undesirable prolonged postures such as holding the telephone to their ear with their shoulder. Based on the premise that the onset of painful and degenerative conditions of the cervical spine is precipitated by deviations in the alignment and movement patterns, this chapter discusses the normal anatomy and kinesiology of the cervical spine to form the basis for understanding and recognizing abnormal motion. The movement system syndromes are then described along with recommendations for rehabilitation.

A common misconception is that because an individual moves in a specific way and because that pattern feels normal, it is an optimal movement pattern. We believe that just as good posture has to be practiced so do optimal movement patterns. Optimal alignment and movement patterns are believed to slow the degenerative process that is associated with arthrokinematic hypermobility.[1] This chapter describes the alterations in alignment and movement patterns that accelerate the degenerative process.

The cervical spine is susceptible to the stresses of daily activities, such as frequently rotating the head and cervical spine to position the eyes and ears[2,3]; flexing, extending, and translating the neck for the same reason; accommodating changes in the alignment of the thoracic spine; and sustaining the weight of the head and upper extremities.[4-6] Malalignment of the cervical spine and adjacent regions can add excessive compressive load onto

the tissues in the cervical region and affect the movement pattern.[7-9] Repetitive upper extremity motions can have the same effect.[10] Appropriate modification of the posture of the cervical, thoracic, and scapular regions can diminish the compressive load on the cervical structure.

Cervical extension secondary to a forward-head posture (Figure 3-1), which is often associated with a thoracic kyphosis, is the most frequently observed alignment impairment of the cervical spine. A forward-head position is described as excessive extension and forward translation of the cervical vertebrae[7,8] (Figure 3-2). Thoracic kyphosis commonly results in increased extension of the cervical spine contributing to the forward-head position[11,12] (Figure 3-3). The extended position of the cervical vertebrae increases the compressive loading on tissues in this region, especially the facet joints.[7]

Other positions of the head and cervical spine can also have an influence on scapular motion. For example, Ludewig et al[13] demonstrated decreased scapular upward rotation and decreased posterior tipping with a flexed neck and head position. The focus of our strategy of alleviating symptoms and improving function of the cervical region is to start with exercises that correct any faults in the alignment of the cervical, thoracic, and scapular regions before focusing on the correction of faulty cervical movements.

Based on clinical observations, the principal movement impairments in the cervical region involve faulty patterns of extension and rotation. If these movements are not performed precisely, the eventual result is pain and limited range of motion (ROM). Correcting the alignment of the thoracic spine, scapulae, and the cervical spine while supporting the arms results in decreased pain and increased ROM during cervical rotation.[9,14] The patient is also instructed to imagine rotating the cervical spine about an axle running through the cervical spine and to avoid any compensatory sidebending and/ or extension. This strategy for performing cervical rotation exercises improves distribution of forces, such as shear and compression, that occur during rotational motions.

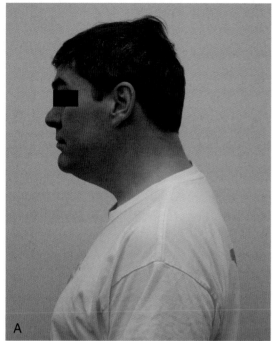

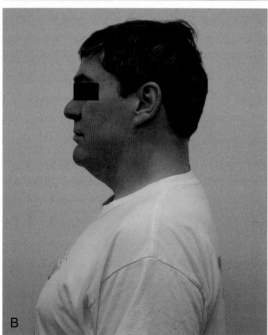

Figure 3-1. **A,** Forward head. **B,** Correction.

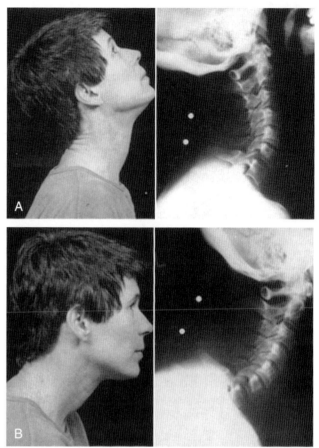

Figure 3-2. **A,** Cervical extension. **B,** Slumping to increase thoracic flexion. Forward head with cervical extension. (From Kendall FP, McCreary EK, Provance PG: *Muscles: testing and function,* ed 4, Philadelphia, 1993, Lippincott Williams & Wilkins.)

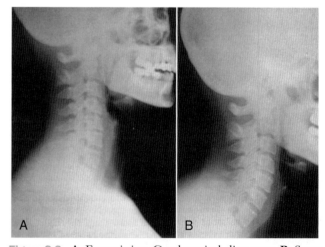

Figure 3-3. **A,** Erect sitting. Good cervical alignment. **B,** Same subject slumping with thoracic flexion. Forward head with cervical extension. (From Kendall FP, McCreary EK, Provance PG: *Muscles: testing and function,* ed 4, Philadelphia, 1993, Lippincott Williams & Wilkins.)

Maintaining precise movement in the cervical region is a challenge because of many factors, including the number of intervening segments, their degrees of freedom, and the influence of the alignment of the thoracic spine and the shoulder girdle musculature. Treatment of the cervical region requires attention to all of these key regions. Treatment strategies include obtaining optimal alignment of the trunk, shoulder girdle, and cervical spine; optimal length and recruitment of the intrinsic muscles of the cervical spine; and optimal movement patterns of the cervical spine and the shoulder girdle and ensuring no compensatory movements of the cervical spine during movement of the upper extremities. The patient should support the upper extremities when sitting by using chairs with armrests that are an appropriate height. Supporting the upper extremities diminishes the downward pull of the limbs that impose compressive forces on the cervical spinal structures, as well as minimizing the tension from the cervicoscapular muscles that can alter the pattern of cervical motion.[5,6,9,14,15]

IDEAL ALIGNMENT OF THE CERVICAL REGION

Ideal alignment of the cervical region allows the head to be positioned with minimal muscular effort.[7,8] Ideal alignment is an inward lordotic curve with both the upper and lower cervical region in a position of slight extension[7,8,16] (see Figure 3-3, *A*). With aging and the inevitable degenerative changes occurring in the cervical discs, the lordotic alignment decreases and there is an increase in forward translation.

As described earlier, the most common alignment impairment observed in the cervical spine is a forward-head posture. The forward-head posture is characterized by forward translation of the lower cervical region and hyperextension of the cervical region with typically, an increased kyphotic curvature in the thoracic region[7,8] (see Figures 3-2 and 3-3, *B*). Patients with chronic neck pain have a decreased ability to maintain a correct alignment when distracted.[17]

The muscular adaptations associated with a forward-head position are shortening of the cervical spine extensors and a lengthening of the intrinsic cervical spine flexors.[8,18] The forward-head position also requires increased activity of the extensor muscles of the cervical spine to counter balance the head against the effects of gravity.[7,19] The muscular adaptations that occur with a forward-head position results in an increase of compressive forces acting on the articular facets.[7,20] In addition, changes may also occur in the ligamentum nuchae that may increase demand on the upper trapezius muscle to stabilize and move the cervical spine.[21]

A forward-head posture is a common physical finding in patients with chronic tension headache and patients with unilateral migraine.[22] Additional alignment faults that we have observed with headache patients include an increase in the degree of upper cervical extension in comparison to that of the lower cervical spine, suggesting possible muscular adaptations in the suboccipital region. These adaptations can include shortness of the suboccipital extensors, superior obliques, inferior obliques, and rectus capitis and lengthened position of the suboccipital flexors, rectus capitis lateralis, and anterior muscles.[18]

We have often observed that body language and deficits in hearing or vision have an influence on a patient's cervical alignment and movement patterns. Patients who use movements and postures of their head and cervical spine as part of their communication strategy can add additional stresses to the cervical region. Common habits that we have observed include excessive extension of upper cervical region and forward translation of the cervical spine during talking, laughing, or reading or while working on a computer. These faults can be exaggerated when the patient wears eyeglasses, especially bifocals.[2] These same patients may also have complaints of pain or headache in the upper cervical region.

Additional alignment faults can result from adaptations arising from asymmetrical use of the eyes or loss of hearing in one ear. Deficits in sight or hearing can result in prolonged posturing in one direction of cervical rotation with associated sidebending in the same direction. The muscular adaptations include unilateral hypertrophy of cervical paraspinals or sternocleidomastoids muscles. These asymmetrical adaptations could cause greater compression forces on the facet joints on one side of the cervical spine. The therapist needs to make the patient aware of these habits to decrease the frequency of the faulty movements and postures while teaching the patient exercises to offset the effects of the postural positions.[3]

MOTIONS OF THE CERVICAL SPINE

The cervical spine consists of seven vertebrae that are divided into two distinct regions: The upper cervical region includes the occiput, C1, and C2 vertebrae and the lower cervical region includes the vertebrae of C3 through to C7. The literature reports a wide variability of available motion in the craniocervical region. With consideration for the large intersubject variability, the typical available motion reported is shown in Table 3-1.[19]

Precise movements in the cervical spine require optimal arthrokinematics and osteokinematics and depend on the muscle length, strength, and recruitment patterns. Motions of the cervical spine are comprised of coupled motions. Coupled motion is defined as a primary

TABLE **3-1**
Distribution of Motion in the Cervical Spine

Motion	Total Motion (Degrees)	Majority of Region Contributing to Motion	Regional Motion (Degrees)
Flexion	45-50	Lower cervical region	35
Extension	85	Lower cervical region	70
Axial rotation	90	Upper cervical region	40-45
		Lower cervical region	45
Lateral flexion	40	Lower cervical region	35

Adapted from Neumann DA: *Kinesiology of musculoskeletal system: foundations for physical rehabilitation*, St Louis, 2002, Mosby.

motion that occurs in one plane that is accompanied automatically by motion in at least one other plane. "Motion in which rotation or translation of a vertebral body about or along one axis is consistently associated with a simultaneous rotation or translation about another axis."[23]

Lysell demonstrated a coupled pattern of motion with cervical flexion and extension.[24] The movement is a combination of translation about a horizontal axis and sagittal plane rotation about a frontal axis of the superior vertebrae.[7] White and Panjabi have reported the total amount of sagittal plane translation to be approximately 3.5 mm at each vertebral level.[23] This would include 1.9 mm in an anterior direction and 1.6 mm in the posterior direction.[23] These reported values represent a small amount of motion and consequently are fairly undetectable to clinical observations, so translation motion observed during the clinical examination can be assumed to be excessive.

Available cervical flexion motion is reported to be 45 to 50 degrees with the lower cervical region contributing approximately 34 degrees. Cervical extension motion is approximately 85 degrees with the majority (about 79 degrees) occurring in the lower cervical region.[19,23] The most common impairment observed during flexion and extension motions is the presence of a relatively greater degree of translation motion as compared to sagittal rotation motion. Observation of the relative amount and timing of upper versus lower cervical motion is also important when assessing the movement pattern of patients with neck pain.

Available rotation motion is comprised of the coupled motions of lateral flexion and rotation in the same direction.[19,23] The observed coupled motion from C2 to C7 demonstrates a gradual decrease in the amount of axial rotation that is associated with lateral flexion as the motion progresses from superior to inferior. This finding has been attributed to the increase in the incline of the orientation of the cervical facet joint.[23] Rotation occurs about a vertical axis with approximately 90 degrees of available motion with 45 degrees attributed to motion at the atlantoaxial joint complex and the remaining 45 degrees from the lower cervical region.[19]

Lateral flexion motion also consists of the coupled motion of lateral flexion and rotation in the same direction. The available lateral flexion motion is approximately 40 degrees, with the majority of motion (35 degrees) contributed by the lower cervical region.[19]

When assessing the active ROM, the therapist should consider the patient's age, with consideration of the possible presence of degenerative changes and decrease in the amount of available ROM.[25] Degenerative disc changes in the cervical spine are observed at a later age than lumbar degenerative changes. Asymptomatic degenerative changes are common on magnetic resonance imaging (MRI) in the cervical spine after 30 years of age with significant changes noted in subjects over 40 years of age.[26-28]

Cervical disc degeneration has been observed in 80% of asymptomatic subjects over the age of 60 years.[29] Disc degeneration is more common in the lower cervical region than in the upper cervical region. The proposed explanation for this phenomena is that the lower cervical region has greater loads imposed on it with daily activities.[7,30,31] In addition, a forward-head alignment with increasing anterior translation of the head increases the flexion moment on the C7-T1 junction.[7]

With aging, there is a decrease in the cervicovertebral ROM of approximately 5 degrees of motion for every 10 years.[25,32] There is also an associated decline in ROM with observed degeneration of the cervical spine, approximately a decrease of 1.2 degrees at the level of the observed degenerative segment with an actual increase in range of 0.8 degrees at the level above the degenerated level.[32] The challenge for the therapist is to attempt to restore the motion at the degenerative segment without causing greater motion at the cervical level above the degenerated segment.

MUSCLE ACTIONS OF THE CERVICAL SPINE

Optimal muscle lengths and recruitment patterns are critical to the performance of cervical motions to allow the ideal ratio of coupled motion to occur. The muscles in the cervical region can be classified into two distinct groups according to the relationship of the attachment of the muscles to the axis of motion of the cervical spine.[7] The **intrinsic muscles** of the cervical spine located close to the axis of motion are felt to provide precise control of motion during movement. The **extrinsic muscles** of the cervical spine are located farther from the axis of motion and provide power to the motion but not necessarily precision of motion. A balance of participation between these two groups is critical for precise and pain-free motion of the cervical spine.

Cervical Flexors

The function of the **cervical intrinsic flexors** is to produce forward sagittal plane rotation or "rolling" of the cervical vertebrae. The muscles producing the sagittal rotation motion in the upper cervical region are the rectus capitis anterior and rectus capitis lateralis[33] (Figure 3-4). In the lower cervical region, forward sagittal rotation is produced by the longus capitis and longus colli. The longus capitis and colli are also active in protecting the anterior structures during forceful extension motions.[7] Impairment of the cervical intrinsic flexors has been reported in patients with cervicogenic headaches and chronic cervical spine pain.[34-38]

The function of the **cervical extrinsic flexors** is to add force to the flexion movement and produce flexion motion associated with forward translation of the cervical vertebrae. The muscles contributing to the forward translatory motion in the cervical region are the

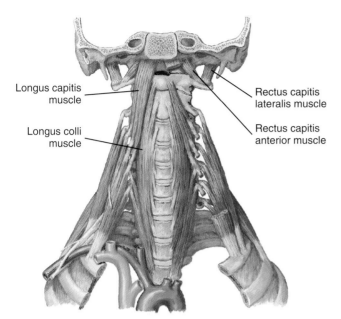

Longus capitis muscle

Longus colli muscle

Rectus capitis lateralis muscle

Rectus capitis anterior muscle

Figure 3-4. Rectus capitis anterior and rectus capitis lateralis muscles. (Reprinted from www.netterimages.com © Elsevier, Inc. All rights reserved.)

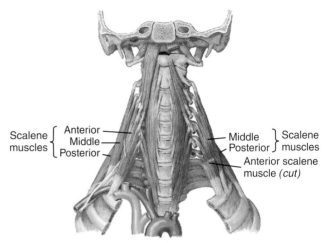

Scalene muscles { Anterior Middle Posterior

Middle Posterior } Scalene muscles

Anterior scalene muscle *(cut)*

Figure 3-6. Anterior and medial scalenes muscles. (Reprinted from www.netterimages.com © Elsevier, Inc. All rights reserved.)

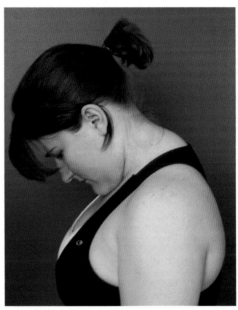

Figure 3-7. Active cervical flexion demonstrating greater translation motion than sagittal rotation.

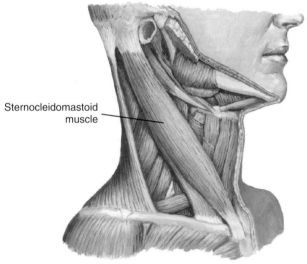

Sternocleidomastoid muscle

Figure 3-5. Sternocleidomastoid muscles. (Reprinted from www.netterimages.com © Elsevier, Inc. All rights reserved.)

sternocleidomastoids and anterior and medial scalenes (Figures 3-5 and 3-6). Commonly, these muscles are the dominant muscle group during flexion movements. The dominant effect of the extrinsic muscles can be attributed to the longer moment arm of this group as compared to the intrinsic muscle group and this may contribute to their increase use during cervical flexion. This faulty movement pattern would result in a movement of anterior translation of the head and cervical spine with diminished anterior sagittal plane rotation[20] (Figure 3-7).

Cervical Extensors

The function of the **intrinsic cervical extensors** is to produce posterior sagittal rotation or backward "rolling" of the cervical vertebrae (Figure 3-8). The muscles attributed to producing the posterior sagittal rotation motion in the upper cervical region are the rectus capitis posterior major and minor, the oblique capitis inferior and superior, and the semispinalis capitis, the splenius capitis, and the longissimus capitis. The muscles in the lower cervical region that produce posterior sagittal rotation are the semispinalis cervicis, the splenius cervicis, and the longissimus cervicis.[20] The cervical multifidus spinae muscles are thought to produce cervical extension, axial rotation, and lateral bending movement, but the total moment-generating capacity is predicted to be less than

1 Nm and therefore not considered to be a clinically significant contribution to movement,[39] although the fascicular attachments of the cervical multifidus to the cervical facet capsules have been proposed to be a possible contributor to neck pain and injury.[39,40]

The function of the **extrinsic cervical extensors** is to produce extension with posterior translation of the cervical vertebrae. The muscles attributed to producing this posterior translatory motion in the cervical region are the upper trapezius and levator scapulae (Figure 3-9). A common faulty recruitment pattern can include greater recruitment of the extrinsic cervical extensors during cervical extension. This faulty recruitment pattern can best be observed in the hands and knees position (Figure 3-10) and the prone position (Figure 3-11). If the patient cannot assume the quadruped position, leaning on the forearms on a counter can be substituted. The objective is to have the scapula in a stabilized position and the head horizontal in relation to gravity.

Cervical Rotators

The **intrinsic cervical rotators** produce rotation about a vertical axis. These muscles include the rectus capitis posterior major, the oblique capitis inferior, the oblique capitis superior, and splenius. The oblique capitis inferior has been demonstrated to have a higher density of muscle

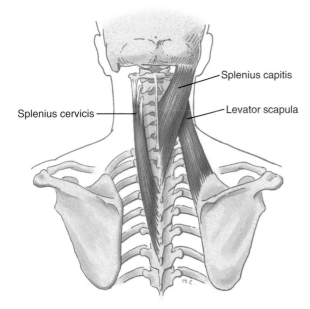

Figure 3-8. Intrinsic cervical extensors. (From Neumann, DA: *Kinesiology of the musculoskeletal system: foundations for rehabilitation*, ed 2, St Louis, 2010, Mosby.)

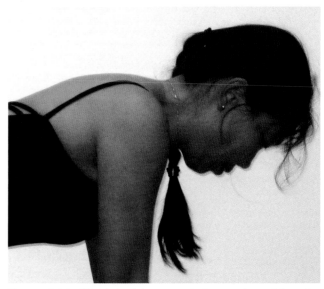

Figure 3-10. Hands and knee cervical extension with active levator scapulae.

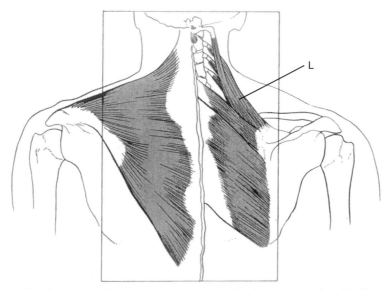

Figure 3-9. Extrinsic cervical extensors—upper trapezius, levator scapulae *(L)*. (From Porterfield JA, DeRosa C: *Mechanical neck pain: perspective in functional anatomy*, Philadelphia, 1995, Saunders.)

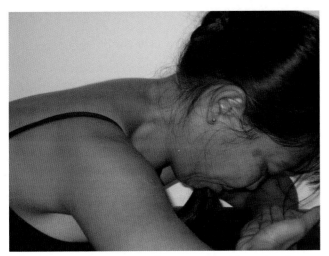

Figure 3-11. Prone cervical extension with active levator scapulae.

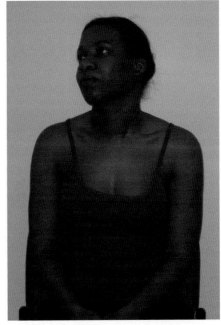

Figure 3-12. Faulty rotation with extension.

spindles compared to other cervical muscles and is thought to be an important contribution to the sensation of cervical rotation.[3]

The **extrinsic cervical rotators** include the sterno-cleidomastoids, the scalenes, the upper trapezii, and the levator scapulae (see Figures 3-5 and 3-6). These muscles all have the action of rotation but also the simultaneous action of lateral flexion. If these groups of muscles are the dominant muscle group during cervical rotation, the precision of movement about a vertical axis may be compromised. The therapist will often observe rotation with concurrent lateral flexion. If the patient uses this strategy for rotation, they may complain of pain when the lateral flexion movement occurs. Repeating the rotation motion while maintaining a rotation movement about a vertical axis without concurrent lateral flexion can result in pain-free ROM.

The therapist may also observe rotation with simultaneous extension (Figure 3-12). This faulty movement pattern may be an indication of dominance of the sterno-cleidomastoid and its influence as an extensor of the upper cervical spine over the poorly recruited intrinsic cervical rotators, which would maintain motion about a vertical axis. The actions of the upper trapezius and/or the levator scapulae can also contribute to cervical extension during rotation.

In addition, the therapist may also observe cervical rotation with simultaneous flexion and/or forward translation of the head and neck (Figure 3-13). This faulty movement pattern may be an indication of dominance of the anterior scalenes, the middle scalenes, and the sterno-cleidomastoids during the movement of rotation. Dominance of these muscles and their propensity to increase translation and shear forces on the lower cervical spine can result in greater movement in the translatory plane rather than rotation about a vertical axis.

As is discussed later in the sections on the appropriate syndromes, manually guiding the patient's pattern of

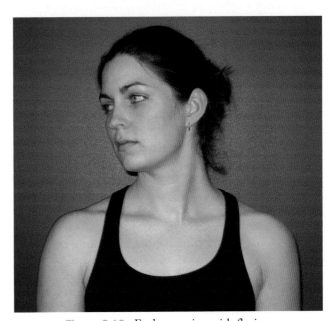

Figure 3-13. Faulty rotation with flexion.

rotation is often necessary. A frequently required intervention is to instruct the patient to turn the head and neck "easily" and with minimal effort to reduce the magnitude of muscular contractions and to encourage a more appropriate muscle recruitment pattern. A strong muscle contraction especially of the extrinsic rotators can add compression of cervical spine structures and favor the use of the muscles with the greatest mechanical advantage.

The upper trapezius and levator scapulae muscles have attachment from the cervical spine region directly to the scapula and clavicle[41] (see Figures 3-5, 3-6, and 3-9). This

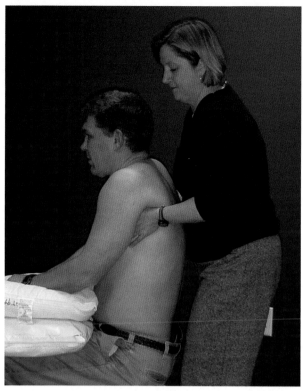

Figure 3-14. Passive support of the upper extremities can reduce the passive stretch of the upper trapezius and levator scapulae.

TABLE 3-2
Cervical Spine Syndromes in Order of Frequency of Observation

Syndrome	Key Findings
Cervical extension-rotation	Forward head with asymmetrical findings: Asymmetry in cervical spinal musculature and/or scapula alignment; pain with rotation-associated sidebending and extension; weak intrinsic cervical flexors; dominance of extrinsic cervical rotators
Cervical extension	Forward head; pain with extension; translation greater than sagittal rotation; weak intrinsic cervical flexors
Cervical flexion-rotation	Decreased cervical lordosis, flat thoracic spine; pain with rotation-associated flexion; excessive recruitment of extrinsic cervical rotators, anterior and middle scalenes
Cervical flexion	Decrease cervical lordosis, flat thoracic spine; pain with flexion; lower cervical flexion greater than upper thoracic flexion; excessive recruitment of extrinsic neck flexors; poor recruitment of intrinsic neck extensors during extension

attachment has clinical significance when examining cervical spine function. Specifically, we have noted in clinical examination that single arm movements can result in compensatory motion of rotation of a cervical spine segment or several segments.[10]

In addition, the attachment of these muscles will influence the ROM during active cervical motions, especially rotation. Examining active cervical rotation with passive support of the weight of the upper extremities can result in increase cervical ROM and decrease pain.[9,14,15] The passive support of the upper extremities can reduce the passive stretch of the upper trapezius and levator scapulae that can potentially decrease the load on the cervical spine structures and permit improved motion and less painful movement[9,14,15] (Figure 3-14).

MOVEMENT SYSTEM SYNDROMES
of the Cervical Spine

Movement system syndromes of the cervical spine are precipitated by deviations in the alignment and movement patterns. Cervical spine syndromes in order of frequency and key findings are included in Table 3-2.

CERVICAL EXTENSION SYNDROME

In individuals with minimal degeneration involving the cervical region, the principal movement impairment in the cervical extension syndrome is imprecise cervical extension that is often associated with pain and limited ROM. There is altered distribution of extension across the cervical region and an imbalance of muscle performance among the cervical extensors and flexors. The extrinsic muscles contribute to excessive horizontal translation of the cervical vertebrae rather than a combination of sagittal rotation produced by the intrinsic cervical muscles and horizontal translation produced by the extrinsic cervical muscles. Contributing factors in the cervical extension syndrome include the weight of the upper extremities, the alignment of the thoracic spine, and the alignment of the scapulae.

Symptoms and History

Pain is typically located in the posterior cervical region with possible radicular symptoms along the cervical nerve root dermatomes and/or scapula region specifically along the vertebral border.[42] The patient complains of pain with cervical spine extension and/or prolonged posturing of a forward-head position (e.g., working at the computer or reading). The patient can commonly have complaints of headaches located in the suboccipital region.

Key Tests and Signs
Alignment Analysis
Alignment faults with cervical extension syndrome include a forward-head position with an increase in the cervical

lordosis and anterior translation (see Figure 3-2). Often, patients with the diagnosis of cervicogenic headaches have an alignment of greater upper cervical spine extension and are positioned in 10 degrees of posterior sagittal extension, as referenced to the vertical plumb line.

Typically, in individuals older than 50 years of age, the forward-head alignment is a position of greater anterior translation in the lower cervical region and greater upper cervical sagittal extension.[26] As described in the literature, degenerative changes are often present with increasing age and will affect the alignment and the loading of the joints. With degeneration of the cervical discs, there is narrowing of the intervertebral foramen and increased approximation and loading of the facet joints.[7,29-31] The changes in alignment observed with degeneration, specifically the approximation of the facet joints, are similar to the same position of physiological extension. Thus a cervical spine with presence of degeneration may have low tolerance to additional extension forces.

The characteristic alignment faults in the adjacent regions include a thoracic kyphosis and scapular malalignment.[11,12,20] An increased thoracic kyphosis is highly correlated with an increase in a forward-head position[11,12,20] (Figure 3-15; see Figure 3-3). Additional alignment faults include the scapulae in a position of excessive depression and/or abduction.[9,14,43]

Movement Impairment Analysis

Individuals with a cervical extension syndrome often complain of pain with movement into active extension (Figure 3-16). During assessment of active cervical extension, the younger spine (15 to 25 years old) may demonstrate a greater amount (or degree) of posterior translation than posterior sagittal rotation and/or an excessive ROM. Older individuals with spinal degeneration may have painful and limited extension because of a starting alignment of a forward-head position with excessive anterior translation. The starting alignment of anterior translation (extended position) limits the available physiological motion into extension. An additional movement impairment with active cervical extension includes a faster rate of upper cervical extension movement compared to that observed in the lower cervical extension movement (Figure 3-17).

Patients with cervical extension syndrome may also demonstrate movement impairments during flexion. Active flexion motion can be limited (Figure 3-18) and painful, particularly when the degree of anterior translation is excessive and relatively greater than the normal anterior sagittal rotation.

The faulty movement of forward translation without the coupled motion of sagittal rotation results in the approximation of the facet joint surfaces. The approximation of the facet joint surfaces during performance of this faulty flexion movement results in similar approximation of the facet joint surfaces as that occurring during cervical

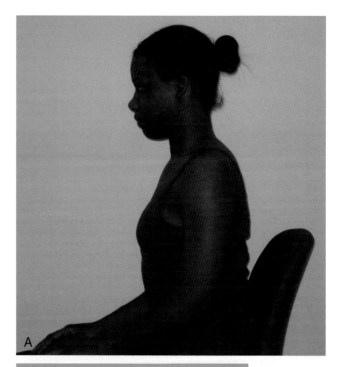

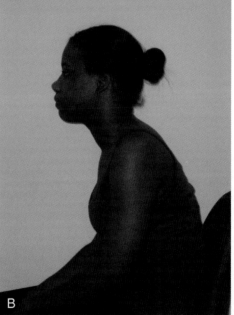

Figure 3-15. A, Good alignment. **B,** Increased thoracic kyphosis is correlated with an increase in a forward head position.

extension, as well as complaints of pain similar to those during active extension (Figure 3-19).

In this system, the primary test is performed by asking the patient to perform the movement in the desired direction such as cervical extension or rotation. During the movement, the therapist asks about symptoms and carefully observes the characteristics of the movement. For the secondary test, the therapist has the patient correct the starting alignment and the movement faults and notes the effect on the symptoms. The corrected alignment and movement pattern is repeated a number

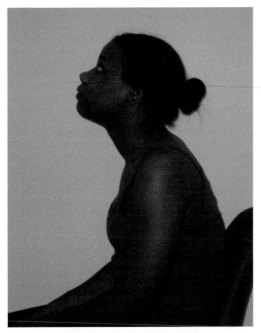

Figure 3-16. Faulty active cervical extension; upper cervical motion is greater than lower cervical motion.

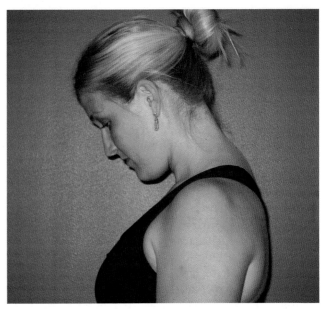

Figure 3-18. Associated limited cervical flexion.

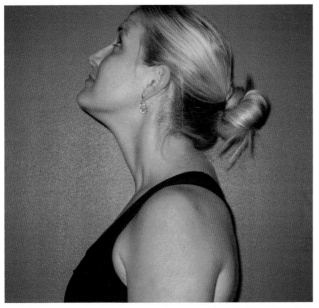

Figure 3-17. Cervical extension movement impairment: Greater upper cervical extension than lower cervical extension (the upper cervical spine is more extended than the lower cervical spine).

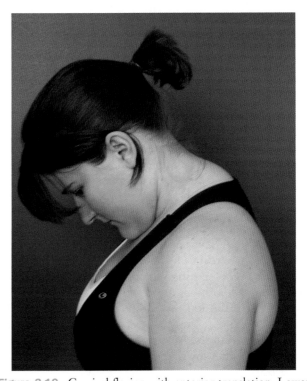

Figure 3-19. Cervical flexion with anterior translation. Lower cervical remains extended.

of times to ensure the improvement in symptoms is consistent. The repetitions also help the patient learn how to move correctly and how to control the symptoms.

Sitting tests. Sitting tests should be performed in active cervical ROM and flexion, extension, and rotation.

Secondary tests. *Correction of alignment:* If there is pain at rest, then correction of the forward-head alignment of the cervical spine may alleviate or decrease the

symptoms. To correct the head and neck alignment, the alignment of the thoracic spine and scapulae must also be corrected.

Passive elevation of the shoulder girdle: Passively elevating the shoulder girdle and/or supporting the weight of the upper extremities before the patient performs active cervical extension, flexion, or rotation may alleviate or decrease the symptoms and often results in increased cervical ROM and typically a decreased level of reported pain during motion[14,15] (see Figure 3-14).

Passive support of the upper extremities can reduce the passive stretch of the upper trapezius and levator scapulae which can potentially reduce the loading and posterior shear forces on the structures of the cervical spine. The passive support typically results in increase ROM and less painful movement.*

Passive elevation of ribcage: Performing the test of passive elevation of the rib cage is indicated in patients with well-developed abdominals, particularly the rectus abdominis. Passive elevation of the rib cage will often improve active cervical ROM and decrease pain.

Elevating the rib cage affects the pain and increases the cervical ROM because well-developed abdominal muscles (rectus abdominis and external oblique) have enough stiffness to passively depress the rib cage. Active contraction of the abdominal muscles would further increase the passive tension and downward pull on the rib cage. The tension would also affect the scalene muscles that attach to the rib cage, thus adding to the compression on the cervical vertebrae and restricting motion. Passive elevation of the rib cage decreases the tension on the scalene muscles, thus decreasing the pain and increasing the cervical rotation ROM.

Supine tests

Active cervical flexion in supine. The primary movement impairment during cervical flexion is excessive anterior translation in relation to the amount of anterior sagittal rotation. The result is a forward-head position and often reports of pain.

Manual muscle test of cervical flexion. The cervical intrinsic flexor muscles will test weak.[8] The patient will be unable to maintain a position of a "neck curl" and will assume an extended forward-head position that is characteristically associated with dominance of the sterno-cleidomastoid and anterior and middle scalenes and weakness of the deep neck flexors[8,35,45] (Figure 3-20).

Secondary test. *Corrected performance of cervical flexion:* Manual assistance provided by the therapist is required to properly perform the "neck curl" movement. When the therapist supports the weight of the head and assists the proper anterior sagittal rotation motion and the patient actively holds the position, there is no pain as long as the patient avoids the extended forward-head position (see Figure 3-20).

Prone and quadruped tests. *Active cervical extension in prone or quadruped:* Active cervical extension can be performed in both the prone and quadruped positions and is characterized by a greater degree of posterior translation as compared to posterior sagittal rotation. During this movement, the examiner will typically observe an increase recruitment of levator scapulae muscles that contribute to posterior translation and

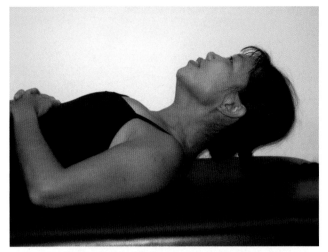

Figure 3-20. Faulty supine neck flexion.

diminished recruitment of the intrinsic cervical extensors that produce posterior sagittal rotation (see Figure 3-10).

Secondary test. *Correction of cervical extension:* Appropriate instruction to initiate the cervical extension movement with posterior sagittal rotation of the head and cervical spine results in decreased pain. Verbal cues can include "roll your head back" or "pretend that there is a pole through your ears and you are rolling around the pole."

Quadruped test. *Active cervical extension in quadruped:* During the quadruped rocking back, the examiner will often observe a compensatory motion of cervical extension. Typically, this movement impairment is not associated with the complaint of pain (Figure 3-21).

The cervical extension during rocking back is believed to be the result of the lengthening or stretching of the levator scapulae, a downward rotator, as the scapula upwardly rotates during the motion of rocking back. The passive lengthening of the levator scapulae muscle causes extension of the cervical spine, which is also associated with posterior translation.

Secondary test. *Correction of cervical extension:* The patient is instructed to repeat the quadruped rocking back with the "chin to the Adam's apple" or the anterior base of the neck to avoid extension of the cervical spine. The patient will commonly report a sensation of diminished pressure in the posterior cervical region during the performance of the secondary test movement. Encouraging the recruitment of cervical flexors during this movement will create the appropriate counteracting force to prevent the cervical extension and translation movements.

Treatment

The goal for treatment of the cervical extension syndrome is to diminish cervical extension movements and forces during daily activities. All exercises and functional instructions include improving the alignment and

---

*References 4, 6, 14, 15, 20, 40, and 43.

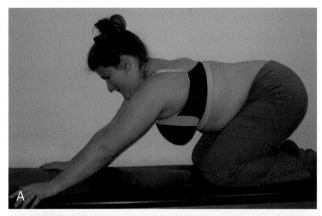

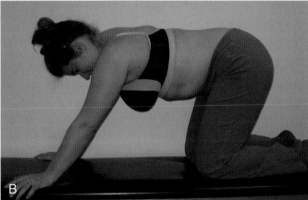

Figure 3-21. **A,** Compensatory cervical extension during quadruped rocking back. **B,** Correction of compensatory cervical extension.

reducing the stress imposed by adjacent regions before initiating cervical movements. Specifically, these instructions include modification of the alignment of the thoracic spine and the shoulder girdle, as well as supporting the upper extremities.

In addition, instructions include strategies to be used during functional activities such as how to support the upper extremities and reduce compensatory motion at the adjacent regions during the day.[5,6] Typical instructions for daily activities would include use of abdominals to maintain neutral position of the lumbar spine and avoiding thoracic flexion or "slumping" especially with sitting activities. The focus of the active exercise program for the cervical region is to improve the strength and motor control of the intrinsic cervical spine flexor muscles along with improving the flexibility of the posterior cervical structures.[33,37,45-47] The active exercise program includes correction of the length, strength, and stiffness of the axioscapular muscles, abdominals, and posterior thoracic spinal musculature.[48]

In addition, upper extremity movements have a direct effect on the cervical spine via the attachment of cervicoscapular muscles. An examination and classification of the associated scapular movement impairments is critical in the management of the patients with cervical pain. Strategies to examine, classify, and manage scapular

movement impairments are clearly described in Sahrmann.[1]

Exercise Program

Sitting with back to the wall—capital flexion. The upper extremities are supported on pillows to diminish the compressive loading of the cervical spine from the transfer of the weight of the upper extremities to the cervical region through the cervicoscapular muscle attachment.[9,15] Each patient needs to be assessed for specific alignment impairments at the lumbar and thoracic spines and scapulothoracic region. The patient is then instructed in strategies to precisely correct alignment faults in these regions before proceeding with cervical movements (Figure 3-22, *A*). These instructions include recruiting the lower abdominal muscles to maintain a neutral lumbar spine alignment and patient-specific instructions to correct scapulae alignment. This will typically include correction of scapular alignment of depression, downward rotation, and/or abduction (internal rotation). The key instruction for faulty alignment of scapulae depression is to "elevate the acromions toward the ears," and the key instruction for the position of the scapulae downward rotation is to "elevate the acromions toward the ears and then slightly adduct the scapulae." Instruction for faulty position of excessive abduction (>3 inches from the spine) would be to "squeeze the shoulder blades together." The ideal position of the scapulae would be (1) the vertebral borders of the scapulae oriented in a vertical position or slight upward rotation, (2) the scapulae positioned 2.5 to 3 inches from the vertebral spine, (3) the scapulae positioned between T2 and T7, (4) 10 degrees of anterior tilt, and (5) 30 to 40 degrees of internal rotation.[1,8,19,43,49]

The patient is instructed to place his or her head close to the wall and perform capital head flexion. The patient is encouraged to "roll" the head and chin toward the base of the anterior neck while trying to maintain the head close to the wall (Figure 3-22, *B*). The verbal cue to "roll" the head is to encourage recruitment of the intrinsic cervical muscle to perform sagittal rotation rather than anterior translation. Many patients report a "tightening" in the front of the cervical spine region while performing this exercise. This sensation is most likely the muscles in the front of the neck being appropriately recruited, and specifically, the muscles are being recruited in a shortened position rather than the lengthened position. In addition, patients also report a "stretch or pull" down the proximal posterior cervical region that can extend into the central upper thoracic region. Again, this is an appropriate stretch to the posterior structures. There should be no pain along the vertebral border of the scapula.

The patient is encouraged to maintain appropriate alignment of the adjacent regions during the movement of the cervical spine. This exercise can best be performed in sitting, but if the patient has difficulty maintaining the

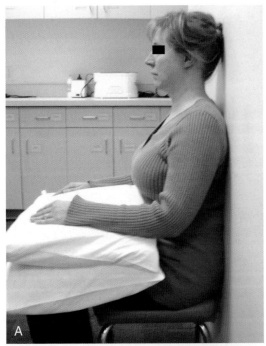

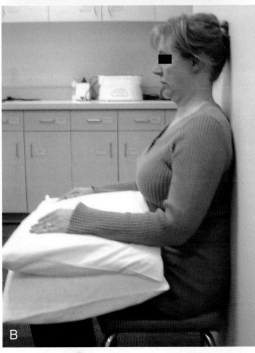

Figure 3-22. **A,** Sitting against the wall, arms supported, correct scapulae position. **B,** Performing capital flexion.

correct postural alignment during the cervical motion, the exercise can be performed in supine. The supine position will not be as challenging on the trunk musculature to maintain the alignment of the adjacent regions, although the demands on the deep neck flexors are greater in the supine position than in sitting.

Any radiation of symptoms to the vertebral border of the scapulae and away from the proximal spine would be considered a possible sign of cervical radiculopathy and an inappropriate response to the movement. If radiation

of symptoms occurs, the therapist should reassess whether this exercise in this position is appropriate for the patient. Radiation of symptoms indicate that the exercise should be made easier by performing the same movement in a supine position with support of the arms with pillows or using the hands to assist with movement of the head and neck.

Strengthening the intrinsic cervical spine flexors in supine. Strengthening the intrinsic cervical spine flexors in supine begins with correcting the alignment of the thoracic spine and shoulders, as well as similar instructions as noted in the previous exercise. Patients are instructed to recruit the lower abdominal muscle to maintain a neutral lumbar spine alignment. Patient-specific instructions are provided to correct the scapulae alignment, typically including correction of scapular alignment of depression, downward rotation, and/or abduction (internal rotation).

The arms should be supported on pillows with the hips and knees in flexion. The patient may require a towel roll under the head. The thickness of the towel roll depends on the patient's thoracic alignment and severity of the forward-head alignment. The greater the kyphosis and forward-head posture the greater the thickness of the towel roll. The following is a progression of exercises from the easiest to the hardest.

Capital flexion without head lift. The patient is instructed to roll the chin toward the front of the cervical spine. The patient should feel a stretch down the central posterior cervical region and muscle recruitment of the anterior intrinsic cervical spine flexors.[33,34,45]

Capital flexion with head lift—with and without assistance. The patient is instructed to roll the chin toward the front of the cervical spine and then continue to roll the cervical spine and head off the supporting surface while maintaining the chin positioned at the anterior cervical spine. Adding the lift of the head is more challenging, and the patient may have trouble maintaining the chin in contact with the anterior cervical spine region.[46,47] Forward translation of the chin or the chin "jutting forward" indicates poor performance of the intrinsic cervical spine flexors and a dominance of the extrinsic cervical spine flexors[8] (see Figure 3-19). If a patient is unable to maintain the head position, he or she can use the hands to lift the head to minimize the load on the cervical spine muscles (Figure 3-23). Patients are encouraged to allow only enough support to permit the appropriate "curl up" position of the head and cervical spine. Progression of the exercise would be to provide less support.

Strengthening the intrinsic cervical spine extensors in prone or quadruped

Prone position. To strengthen the intrinsic cervical spine extensors in prone, the patient is positioned with the forehead on the palms of the hands (Figure 3-24). The patient is then instructed to "roll" the head back in a pain-free range. The instruction of rolling the head

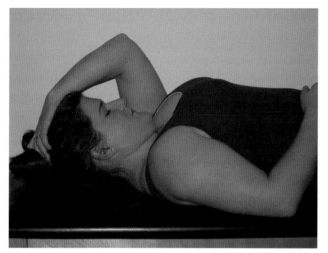

Figure 3-23. Supine: Strengthening of deep cervical flexors with assistance.

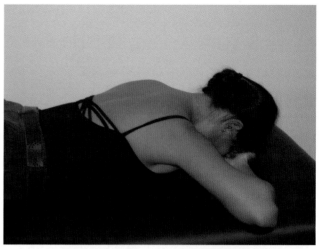

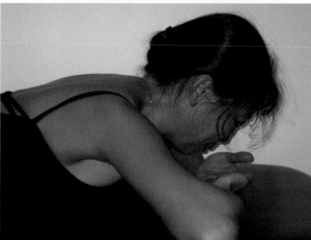

Figure 3-24. Prone cervical extension with emphasis of sagittal rotation.

back is to encourage recruitment of intrinsic cervical spine muscles (splenius/semispinalis) to produce posterior sagittal rotation and diminish recruitment of the extrinsic cervical spine muscles (levator scapulae/upper trapezius) and the movement of the posterior translation. The therapist should observe the appropriate muscle recruitment of the intrinsic cervical spine muscles and diminished recruitment of the extrinsic muscles.

Quadruped position. To strengthen the intrinsic cervical spine extensors in quadruped, the patient is instructed to flatten the thoracic spine like a "table top" and align the head and cervical spine with the thoracic and lumbar spine. The patient is instructed to "roll" the head down and then roll the head back while imagining that there is a rod running through the middle of the neck and rotating about the rod. The instruction of rolling the head back encourages recruitment of intrinsic cervical spine muscles (suboccipitals, semispinalis, and splenius) to produce posterior sagittal rotation and diminish recruitment of the extrinsic cervical spine muscles (levator scapulae/upper trapezius) and posterior translation. The patient should be instructed to perform the movement in the "middle-third" of the range to avoid end-ranges. The therapist should observe the appropriate muscle recruitment of the intrinsic cervical spine muscles and diminished recruitment of the extrinsic muscles. Performing this movement in the quadruped position is a greater challenge because the patient must maintain proper trunk and scapulothoracic position in an upper extremity weight-bearing position during the movement of the cervical spine (Figure 3-25).

Sitting with back to wall—shoulder abduction lateral rotation. Sitting with back to wall—shoulder abduction lateral rotation exercise is a progression of the back to wall—capital flexion exercise. The patient assumes the position as described in the first exercise, which includes correct positioning of the lumbar spine, thoracic spine, scapulae, and cervical capital flexion. The patient

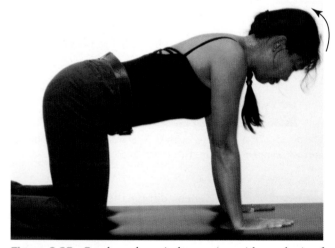

Figure 3-25. Quadruped cervical extension with emphasis of sagittal rotation in midrange.

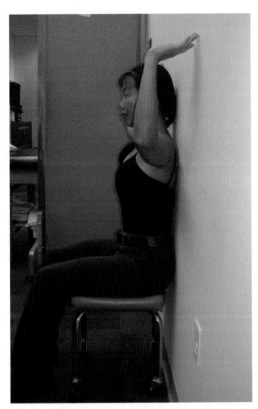

Figure 3-26. Sitting back to wall, shoulder abduction lateral rotation.

then performs bilateral shoulder abduction and lateral rotation so that the arms are against the wall without compensatory thoracic, lumbar, or cervical extension. The patient slides the arms up the wall, maintaining spinal alignment, especially capital flexion. A typical response from the patient is a report of increased muscle activity in the midthoracic region, indicating increased recruitment of trapezius, rhomboid, and thoracic spinal musculature (Figure 3-26).

Modification: The arms do not make full contact with the wall. The arms can be parallel to the wall.

Modification: The fingertips can be placed on the wall with the elbows away from the wall.

Progression: When adding resistance with free weights or resistance bands, the patient is instructed to position the trunk, neck, and arms as described previously, then move through shoulder abduction with resistance. The patient continues to maintain the lumbar spine against the wall and capital cervical flexion during the shoulder movement.

Sitting with back to wall performing shoulder flexion. Sitting with the back to the wall performing shoulder flexion exercise is a progression of the back to wall—capital flexion exercise program. The patient assumes the same head and trunk alignment, as described, of correct positioning of the lumbar spine, scapulae, and cervical capital flexion. The patient performs shoulder flexion and lateral rotation to 90 degrees with the elbows

flexed and the "palms facing you." The patient is then instructed to perform shoulder flexion by "reaching up toward the ceiling." The patient should maintain the lumbar spine against the wall and the cervical spine in the position of capital flexion. Since the movement of shoulder flexion is increased, there is a stretch to the latissimus dorsi and avoiding lumbar extension will be difficult if the muscle is short or stiffer than the abdominal muscles. In addition, during shoulder flexion, maintaining the humeral position of lateral rotation will also be difficult and the therapist should monitor the elbow position for indication of compensatory medial rotation. A verbal cue of "elbows in" can assist in preventing medial rotation. Also, as shoulder flexion motion increases, there often is associated cervical extension because of the stretch of the levator scapulae as the scapula upwardly rotate. Again, the patient should be encouraged to maintain capital cervical flexion and avoid compensatory cervical extension. Maintaining the position of cervical flexion during the movement of the arms encourages recruitment of the intrinsic cervical flexors to maintain cervical alignment (Figure 3-27).

Modification: Position the humeri/arms in the scapular plane: 30 degrees of horizontal abduction.

Modification: Position the humeri in less lateral rotation: "Palms face each other, elbows in."

Progression: When adding resistance with free weights or resistance bands, the patient is instructed to position the trunk, neck and arms as described previously then move through movement of shoulder flexion with resistance. The patient continues to maintain the lumbar spine against the wall and will find it a challenge to maintain capital cervical flexion and avoid cervical extension during the shoulder movement (Figure 3-28).

Wall slides: facing the wall—shoulder flexion. The patient is instructed to face the wall and place the ulnar side of the hands on the wall with the shoulders in flexion. The patient is instructed in the correct scapulae position and to bring the chin down toward the front of the neck. The patient is then instructed to slide the arms up the wall while maintaining the cervical spine position, avoiding any compensatory cervical extension during the movement of shoulder flexion and returning to the starting position (Figure 3-29).

Modification: Position the shoulders in the scapular plane.

Progression: When adding resistance with resistance bands, the patient is instructed to maintain the cervical position and to avoid any compensatory cervical extension during the movement of the shoulder flexion wall slide (Figure 3-30).

Functional Instructions

The goal in modification of functional activities of the cervical extension syndrome is to diminish cervical extension and forward translation movements of the cervical spine during daily activities. The most common activities

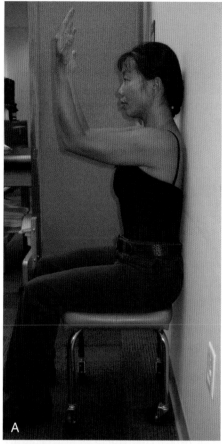

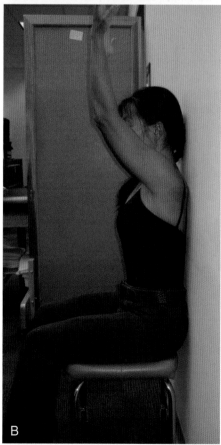

Figure 3-27. Back to wall sitting, shoulder flexion with lateral rotation. **A,** Start position. **B,** Shoulder flexion.

that require instruction are prolonged sitting, especially at the computer, and the use of eyeglasses, in particular, multifocal lenses.

When sitting at the computer, patients are instructed to have a supportive chair that will reduce thoracic flexion and assist in maintaining good thoracic alignment. They should support their forearms either on the desk or an extended tray for a keyboard. The desk or tray should be at the appropriate height so that the patient does not need to "slouch" for the arms to be supported. Commonly, if the support is too low, the patient may increase thoracic flexion and/or scapular depression to position the arms for support. Raising the supporting surface or adding armrests can be helpful.

The therapist should observe the patient using his or her eyeglasses. Frequently, the patient can be observed assuming a forward-head position and/or increase upper cervical extension when using eyeglasses, especially multifocal lens.[2] Alignment correction when wearing glasses should follow the same sequence that has been demonstrated in the sitting back to wall exercises: Start with correction of lumbar, thoracic, and scapular alignment and then neck and head position.

CERVICAL EXTENSION-ROTATION SYNDROME

Cervical extension-rotation syndrome is characterized by pain associated with cervical extension and rotation. This syndrome is the most common cervical syndrome seen in our clinic. The principal movement impairment in this syndrome is imprecise cervical rotation with associated cervical extension and/or sidebend, which is often associated with pain, limited ROM and altered distribution of rotation motion across the cervical region. An imbalance of muscle performance among the cervical rotator muscles and the extrinsic muscles contributes to multiplanar movements rather than precise uniplanar motion produced by the intrinsic rotators. In addition, an imbalance of muscle performance of the intrinsic cervical extensors with the extrinsic extensors contributes to a compensatory extension movement during performance of rotation. The contributing factors in the cervical extension-rotation syndrome include weight of the upper extremities and alignment of the thoracic spine and scapulae. There may also be asymmetries in the appearance of the cervical spine, thoracic spine, and scapular regions.

Symptoms and History

Symptoms and history can be similar to the findings found in cervical extension syndrome. In addition, the patient with this syndrome may report a history of vision or hearing deficits that may require frequent movement of cervical rotation or sustained postures of cervical rotation to accommodate for the deficits. Symptom location is typically located more unilaterally.

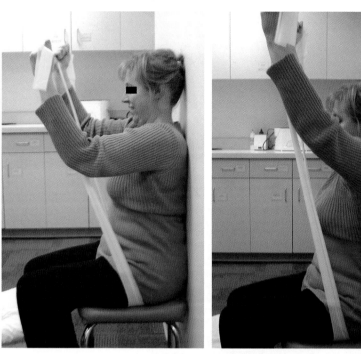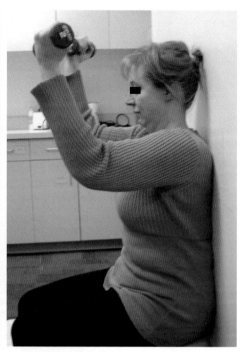

Figure 3-28. Progression of wall exercises with resistance bands and free weights.

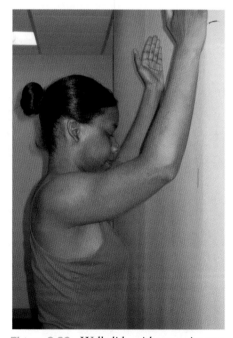

Figure 3-29. Wall slide without resistance.

Key Tests and Signs

Alignment Analysis

Alignment faults can be similar to the findings seen in cervical extension syndrome. Additional alignment faults include an asymmetry in muscle size of the cervical extensors. The asymmetry may be associated with the vision or hearing deficits as described earlier. Also, the asymmetry may be associated with activities that require repetitive resisted one arm activities or other work activities that required prolonged posturing in one direction of rotation. Patients who have the habit of posturing in one direction of rotation during an activity may also maintain the same position of slight rotation with activities that do not require the posture of rotation. Many times patients do not realize they are assuming this position because their eyes have adjusted to the altered head position. When patients use a mirror to monitor head alignment, they can easily correct the position and often alleviate the symptoms. Patients will initially need to practice alignment correction in front of a mirror to achieve a natural position of correct alignment.

Similar alignment faults of the adjacent regions observed in the cervical extension syndrome can also be observed with this syndrome. In addition, we have noted unilateral impairments in the thoracic and scapulothoracic region. In the thoracic region, asymmetry may be noted with the rib cage rotated in one direction or increased spinal musculature on one side. In the scapulothoracic region one scapula can be positioned in excessive depression or downward rotation and impose an unbalanced stress on the cervical spine through the attachment of the scapulocervical muscles (Figures 3-31 and 3-32).

Movement Impairment Analysis

Movement impairments that are characteristic of cervical rotation extension syndrome include complaints of pain and limitation of motion during active rotation. During active rotation, there is imprecise cervical rotation with associated compensatory cervical extension and/or lateral

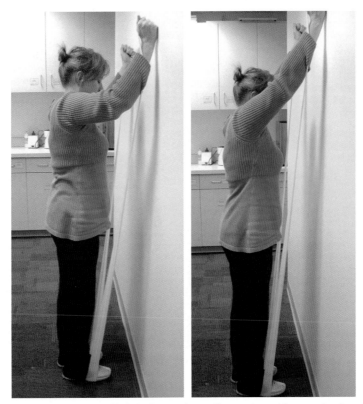

Figure 3-30. Progression of wall slide facing the wall exercise with scapula elevation adding resistance with elastic band. Patient instructed to look down and avoid any compensatory cervical extension.

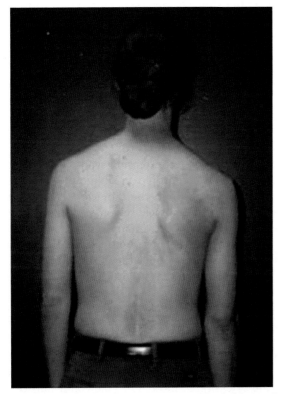

Figure 3-31. Right scapula in a greater position of depression.

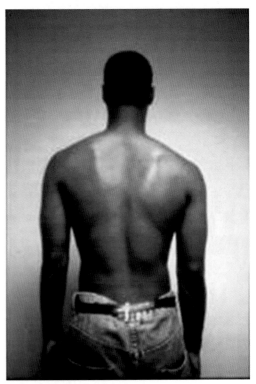

Figure 3-32. Right scapula in a position of greater downward rotation and depression than the left.

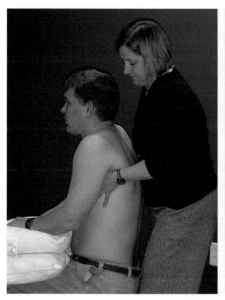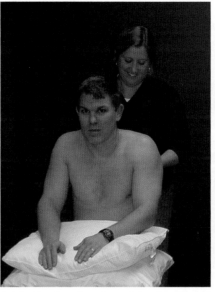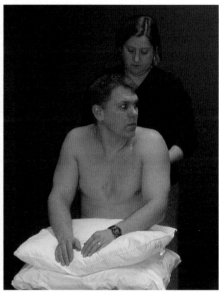

Figure 3-33. Passive elevation of the shoulder girdle test.

flexion that is often associated with pain and limited ROM.

Sitting tests

Active cervical range of motion/rotation. The primary tests are the same as for the extension syndrome with the additional findings of painful and/or limited rotation often associated with concurrent cervical extension or lateral flexion as an associated movement direction. Performance of primary tests considers adjacent regions and the precision of movement.

Secondary tests. Correction of alignment and observed compensatory motions are key to diminishing pain and improving ROM. Passive elevation of the shoulder girdle and/or supporting the weight of the upper extremities results in an increase in rotation ROM and a decrease in pain[14,15] (Figure 3-33).

Correction of alignment before movement. Correction of thoracic kyphosis and/or a forward-head posture before the initiation of active rotation motion results in increased rotation ROM and diminished symptoms.

Correction of compensatory movement. Correction of the movement fault of compensatory of cervical extension and lateral flexion during active rotation diminishes symptoms and increases ROM. The therapist guides the patient to maintain precise rotation about a vertical axis, and the ROM and the symptoms are reassessed.

Additional sitting tests. Single shoulder flexion/monitoring cervical spinous processes: During active single-arm flexion, rotation of a single or multiple vertebrae is noted via palpation of the cervical spinous processes.[10] Patients do not typically complain of pain during this test. An alternative finding during single-arm flexion is compensatory sidebending of the cervical spine.

Secondary tests. Correction of this rotation movement impairment can be difficult. There are several strategies that can be attempted, as follows:

- Instruct the patient to recruit the intrinsic cervical flexors by actively maintaining capital flexion during single arm flexion.
- Assist the patient in correcting the associated scapular movement impairment during the single-arm shoulder flexion movement.
- Instruct the patient to perform bilateral shoulder flexion and note if the movement impairment improves.

The patient's individual response to the secondary tests assists the therapist in choosing the appropriate intervention strategies.

Supine test. Supine active cervical flexion: In supine, active cervical rotation is limited and painful.

Secondary test. Correction and assistance of movement: Correct positioning of the cervical spine in neutral, passively elevating the shoulders, and manually guiding the cervical rotation so that the motion is precise decreases the symptoms and increases the range of pain-free motion.

Quadruped test. Active cervical rotation: In the quadruped position, active cervical rotation is limited and painful.

Secondary test. Correction of alignment, movement—verbal and manual cues: In quadruped, correcting the alignment of the thoracic spine, cervical spine, and head and manually guiding the motion to ensure precision rotation will increase the pain-free ROM. The verbal cues during this secondary test in quadruped include "keeping the head and neck in line with the thorax" and "keeping the chin rotated into the front of the neck."

From the back, the therapist places the fingers around the patient's neck and guides the active rotation motion. The guidance alleviates the faulty extension or sidebending motions. This secondary test movement results in improved ROM and diminished symptoms.

Treatment

In addition to the strategies described previously in the section on cervical extension syndrome, the goal for treatment of the cervical rotation-extension syndrome is to decrease the compensatory cervical extension and lateral flexion during active cervical rotation. Correction of the pattern of movement during daily activities is particularly important. Instruction in strategies to be used during functional activities, such as supporting the upper extremities, is important. Additional strategies to manage the rotation impairment include using minimal effort to rotate the head and neck to diminish the disproportionate recruitment of the extrinsic cervical rotators (scalene and sternocleidomastoid) and correcting any sustained asymmetrical positions of the head and neck. Educating the patient and diminishing movements of the head and neck as part of the patient's body language are essential.[4,6,14,15] The focus of the active exercise program in the cervical region is to improve the strength and motor control of the intrinsic cervical spine rotators.

As noted in the description of the cervical extension syndrome, upper extremity movements have a direct effect on the cervical spine via the attachment of cervicoscapular muscles. An examination and classification of the associated scapular movement impairments is critical in the management of the patients with cervical pain. Strategies to examine, classify, and manage scapular movement impairments are clearly described in Sahrmann.[1]

Exercise Program

Sitting with back to wall performing cervical rotation. The initial positioning for the sitting with back to wall performing cervical rotation exercise is the same as the first exercise described in the section on cervical extension syndrome. The initial instructions address impairments in adjacent regions. The upper extremities are supported on pillows to diminish the compressive loading of the cervical spine from the transfer of the weight of the upper extremities to the cervical region through the cervicoscapular muscle attachment.[9,15] Each patient needs to be assessed for specific alignment impairments at the lumbar and thoracic spines and scapulothoracic region. The patient is then instructed in strategies to precisely correct individual alignment faults in these regions before proceeding with the exercise (see Figure 3-22).

The patient is then instructed to perform cervical rotation about a "vertical axis" and to avoid the compensatory movements of extension and sidebending. The therapist should encourage the patient to "easily" turn the head and neck to minimize the recruitment of the extrinsic cervical rotators. Specific instructions include "keep the chin down" and "do not lean the head and neck toward the side you are rotating toward." Additional instructions to sidebend in the opposite direction that the patient is rotating the head, typically result in a vertical position of the head and neck and diminished ipsilateral sidebending. Maintaining the precise motion of rotation without compensatory sidebending or extension promotes an increased use of the intrinsic rotators and diminished use of the extrinsic rotators, thus reducing shear forces on the cervical spine.

As described in cervical extension syndrome, the patient is encouraged to maintain appropriate alignment of the adjacent regions during this movement of the cervical spine. This exercise can be ideally performed in sitting, but if the patient has difficulty maintaining the correct postural alignment during the cervical motion, the exercise can be performed in supine. The supine position will not be as challenging on the trunk musculature to maintain the alignment of the adjacent regions.

Supine active cervical rotation. Performance of precise cervical rotation in supine can be performed if sitting cervical rotation is too difficult or painful. The patient assumes a hook lying position with the arms supported on pillows (Figure 3-34). The patient may require a towel roll under the head. The thickness of the towel roll depends on the patient's thoracic alignment and severity of the forward-head alignment. The greater the kyphosis and forward-head posture the greater the thickness of the towel roll. The same initial instructions to address the adjacent regions impairments as explained in the sitting exercises. The patient is then instructed in strategies to precisely correct individual alignment faults in the adjacent regions—lumbar and thoracic spines and scapulothoracic region—before proceeding with the exercise. The patient is then instructed to perform cervical rotation about a "vertical axis" and to avoid the movements of cervical extension and sidebending.

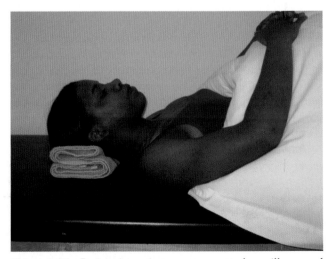

Figure 3-34. Patient in supine, arms supported on pillows, and head on folded towel.

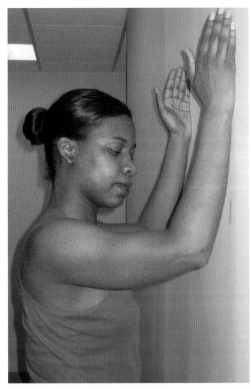

Figure 3-35. Facing wall, arms overhead and supported on the wall.

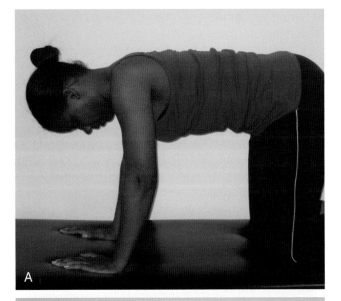

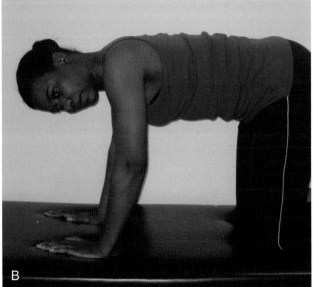

Figure 3-36. Corrected quadruped **(A)** and quadruped cervical rotation **(B)**.

Facing wall, arms supported—active cervical rotation. An additional position of facing the wall with the arms overhead supported on the wall can be used to perform precise cervical rotation with support to the upper extremities. The patient is instructed to rest his or her forearms on the wall, allowing the wall to support the upper extremities and relaxing the upper trapezius muscles (Figure 3-35). The patient is instructed to roll the chin down slightly and then perform precise cervical rotation about a vertical axis and to avoid movements of cervical extension and sidebending.

Quadruped active cervical rotation. The alternative position of quadruped can be used to perform precise cervical rotation if the previously described positions of sitting or supine are too difficult or painful with cervical rotation motion (Figure 3-36). The patient is instructed to flatten the spine like a "table top," align the head and cervical spine with thoracic and lumbar spine and then rotate the head and neck about an axis of motion. The patient is instructed to avoid movements of cervical extension and sidebending.

Functional Instructions

The goal for instruction in modification of functional activities of the cervical extension-rotation syndrome is to diminish cervical extension and forward translation movements, as described in the cervical extension syndrome, and to minimize asymmetrical stresses of the

cervical spine during daily activities. Asymmetrical stresses may come from posturing of the cervical and/or thoracic spine in sidebend or rotation, especially during sitting activities. Asymmetrical stresses may also be imposed by unilateral movements of an upper extremity via the attachment of the cervicoscapular muscles.[10]

When sitting at the computer, patients are instructed to have a supportive chair with armrests that will reduce thoracic flexion and assist in maintaining good thoracic alignment. They should support their forearms on the armrests, the desk, or an extended tray for a keyboard. The armrests, desk, or tray should be at the appropriate height so that the patient does not need to "slouch" for the arms to be supported. The computer or work station should be centered to the chair so there is no prolonged posturing in rotation or sidebend of the cervical or thoracic spine.

The patient should be instructed to avoid prolonged positions of rotation or sidebend of the cervical or thoracic spine during daily activities. These positions can commonly occur while watching TV, playing video games, and so on, without the patient being aware of the posturing. Using the telephone in a prolonged cervical sidebend position is common, and the patient should be encouraged to consider the use of a head set or "blue tooth" apparatus to diminish use of the prolonged cervical sidebend position.

Additional activities on which to counsel the patient include avoiding repetitive and/or resistive one arm activities. These activities can inflict asymmetrical stresses on the cervical spine via the attachment of the cervicoscapular muscles. If the patient must continue with one-arm activities, it will be very important that he or she maintains proper alignment of the thoracic and cervical spines, especially avoiding cervical extension and/or a forward-head position during the activity. Instructing the patient to "keep the chin and nose down" will recruit the intrinsic cervical neck flexors to support the cervical spine during the one arm activities.

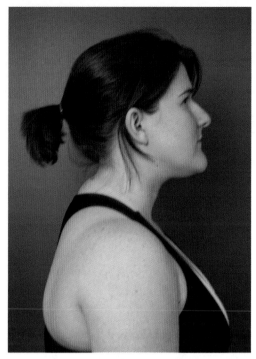

Figure 3-37. Alignment side view.

CASE PRESENTATION
Cervical Extension-Rotation Syndrome

Symptoms and History

A 24-year-old female student presents with a complaint of neck pain that has worsened in the last 4 months. Pain is located in the bilateral upper cervical region, right lower cervical region, and right upper trapezius muscle. She also complains of occasional numbness and tingling in the right forearm and hand. She rates her average daily pain 4/10. Pain can increase to 7/10 with prolonged sitting, working on the computer, and studying. Her neck disability index (NDI) score = 23 indicating moderate disability.[50] Radiographs of the cervical spine were unremarkable.

She reports a history of chronic migraines since she was 16 years old. She averages about one migraine a month and manages the migraines with Imitrex and rest. In the last 4 months, as her neck pain has worsened, she has noted an increase frequency of migraines to 2 to 3 per month.

Alignment Analysis

In standing, she presents with a position of forward head with upper cervical extension, increased flexion at the upper thoracic region with a flat thoracic spine below and lumbar lordosis (Figure 3-37). The scapulae are positioned in abduction and slight depression. The right scapula is positioned 4 inches lateral from the spine, and the left scapula is positioned 3.5 inches lateral from the spine.

Movement Analysis and Active Range of Motion Findings

	ROM (Degrees)	Movement Analysis	Symptoms
Flexion	49	Lower cervical spine remains extended	
Extension	80		Pain in the upper cervical region
Rotation R	49	Compensatory cervical extension	Painful in right lower cervical, correction of extension > decrease pain
Rotation L	60		
Lateral flexion R	40		
Lateral flexion L	55		
PASSIVE ELEVATED SHOULDER GIRDLE			
Flexion	60	Decrease cervical extension at end-range	
Extension	80		No complaint of pain
Rotation R	80		No complaint of pain
Rotation L	80		

ROM, Range of motion; *R,* right; *L,* left.

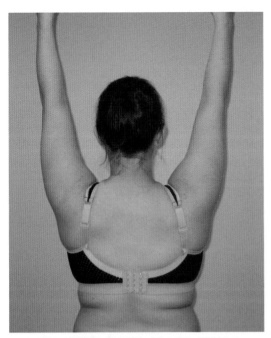

Figure 3-38. Standing shoulder flexion.

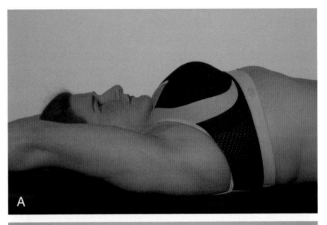

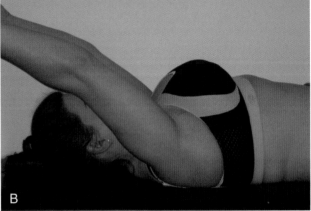

Figure 3-39. **A,** Supine shoulder flexion with rib cage elevation. **B,** Supine shoulder flexion with correction.

Passive mobility findings

Inspection of the posterior cervical region reveals that the left articular pillar appear more prominent than right. Central posterior to anterior (PA) pressures performed on the C5/6 and C6/7 spinous process indicate that they are hypomobile, and she complains of pain over the local area. Unilateral PA pressures on the left C5/6 and C6/7 articular pillar indicate that they are hypomobile, and she complains of pain over the local area.

Active shoulder movements

Shoulder flexion demonstrated a decreased upward rotation of scapulae: <60 degrees.[49] Patient also demonstrates compensatory cervical extension and complaint of cervical pain (Figure 3-38).

Secondary Tests. The therapist corrects the starting alignment of the abducted scapulae and cervical spine extension position, then during active shoulder flexion, the therapist manually assists the scapulae into the greater upward rotation and instructs the patient to avoid compensatory cervical extension. The corrections resulted in greater scapular upward rotation and no complaint of neck pain.

Additional impairments

Supine shoulder flexion demonstrates limited shoulder motion with compensatory rib cage elevation, lumbar extension, and cervical extension (Figure 3-39).

Secondary Tests. The patient was then instructed to correct the starting scapular alignment by actively adducting the scapulae; to recruit lower abdominals to maintain lumbar spine alignment, and to avoid rib cage elevation and cervical extension. The patient was then instructed to actively perform shoulder flexion without

compensatory motions. Shoulder flexion ROM is decreased, but she able to perform movement without compensatory motion. Passive length assessment of the latissimus dorsi bilaterally was determined to be short.[8]

Length test of the pectoralis minor: Passive length assessment of the pectoralis minor was determined to be short bilaterally with the right shorter than the left.[8] Also noted was compensatory cervical rotation in the direction of the muscle being tested.

Manual muscle testing (MMT): The lower abdominal muscles were weak at a 2/5 level, with compensatory rib cage elevation and cervical extension during testing.[1] The deep neck flexors were 2/5 muscle grade.[8] The strength of the middle trapezius was determined to be 3/5 on both right and left.[8]

Diagnosis and Staging

The patient's diagnosis is cervical extension-rotation syndrome with scapula abduction.[1] The stage for rehabilitation is Stage 2. Her prognosis is good to excellent. Her positive moderators include her young age, overall good health, and moderate duration of symptoms. Her negative moderators include her reports of radiculopathy and long history of migraines.

Diagnosis	Key Tests
Cervical extension-rotation	Alignment of cervical spine: Forward head with upper cervical extension. AROM: Painful limited cervical rotation with compensatory extension, correction of compensatory extension movement diminishes symptoms. Passive elevation of the scapulae increases ROM and decreases pain. Compensatory movements of the neck in the direction of extension with movements of the upper extremities and during muscle length testing.
Scapular abduction	Alignment: Scapula position is 4 inches from spine. AROM: Excessive abduction and decreased upward rotation with shoulder flexion.

AROM, Active range of motion; *ROM,* range of motion.

Treatment

The patient was seen once a week for 4 weeks and then once every other week for 4 weeks. Each treatment session lasted approximately 30 minutes. The treatment included instruction in a specific home exercise program to improve cervical spine function and functional instructions to diminish excessive forces on the cervical spine during her daily activities.

Exercise program

Initially, the patient was instructed in active cervical ROM exercises. The initial "set up" for the patient was sitting in a chair with the back against the wall and the arms supported on pillows. This type of positioning diminished thoracic flexion and provided the patient with tactile feedback of "correct alignment." The pillows allow support of the weight of the upper extremity and diminish the downward pull on the cervical spine via the attachment of the cervicoscapular muscles.[9] The patient was then instructed in the following cervical exercises:

Capital flexion in sitting (see Figure 3-40): The patient was instructed to recruit the lower abdominal muscles to maintain a neutral lumbar spine alignment then correct her faulty scapular position of scapula depression and abduction. She was instructed to slightly elevate the shoulders toward the ears and then adduct the scapulae. Once she had corrected her starting alignment of her lumbar spine, thoracic spine, cervical spine, and scapulae, she was instructed to place her head close to the wall and perform capital head flexion. The patient was encouraged to "roll" the head and chin toward the base of the anterior neck while trying to maintain the head close to the wall. The verbal cue to "roll" the head is to encourage recruitment of the intrinsic cervical muscle to perform sagittal rotation rather than anterior translation. The patient reported a "tightening feeling" in the front of the neck

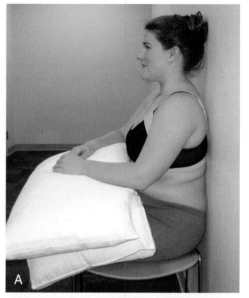

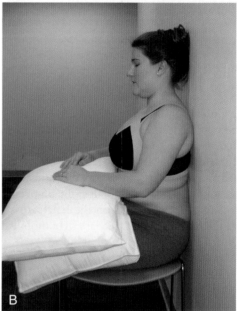

Figure 3-40. **A** and **B,** Sitting capital flexion arms supported.

and stretching in the back of the neck. She did not have complaints of reproduction of cervical spine pain or any complaints of peripheralization of symptoms into her arm. She was instructed to repeat the movement five times. At the completion of the repetitions, the patient reported that the exercise was difficult, but there was no increase or peripheralization of her symptoms. She reported that her neck felt "looser," and she felt a decrease in her headache pain. She was instructed to repeat the exercise an additional five repetitions. She again reported a positive response.

Cervical rotation in sitting: The patient was instructed to position herself in the same position as in the previous exercise. This incorporated support of the upper extremities and correction of spinal and scapulae alignment, including rolling the head and chin down to the correct cervical spinal extension position. Once positioned, the patient was instructed to perform rotation. The patient was then instructed to perform cervical rotation about a "vertical axis" and to avoid the movements of extension and sidebending. Specific instructions included "keep the chin down" and "do not lean the head and neck toward the side of rotation." Additional instructions included to sidebend in the opposite direction of the rotation, which results in a vertical position of the head and neck and diminished ipsilateral sidebending. Maintaining the precise motion of rotation without compensatory side-bending or extension promotes increased use of the intrinsic rotators and diminished use of the extrinsic rotators, thus diminishing shear and translatory forces on the cervical spine. Initially, the patient was able to perform approximately 60 degrees of pain-free rotation without compensatory cervical extension. She was reminded to keep her "nose down" during the rotation movement. Practice during the first session resulted in approximately 70 degrees of pain-free rotation without compensatory extension.

Sitting—shoulder abduction lateral rotation (see Figure 3-41, A): The patient was instructed to position herself in the same position as the previous exercises. She correctly positioned her lumbar spine, scapulae and cervical spine (capital flexion). The patient then performed shoulder abduction and lateral rotation and maintained the position by placing her arms against the wall. The patient then slid the arms up the wall (abduction-elevation), maintaining spinal alignment, especially capital flexion. The patient reported and increased muscle activity in the midthoracic region, indicating increased recruitment of trapezius, rhomboid, and thoracic spinal musculature.

Sitting—shoulder flexion (see Figure 3-41, B): The patient was instructed to position herself as noted in the first two exercises. The patient then performed 90 degrees of shoulder flexion and lateral rotation of the humerus "palms facing each other." The patient was then instructed to perform shoulder flexion: "reach up toward the ceiling." The patient was instructed to "keep elbows in" to prevent humeral medial rotation, and to maintain the lumbar spine against the wall and the cervical spine in the position of capital flexion.

Supine capital flexion without head lift: In a supine position with the arms supported on pillows, the patient was instructed to recruit the lower abdominals to maintain the lumbar spine position, adduct the scapula to properly align the scapulae, and then perform capital cervical flexion without a head lift. The patient was instructed to maintain the lumbar spine and scapulae alignment during the movement of the neck. The patient should feel a stretch in the posterior neck region and a recruitment of the intrinsic cervical flexor muscles.

Supine neck flexor strengthening—with assisted head lift (Figure 3-42): The patient was instructed to roll the chin toward the front of the cervical spine and assist with her

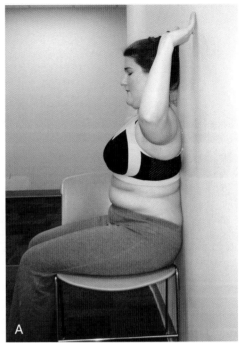

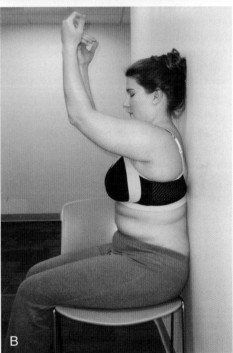

Figure 3-41. **A,** Sitting-shoulder abduction with lateral rotation. **B,** Sitting-shoulder flexion with lateral rotation.

hand to roll the cervical spine off the supporting surface while maintaining the chin positioned at the anterior cervical spine. The assisting hand should be placed at the back of the head to help direct the movement of capital flexion and assist in lifting the weight of the head. The patient was encouraged to only allow enough support that permits the appropriate "curl up" position of the head and cervical spine. Progression of the exercise would be to provide less support.

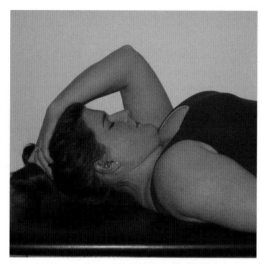

Figure 3-42. Assisted neck flexion.

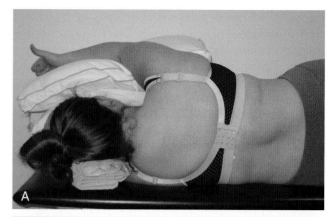

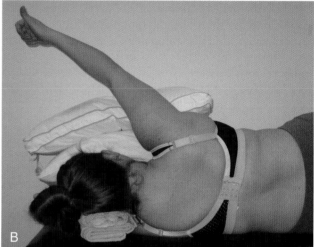

Figure 3-43. **A** Starting position for trapezius exercises. **B,** Final position.

Trapezius exercises in sidelying (Figure 3-43): The patient is positioned in sidelying with her head supported on a towel roll and her arm overhead. The therapist supports the arm with one hand and guides the scapula into adduction, external rotation and posterior tilt with the other hand. The patient is asked to adduct the scapula, and at the end of the scapula adduction ROM, the therapist instructs the patient to hold the weight of the arm while keeping the scapula adducted and avoiding any position of neck extension. The therapist should observe appropriate recruitment of the trapezius muscle. The patient can perform this exercise at home with her arms supported on pillows.

Wall slides: Facing the wall—shoulder flexion: The patient is instructed to face the wall and place the ulnar side of the hands on the wall with the shoulders in the flexion plane. The patient is instructed how to use correct scapulae position and bring the chin down toward the front of the neck. The patient is then instructed to slide the arms up the wall and gently push into the wall to recruit the serratus anterior while maintaining the cervical spine position. The patient should avoid any compensatory cervical extension during the movement of shoulder flexion and return from shoulder flexion.

Facing wall, arms supported—active cervical rotation (Figure 3-44): An additional position of facing the wall with the arms overhead and supported on the wall can be used to perform precise cervical rotation with support to the upper extremities. The patient is instructed to rest the forearms on the wall, allow the wall to support the upper extremities, and relax the upper trapezius muscles. The patient is instructed to roll the chin down slightly, perform precise cervical rotation about a vertical axis, and avoid movements of cervical extension and sidebending. These instructions are similar to the instructions used in cervical rotation in sitting.

Quadruped rocking back without associated extension (Figure 3-45): The patient was instructed to assume the quadruped position, flatten the spine like a "table top," and align the head and cervical spine with thoracic and lumbar spine. She was then instructed to rock back on to her heels while maintaining a "flat spine" and "chin rolled in toward the front of the neck." She was instructed to avoid cervical extension during the movement of rocking back. The patient had difficulty maintaining the thoracic and cervical spine position as she rocked back. Her rocking back range was limited to the range in which there was no spinal movement.

Functional Instruction

The patient was encouraged during sitting activities to support the arms and periodically recruit abdominals and scapular posterior tilt and external rotation muscles, while maintaining neutral neck position with the chin and nose slightly down.[5] She was encouraged to use a chair that would support her thoracic spine and not allow thoracic flexion.[11] She was instructed in proper use of eyeglasses to allow a neutral neck position during computer use. The instructions were directed to diminish upper cervical extension and forward translation.[2] She was also instructed in the typical "gestures" and "habits" of cervical extension that she demonstrated during the

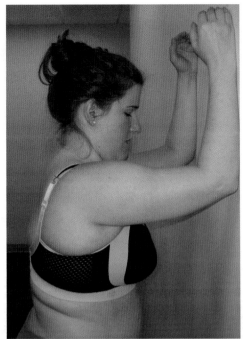

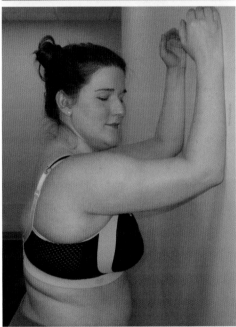

Figure 3-44. Arms supported on wall; capital flexion and rotation.

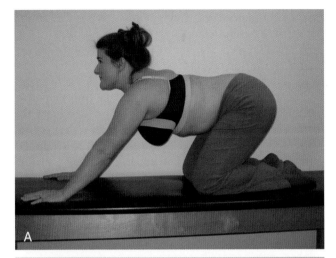

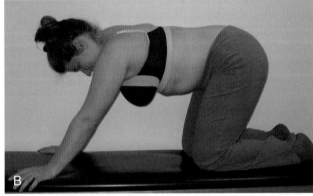

Figure 3-45 **A,** Rocking back with compensatory extension. **B,** Correctional exercise—rocking back without associated extension.

examination while she was communicating and expressing herself. She was instructed in strategies to diminish these habits during her day.

At the end of 4 weeks of treatment (4 treatment sessions), the patient reported no episodes of numbness/tingling in her forearm or hand. She reported only 1 migraine headache during the 4-week period (previously 2 to 3 a month). She rated her daily average pain 2/10 and also 2/10 with prolonged sitting at a computer. Her NDI score was 14, indicating minimum disability. At the end of 8 weeks of treatment (6 treatment sessions), she reported

her daily average pain 0/10 and occasional pain (2/10) if she sat more than 2 hours at the computer without a break or did not support her arms during the sitting activity. Her headache behavior was now typical of what she experienced before the recent neck pain flare-up, or one migraine a month. She reported that she was using her eyeglasses properly while working on her computer and had become more "aware" of her gestures and habits that contribute to stress on her cervical spine. She was making an effort to diminish cervical extension movements during her daily activities. She continued to remind herself to keep her "nose down" to avoid excessive extension.

This case is a useful illustration of the importance of addressing the adjacent regions, shoulders and thoracic spine, when treating a patient with cervical extension-rotation syndrome and associated headache. Alignment, length, and strength of muscles in the adjacent region are critical to address before attending to the cervical movement impairments. In addition, demonstrating to the patient that she had a tendency to frequently move in the direction of extension rotation and teaching her that this movement needed to be reduced during her daily activities helped alleviate her pain. Patient awareness of her daily movement habits and postures is essential in managing her symptoms and possible future flare-ups. Essential components for management of her problem included (1) improving the strength of her scapula posterior tilt and external rotator muscles, serratus anterior, rhomboids, and middle trapezius to maintain appropriate alignment of her scapula. Improving the participation of the serratus anterior muscle reduces the loading from the cervicoscapular muscles on the cervical spine and increases the support from the axioscapular muscle for the weight of her upper extremities. Proper support of her upper extremities is necessary for decreasing the compressive load on the cervical spine structures and allows pain-free motion of the cervical spine.[44] Improving the strength and recruitment of her abdominal muscles supports the appropriate alignment of her lumbar spine and rib cage during movements of the extremities and neck. Education in the patient's preferred daily habits and postures contribute to stress on cervical spine structures. All of these components contributed to a successful outcome and enabled her to manage her symptoms.

CERVICAL FLEXION SYNDROME

The principal movement impairment in cervical flexion syndrome is imprecise cervical flexion that is often associated with pain and limited ROM. There is an altered distribution of flexion across the cervical and thoracic regions, with the lower cervical region flexing more than the upper thoracic region. The imbalance of muscle performance of the cervical flexors with dominance of intrinsic cervical flexors can create a kyphotic position of the cervical spine and/or insufficient recruitment of cervical extensors during cervical extension movements.

History and Symptoms

Symptom location can be similar to the findings in cervical extension syndrome. The patient complains of pain with flexion. This syndrome is typically seen in younger patients because their spines have the flexibility and extensibility to move in the direction of flexion. The patients that demonstrate this syndrome characteristically have a history of activities that require repetitive positioning in "correct alignment." They may be required to maintain a "military posture" or a ballet position that may necessitate extreme "straightening" or flexing of the cervical spine.

Key Signs and Symptoms

Alignment Analysis

Alignment faults for cervical flexion include a decrease of the normal cervical inward curve. The cervical spine may appear flat (Figure 3-46). The patients with this syndrome may also have associated thoracic alignment fault of a decreased thoracic curve. The reduced flexion curve in the thoracic spine is typically associated with loss of flexion ROM in the thoracic region. The reduced

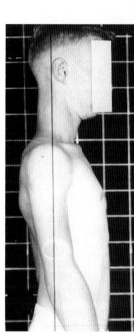
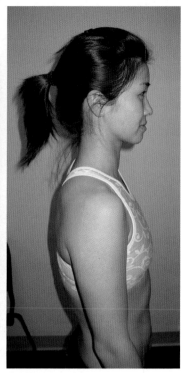

Figure 3-46. Decreased cervical inward curve. (**A** from Kendall FP, McCreary EK, Provance PG: *Muscles: testing and function,* ed 4, Philadelphia, 1993, Lippincott Williams & Wilkins.)

thoracic flexion curve may influence or require greater flexion motion in the cervical region. There may also be scapular alignment faults, including scapular depression and/or downward rotation. Frequently, specific verbal cueing and manual assistance to promote thoracic flexion and cervical extension can diminish symptoms during standing. The patient can be encouraged to assume a "slumped position" to promote an increase in thoracic flexion and instructed to slightly lift the chin and nose to encourage a position of less cervical flexion. These directions can result in a normal curve of the thoracic spine and a normal inward curve of the cervical spine, which can result in a decrease in symptoms in standing or sitting.

Movement Impairment Analysis

During the performance of active cervical flexion in standing, patients complain of pain and demonstrate greater motion of flexion in the lower cervical region than the upper thoracic region (Figure 3-47).

Secondary test. *Correction by increasing thoracic flexion:* During active cervical flexion the therapist encourages greater flexion motion in the upper thoracic region and limits the amount of cervical flexion ROM, resulting in decreased pain. One strategy to achieve greater thoracic flexion can include an instruction to the patient to "slump" or flex the thoracic spine before initiating active cervical flexion.

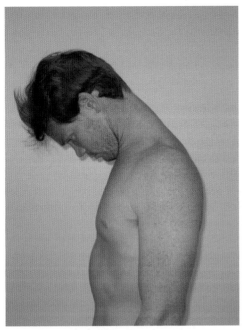

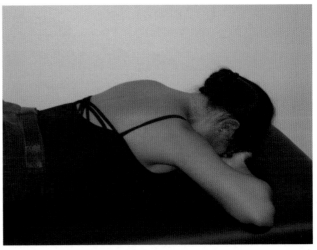

Figure 3-48. Prone position.

Figure 3-47. Movement impairment: Lower cervical flexion greater than upper thoracic flexion.

Muscle Strength and Performance

Poor performance and recruitment of the intrinsic cervical extensors are primarily demonstrated in the prone and/or quadruped position. During performance of active cervical extension, there is poor recruitment of the intrinsic cervical extensors and dominant recruitment of the extrinsic cervical extensors, primarily the levator scapulae. The cervical extension movement results in greater posterior translation and diminished posterior sagittal rotation.

Secondary tests. *Correction by increasing recruitment of intrinsic cervical extensors:* Repeating the movement of cervical extension in prone or quadruped position with verbal cues to "roll the head back" typically results in improved recruitment of the intrinsic cervical spinal extensors and diminished recruitment of the extrinsic cervical extensors. The modified extension movement results in greater posterior sagittal rotation and less pain.

Performance of cervical flexors: There is excessive recruitment of all neck flexors, particularly the recruitment of anterior and middle scalene during use of the arms or during daily activities or personality gestures. The therapist observes excessive straightening of the cervical spine.

Correction by improving recruitment of intrinsic cervical extensors: Instruct the patient to lift the chin and nose to promote the appropriate recruitment of cervical extensors and assumption of a normal inward curve during arm movements.

Treatment

The primary goals in the treatment of cervical flexion syndrome are to restore a normal inward cervical curve, improve function of the intrinsic cervical extensors, and

to avoid positions and movements that would encourage excessive cervical flexion. A common alignment fault associated with cervical flexion is a reduced thoracic curve. The straight thoracic spine has decreased flexibility in the direction of flexion, which potentially results in compensatory flexion in the cervical flexion. Treatment strategies include instructing the patient on how to increase thoracic flexion or encouraging the patient to "slump," which is not a typical functional instruction but appropriate if the patient's thoracic impairments necessitate these instructions.

Exercise Program

The key exercises to improve intrinsic cervical extensor function include exercises that can be performed in prone and/or quadruped.

Prone active cervical extension. In prone or in quadruped, the patient is instructed to "roll" head and neck back in the direction of extension (Figure 3-48). The verbal cue of rolling is to facilitate the recruitment of the intrinsic neck extensors and reduce recruitment of the extrinsic neck extensors. The patient is encouraged not to reach full end-range extension to avoid excessive compression on the cervical facets and discs.

Quadruped active cervical extension. The quadruped position can be a more difficult exercise because the exercise requires good axioscapular muscle function while weight bearing through the upper extremities (Figure 3-49). When performing the cervical extension exercise in the quadruped, the patient is encourage to perform the movement in the middle third of the ROM to avoid end-range extension or flexion.

The description of treatment for the previous diagnoses indicates that examination and classification of associated scapular movement impairments is critical in the management of the patients with cervical pain. Strategies to examine, classify, and manage scapular movement impairments are clearly described in Sahrmann.[1]

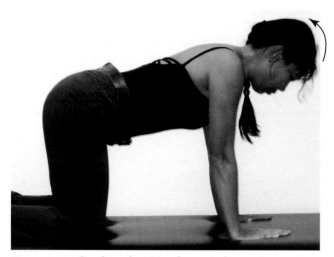

Figure 3-49. Quadruped position for cervical extension exercise.

Functional Instructions

Instructions during key functional activities of patients with the cervical flexion syndrome include encouraging flexion in adjacent regions to minimize the amount of cervical flexion that is required during daily activities. This includes encouraging the patient to "slump" or increase thoracic flexion to diminish the amount of cervical flexion that is required. This strategy is the opposite instruction and effect that the therapist would use with a patient with cervical extension syndrome with a thoracic kyphosis. When the patient attempts to slump, it may initially feel very awkward and unfamiliar. The patient may have conscientiously worked to maintain correct alignment, but overcompensated with excessive thoracic extension that then required excessive cervical flexion to maintain the eyes and head in a functional position. Allowing greater flexion in the thoracic spine will reduce the cervical flexion. The instructions of "slumping" can make the patient feel self-conscious about his or her appearance. Using a mirror to demonstrate that the strategy does not result in excessive thoracic flexion or kyphosis can be very useful in reassuring the patient that he or she is not going to develop the type of alignment characteristic of the elderly.

To avoid excessive cervical flexion and translation during sitting activities, the patient can be encouraged to lean forward by increasing the degree of hip flexion.

Strategies to diminish excessive cervical flexion during daily activities include raising the computer screen or using a book holder to raise the work items so that the patient does not have to flex the cervical spine as far.

Additional functional instructions include use of cervical pillow or towel to support the cervical spine in a cervical lordosis. This can be helpful with sleeping or prolonged sitting and computer work. The support of the cervical spine should be provided in both the supine and sidelying positions.

The therapist should review use of eyeglasses. The habit the patient may demonstrate is excessive flexion to position his or her eyes with the use of reading glasses. The patient will be encouraged to properly position the glasses on the nose that will allow a neutral position of the neck so the patient has to raise the nose and chin when using the glasses.

Cervical Flexion-Rotation Syndrome

The principal movement impairment in cervical flexion-rotation syndrome is imprecise cervical rotation with associated compensatory cervical flexion, which is often associated with pain and limited ROM. The imbalance of muscle performance among the cervical rotator muscles with extrinsic muscles contributes to multiplanar movements rather than precise uniplanar motion produced by the intrinsic rotators. An imbalance of muscle performance of the cervical flexors contributes to compensatory flexion movement during performance of rotation. The contributing factors in the cervical rotation-flexion syndrome include weight of the extremities and alignment of the thoracic spine and the scapulae. There may also be asymmetries in the appearance of the neck and scapula region.

Symptoms and History

Symptoms and history can be similar to the findings found in cervical flexion syndrome. In addition, the patient with this syndrome may report pain with rotation movements.

Key Tests and Signs

Alignment Analysis

In addition to the alignment faults that were noted in the cervical flexion syndrome, the cervical spine may also be in a sidebend and/or rotated position. Commonly, this position may be an indication of a hearing or vision impairment, as discussed in the section on cervical extension-rotation syndrome. The therapist should obtain this information when taking the history. Asymmetrical alignment of the scapulae may also be present. Verbal cueing and manual assistance to correct alignment of the cervical spine position and scapulae position can decrease symptoms. Use of a mirror is also a helpful tool for patient feedback and independent correction.[2]

Movement Impairment Analysis

In addition to the movement impairments noted in the section on the cervical flexion syndrome, the patient can complain of pain with rotation and demonstrate associated cervical flexion and sidebending movements during rotation.

Secondary tests. Secondary follow-up tests can include several strategies, including repeating active rotation without associated flexion and/or sidebending movement. In addition, instructing the patient to "slump" before performing active rotation can promote an improved starting alignment of the cervical spine with reduced cervical flexion. Other corrections include passive support of the upper extremities during performance of active rotation and/or the therapist can passively assist the cervical vertebrae and guide precise rotation motion.

During active single arm flexion, rotation of a single or multiple vertebrae are noted via palpation of the cervical spinous process. The patient does not typically complain of pain. An alternative finding during single-arm flexion is compensatory sidebending or rotation of the cervical spine.[10]

Correction of this rotation movement impairment can be difficult. Several strategies can be attempted, as follows:

- *Correct cervical alignment:* Instruct the patient to correct the cervical alignment as previously described by lifting the nose and chin to assume a normal inward curve and lessen the recruitment of the cervical flexors. Encourage the patient to actively maintain the corrected alignment during single arm flexion.
- *Correct scapular movement impairment:* The therapist can assist the patient in correcting the associated scapular movement impairment during the single arm shoulder flexion movement. The patient can perform bilateral shoulder flexion and note if the movement impairment improves. The patient's individual response to the secondary test will assist the therapist in developing the appropriate intervention strategies.

Treatment

The primary goals of treatment for cervical flexion-rotation syndrome are similar to the goals of cervical flexion syndrome, which are to restore the normal cervical inward curve, instruct the patient in strategies to avoid excessive flexion in the cervical spine, and encourage increase flexion movements in other regions, usually the thoracic spine. Additional treatment includes restoration of precise motion of active cervical rotation by performing motion without associated flexion and using minimal effort to rotate the head and neck. The focus of the active strengthening exercise program in the cervical region is to improve the strength and motor control of the intrinsic cervical spine rotators. Correcting sustained asymmetrical positions of the head and neck and avoiding movements of the head and neck as part of body language is essential.

Additionally, as described in the treatment section for cervical extension syndrome, the patient is instructed in functional activities such as supporting the upper extremities.[5,6,14,15] Correction of the pattern of movement during daily activities is particularly important. An examination and classification of the associated scapular movement impairments is critical in the management of the patients with cervical pain. Strategies to examine, classify, and manage scapular movement impairments are clearly described in Sahrmann.[1]

Exercise Program

Sitting Cervical Rotation. The patient may not need to assume the position of sitting with the back to the wall as has been previously described for the cervical extension syndrome. Sitting in a chair with good thoracic spine support may be appropriate and may encourage a normal thoracic alignment of slight flexion and discourage a flat thoracic spine. As described in cervical flexion syndrome, an exaggerated straightening or reduced flexion of the thoracic spine may result in compensatory flexion of the cervical spine. Initial instructions address the impairments of adjacent regions, which were previously described. The upper extremities are supported on pillows to diminish the compressive loading of the cervical spine from the transfer of the weight of the upper extremities to the cervical region through the cervicoscapular muscle attachment.[9,15] Each patient needs to be assessed for his or her specific alignment impairments at the lumbar and thoracic spines and scapulothoracic region. The patient is then instructed in strategies to precisely correct his or her individual alignment faults in these regions before proceeding with the exercise.

The patient is then instructed to perform cervical rotation about a "vertical axis" and to avoid the movements of flexion and sidebending. Specific instructions include "raise the chin up slightly" to avoid compensatory flexion during rotation and "do not lean the head and neck toward the side to which you are rotating." Additional instructions to sidebend in the opposite direction that the patient is rotating his or her head typically result in a vertical position of the head and neck and diminished ipsilateral sidebending. Maintaining the precise motion of rotation without compensatory sidebending or flexion promotes increased use of the intrinsic rotators and diminished use of the extrinsic rotators, thus diminishing shear and translatory forces on the cervical spine.

The patient is encouraged to maintain appropriate alignment of the adjacent regions during this movement of the cervical spine. This exercise can be ideally performed in sitting, but if the patient has difficulty maintaining the correct postural alignment during the cervical motion, the exercise can be performed in supine. The supine position will not be as challenging as control by the trunk musculature in maintaining alignment of the adjacent regions.

Supine active cervical rotation. Performance of precise cervical rotation in supine can be performed if sitting cervical rotation is too difficult or painful. The patient assumes a hooklying position with the arms supported on pillows. The patient may require a towel roll under the cervical spine to support a normal cervical curve and prevent a position of excessive flexion. The same instructions used for the sitting exercises can be used to address the adjacent regions impairments. The patient is then instructed in strategies to precisely correct his or her individual alignment faults in the adjacent regions (lumbar and thoracic spines and scapulothoracic region) before proceeding with the exercise. The patient is then instructed to perform cervical rotation about a "vertical axis" and to avoid the movements of cervical flexion and sidebending. Other key verbal cues are similar to ones used for the sitting exercises: "raise the chin up slightly" to avoid compensatory flexion during rotation and "do not lean the head and neck toward the side you are rotating toward."

Quadruped active cervical rotation. The alternative position of quadruped can be used to perform precise cervical rotation if the previously described positions of sitting or supine are too difficult or painful with cervical rotation motion (see Figure 3-36). The patient is instructed to allow the thoracic spine to be slightly flexed. The patient should raise the head and chin slightly to avoid a position of excessive flexion of the cervical spine. The patient is instructed to rotate the head and neck about an axis of motion. The patient is instructed to avoid movements of cervical flexion and sidebending.

Facing wall, arms supported—active cervical rotation. An additional position of facing the wall with the arms overhead supported on the wall can be used to perform precise cervical rotation (see Figure 3-35). The patient is instructed to rest the forearms on the wall, allow the wall to support the upper extremities, and relax the upper trapezius muscles. The patient is then instructed to raise the head and chin slightly to avoid the position of excessive cervical flexion, then perform precise cervical rotation about a vertical axis, and to avoid movements of cervical flexion and sidebending.

Functional Instructions

Key functional instructions for cervical flexion rotation syndrome include the strategies described in the section on cervical flexion syndrome to encourage flexion in the thoracic spine, which can minimize the amount of cervical flexion that is required during daily activities. In addition, strategies should be implemented to minimize asymmetrical stress on the cervical spine through decreasing repetition of one arm activities or prolonged positioning in sidebend or rotation (see section on Cervical Extension-Rotation Syndrome).

CASE PRESENTATION
Cervical Flexion-Rotation Syndrome

History and Symptoms

A 26-year-old male complains of lower cervical neck and right upper trapezius pain that is increased with sustained sitting postures working at the computer. He rates his pain 2/10 at rest and 4/10 with neck movements. His NDI score = 14, indicating mild disability. He reports that in high school he was a competitive swimmer and presently enjoys surfing.

Alignment

In standing, he has a swayback posture, with the thoracic region swayed posterior.[8] The spinal alignment was

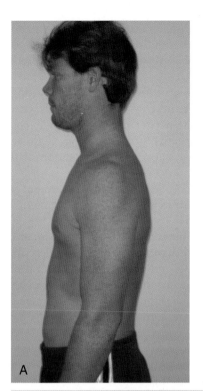

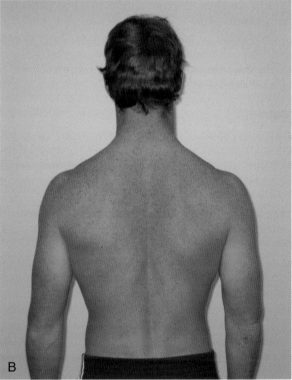

Figure 3-50. **A,** Reduced cervical curve from thoracic spine. **B,** Depressed shoulders.

remarkable for a reduced curve in the cervical region and also a reduced curve or "flat" thoracic spine (Figure 3-50, *A*). The clavicular alignment appears horizontal with a diminished upward slope of the distal end of the clavicle. The scapulae were in a position of depression with the superior angle of scapula positioned below T2[8] (see Figure 3-50, *B*).

Reduced muscle bulk was noted in the cervical paraspinal musculature. He also complained of pain on palpation of right upper trapezius and levator scapulae muscles.

Movement Analysis and Active Range of Motion Findings

Active ROM test results are given in the following table.

	ROM (Degrees)	Movement Analysis	Symptoms
Flexion	70		Painful in the lower cervical region
Extension	70		
Rotation R	70		
Rotation L	60	Associated cervical flexion	Painful in the lower cervical region
Lateral flexion R	50		
Lateral flexion L	55		
PASSIVE ELEVATED SHOULDER GIRDLE			
Flexion	70		No complaint of pain
Extension	70		
Rotation R	80		
Rotation L	80	No associated cervical flexion	No complaint of pain

ROM, Range of motion; *R*, right; *L*, left.

Passive mobility findings
Central PA pressure performed on the C4/5 and C5/6 spinous process indicated they were hypomobile and painful over the local area. Unilateral PA pressures on the right C4/5 and C5/6 articular pillar indicated that these areas were hypomobile and caused pain over the local area.

Active shoulder movements
Shoulder flexion demonstrated decreased scapulae elevation with the result of decrease upward rotation of the scapulae. Also noted was associated cervical flexion with active shoulder flexion and an increase of the posterior thoracic sway.

Secondary tests. The therapist corrected the cervical starting alignment by having the patient lift the chin and nose slightly and maintain head and neck position during shoulder flexion. In addition, the starting scapulae alignment and thoracic sway were corrected, and he was cued to maintain the thoracic position and elevate the scapulae during shoulder flexion. The patient was able to correct

the movement impairments during shoulder flexion but he reported difficulty performing this motion.

Single-arm flexion monitoring cervical spine: Palpation of the lower cervical vertebrae during left shoulder flexion demonstrated compensatory rotation of the spinous process to the left. These findings indicated relative flexibility of the lower cervical segments in the direction of rotation with left arm movements. No compensatory motion of lower cervical rotation was noted with right arm movements. There was no complaint of neck pain with either arm movements. Bilateral shoulder flexion did not cause cervical rotation.

Diagnosis and Staging
The patient's diagnosis is cervical flexion rotation with scapula depression and the stage for rehabilitation is Stage 3. His prognosis is excellent. His positive moderators include young age, good health, minimal duration of symptoms, and low NDI score.

Diagnosis	Key Tests
Cervical flexion rotation	Alignment of cervical spine: Cervical flexion/flat cervical and thoracic spine alignment. AROM: Pain with flexion and rotation. Excessive flexion ROM. Compensatory flexion with rotation ROM. Compensatory movements of the neck in the direction of flexion with shoulder flexion movements. Compensatory lower cervical rotation with left arm movements.
Scapular depression	Alignment: Scapulae position in depression—superior angle of scapulae below T2. AROM: Decrease elevation of scapulae during shoulder flexion motion. Elevating scapulae results in decreased pain and improved range of cervical motions.

AROM, Active range of motion; *ROM*, range of motion.

Treatment
The patient was seen once a week for 2 weeks and then once every other week for 4 weeks. Each treatment session lasted approximately 30 minutes. The treatment included instruction in a specific home exercise program to improve cervical spine function and functional instructions to diminish excessive forces on the cervical spine during daily activities.

Exercise program
Initially, the patient was instructed in active cervical ROM exercises. The initial "set up" for the patient was sitting a chair but not with his back against the wall as was described in the cervical extension case presentation. The patient arms were supported on pillows to decrease the downward pull on the neck and to improve

scapulothoracic alignment by diminishing the amount of scapulae depression. The patient was also instructed to "relax" the thoracic spine to allow greater thoracic flexion.

Cervical rotation: The patient was instructed to support his arms on the pillows and relax the trapezius muscles. The patient was then instructed to rotate the head and neck about a vertical axis. The patient was instructed to imagine that there is "a pole" down his spine and rotate about that pole. The patient was also instructed to keep his nose and chin up to avoid compensatory flexion during active cervical rotation and to minimize the effort during the rotation to diminish recruitment of the extrinsic neck rotators (sternocleidomastoid and scalene) and compressing on the stabilizing force of the contracting muscles.

Additional exercises

Additional exercises to improve intrinsic cervical extensor muscle function include the following:

Prone cervical extension to improve the strength and recruitment of the intrinsic cervical extensors (see Figure 3-48): The patient is positioned prone with his forehead resting in the palm of his hands. The patient is to perform active cervical extension by "rolling" the head and neck back in the direction of extension but not to end-range. The patient is instructed to imagine an "axial running through the middle of his cervical spine" and rotate about the axial as he performs active extension. The therapist should observe if the patient is properly recruiting the intrinsic neck extensors and not excessively recruiting the extrinsic muscles (levator scapulae and upper trapezius).

Quadruped active cervical extension (see Figure 3-49): An alternative exercise that can improve cervical extensor function is to perform the previously described motion in the quadruped position. The patient is encouraged to avoid excessive thoracic extension and assume slight thoracic flexion. The patient is to perform active cervical extension by "rolling" the head and neck back in the direction of extension but not to end-range. The patient is instructed to imagine an "axial running through the middle of his cervical spine" and rotate about the axial as he performs active extension. The therapist should observe if the patient is properly recruiting the intrinsic neck extensors and not excessively recruiting the extrinsic muscles (levator scapulae and upper trapezius). The patient is also instructed to "roll" his head and neck forward as he returns from cervical extension. The patient is instructed to perform the movement of flexion and extension with precision and in the middle-third of the range, avoiding end-range extension or flexion.

Facing the wall—shoulder flexion with scapula elevation (Figure 3-51): This exercise improves strength and length of the upper trapezius and serratus anterior muscles.[51] The patient's scapulae position was determined to be in a position of depression, which results in a lengthened upper trapezius muscle. The objective of the exercise is to strengthen the upper trapezius muscle in a shortened position. The patient is instructed to face the wall and

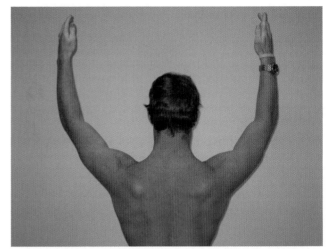

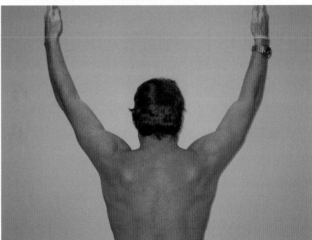

Figure 3-51. Facing the wall, shoulder flexion with scapula elevation.

rest his hands on the wall just above shoulder level. As he slides his hands up the wall, he is instructed to elevate the scapula/acromion toward his ears. He is instructed to "keep his nose and chin slightly up" to avoid cervical flexion. In addition, he can return from flexion, slide his hands down while maintaining the scapulae in an elevated position and not allow excessive depression while returning from the flexion position.

Functional Instruction

During sitting activities, the patient is encouraged to "Slump!" He is encouraged not to attempt to have a very straight thoracic spine and to relax the neck position. He is encouraged to allow the chin and nose to be slightly up. The patient may feel that he is excessively slumped because he is accustomed to being very straight. A mirror can provide visual feedback that the correction does not result in excessive slumping but rather appropriate alignment of thoracic and cervical spines. In addition, the patient is encouraged to support the arms on pillows or the desk to minimize the downward pull on the upper trapezius and levator scapulae muscles. The patient is instructed in a strategy of allowing the thoracic spine to flex, which will also minimize excessive flexion in the cervical spine.

The patient was also instructed in the appropriate cervical and head positions when using his eyeglasses. The patient is to position his eyeglasses to allow a neutral neck position during computer use and should exaggerate a flexed cervical position.

The patient was also instructed to minimize one-arm activities with the left arm to avoid compensatory lower cervical rotation. When possible, he should consider using the right arm or both arms with functional activities.

At end of 6 weeks of treatment (4 treatment sessions), the patient reported 0/10 pain at rest and with movements of the neck. His neck disability index score = 4, indicating no disability. He also reported that he was doing his exercises several times a week, but he found that the functional instructions were the most helpful in managing his symptoms. He found that supporting his arms during the day, relaxing his upper back, and trying not to sit up too straight decreased the stress through his neck region.

This case is an illustration of how excessive motion in one region of the spine and lack of motion in adjacent regions can increase stress on the spinal tissue that demonstrates excessive motion. This patient's attempts for "correct" posture were exaggerated. The flat thoracic spine and loss of a normal thoracic curve did not permit proper neck alignment. Relaxing the upper back to allow some flexion also allows the cervical spine to acquire a normal lordotic curve of the cervical spine. It was important that the patient avoid excessive flexion and encourage extension or a normal inward curve of the cervical spine. This acquired posture allows appropriate distribution of stresses across the spine. In addition, support of the upper extremities and improving the alignment of the scapulae into an elevation out of a depressed position also decreased the compressive load on the cervical spine structures.

REFERENCES

1. Sahrmann SA: *Diagnosis and treatment of movement impairment syndromes*, St Louis, 2002, Mosby.
2. Willford CH, Kisner C, Glenn TM, et al: The interaction of wearing multifocal lenses with head posture and pain, *J Orthop Sports Phys Ther* 23:194-199, 1996.
3. Bexander CS, Mellor R, Hodges PW: Effect of gaze direction on neck muscle activity during cervical rotation, *Exp Brain Res* 167:422-432, 2005.
4. Schuldt K, Ekholm J, Harms-Ringdahl K, et al: Effects of changes in sitting work posture on static neck and shoulder muscle activity, *Ergonomics* 29:1525-1537, 1986.
5. Schuldt K, Ekholm J, Harms-Ringdahl K, et al: Effects of arm support or suspension on neck and shoulder muscle activity during sedentary work, *Scand J Rehabil Med* 19:77-84, 1987.
6. Straker L, Burgess-Limerick R, Pollock C, et al: The effect of forearm support on children's head, neck and upper limb posture and muscle activity during computer use, *J Electromyogr Kinesiol* 19(5):965-974, 2008.
7. Otis CA: *Kinesiology: the mechanics and the pathomechanics of human movement*, Philadelphia, 2004, Lippincott Williams & Wilkins.
8. Kendall FP, McCreary EK, Provance P: *Muscles: testing and function*, ed 4, Baltimore, 1993, Williams & Wilkins.
9. McDonnell MK, Sahrmann SA, Van Dillen LR: A specific exercise program and modifications of postural alignment for treatment of cervicogenic headache: a case report, *J Orthop Sports Phys Ther* 35(1):3-15, 2005.
10. Takasaki H, Hall T, Kaneko S, et al: Cervical segmental motion induced by shoulder abduction assessed by magnetic resonance imaging, *Spine* 34(3):E122-E126, 2009.
11. Black KM, McClure P, Polansky M: The influence of different sitting positions on cervical and lumbar posture, *Spine* 21(1):65-70, 1996.
12. Kebaetse M, McClure P, Pratt NA: Thoracic position effect on shoulder range of motion, strength, and three-dimensional scapular kinematics, *Arch Phys Med Rehabil* 80:945-950, 1999.
13. Ludewig PM, Cook TM: The effect of head position on scapular orientation and muscle activity during shoulder elevation, *J Occup Rehab* 6(3):147-158, 1996.
14. Van Dillen LR, McDonnell MK, Susco TM, et al: The immediate effect of passive scapular elevation on active cervical rotation range of motion and symptoms in patients with neck pain, *Clin J Pain* 23(8):641-647, 2007.
15. Andrade GT, Azevedo DC, Lorentz ID, et al: Influence of scapular position on cervical rotation range of motion, *J Orthop Sports Phys Ther* 38(11):668-673, 2008.
16. Harrison DD, Harrison DE, Janik TJ, et al: Modeling of the sagittal cervical spine as a method to discriminate hypolordosis: results of elliptical and circular modeling in 72 asymptomatic subjects, 52 acute neck pain subjects, and 70 chronic neck pain subjects, *Spine* 29(22):2485-2492, 2004.
17. Falla D, Jull G, Russell T, et al: Effect of neck exercises on sitting posture in patients with chronic neck pain, *Phys Ther* 87:4, 2007.
18. Fernandez-de-las-Penas C, Alonso-Blanco C, Cuadrado ML, et al: Forward head posture and neck mobility in chronic tension-type headache: a blinded, controlled study, *Cephalagia* 26:314-319, 2005.
19. Neumann DA: *Kinesiology of the musculoskeletal system: foundations of rehabilitation*, St Louis, 2002, Mosby.
20. Porterfield JA, DeRosa C: *Mechanical neck pain: perspectives in functional anatomy*, Philadelphia, 1995, WB Saunders.
21. Allia P, Gorniak G: Human ligamentum nuchae in the elderly: its function in the cervical spine, *J Man Manip Therapy* 14(1):11-21, 2006.
22. Fernandez-de-las-Penas C, Cuadrado ML, Pareja JA: Myofascial trigger points, neck mobility and forward head posture in unilateral migraine, *Cephalagia* 26:1061-1070, 2006.
23. White AA, Panjabi MM: Kinematics of the spine. In Cooke DB, ed: *Clinical biomechanics of the spine*, Philadelphia, 1990, JB Lippincott.
24. Lysell E: Motion in the cervical spine, *Acta Orthop Scand* 123[Suppl]: 1-61, 1969.

25. Salo PK, Hakkinen AH, Kautiainen H, et al: Quantifying the effect of age on passive range of motion of the cervical spine, *J Orthop Sports Phys Ther* 39(6):478-483, 2009.

26. Lehto IJ, Tertti MO, Komu ME, et al: Age-related MEI changes at 0.1 T in cervical discs in asymptomatic subjects, *Neuroradiology* 36(1):49-53, 1994.

27. Dvorak J, Antinnes J, Panjabi M, et al: Age and gender related normal motion of the cervical spine, *Spine* 17:393-398, 1992.

28. Netzer O, Payne VG: Effects of age and gender on functional rotation and lateral movements of the neck and back, *Gerontology* 39:320, 1993.

29. Matsumoto M, Fujimura Y, Suzuki N, et al: MRI of cervical intervertebral discs in asymptomatic subjects, *J Bone Joint Surg Br* 80:19-24, 1998.

30. Joosab M, Torode M, Rao PV: Preliminary findings on the effect of load-carrying to the structural integrity of the cervical spine, *Surg Radiol Anat* 16:393-398, 1994.

31. Moroney S, Schultz AB, Miller JA: Analysis and measurement of neck loads, *J Orthop Res* 6:713-720, 1988.

32. Simpson AK, Biswas DBA, Emerson JW, et al: Quantifying the effects of age, gender, degeneration, and adjacent level degeneration on cervical spine range of motion using multivariate analyses, *Spine* 33(2):183-186, 2008.

33. Falla D, Jull G, Dall'Alba P, et al: An electromyographic analysis of the deep cervical flexor muscles in performance of craniocervical flexion, *Phys Ther* 83:899-906, 2003.

34. Beazell JR: Dysfunction of the longus colli and its relationship to cervical pain and dysfunction: a clinical case presentation, *J Man Manipulative Ther* 6(1):12-16, 1998.

35. Watson DH, Trott PH: Cervical headache: an investigation of natural head posture and upper cervical flexor muscle performance, *Cephalalgia* 13:272-284, 1993.

36. Placzek J: The influence of the cervical spine on chronic headache in women: a pilot study, *J Manual Manipulative Ther* 7(1):33-39, 1999.

37. Jull G, Kristjansson E, Dall'Alba P: Impairment in the cervical flexors: a comparison of whiplash and insidious onset cervical spine pain patients, *Manual Ther* 9:89-94, 2004.

38. Falla D, Jull G, Hodges P, et al: An endurance-strength training regime is effective in reducing myoelectric manifestations of cervical flexor muscle fatigue in females with chronic cervical spine pain, *Clin Neurophysiol* 117:828-837, 2006.

39. Anderson JS, Hsu AW, Vasavada AN: Morphology, architecture and biomechanics of human cervical multifidus, *Spine* 30(4):E86-E91, 2005.

40. Siegmund GP, Blouin JS, Carpenter MG, et al: Are cervical multifidus muscles active during whiplash and startle? An initial experimental study, *BMC Musculoskel Disord* 9:80, 2008.

41. Johnson G, Bogduk N, Nowitzke A, et al: Anatomy and actions of the trapezius muscle, *Clin Biomech* 9:44-50, 1994.

42. Dwyer A, April C, Bogduk N: Cervical zygapophyseal joint pain patterns, *Spine* 15:453-457. 1990.

43. Sobush DC, Simoneau GG, Dietz KE, et al: The Lennie test for measuring scapular position in healthy young adult females: a reliability and validity study, *J Orthop Sports Phys Ther* 23:39-50, 1996.

44. Azevedo D, de Lima Pires T, de Souza Andrade F, et al: Influence of scapular position on the pressure pain threshold of the upper trapezius muscle, *Eur J Pain* 12(2):226-232, 2007.

45. Jull G, Barrett C, Magee R, et al: Further clinical clarification of the muscle dysfunction in cervical headache. *Cephalalgia* 19:179-185, 1999.

46. O'Leary S, Jull G, Kim M, et al: Specificity in retraining craniocervical flexor muscle performance, *J Orthop Sports Phys Ther* 37:3-9, 2007.

47. O'Leary S, Falla D, Elliott JM, et al: Muscle dysfunction in cervical spine pain: implications for assessment and management, *J Orthop Sports Phys Ther* 39(5):324-333, 2009.

48. Jull G, Trott P, Potter H, et al: A randomized controlled trial of exercise and manipulative therapy for cervicogenic headache, *Spine* 27:1835-1843, 2002.

49. Ludewig PM, Phadke V, Braman JP, et al: Motion of the shoulder complex during multiplanar humeral elevation, *J Bone Joint Surg Am* 91:378-389, 2009.

50. Vernon H, Mior S: The neck disability index: a study of reliability and validity, *J Manipulative Physiol Ther* 14:409-415, 1991.

51. Hardwick DH, Beebe JA, McDonnell MK, et al: A comparison of serratus anterior muscle activation during a wall slide exercise and other traditional exercises, *J Orthop Sports Phys Ther* 36(12):903-910, 2006.

APPENDIX

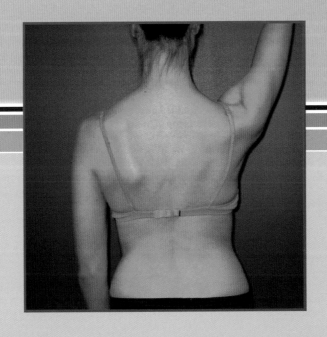

Cervical Extension Syndrome

The principal movement impairment in cervical extension syndrome is imprecise cervical extension and flexion that is often associated with pain and limited ROM. There is an altered distribution of extension across the cervical region and an imbalance of muscle performance among the cervical extensors and flexors, with the extrinsic muscles

Symptoms and History

- Pain location: Cervical region
- Radicular symptoms along the vertebral border, arm, and/or scapular region
- Pain with neck extension
- History of whiplash injury

Common Referring Diagnoses
- Cervical radiculopathy
- Degenerative disc disease
- Herniated cervical disc
- Facet syndrome
- Spondylosis

Key Tests and Signs for Movement Impairment

Alignment Analysis
Cervical Alignment
- Forward-head posture: Increased lordosis of the upper and lower cervical spine
- Older spine: Lower cervical vertebral bodies in a position of anterior translation with upper cervical extension
- Headache patients: The upper cervical spine (head on neck) positioned in 10 degrees of extension

Thoracic Alignment
- Thoracic kyphosis with increased cervical extension/translation

Scapular Alignment
- Resting alignment of scapular depression or abduction

Movement Impairment Analysis
Standing/Sitting
- Cervical extension range of motion (ROM) is painful
- Younger spine: During active extension excessive posterior translation is observed
- Older degenerative spine: Limited extension because of excessive anterior translation
- The rate of movement of upper cervical extension is greater than the rate of lower cervical extension
- Correction of thoracic kyphosis alignment improves extension ROM and decreases pain

Unloading Tests
- Passive elevation of the shoulder girdle and/or supporting the weight of the limbs decreases pain and improves cervical extension
- In patients with well-developed abdominals who are physically active, passive elevation of the rib cage decreases pain and improves cervical extension
- Cervical flexion ROM is painful
  - Cervical flexion: Greater anterior translation than sagittal rotation
  - Correction of thoracic kyphosis alignment improves flexion ROM and decreases pain

Unloading Tests
- Passive elevation of the shoulder girdle and/or supporting the weight of the limbs decreases pain and improves cervical flexion
- In patients with well-developed abdominals who are physically active, passive elevation of the rib cage decreases pain and improves cervical flexion

Supine
- Active cervical flexion: Greater anterior translation than sagittal rotation and painful
- Intrinsic cervical flexors test weak
  - Manual assistance to diminish translation and encourage sagittal rotation decreases pain

Prone
- Active cervical extension: Greater posterior translation than sagittal rotation and painful; poor recruitment of cervical paraspinals noted
  - Verbal instruction to improve posterior sagittal cervical rotation and diminish cervical posterior translation results in improved recruitment of cervical paraspinals and less pain

Quadruped
- Active cervical extension: Greater posterior translation than sagittal rotation and painful; observe increased recruitment of levator scapulae and diminished intrinsic neck extensor recruitment
  - Instruction to increase posterior sagittal rotation results in improved recruitment of intrinsic cervical extensors and less pain
- Active neck flexion: Poor control of movement
  - Instruction to increase anterior sagittal rotation improves quality of motion
- Rocking back: Cervical spine extends
  - Instruction to maintain "chin to Adam's apple" results in a neutral cervical spine position with quadruped rocking; other observations can include a "shortening" of the cervical region or compression of the cervical region

Muscle Strength/Performance Impairments
- Weak intrinsic cervical flexors

Muscle Length Impairments
- Short, stiff posterior cervical structures

Joint Integrity
- Accessory motion ligamentous test, active and passive ROM

contributing to excessive horizontal translation of the cervical vertebrae rather than a combination of sagittal rotation produced by the intrinsic cervical muscles and horizontal translation produced by the extrinsic cervical muscles. The contributing factors in the cervical extension syndrome include the weight of the extremities and alignment of the thoracic spine and the scapulae.

Associated Signs or Contributing Factors

- Thoracic kyphosis
- Heavy upper extremities and/or heavy breasts
- Resistance to passive elevation of the scapula
- Well-developed abdominals in physically active individuals (limited chest expansion of 1 inch or less)
- Cervical extension with active contraction of abdominals
- Cervical extension with active shoulder flexion
- Use of head for body language

Differential Diagnosis

Movement System Diagnoses
- Cervical extension rotation
- Scapula depression
- Scapula downward rotation
- Scapula abduction

Potential Diagnoses Requiring Referral Suggested by Signs and Symptoms

Neuromusculoskeletal
- Metastatic tumor in the cervical spine
- Fracture
- Frank neurological signs
- Vertebrobasilar insufficiency (VBI)

Systemic
- Cardiac
- Pulmonary
- Liver
- Gall bladder
- Tracheobronchial referral
- Neoplasms
- Metastatic tumors in the cervical spine

Treatment

The goal for treatment of the cervical extension syndrome is to diminish cervical extension movements and extension forces on the cervical spine during daily activities. All exercises and functional instructions include considerations of the adjacent regions before initiating cervical movements and specifically, modification of compensatory motion of the adjacent regions and support of the upper extremities.

In addition, instructions are given for strategies to be used during functional activities such as how to support the upper extremities and reduce compensatory motion at the adjacent regions during the day.[1,2] The focus of the active exercise program for the cervical region is to improve the strength and motor control of the intrinsic cervical spine flexor muscles along with improving the flexibility of the posterior cervical structures. The focus of the active exercise program in the adjacent regions includes strengthening of the scapulothoracic muscles, abdominals, and posterior thoracic spinal musculature.

In addition, upper extremity movements have a direct effect on the cervical spine via the attachment of cervicoscapular muscles. An examination and classification of the associated scapular movement system syndromes are critical in the management of the patients with cervical pain. Strategies for examination, classification, and management of scapular movement impairments are clearly described in Sahrmann.[3]

Key Exercises

A. *Sitting with back to wall—capital flexion:* Position: The upper extremities are supported on pillows to diminish the compressive loading of the cervical spine from the transfer of the weight of the upper extremities to the cervical region through the cervicoscapular muscle attachment. The patient is then instructed to place his or her head close to the wall and perform capital head flexion. The patient is encouraged to "roll" the head and chin toward the base of the anterior neck while trying to maintain the head close to the wall. This exercise can be ideally performed in sitting, but if the patient has difficulty maintaining the correct postural alignment during the cervical motion, the exercise can be performed in supine.

B. *Strengthening of the intrinsic cervical spine flexors in supine:* Position: The arms should be supported on pillows with the hips and knees in flexion. The patient may require a towel roll under the head.
   1. *Capital flexion without head lift:* The patient is instructed to roll the chin toward the front of the cervical spine. The patient should feel a stretch down the central posterior cervical region and muscle recruitment of the anterior intrinsic cervical spine flexors.
   2. *Capital flexion with head lift—with and without assistance:* The patient is instructed to roll the chin toward the front of the cervical spine and then continues to roll the cervical spine and head off the supporting surface while maintaining the chin positioned at the anterior cervical spine. Adding the lift of the head is more challenging, and the patient may have trouble maintaining the chin in contact with the anterior cervical spine region.

C. *Strengthening of the intrinsic cervical spine extensors in prone or quadruped.*
   1. In prone: The patient is instructed to place the forehead on the palms of his or her hand. The patient is then instructed to "roll" the head back in a pain-free range.
   2. In quadruped: The patient is instructed to flatten the spine like a "table top," align the head and cervical spine with the thoracic and lumbar spines, and "roll" the head down, then roll the head back. The patient is to imagine that there is a rod running through the middle of his or her neck and rotate about the rod.

D. *Sitting with back to wall—shoulder abduction lateral rotation:* This exercise is a progression of exercise A (back to wall—capital flexion). The patient positions the arms in shoulder abduction and lateral rotation. The patient then slides the arms up the wall, maintaining spinal alignment, especially capital flexion.
   1. *Modifications:* The arms do not make full contact with the wall, the arms can be parallel to the wall, or the fingertips can be placed on the wall with the elbows away from the wall.
   2. *Progression:* After adding resistance with free weights or resistance bands, the patient is instructed to position the trunk, neck, and arms as described previously and then move through shoulder abduction with resistance. The patient continues to maintain the lumbar spine against the wall and capital cervical flexion during the shoulder movement.

E. *Sitting with back to wall performing shoulder flexion:* This exercise is a progression of the exercise A (back to wall—capital flexion). The patient position the arms in 90 degrees of shoulder flexion and lateral rotation ("palms facing you"). The patient is then instructed to perform shoulder flexion ("reach up toward the ceiling"). The patient should be encouraged to maintain capital cervical flexion and avoid compensatory cervical extension.
   1. *Modifications:* Position the humeri/arms in the scapular plane: 30 degrees of horizontal abduction *or* position the humeri in less lateral rotation ("palms face each other, hands slightly medial to the elbows").
   2. *Progression:* After adding resistance with free weights or resistance bands, the patient is instructed to position the trunk, neck, and arms as described previously and then move through shoulder flexion with resistance. The patient continues to maintain

the lumbar spine against the wall; it will be a challenge to maintain capital cervical flexion during the shoulder movement.

F. *Wall slides: Facing the wall—shoulder flexion:* The patient is instructed to face the wall and place the ulnar side of the hands on the wall with the shoulders in the flexion plane. The patient is instructed to correct scapulae position and bring chin down toward the front of the neck. The patient is then instructed to slide the arms up the wall while maintaining the cervical spine position and avoid any compensatory cervical extension during the movement of shoulder flexion and return from shoulder flexion.

1. *Modifications:* Position the shoulders in the scapular plane.
2. *Progression:* After adding resistance with resistance bands, the patient is instructed to maintain the cervical position and avoid any compensatory cervical extension during the movement of the shoulder flexion wall slide.

Functional Instructions

The goal for instruction in modification of functional activities of the cervical extension syndrome is to diminish cervical extension and forward translation movements of the cervical spine during daily activities.

In addition, strategies to support the upper extremities to diminish the load on the cervical spine are critical. The most common activity that we instruct our patients in is prolonged sitting, especially at the computer, and use of eyeglasses, particular multifocal eyeglasses for reading.

When sitting at the computer, patients are instructed to have a supportive chair that will reduce thoracic flexion and assist in maintaining good thoracic alignment. They should support their forearms either on the desk or an extended tray for a keyboard. The desk or tray should be at the appropriate height so that the patient does not need to "slouch" for the arms to be supported. Commonly, if the support is too low, the patient may increase thoracic flexion and/or scapular depression to position the arms for support. Raising the supporting surface or adding armrests can be helpful.

The therapist should observe the patient using his or her eyeglasses. Frequently, the patient can be observed assuming a more forward-head position and/or increasing upper cervical extension when using eyeglasses, especially multifocal lenses. Alignment correction when wearing eyeglasses should follow the same sequence that has been demonstrated in the sitting back to wall exercises. Start with correction of lumbar, thoracic, and scapular alignment and then neck and head position.

Cervical Extension-Rotation Syndrome

Cervical extension-rotation syndrome is characterized by pain associated with cervical extension and rotation. The principal movement impairment in this syndrome is imprecise cervical rotation with associated compensatory cervical extension and/or sidebend, which is often associated with pain and limited ROM. There is an altered distribution of rotation motion across the cervical region and an imbalance of muscle performance among the cervical rotator muscles, with extrinsic muscles contributing to multiplanar movements rather than the precise uniplanar motion

Symptoms and History

- Pain location: Cervical region
- Radicular symptoms along the vertebral border, arm, and/or scapular region
- Pain with cervical rotation
- Pain is earlier in the range if spine is extended, and pain onset is delayed if spine remains neutral
- Pain can be located in the neck, upper trapezius, and/or arm
- Performance of activities that require frequent cervical rotation such as:
  - Driving
  - Talking on the phone
  - Golfing
- May have clicking during rotation
- Pain with repetitive single arm activities, particularly activities with single arm movements that involve lifting or carrying heavy objects
- Eye and hearing deficits should be assessed

Common Referring Diagnoses
- Cervical radiculopathy
- Degenerative disc disease
- Herniated cervical disc
- Facet syndrome
- Spondylosis

Key Tests and Signs for Movement Impairment

Alignment Analysis
Cervical Alignment
- Forward-head posture may be sidebent or rotated
- Asymmetry in muscles in the cervical region
- Resting alignment of scapular depression or elevation, depressed chest, and may be asymmetrical
- Thoracic kyphosis with increased cervical extension/translation

Movement Impairment Analysis
Standing/Sitting
- Cervical rotation ROM is limited and painful
- Observe cervical sidebending and extension during rotation
- Performing precise active rotation with correction of cervical sidebending and extension movement impairment results in diminished symptoms and/or improved cervical rotation ROM
- Passive assistance of rotation of cervical vertebrae decreases pain
- Correction of thoracic kyphosis alignment improves rotation ROM and decreases pain

Unloading Tests
- Passive elevation of the shoulder girdle and/or supporting the weight of the limbs decreases pain and improves cervical rotation
- In patients with well-developed abdominals who are physically active, passive elevation of the rib cage decreases pain and improves cervical rotation
- During single arm flexion rotation of a single or multiple vertebrae are noted. Patient does not typically complain of pain
- Many times correction of this fault is difficult. Several of the following strategies can be utilized:
  - Have the patient recruit the intrinsic cervical flexors by maintaining capital flexion during single arm flexion

    or
  - Correct associated scapular movement system syndromes during single arm flexion

    or
  - Perform bilateral shoulder flexion and note if the movement impairment improves

Supine
- Active cervical rotation is painful and possibly limited
- Passive elevation of the shoulder girdle results in diminished symptoms and/or improved rotation ROM
- Passive assistance in maintaining precise cervical rotation results in diminished symptoms and/or improved rotation ROM
- Active cervical flexion: Greater anterior translation than sagittal rotation and painful; intrinsic cervical flexors test weak
  - Manual assistance to diminish translation and encourage sagittal rotation decreases pain

Prone
- Active cervical extension: Greater posterior translation than sagittal rotation and painful; poor recruitment of cervical paraspinals noted
  - Verbal instruction to improve posterior sagittal cervical rotation and diminish cervical posterior translation results in improved recruitment of cervical paraspinals and less pain

Quadruped
- Active cervical rotation in quadruped is painful and associated with extension
  - Correction of the faulty alignment and pattern of movement results in diminished symptoms and/or improved rotation ROM
- Active cervical extension: Greater posterior translation than sagittal rotation and painful; observe increased recruitment of levator scapulae and diminished intrinsic neck extensor recruitment
  - Instruction to increase posterior sagittal rotation results in improved recruitment of intrinsic cervical extensors and less pain
- Active neck flexion: Poor control of movement
  - Instruction to increase anterior sagittal rotation improves quality of motion
- Rocking back: Cervical spine extends
  - Instruction to maintain "chin to Adam's apple" results in a neutral cervical spine position with quadruped rocking; other observations can include a "shortening" of the cervical region or compression of the cervical region

Muscle Length/Strength Impairments
- Weak intrinsic cervical flexors: Longus colli capitis and cervicis
- Short, stiff posterior cervical structures
- Dominant extrinsic cervical rotators: Sternocleidomastoid and scalene muscles

produced by the intrinsic rotators. There is also an imbalance of muscle performance of the cervical extensors, with the extrinsic extensors contributing to a compensatory extension movement during performance of rotation. The contributing factors in the cervical rotation extension syndrome include weight of the extremities and alignment of the thoracic spine and the scapulae. There may also be asymmetries in the appearance of the neck and scapular regions.

Associated Signs and Contributing Factors

- Prolonged sidebending (i.e., telephone holding)
- Repeated overhead shoulder flexion usually with resistance
- Golf, racquetball
- Prolonged position of a forward head posture
- Sleeping with arms overhead and head turned to side
- Sustained postures in rotation
- Hearing or visual impairments requiring frequent cervical rotation
- History of whiplash injury

Differential Diagnosis

Movement System Diagnoses
- Scapula depression
- Scapula downward rotation
- Scapula abduction

Musculoskeletal
- Fracture
- Cervical disc disease
- Spondylosis—degenerative arthritis
  - Consider visceral organ referral
- Vertebrobasilar insufficiency (VBI)
- Cervical radiculopathy
  - Degenerative disc disease
  - Herniated cervical disc
  - Facet syndrome

Systemic
- Cardiac
- Pulmonary
- Liver
- Gall bladder
- Tracheobronchial referral
- Neoplasms
- Metastatic tumors in the cervical spine

Treatment

In addition to the strategies described in cervical extension syndrome, the goal for treatment of the cervical rotation extension syndrome is to decrease the compensatory cervical extension and lateral flexion during active cervical rotation. Correction of the pattern of movement during daily activities is particularly important. As described in treatment for cervical extension, instruction in strategies to be used during functional activities, such as supporting the upper extremities, is important. Additional strategies used to manage the rotation impairment include using minimal effort to rotate the head and neck, correcting any sustained asymmetrical positions of the head and neck, and avoiding movements of the head and neck as part of body language. The focus of the active exercise program in the cervical region is to improve the strength and motor control of the intrinsic cervical spine rotators.

Key Exercises

A. *Sitting with back to wall performing cervical rotation:* Position: The initial positioning for this exercise is the same as in Exercise A described in "Cervical Extension Syndrome." As described previously, the initial instructions address impairments in the adjacent regions. The upper extremities are supported on pillows to diminish the compressive loading of the cervical spine from the transfer of the weight of the upper extremities to the cervical region through the cervicoscapular muscle attachment. The patient is then instructed to perform cervical rotation about a "vertical axis" and to avoid the compensatory movements of extension and sidebending and is encouraged to "easily" turn the head and neck to minimize the recruitment of the extrinsic cervical rotators. Specific instructions include "keep the chin down" and "do not lean the head and neck toward the side you are rotating toward." Additional instructions to have the patient sidebend in the opposite direction in which the patient is rotating the head typically results in a vertical position of the head and neck and diminished ipsilateral sidebending.

B. *Supine active cervical rotation:* Performance of precise cervical rotation in supine can be performed if sitting cervical rotation is too difficult or painful. The patient assumes a hooklying position with the arms supported on pillows. The patient may require a towel roll under the head; the thickness of the towel roll depends on the patient's thoracic alignment and severity of the forward head alignment. The same initial instructions as explained in the sitting exercises address the impairments in the adjacent regions. The patient is then instructed in strategies to precisely correct his or her individual alignment faults in the adjacent regions: lumbar and thoracic spines and scapulothoracic region before proceeding with the exercise. The patient is then instructed to perform cervical rotation about a "vertical axis" and to avoid the movements of cervical extension and sidebending.

C. *Facing wall, arms supported—active cervical rotation:* An additional position of facing the wall with the arms overhead and supported on the wall can be used to perform precise cervical rotation with support to the upper extremities. The patient is instructed to rest the forearms on the wall, allow the wall to support the upper extremities, and relax the upper trapezius muscles. The instructions instruct the patient to roll the chin down slightly, perform precise cervical rotation about a vertical axis, and avoid movements of cervical extension and sidebending.

D. *Quadruped active cervical rotation:* The alternative position of quadruped can be used to perform precise cervical rotation if the previously described positions of sitting or supine are too difficult or painful with cervical rotation motion. The patient is instructed to flatten the spine like a "table top," align the head and cervical spine with thoracic and lumbar spines and then rotate the head and neck about an axis of motion. The patient is instructed to avoid movements of cervical extension and sidebending.

Functional Instructions

The goal for instruction in modification of functional activities of the cervical extension-rotation syndrome is to diminish cervical extension and forward translation movements as described in the cervical extension syndrome. Another goal is to minimize asymmetrical stresses of the cervical spine during daily activities. Asymmetrical stresses may come from posturing of the cervical and/or thoracic spines in sidebend or rotation, especially during sitting activities. Asymmetrical stresses may also be imposed by unilateral movements of an upper extremity via the attachment of the cervicoscapular muscles.

When sitting at the computer, patients are instructed to have a supportive chair that will reduce thoracic flexion and assist in maintaining good thoracic alignment. They should support their forearms either on the desk or an extended tray for a keyboard. The desk or tray should be at the appropriate height so that the patient does not need to "slouch" for the arms to be supported. The computer or work station should be centered to the chair so there is no prolonged posturing in rotation or sidebend of the cervical or thoracic spine.

The patient should be instructed that prolonged positions of rotation or sidebend of the cervical or thoracic spines during daily activities should be avoided. This can commonly occur while watching TV, playing video games, and so on, without the patient being aware of the posturing. Using the telephone in a prolonged cervical sidebend position is common, and the patient should be encouraged to consider the use of a head set or "blue tooth" apparatus to diminish use of a prolonged cervical sidebend position.

Additional activities on which to counsel the patient include avoiding repetitive and/or resistive one-arm activities. These activities can inflict asymmetrical stresses on the cervical spine via the attachment of the cervicoscapular muscles. If the patient must continue with one-arm activities, it will be very important that he or she maintains proper alignment of the thoracic and cervical spines, especially avoiding cervical extension and/or a forward-head position during the activity. Instructing the patient to "keep the chin and nose down" will recruit the intrinsic cervical neck flexors to support the cervical spine during the one-arm activities.

Cervical Flexion Syndrome

The principal movement impairment in this syndrome is imprecise cervical flexion that is often associated with pain and limited ROM. There is an altered distribution of flexion across the cervical and thoracic regions, with the lower cervical region flexing more than the upper thoracic region. There is an imbalance of muscle performance of the cervical flexors with dominance of intrinsic cervical flexors that can create a kyphotic position of the cervical spine and/or insufficient recruitment of cervical extensors during cervical extension movements.

Symptoms and History

- Pain location: Cervical region
- Radicular symptoms along the vertebral border, arm, and/or scapular region
- Pain with neck flexion
- Typically a younger spine
- Performance of activities that require repetitive positioning in "correct alignment" (e.g., military posture, ballet activities)

Common Referring Diagnoses

- Cervical radiculopathy
- Degenerative disc disease
- Herniated cervical disc
- Facet syndrome
- Spondylosis

Key Tests and Signs for Movement Impairment

Alignment Analysis

Cervical Alignment

- Decreased cervical inward curve
  - Increasing the inward curve of the cervical spine decreases symptoms

Thoracic Alignment

- Decreased thoracic kyphosis

Scapular Alignment

- Resting alignment of scapular depression or downward rotation

Movement Impairment Analysis

Standing/Sitting

- Cervical flexion ROM is painful
- Impairments: Lower cervical flexes more readily than the upper thoracic region
  - Correction encourages greater flexion movement in the upper thoracic region and limits lower cervical flexion
  - Passive elevation of the shoulder girdle encourages greater flexion in the upper thoracic region
  - Instruct patient to increase thoracic flexion: "Slump" before performing flexion

Prone

- Active cervical extension: Greater posterior translation than sagittal rotation; poor recruitment of cervical paraspinals noted
  - Verbal instruction to improve posterior sagittal cervical rotation and diminish cervical posterior translation results in improved recruitment of cervical paraspinals

Quadruped

- Active cervical extension: Greater posterior translation than sagittal rotation and painful. Observe increased recruitment of levator scapulae and diminished intrinsic neck extensor recruitment
  - Instruction to increase posterior sagittal rotation results in improved recruitment of intrinsic cervical extensors and less pain

Muscle Strength/Performance Impairments

- Dominance of intrinsic cervical flexors creates kyphotic curve
- Excessive length of neck extensors

Associated Signs or Contributing Factors

Structural Variations

- Decreased thoracic kyphosis
- Heavy upper extremities and/or heavy breasts
- Resistance to passive elevation of the scapula

Acquired Faults

- Straightening of the cervical spine and depression of the shoulders (i.e., ballet, modern dance, and gymnastics)
- Habits of maintaining a straight spine, such as sleeping with a large pillow or habitually lying with the head propped
- Sustained postures in flexion

Differential Diagnosis

Movement System Diagnoses

- Cervical flexion rotation
- Thoracic extension
- Scapula depression
- Scapula downward rotation
- Scapula abduction

Potential Diagnoses Requiring Referral Suggested by Signs and Symptoms

Neuromusculoskeletal

- Metastatic tumor in the cervical spine
- Fracture
- Frank neurological signs
- Vertebrobasilar insufficiency (VBI)

Systemic

- Cardiac
- Pulmonary
- Liver
- Gall bladder
- Tracheobronchial referral
- Neoplasms
- Metastatic tumors in the cervical spine

Treatment

The primary goals in the treatment of cervical flexion syndrome are to restore a normal lordotic cervical curve, improve function of the intrinsic cervical extensors, and to avoid positions and movements that would encourage excessive cervical flexion. A common alignment fault associated with cervical flexion is a reduced thoracic curve. The straight thoracic spine has decrease flexibility in the direction of flexion, which potentially results in compensatory flexion in the cervical flexion. Treatment strategies include instructing the patient on how to increase thoracic flexion or encouraging the patient to "slump," which is not a typical functional instruction but appropriate if the patient's thoracic impairments necessitate these instructions.

Key Exercises

A. *Prone active cervical extension:* In prone position with the patient's forehead resting in the palms of the hands, the patient is instructed to "roll" head and neck back in the direction of extension. The verbal cue of rolling is to facilitate the recruitment of the intrinsic neck extensors and reduce recruitment of the extrinsic neck extensors. The patient is encouraged not to reach full end-range extension to avoid excessive compression on the cervical facets and discs.

B. *Quadruped active cervical extension:* The quadruped position can be a more difficult exercise because the exercise requires good scapulothoracic muscle function while weight bearing through the upper extremities. The same instruction is to "roll" the head and neck both into flexion and then extension. When performing the cervical extension exercise in the quadruped, the patient is encourage to perform the movement in the "middle third" of the ROM to avoid an end-range extended or flexed position.

Functional Instruction

Key functional instructions for cervical flexion syndrome include encouraging flexion in adjacent regions to minimize the amount of cervical flexion that is required during daily activities. This will include encouraging the patient to "slump" or increase thoracic flexion, which may diminish the amount of cervical flexion that is required. This strategy is the opposite instruction and opposite effect that the therapist would have used with a patient with cervical extension syndrome with kyphosis. When the patient attempts to slump, it may initially feel very awkward and unfamiliar. The instruction to "slump" can make the patient feel self-conscious about his or her appearance. Using a mirror to demonstrate that the strategy does not result in excessive flexion or kyphosis can be very useful in reassuring patients that they are not going to end up like their osteoporotic grandmother!

The hip joint is an additional adjacent region in which the therapist can encourage flexion motion to reduce the amount cervical flexion with forward-bend movements. During sitting activities, patients may be encouraged to lean toward the object that they are looking at by flexing at the hips rather than increasing cervical flexion.

Additional instructions can include different strategies to diminish excessive cervical flexion during daily activities. Suggestions at a patient's work station may include raising the computer screen or using of a book holder to raise the work items closer to the patient rather than the patient flexing the cervical spine. Also, use of a cervical pillow or towel to support the cervical spine during sleeping can be helpful.

The therapist should review the use of eyeglasses. The patient may demonstrate the common habit of excessive flexion to position the eyes with the use of reading glasses. The patient will be encouraged to properly position the glasses on the nose that allows a neutral position of the neck so that the patient raises the nose and chin when using the glasses.

NOTES

Cervical Flexion-Rotation Syndrome

The principal movement impairment in cervical flexion-rotation syndrome is imprecise cervical rotation with associated compensatory cervical flexion, which is often associated with pain and limited ROM. There is an imbalance of muscle performance among the cervical rotator muscles, with extrinsic muscles contributing to multiplanar movements rather than the precise uniplanar motion produced by the intrinsic rotators. There is also an imbalance of muscle performance of the cervical flexors contributing to compensatory flexion movement during performance of rotation. The contributing factors in the cervical rotation flexion syndrome include weight of the extremities and alignment of the thoracic spine and the scapulae. There may also be asymmetries in the appearance of the neck and scapular regions.

Symptoms and History

- Pain location: Cervical region
- Radicular symptoms along the vertebral border, arm, and/or scapula region
- Pain with neck flexion and/or rotation
- Pain with cervical rotation
- Pain is earlier in the range if spine is in flexion and pain onset delayed if spine remains neutral
- Typically a younger spine
- Performance of activities that require repetitive positioning in "correct alignment" (e.g., military posture, ballet activities)
- Pain with driving: Rotating head

Common Referring Diagnoses

- Cervical radiculopathy
- Degenerative disc disease
- Herniated cervical disc
- Facet syndrome
- Spondylosis

Key Tests and Signs for Movement Impairment

Alignment Analysis
Cervical Alignment
- Decreased cervical inward curve with a position of sidebend or rotation
  - Increasing the inward curve of the cervical spine and/or position of sidebend or rotation decreases symptoms
- Asymmetry of muscles in the cervical region

Thoracic Alignment
- Decreased thoracic kyphosis
- Resting alignment of scapular depression or downward rotation

Movement Impairment Analysis
Standing/Sitting
- Cervical flexion ROM is painful
- Impairments: Lower cervical flexes more readily than the upper thoracic region
  - Correction encourages greater flexion movement in the upper thoracic region and limits lower cervical flexion
  - Passive elevation of the shoulder girdle encourages greater flexion in the upper thoracic region
  - Instruct patient to increase thoracic flexion: "Slump" before performing flexion
  - Passive elevation of the shoulder girdle and/or supporting the weight of the limbs decreases pain and improves cervical flexion
- Cervical rotation ROM is painful
- Cervical flexion during performance of rotation:
  - Correction of cervical flexion movement results in diminished symptoms and/or improved cervical rotation ROM
  - Instruct patient to increase thoracic flexion: "Slump" before performing rotation
  - Passive assistance of rotation of cervical vertebrae decreases pain
  - Passive elevation of the shoulder girdle and/or supporting the weight of the limbs decreases pain and improves cervical rotation
- During single-arm flexion, rotation of a single or multiple vertebrae is noted. Patient does not typically complain of pain
  - Many times correction of this fault is difficult. Several strategies can be used:
  - Have the patient assume ideal alignment of the cervical spine by avoiding excessive flexion and assume a position of slight extension
    or
  - Correct associated scapular movement system syndromes during single-arm flexion
    or
  - Perform bilateral shoulder flexion and note if the movement impairment improves

Prone
- Active cervical extension: Greater posterior translation than sagittal rotation; poor recruitment of cervical paraspinals noted
  - Verbal instruction to improve posterior sagittal cervical rotation and diminish cervical posterior translation results in improved recruitment of cervical paraspinals

Quadruped
- Active cervical extension: Greater posterior translation than sagittal rotation and painful; observe increased recruitment of levator scapulae and diminished intrinsic neck extensor recruitment
  - Instruction to increase posterior sagittal rotation results in improved recruitment of intrinsic cervical extensors and less pain

Muscle Strength/Performance Impairments
- Dominance of intrinsic cervical flexors creates kyphotic curve
- Excessive length of neck extensors

Associated Signs or Contributing Factors

Structural Variations

- Decreased thoracic kyphosis
- Heavy upper extremities and/or heavy breasts
- Resistance to passive elevation of the scapula

Acquired Faults

- Straightening of the cervical spine and depression of the shoulders, i.e., ballet, modern dance and gymnastics
- Habits of maintaining a straight spine, sleeping with a large pillow or habitually lying with head propped
- Sustained postures in flexion
- Sustained postures in rotation
- Hearing or visual impairments requiring frequent cervical rotation

Differential Diagnosis

Movement System Diagnoses

- Cervical flexion rotation
- Thoracic extension
- Scapula depression
- Scapula downward rotation
- Scapula abduction

Potential Diagnoses Requiring Referral Suggested by Signs and Symptoms

Neuromusculoskeletal

- Metastatic tumor in the cervical spine
- Fracture
- Frank neurological signs
- Vertebrobasilar insufficiency (VBI)

Systemic

- Cardiac
- Pulmonary
- Liver
- Gall bladder
- Tracheobronchial referral
- Neoplasms
- Metastatic tumors in the cervical spine

Treatment

The primary goals of treatment for cervical flexion-rotation syndrome are similar to those of cervical flexion syndrome: to restore the normal cervical lordotic curve, to avoid excessive flexion in the cervical spine, and encourage increase flexion movements in other regions, usually the thoracic spine. Additional strategies include instructing the patient in restoration of precise motion of active cervical rotation by performing motion without associated flexion and using minimal effort to rotate the head and neck. Other strategies include correcting any sustained asymmetrical positions of the head and neck and avoiding movements of the head and neck as part of body language. The focus of the active exercise program in the cervical region is to improve the strength and motor control of the intrinsic cervical spine rotators. Additionally, as described in previous syndromes, instruction in strategies to diminish the load of the upper extremities, such as supporting the upper extremities, is important.

Key Exercises

A. *Sitting cervical rotation:* The patient may not need to assume the position of sitting with the back to the wall as have been previously describe in cervical extension syndrome. Sitting in a chair with good thoracic spine support may be more appropriate and may encourage a normal thoracic alignment of slight flexion and discourage a flat thoracic spine. The upper extremities are supported on pillows to diminish the compressive loading of the cervical spine. The patient is then instructed to perform cervical rotation by rotating with minimal effort and rotating about a "vertical axis" to avoid the movements of flexion and sidebending. Specific instructions include "raise the chin up slightly" to avoid compensatory flexion during rotation and "do not lean the head and neck toward the side you are rotating toward." Additional instructions to sidebend in the opposite direction that the patient is rotating the head typically result in a vertical position of the head and neck and diminished ipsilateral sidebending.

B. *Supine active cervical rotation:* Precise cervical rotation in supine can be performed if sitting cervical rotation is too difficult or painful. The patient assumes a hooklying position with the arms supported on pillows. The patient may require a towel roll under the cervical spine to support a normal cervical and prevent a position of excessive flexion of the cervical region. The same initial instructions to address impairments in the adjacent regions are used, as explained in the sitting exercises. The patient is then instructed to perform cervical rotation with minimal effort about a "vertical axis" to avoid the movements of cervical flexion and sidebending. Other key verbal cues are similar to cues that were used in sitting exercises: "raise the chin up slightly" to avoid compensatory flexion during rotation and "do not lean the head and neck toward the side you are rotating toward."

C. *Quadruped active cervical rotation:* The alternate position of quadruped can be used to perform precise cervical rotation if the previously described positions of sitting or supine are too difficult or painful. The patient is instructed to allow the thoracic spine to flex slightly, align the head and cervical spine with the thoracic spine, but the patient should be instructed to raise the head and chin slightly to avoid a position of excessive flexion of the cervical spine. The patient is instructed to rotate the head and neck about an axis of motion that follows the spine. The patient is instructed to avoid movements of cervical flexion and sidebending.

D. *Facing wall, arms supported—active cervical rotation:* An additional position of facing the wall with the arms overhead supported on the wall can be used to perform precise cervical rotation with support to the upper extremities. The patient is instructed to rest the forearms on the wall, allow the wall to support the upper extremities, and relax the upper trapezius muscles. The patient is then instructed to raise the head and chin slightly to avoid the position of excessive cervical flexion, then perform with minimal effort precise cervical rotation about a vertical axis, and to avoid movements of cervical flexion and sidebending.

Functional Instructions

Key functional instructions for cervical flexion rotation syndrome include the strategies described in the cervical flexion syndrome, which encourage flexion in adjacent regions to minimize the amount of cervical flexion that is required during daily activities (see "Cervical Flexion Syndrome"). In addition, strategies should be implemented to minimize asymmetrical stress on the cervical spine through decreasing repetition of one arm activities or prolonged positioning in sidebend or rotation (see "Cervical Extension-Rotation Syndrome").

REFERENCES

1. Schuldt K, Ekholm J, Harms-Ringdahl K, et al: Effects of arm support or suspension on neck and shoulder muscle activity during sedentary work, *Scand J Rehabil Med* 19:77-84, 1987.

2. Straker L, Burgess-Limerick R, Pollock C, et al: The effect of forearm support on children's head, neck and upper limb posture and muscle activity during computer use, *J Electromyogr Kinesiol* 19(5):965-974, 2008.

3. Sahrmann SA: *Diagnosis and treatment of movement impairment syndromes*, St Louis, 2002, Mosby.

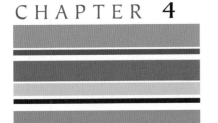

Movement System Syndromes of the Thoracic Spine

Theresa Spitznagle, Renee Ivens

INTRODUCTION

Thoracic spine pain syndromes are most commonly the result of cumulative microtrauma caused by impairments in alignment, stabilization, and movement patterns. In a normal thoracic spine, balance of the trunk musculature and other contributing tissues (bone, nerve, ligaments, and discs) provides support and control of movement to prevent impairments. The major objective for diagnosis, prognosis, and treatment of thoracic movement system syndromes is to identify all factors that create impairments of the tissues. Thoracic spine diagnoses are determined by direction and magnitude of postural alignment and movements of the thoracic spine that consistently elicit or increase the patient's symptoms. Individual differences in age, activity level, anthropometrics, and gender assist the physical therapist in (1) understanding the status of the tissues and (2) precisely determining treatment and prognosis.

When a system is multisegmented, as is the case of the human movement system, the greatest degree of motion occurs at the most flexible segment.[1] The distribution of motion in the thoracic spine is determined by the mechanical characteristics of the region.[2] Following the basic law of physics, movement takes place along the path of least resistance. Thus, because of the increased length of the region (creating a long lever arm) and the angle of the facets (facilitating superior glide and rotation),[3] the thoracic region of the spine easily moves into flexion and rotation. To illustrate this concept, consider a young female with a long trunk who develops the habit of bending down to converse with her peers. Thus she develops the movement "habit" of thoracic flexion early in her life. At a later time in this woman's life, thoracic flexion, coupled with the degenerative process of the aging female spine, creates a structural kyphosis. In the last decades of her life, the unchecked kyphosis becomes so severe that she is predisposed to compression fractures.[4-6] Thus the uncorrected habit of thoracic flexion can develop over time into permanent alignment changes.

The most common movement impairments contributing to thoracic spine pain syndromes are related to an imbalance of the trunk and limb musculature creating alterations in the relative flexibility of the thoracic spine. Sustained positions or repetitive movements of the thoracic spine cause microtrauma to the tissues. This microtrauma, if sustained over time, will progress to macrotrauma of the associated spinal structures. Pathology, such as intercostal nerve compromise, disc herniation, osteophyte formation, or compression fracture, will eventually develop as the result of impairments of thoracic spine stability or movement. In addition, upper or lower extremity limb movements during functional activities can impose stress across the thoracic spine. Typically, the movement impairments of the thoracic spine present as excessive or incorrect timing of one or more of the normal motions and positions of flexion, rotation, and extension.

Pain syndromes that develop from movement-related tissue injury require consideration of the mechanisms that cause tissue injury. Factors that affect movement-related tissue injury include (1) excessive joint mobility; (2) impaired timing of the movement relative to the functional requirements; or (3) excessive frequency, duration, or intensity of movement, thus exceeding the tissue's tolerance to stress.[7] Excessive joint mobility will require a precise neuromuscular training program that may include strength training,[8] in addition to correction of the impaired movement at the site of pain and the adjoining regions. Patient education for strength training must focus on teaching the patient to control movement within the optimal range of motion (ROM),[9] while avoiding excessive frequency of motion for all activities and exercise. Impaired timing of movements present in an individual who moves primarily in the thoracic region without distribution of the motion to other regions of the spine (cervical or lumbar). For example, during forward bending the thoracic spine moves into flexion more rapidly than the lumbar spine (Figure 4-1). Treatment in this circumstance focuses on education regarding reduction of thoracic spine motion by redistribution of the motion to other regions by increasing hip and knee flexion (Figure 4-2).

Finally, excessive frequency, duration, or intensity of movement creates an imbalance of stress on tissues so

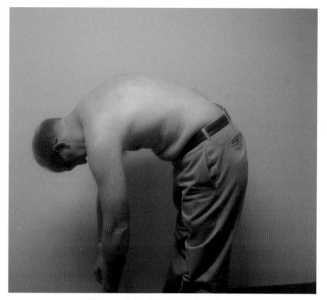

Figure 4-1. Forward bending.

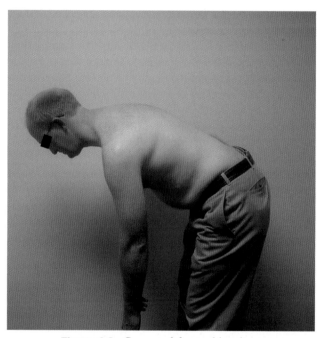

Figure 4-2. Corrected forward bending.

that tissue recovery is impaired and pain develops. Treatment in this case necessitates reduction of one or more of these factors to protect the tissues. Consideration of the frequency, duration, and intensity of the motion allows the physical therapist to individualize patient education regarding all activities, whether recreational, occupational, or functional. For example, excessive performance of trunk curl exercises increases the stiffness and shortens the abdominal musculature, while simultaneously increasing the length and possibly weakening the thoracic trunk extensors. Weakness of the back extensors has been associated with kyphosis.[10-12] Thus reducing the

frequency of performance or elimination of trunk curling exercises may be necessary in an individual with a thoracic kyphosis. Likewise, the amount of time spent in a specific position that would flex the spine will contribute to development of a kyphosis. Questioning the individual regarding typical daytime activities can give insight into the amount of time spent sitting or standing. Observation of the patient during "nonclinical" examination times, such as sitting in the waiting room, waiting for the home program to print, or bending down to pick up her purse as she is leaving the clinic, is helpful to determine the presence of habits or body language that perpetuates impaired movement patterns. Some individuals with an overdeveloped and short rectus abdominis (RA) muscle demonstrate thoracic flexion even when they laugh.

The keys to prevention and correction of thoracic spine movement system syndromes are (1) to have the trunk musculature hold the vertebral column in the optimal alignment, (2) to address limb movements that perturb the vertebral column, and (3) to prevent repeated movement at the most flexible thoracic segments during functional activities. To achieve these aims, the impairments in muscle length, stiffness, and performance are addressed. Movement education is provided for motor learning during both trunk and limb motions. In the case of excessive thoracic flexion, the movement of the trunk into forward flexion would be redistributed to increase the motion across the hips instead of across the thoracic region. The habit of flexing primarily in the thoracic region during forward bending needs to be addressed during education regarding common functional activities such as bending, dressing, and lifting tasks. Finally, functional activities are modified to reduce stresses on the thoracic spine segments. For example, sitting alignment is corrected to avoid the position of thoracic flexion, thus decreasing the resting length of the thoracic paraspinal musculature and increasing the resting length of the abdominal musculature.

This chapter presents key principles for examining alignment and movement, determining muscle length, and testing the strength of the musculature of the thoracic spine. The diagnostic categories for the thoracic region are described (Table 4-1). Case examples are provided for the most common movement system syndromes. Associated cervical, scapular, and lumbar region movement system syndromes are mentioned. Syndrome-specific treatment suggestions are provided, including movement system impairment exercises and patient education for functional activities and personal habits.

ALIGNMENT OF THE THORACIC SPINE

Normal Standing Alignment

In standing, the normal alignment of the thoracic spine is a flexion curve of 40 degrees, as measured using a Cobb angle.[3,13-23] Clinically, a normal thoracic spine has a mild posterior convexity and even distribution of flexion

TABLE 4-1
Thoracic Spine Movement Impairment Syndromes

Syndrome	Key Findings
Rotation-flexion	Pain with postures or motion that flex and rotate the thoracic spine.
Flexion	Pain with postures or motion that flex the thoracic spine. In the case of increased kyphosis, pain may occur with correction of the alignment.
Rotation-extension	Pain with postures or motion that extend and rotate the thoracic spine.
Rotation	Pain with postures or motion that rotate the thoracic spine.
Extension	Pain with postures or motion that extend the thoracic spine.

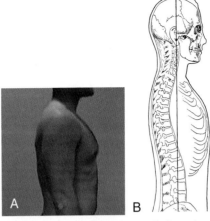

Figure 4-3. **A** and **B**, Normal thoracic alignment. (**B**, From Kendall FP, McCreary EK, Provance PG: *Muscles: testing and function*, ed 4, Philadelphia, 1993, Lippincott Williams & Wilkins.)

(Figure 4-3). The shape of the thoracic curve is attributed to a slight wedging of the vertebrae.[96] A lateral view of a chest x-ray shows that the anterior aspects of the vertebral bodies are slightly smaller than the posterior aspect[24] (Figure 4-4). There are no known sex differences in the overall amount of normal thoracic flexion alignment[17,25,26]; however, with aging, there is an increase in thoracic flexion, with females demonstrating a greater increase than males.[17,25]

The normal rib cage is slightly rounded in circumference—the superior aspect of the rib cage is more narrow than the inferior aspect. The rib cage is normally symmetrical from side to side. The shape of the rib cage can be attributed to the variation in the length and curvature of the ribs and their anterior attachment to the sternum. The angle formed by the costal margins of ribs 7 to 10 is referred to as the *subcostal margin*. An ideal subcostal angle of approximately 90 degrees is considered to be a reflection of balance between the length of the internal and external oblique muscles.[1-27] Age-related changes of the rib cage have not been well studied; clinical observations indicate that individuals with a thoracic kyphosis, as well as individuals with central obesity, will have a flaring of the lower ribs. Reported sex differences of the rib cage indicate that males tend to have a narrower anterior-to-posterior dimension and a broader medial-to-lateral dimension, whereas females tend to have a more rounded chest wall with a narrower overall diameter[28] (Figure 4-5).

Impaired Standing Alignment

Alignment impairments of the thoracic spine can be both postural and structural. Postural impairments are flexible and respond to positional changes or cues to change alignment. Structural alignment impairments are fixed alignments of the boney structures that persist, regardless of the position of the individual. Though structural

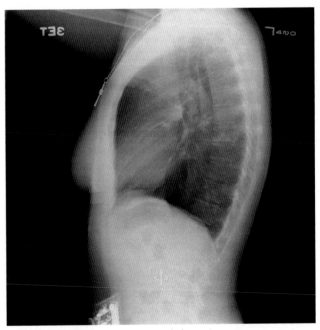

Figure 4-4. Normal thoracic curve.

changes are present, some correction may be possible if connective tissues are extensible. Genetic variation in tissue mobility is a factor in determining the magnitude of alignment change. A structural impairment can be demonstrated with radiographic studies. Attempts to change a structural alignment may increase stress across a region and may worsen a pain syndrome by forcing motion above or below the malaligned segments. For example, cueing an individual with a structural kyphosis to extend the thoracic spine often results in an increase in lumbar or cervical extension. Recognition of a structural impairment and accommodation for the fixed impairment must be made to reduce mechanical stresses

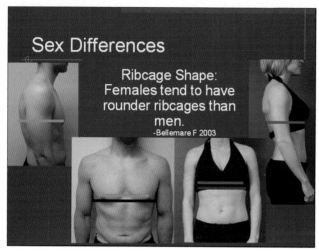

Figure 4-5. *Male:* Greater medial to lateral width (*black line*) than anterior posterior width (*gray line*). *Female:* Medial to lateral width (*red line*) is similar to anterior posterior width (*pink line*).

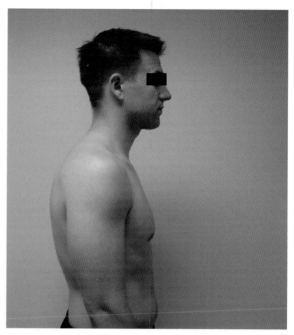

Figure 4-6. Kyphosis.

and pain. Patients may also present with a combination of structural and postural alignment impairments. In this case, attempts at postural correction may be only partially successful.

There are five categories of impaired thoracic alignment: kyphosis, posterior trunk sway, flat back, rotation, and scoliosis. Thoracic kyphosis is defined as an increase in the flexion curve in the thoracic region[3,29] (Figure 4-6). With a sustained postural kyphosis, structural accommodation to the persistent anterior forces on the vertebral bodies results in increasing disc and vertebral body loading, causing a wedging of the thoracic vertebrae.[5] In this case, kyphosis that started as a postural fault becomes a structural impairment according to the principles of Wolff's law. This phenomenon commonly is not painful until a severe kyphosis has developed.

Individuals with a thoracic kyphosis commonly have a lumbar lordosis.[29] Specific movement testing may help to determine if the kyphosis-lordosis alignment is (1) structural (fixed), (2) caused by weakness or excessive length of thoracic extensor muscles, or (3) caused by passive stiffness or frequent (habitual) contraction of the abdominal musculature, specifically the RA. Usually, when the kyphosis is structural, the thoracic curvature does not change when the patient is examined in the supine, prone, and quadruped position even when instructed to straighten the thoracic spine. Although a structural kyphosis can occur at any age, older individuals with degenerative changes and osteoarthritis are more likely to have a structural kyphosis.

Scheuermann's disease, or juvenile kyphosis, is a structural impairment believed to occur as the result of a variation in the growth of the endplates of the vertebral bodies.[30] However, the etiology of Scheuermann disease is still unknown. The structural change is a wedge deformity of 5 degrees or more across three consecutive

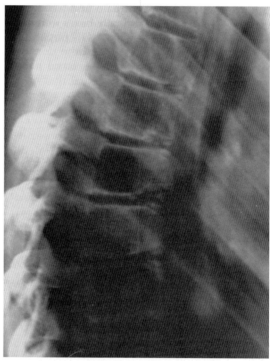

Figure 4-7. X-ray of Scheuermann's disease. (Courtesy of Dr. R. Cairns. From Cassidy JT, Petty RE: *Textbook of pediatric rheumatology*, ed 5, Philadelphia, 2005, Saunders.)

vertebrae[31] (Figure 4-7). The lower thoracic or high lumbar regions are most commonly involved, and the thoracic kyphosis is typically greater than 45 degrees.[30,32] Individuals with Scheuermann's disease should avoid positions or exercises that contribute to thoracic flexion. Attempts to overcorrect the thoracic flexion could result

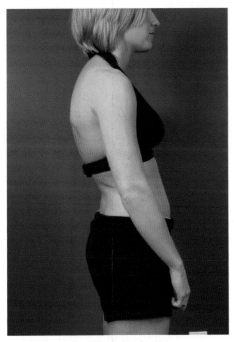

Figure 4-8. Swayback alignment.

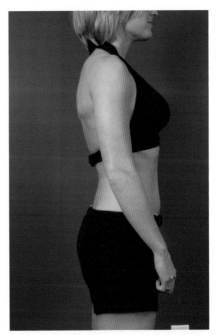

Figure 4-9. Corrected swayback alignment.

in increased lumbar extension. Patient education is important regarding the effect of anterior compressive forces on the spine and minimizing activities that would worsen the condition such as unsupported sitting, trunk curl exercises, and even various weight-training exercises. The patient should also avoid activities that require prolonged trunk flexion.

Osteoporosis is another condition that often results in a thoracic kyphosis because of vertebral compression fractures that result in wedge deformities of the thoracic vertebral bodies.[5] The greatest risk factor for development of a compression fracture in an osteoporotic spine is a previous fracture in the same region.[33,34] Kyphosis as a result of osteoporotic compression fractures has been reported to be associated with decreased function and quality of life[35] and an increased risk for falls.[36,37]

Posterior trunk sway of the thoracic spine occurs when the upper back is shifted backward and the hips are swayed forward so that typically the shoulders are posterior to the hip joints.[29] Generally, individuals with this type of posture have a long kyphosis[29]; however, the amount and location of the thoracic flexion may vary. Posterior trunk sway results in decreased participation of the trunk extensors and an increase in the use of the RA as an antigravity muscle to control the trunk.[38] In this alignment impairment, a thoracic kyphosis can be masked by the change in alignment of the both the lower thoracic spine at the region of the thoracolumbar junction (posterior glide of the vertebrae) and the upper body sway behind the hip joint axis (Figures 4-8 and 4-9).

The flat back posture is one in which the thoracic spine is straight or the degree of flexion is notably less than normal. In severe cases of a flat thoracic spine, there

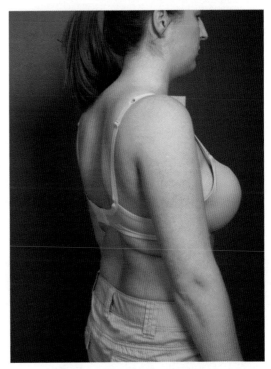

Figure 4-10. Flat thoracic spine.

can be the appearance of a thoracic lordosis (Figures 4-10 and 4-11). The flattened thoracic spine can be an assumed posture or structural variation. When the thoracic spine is extended, structural changes are more likely. The individual with a postural flat back will be able to achieve some thoracic flexion. Those with a structural flat back usually cannot achieve full flexion, even with an active effort to curl the trunk.

There is a lack of normal rib cage contour in a structural flat back alignment, which often makes the scapulae more prominent on the thorax. The prominence of the vertebral border of the scapulae can be mislabeled as winging. Grieve[39] notes that a flat thoracic spine is common in individuals with a "painful stiffening" of the cervical region, as well as increased complaints of neck and shoulder pain. Individuals with a flat thoracic spine are more likely to have pectus excavatum.[40]

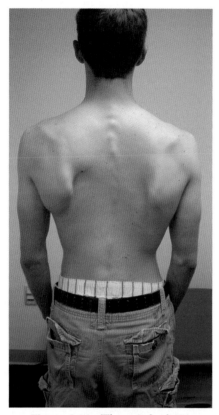

Figure 4-11. Thoracic lordosis.

Rotation of the thoracic spine is almost always an acquired problem that results from repeated movements in one direction. Activities requiring rotation associated with throwing or one-handed sports such as in baseball, softball, volleyball, or tennis can cause rotation of the thorax. Even less vigorous activities such as sitting at a desk and rotating frequently to one side to work on a computer or to answer the phone can also contribute to the thoracic spine becoming rotated. In these individuals, the rotation of the rib cage can be evident in the front view by asymmetry of the rib cage with the side contralateral to the rotation being more prominent. In this type of rotation, there is not the compensatory rotation in the opposite direction with the S-type curve that is the prevailing feature of scoliosis as described below. Some clinicians may refer to this form of rotation which is usually in only one plane as a functional scoliosis though most often the rib deformity is not as marked nor is the lateral flexion of the trunk present.

The last category of impaired thoracic alignment, scoliosis, is present when the thoracic spine and rib cage are rotated. Rotation of the rib cage and/or the thoracic vertebrae may be localized to a few vertebrae or can involve the whole thoracic spine.[3] An asymmetrical contour of the rib cage is usually evident from a posterior view and becomes even more obvious in forward bending. The asymmetry may also be evident from an anterior view (Figure 4-12). The asymmetry of the rib cage usually causes an asymmetry in the position of the scapulae. Scoliosis can be postural or structural or a combination of both. Postural scoliosis, sometimes referred to as *functional scoliosis*,[29,41] is considered present when there is an asymmetry in the alignment of the thoracic spine or rib cage that is not fixed. Similar to other alignment impairments, postural scoliosis can be distinguished from structural based on the ability to restore symmetrical alignment. Postural scoliosis can occur as the result of an activity,

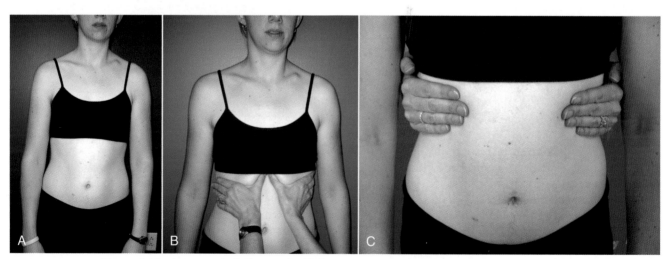

Figure 4-12. Asymmetrical rib cage. **A,** Slight appearance and asymmetry. Note arm position in relation to rib cage and pelvis. **B,** Right side of rib cage more prominent than left. **C,** Another method demonstrating right rib cage prominence.

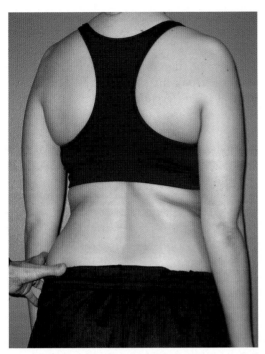

Figure 4-13. Postural scoliosis with right rotation of rib cage.

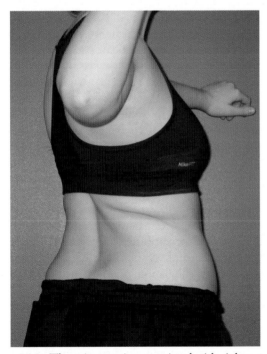

Figure 4-14. Throwing motion associated with right rotation.

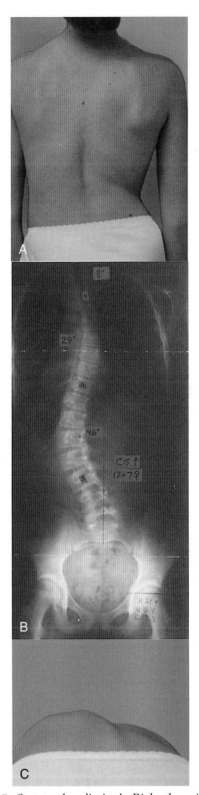

Figure 4-15. Structural scoliosis. **A,** Right thoracic convexity and left lumbar convexity. **B,** X-ray of similar curvature. **C,** Forward bending demonstrating left lumbar convexity.

such as throwing, that would habitually rotate the thoracic spine (Figures 4-13 and 4-14). In a postural scoliosis, there are no structural changes in the shape of the vertebral bodies or ribs.

Structural scoliosis is defined as a structural impairment of the vertebrae that affects all three planes: frontal, sagittal, and transverse[3] (Figure 4-15). Structures that are affected by this asymmetry include not only the vertebral body but also the corresponding ribs and soft tissue structures. Idiopathic scoliosis most commonly presents in adolescence and is believed to have a familial pattern.[42] The etiology of idiopathic scoliosis is believed to be multifactorial; possible contributing factors are hormones,[43-46] biomechanics,[47-50] and motor control.[51-55] Increased height and hypokyphosis, or flat spine, which potentially causes improper loading of the spine and thus asymmetrical growth patterns, have also been reported in individuals with idiopathic adolescent scoliosis.[47] Locomotor skills, including lateral step, balance strategies, and vibratory sense, have been reported as impaired in individuals with a structural scoliosis.[51-55] Currently, it remains unclear if the motor control impairments contribute to the spine malalignment or if the spine malalignment contributes to the motor control impairments.

Rib Cage Alignment Impairments

The most common rib cage alignment impairments are rotational asymmetry or altered rib cage circumference. In the presence of either impairment, the subcostal angle will show a deviation from the normal symmetrical angle of approximately 90 degrees. Widening of the subcostal angle is often accompanied by an outward flare of the lower ribs in obese individuals or those with poor abdominal muscle tone. Overdevelopment of the pectoral muscles in an individual with poor abdominal muscle control can contribute to rib cage malalignment because every time the pectoral muscles are contracted the rib cage is elevated. Conversely, overdevelopment of abdominal musculature can result in narrowing of the subcostal margin; these concepts are discussed in the "Abdominal Muscle Length" section later in the chapter.

Obesity causes increased fat distribution within the chest and abdomen, which can lead to the long-term development of a barrel-shaped chest (Figure 4-16). Changes in trunk shape can be seen even in individuals who have lost weight.[56] This change in the contour of the chest wall may cause the scapulae to appear more internally rotated; however, overcorrection of scapular

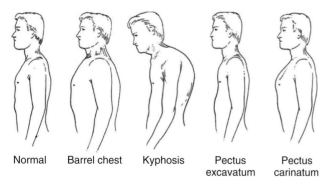

Figure 4-16. Variations in trunk shape. (From Frownfelter D, Dean E: *Cardiovascular and pulmonary physical therapy*, ed 4, St Louis, 2006, Mosby.)

Normal   Barrel chest   Kyphosis   Pectus excavatum   Pectus carinatum

alignment should be avoided because of this change in chest wall shape.

Rib cage asymmetry is commonly caused by changes in thoracic spine alignment, as well as muscle length changes in the trunk and shoulder girdle. Thoracic spine rotation will create asymmetry in the subcostal angle, with one side appearing to be closer to midline than the other. As with scoliosis, subcostal angle asymmetry can be structural, postural, or both. Asymmetry of the rib cage can cause approximation of two adjacent ribs, resulting in compression of the intercostal nerves or increased tension at the rib insertion along the sternum or costal cartilage. Common conditions that could result include intercostal neuritis or neuralgia,[57-61] costochondritis,[62,63] and slipping rib syndrome.[63-65] The alignment of the lower ribs is greatly affected by muscular interaction of the external oblique, internal oblique, transversus abdominis, and diaphragm (see the following sections, "Abdominal Muscle Length" and "Muscle Performance").

Assessment of the upper extremity muscle length and function is needed to determine if muscle imbalance in the shoulder girdle is contributing to upper rib cage postural malalignment.[29]

Other structural impairments of the rib cage include pectus excavatum, or funnel chest, and pectus carinatum, or pigeon chest (see Figure 4-16). When severe, these conditions can require surgical intervention. Rib cage depression compromising the heart and lungs occurs with severe pectus excavatum.[67] Cosmesis is the most common reason for surgery with pectus carinatum.[66] Both conditions commonly present with a hypokyphosis and scoliosis[67] and are theorized to occur because of overgrowth of costal cartilage.[68]

Only limited information is available on conservative management of pectus excavatum and pectus carinatum.[67,69,70] Physical therapy is believed to be helpful if thoracic or chest wall pain is present in someone with either of these conditions.[69,70] Understanding the biomechanical effect of the structural changes on movement may help guide expectations for treatment. With pectus excavatum because there is a fixed depression of the sternum, during inhalation there is insufficient sternal elevation resulting in decreased pump handle motion of the ribs.[29,56] On the other hand, pectus carinatum is a deformity of the chest characterized by a protrusion of the sternum and ribs. With pectus carinatum there may be insufficient sternal and rib depression during exhalation. Thus, in both cases, there is the potential to develop a secondary ventilatory impairment as well as affect the length of the abdominal and intercostal musculature. In the case of pectus excavatum, the abdominal and intercostal muscles may be shortened, whereas in the case of pectus carinatum, they may be lengthened. Breathing exercises with emphasis on the specific mechanical deficit can be used to improve ventilatory mechanics in either case.[66,70]

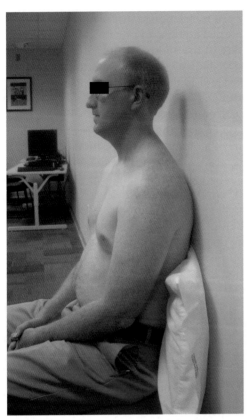

Figure 4-17. Kyphosis, sitting with lumbar support.

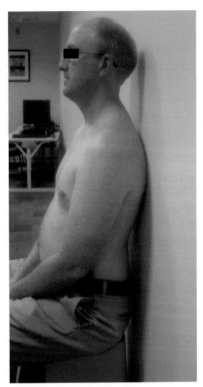

Figure 4-18. Kyphosis, sitting without lumbar support.

Normal Sitting Alignment

Ideal sitting alignment for most people is with the spine erect and supported, the shoulders aligned over the hips, the feet supported, and the hips flexed to 90 degrees.[1,29] In unsupported sitting, normally, the pelvis is in a slight posterior tilt, resulting in flat lumbar spine but relatively unchanged thoracic and cervical spinal alignment when compared to the standing position.[3] Because of the variation in posture and anthropometrics among individuals, no chair or sitting surface is perfect for everyone. For example, a person with a long trunk will require a chair back that is higher than average to maintain adequate support of the spinal column. An individual with a fixed kyphosis should have extra support at the base of the chair back to support the lumbar spine and allow the thoracic spine to rest against the back of the chair (Figures 4-17 and 4-18). In this position, the thorax assumes a vertical alignment, which facilitates good alignment of the cervical spine. Note also that the support at the lumbar spine should not contribute to lumbar extension.[1] In an erect unsupported sitting position, there is a significant increase in the activity of internal obliques and thoracic and lumbar paraspinal musculature as compared to the slumped sitting position.[38] With prolonged slumped sitting, there is a "flexion relaxation phenomenon" that occurs in the thoracic erector spinae muscles.[71,72] Thus, as an individual deviates from an ideal erect position to a more flexed thoracic spine, there is an increased dependence on the passive structures of the spine. Because both erect and relaxed unsupported sitting can be difficult for an individual to maintain, a chair with a back support should be used for prolonged sitting.

Impaired Sitting Alignment

Impaired sitting alignment can be the result of postural alignment impairments, anthropometric variations, and improper environmental factors, including seating surface and work-station configurations. Postural alignment impairments in sitting include a combination of excessive thoracic flexion, rotation, or extension, depending on the habits and alignment of the patient. A patient with thoracic rotation-flexion syndrome may habitually sit with the hips away from the chairback and leaning over onto the armrest. Sitting on one foot or sitting with your legs crossed is a common habit that can contribute to a postural scoliosis and thoracic rotation movement system syndrome. Sitting on the edge of the seat while maintaining the trunk in too erect a position may be noted in individuals with a flat thoracic spine and thoracic extension syndrome. Individuals with a long trunk and short arms are susceptible to leaning over on an armrest because of lack of support while sitting. Individuals with long legs may sit with their knees higher then their hips, causing excessive lumbar and thoracic flexion. Specific seating surface issues need to consider the effect on the thoracic spine. For example, a recliner or low couch may contribute to thoracic flexion. Habitually practicing the piano on a bench without back support may contribute to thoracic extension. The configuration of an office may contribute to thoracic rotation if the patient habitually turns to one side to file, answer the phone, or read the computer monitor. Treatment suggestions for correction of specific sitting postures can be found in the descriptions of the thoracic movement system syndromes and treatment.

MOTION OF THE THORACIC SPINE

Clinical examination of thoracic spine and rib cage motion is critical to determine key components of the syndrome and subsequent treatment. Development of a "clinical eye" for impaired thoracic spine and rib cage motion starts with understanding the kinematic principles related to normal motion. Essential aspects of movement that should be considered include the path of instantaneous center of rotation (PICR) for each motion, the normal amount of accessory and physiological motion available at each joint/region, and specific anatomical considerations unique to the thoracic spine and rib cage.

Thoracic Spine Motion

Across the twelve thoracic vertebrae, motion is cumulative, with each segment contributing relatively small degrees of movement for each direction. In comparison, sagittal plane motion of the thoracic spine segments is more limited than in the cervical and lumbar regions. The amount of motion that is available in the upper and middle thoracic regions is limited by the ribs and sternum. The lower thoracic segments have floating ribs that do not limit mobility as much as true ribs, thus contributing to increased sagittal plane motion in the lower thoracic segments.[2]

During active thoracic flexion and extension, motion should be occurring in all segments; however, the distribution of motion should gradually increase from T1 to T12. Currently, it is accepted that normal thoracic flexion ROM is 30 to 40 degrees, while thoracic extension is 20 to 30 degrees with a combined ROM of 50 to 70 degrees.[3] According to White and Panjabi,[2] for flexion and extension the contribution of motion from each segment is as follows: The upper thoracic spine (T1 to T5) contributes approximately 4 degrees of motion, the middle thoracic spine (T6 to T10) contributes approximately 6 degrees of motion, and the lower thoracic spine (T11 and T12) contributes 12 degrees of motion (Figure 4-19). According to Panjabi et al,[73] the PICR for flexion and extension of the thoracic spine is centered in the body of the inferior vertebrae. During thoracic flexion, there is an anterior-superior translation of the inferior facet of the superior segment, and during extension, there is a posterior-inferior translation of the inferior facet of the superior segment (Figures 4-20 and 4-21). Observation of increased motion at any segment is probably indicative

of increased translation at that segment. Research related to the normal amount of in vivo motion is very limited.

Because of the approximation of the ribs and the orientation of the facets, the amount of lateral bending in the upper and middle thoracic spine is relatively small. The upper and middle regions of the thoracic spine contribute 6 degrees of motion, whereas the lower segments T11 and T12 contribute 8 to 9 degrees of motion at each segment.[2] The total amount of thoracic lateral bending is 25 degrees.[3] The PICR for lateral bending is centered in the lateral half of the body of the inferior nonmoving segment, contralateral to the direction of the motion.[2] For example, during right lateral flexion, as T8 moves to the right, the PICR will be in the left lateral aspect of T9 vertebral body.

In contrast to lateral flexion, there is a greater amount of rotation ROM available in the thoracic spine. In addition, compared to the lumbar spine, the motion of rotation is greater in the thoracic region. Total amount of unilateral rotation in the thoracic region is 30 to 40 degrees.[3,74-76] The upper and middle regions of the thoracic spine demonstrate more rotation ROM than in the lower thoracic region (see Figure 4-19). The angle of the thoracic facets allows increased motion into rotation, especially in the upper and middle thoracic region.[2] White and Panjabi report the following values for rotation: T1 to T10 contributes 8 to 9 degrees of motion from each segment, whereas at the thoracolumbar junction, T11 and T12 only contribute 2 degrees of motion per segment.[2]

Description of the PICR for thoracic rotation differs between sources depending on the study methodology. White and Panjabi's conclusion that the PICR for rotation is located on the endplate and spinal canal of the inferior vertebrae is based on their literature review.[2] Most of the studies included in their review used cadavers with the rib cages removed. Molnar et al[77] used geometric modeling of the thoracic spine with ribs attached and concluded that the PICR is in the anterior portion of the spinal canal. Placement of the PICR for rotation in a more anterior location or lateral location would create spinal cord displacement, which is known as the cigar-cutting effect. Because of these relative small axes of motion, when observing the motions of lateral flexion and rotation, one should observe motion being equally distributed across each segment. Rotation of the thoracic spine should be symmetrical and maintain a relatively vertical axis with minimal lateral movement. Any significant lateral "off axis" translation observed during active thoracic rotation would be considered an impairment. Clinically, thoracic rotation is the most common cause of pain syndromes in the thoracic region.[2,78-80]

The upper thoracic region is believed to demonstrate an ipsilateral coupling pattern of lateral flexion and rotation, similar to the cervical spine, whereas the middle and lower segments demonstrate an inconsistent pattern of coupling.[2,3,81] Recent investigators, however, have noted

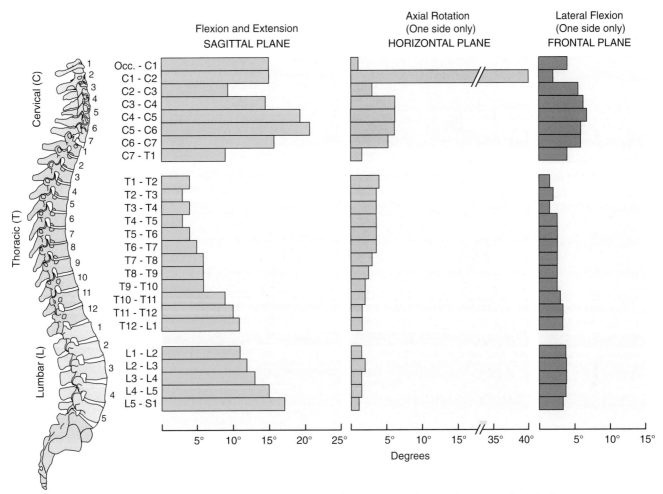

Figure 4-19. Distribution of motion across each segment of the spinal column. (Styled after White AA, Panjabi MM: Kinematics of the spine. In White AA, Panjabi MM, eds: *Clinical biomechanics of the spine*, ed 2, Philadelphia, 1990, Lippincott. In Neumann, DA: *Kinesiology of the musculoskeletal system: foundations for rehabilitation*, ed 2, St Louis, 2010, Mosby.)

that the coupling pattern of lateral flexion and rotation of the thoracic region remains inconsistent across all regions.[82] Generally, end-range of flexion or extension of the thoracic spine will decrease the amount of rotation that is available, resulting in compensatory lateral flexion to gain ROM.[39,74] The ease of motion into flexion and anterior translation causes joint surface approximation and soft tissue tension; subsequently, either rotation or lateral flexion can cause relatively large stresses on the soft tissues in the region of the thoracic spine. A movement examination should include the observation of (1) the starting position of the thoracic spine and (2) the relative segmental contributions for rotation and lateral flexion. Based on these observed movement impairments and the effect on the symptoms, a specific treatment program can be developed.

Incidence of degeneration of the thoracic spine is relative low when compared to the lumbar and cervical spines.[83,84] This difference in the thoracic region has been attributed to a relatively small PICR for the thoracic

spine motions, the load-bearing capacity of the ribs, and the relative small size of the intervertebral discs.[83] Lower segments of the thoracic spine are the most common site of degeneration and disc herniation.[83,84] Atypical symptoms related to neural compromise have been reported in individuals with thoracic herniation, including extremity, abdominal, pelvic, and chest pain.[85-92]

Rib Cage Motion

During ventilation, there is a simultaneous change in the rib cage shape across three planes of motion. During maximum inhalation, there is a slight superior and posterior motion of the thoracic vertebrae causing very slight extension, as well as superior anterior expansion of the rib cage[81,93] (Figure 4-22). Rotation of the ribs occurs during this superior motion along a 35- to 45-degree axis from the demifacets located on the vertebral bodies and discs. During exhalation, there is a reversal of these motions. Pump-handle motion is the sagittal plane or anterior superior motion of the ribs. Bucket-handle

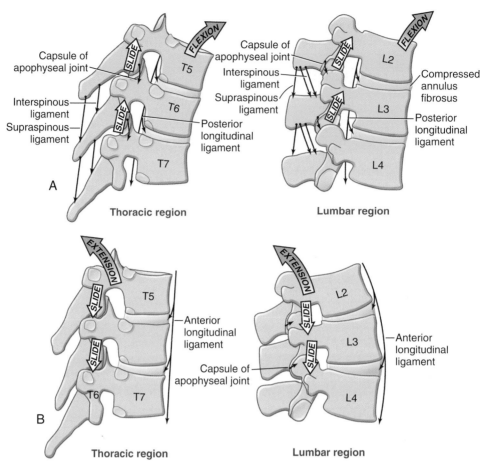

Figure 4-20. A, Thoracic flexion. **B,** Thoracic extension. (Modified from Neumann, DA: *Kinesiology of the musculoskeletal system: foundations for rehabilitation,* ed 2, St Louis, 2010, Mosby.)

motion is the frontal plane or superior lateral motion of the ribs. Clinical assessment of ventilatory motion should include observation of the lateral and anterior aspects of the rib cage and a posterior view of the thoracic spine. The alignment of the trunk and the flexibility of specific vertebral segments contribute to the development of common movement system syndromes. For example, during inhalation, individuals with a thoracic flexion syndrome and a kyphosis have decreased superior motion of the spine, sternum, and anterior rib cage, with an increase in the lateral motion of the rib cage. Individuals with a swayback alignment have excessive posterior motion of the thoracic spine during ventilation. Individuals with a thoracic extension syndrome with a flat thoracic spine have an increase in the superior posterior motion of the spine and superior anterior motion of the sternum and anterior rib cage. Rotation of the thoracic vertebrae causes rotation of the rib cage. Thus, in the case of scoliosis, the rib cage is asymmetrical. Asymmetrical breathing patterns are common in individuals with scoliosis and have been suggested as contributing to imbalances of the trunk musculature.[94]

MUSCULATURE OF THE THORACIC SPINE AND RIB CAGE

Muscles of thoracic spine and rib cage are described by their anatomical location: posterior and anterior. Most of the musculature of the thorax is continuous with other regions, specifically the lumbar spine and the upper extremities; however, this discussion is based on the primary role of a muscle or muscle group as it pertains to the thorax.

Posterior Musculature

Muscles Responsible for Thoracic Motion and Stability

The erector spinae muscle group is the most superficial of the spinal extensors. The muscles of the erector spinae are a complex arrangement of muscle that originates from a common tendinous aponeurosis attached to the sacrum and spinous process of the lumbar and lower thoracic spines.[95] The erector spinae divides into ascending sections by muscle fibers that blend from section to section, terminating at the cervical spine. The mass of

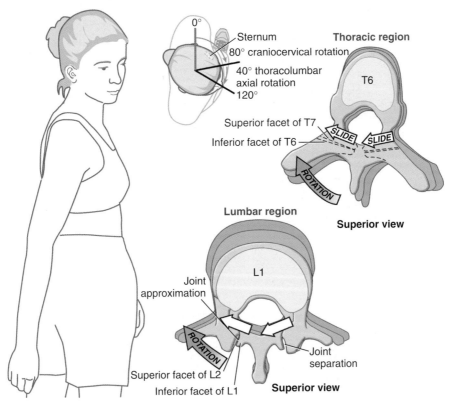

Thoracolumbar axial rotation

Figure 4-21. Rotation. (From Neumann, DA: *Kinesiology of the musculoskeletal system: foundations for rehabilitation*, ed 2, St Louis, 2010, Mosby.)

the erector spinae muscle is greatest in the lumbar and thoracic regions. The three thoracic sections of the erector spinae muscles are iliocostalis thoracis, longissimus thoracis, and spinalis thoracis. The iliocostalis thoracis, the most lateral of the thoracic erector spinae muscles, originates not only from the tendinous origin of the sacrum but also from muscle slips that run from the transverse processes of the lumbar and thoracic regions and ribs. Specifically, the iliocostalis thoracis originates from the lower six ribs, ascending to insert into the upper six ribs. The longissimus thoracis, the intermediate muscle of the thoracic erector spinae, has the largest cross-sectional area of the spinal extensors and originates from the erector spinae aponeurosis and spinous processes of lumbar vertebrae and inserts into the transverse processes and ribs of the lower nine ribs. Finally, the spinalis thoracis, the most medial muscle of the erector spinae group, arises from the vertebral spines of the upper lumbar and lowest thoracic vertebrae. The spinalis thoracis muscle fibers blend with the iliocostalis thoracis laterally and semispinalis thoracis superiorlaterally before inserting on the spinous processes of the upper thoracic vertebrae.

The complexity of this anatomical arrangement provides insight into the motor control requirements specific to the thoracic erector spinae. In standing, isolated contraction of the thoracic erector spinae extends the thoracic spine without necessarily extending the lumbar spine. Contraction of the lumbar erector spinae without simultaneous contraction of the thoracic erector spinae, contributes to lumbar extension and/or a posterior lower thoracic trunk sway. Thus the thoracic spine can be flexed while the lumbar spine is extended. Another possibility is flexion of the upper thoracic spine with posterior translation/extension at the thoracolumbar junction. Clinically, the differences in regional control of the erector spinae muscles enable the patient to hold the lumbar spine and thoracolumbar junction stable while moving the thoracic spine out of flexion.

From the upright position, bilateral erector spinae contraction extends the spine. When bending forward, the erector spinae work eccentrically until approximately two thirds into the range,[96] at which point their activity normally subsides and the trunk motion is controlled by the eccentric activity of the hip extensors. A similar pattern in reverse occurs with the return to the upright position. Erector spinae activity is necessary in the upright position to counter the force of gravity. The thoracic erector spinae have a greater percentage of type I muscle fibers than lumbar erector spinae muscles,

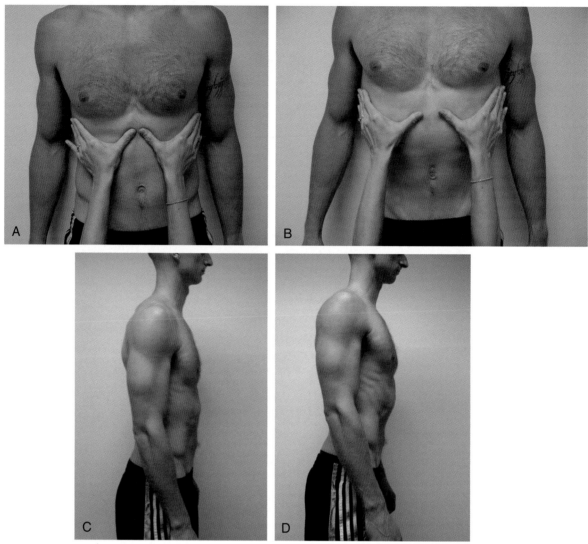

Figure 4-22. Ventilation. Four views: **A,** Subcostal angle at rest. **B,** Subcostal angle with inhale. **C,** Side view at rest. **D,** Elevation of rib cage with inhale.

suggesting a greater reliance on the thoracic erector spinae for postural support.[96,97] Not all authors agree on the contribution of the unilateral erector spinae to thoracic rotation or lateral flexion[3,29,80,96]; however, recent work using intramuscular electromyography (EMG) has demonstrated that the longissimus thoracis is active during seated ipsilateral trunk rotation and lateral flexion.[80,99] The capacity of the longissimus thoracic for torque production during rotation may be greater in the upper thoracic spine than in the lower thoracic spine.[80]

Contraction of the right longissimus thoracis during left arm movement would help offset the trunk flexion, rotation, and lateral flexion moments.[100] Thus, using arm motions to help promote thoracic muscle activity is a useful treatment strategy. Instructions are given to the patient to maintain thoracic spine and rib cage stability while flexing the shoulder. Initially the patient may need to perform this with the elbow flexed to shorten the lever arm and reduce the load. As control improves, the shoulder can be flexed with the elbow in extension or an elastic band can be used for added resistance to the shoulder motion. Alternatively, the patient could lift a weight from counter height and hold it in his hands while maintaining the appropriate thoracic alignment; this could be done using one or both hands, depending on the ability to control the rotatory force.

Thoracic kyphosis creates a shorter lever arm for the erector spinae while placing the muscles in lengthened position, forcing them to generate large extension moments to counter the effects of gravity.[101] These large extension moments create increased spinal compression. In addition to the change in muscle force, the center of gravity moves anterior as a result of the thoracic kyphosis, further compounding the situation.[101] Clinically, the implications of this are that we must help our patients correct their postural kyphosis and minimize progression, if structural. The patient with structural kyphosis will require greater finesse in exercise and postural correction because compensatory extension in the other areas of the spine must be avoided.

The intermediate layer of spinal extensor muscles is comprised of semispinalis thoracis, the multifidi, and the rotatores. In each of these muscle groups, the number of spinal segments crossed by the muscles progressively decreases when moving from superficial to deep. For example, the semispinalis thoracis will cross six to eight spinal segments, the multifidi cross two to four segments, and the rotatores usually span only one to two segments.[3,95] This arrangement permits the smaller muscles to have more precise control over their respective segments. The thoracic rotatores are most developed compared to the other regions in the spine, yet their exact purpose is not fully understood.[3,96] These muscles are thought to be more "position sensors than torque producers,"[96] so their contribution to motor control in the thoracic spine is important.

Multiple studies have investigated lumbar muscle EMG activity in both normals and subjects with low back pain; however, by comparison, there are very few publications that have examined the muscle activity in the thoracic region. Despite the regional proximity, assumptions that the thoracic spine musculature would behave similarly to the lumbar should not be made because the thoracic spine motion and muscle activity are complicated by the rib cage[80] and differences in facet joint orientation.[2] In response to arm movement, the multifidus activity in the lumbar spine was independent of force direction[102]; however, the activity of the thoracic multifidus was dependent on the direction of arm motion so that right arm movement was associated with electromylographic (EMG) activity in the right thoracic multifidus muscles.[80] During sitting trunk rotation, the activity of the thoracic multifidus was variable. Bilateral activity of the multifidus occurred in upper thoracic segments during trunk rotation, but no consistent pattern of activity was found for the multifidus in the middle and lower thoracic spine.[80] The authors suggest that the multifidus function in the middle and lower thoracic spine may be to control rotational forces.[80]

The interspinales and intertransversarii are the deepest layer of the posterior spinal muscles. This muscle group is thought to be absent in the thoracic region by some,[3] and others report the presence of these muscles in only the upper and lower segments of the thoracic spine.[29,95] The significance of these muscles in the thoracic spine is not known.

Although the quadratus lumborum muscle attaches to the twelfth rib, its influence on the thoracic spine is mainly through the stabilization that it provides to the pelvis and lumbar spine.

Extremity Muscles with Spinal Origin

The latissimus dorsi muscle originates from the lumbodorsal fascia; the last three or four ribs; and spinous processes of the sacral, lumbar, and the lower six thoracic vertebrae. The muscle traverses laterally and superiorly to insert on the humerus. With the insertion of the latissimus held relatively stable, bilateral contraction of the muscle will assist with anterior pelvic tilt and spinal extension. If acting unilaterally, contraction of the latissimus produces a rotation moment on the lumbar and lower half of the thoracic spine. According to Porterfield and DeRosa,[104] the latissimus dorsi muscle has a long moment arm, thus small forces generated from this muscle can easily influence the mechanics of the spine. Passive tension from the latissimus dorsi muscle should also be considered. Shortness or stiffness of the muscle may induce spinal rotation with unilateral arm motion or spinal extension with bilateral shoulder flexion. Because the latissimus muscle originates from the lower half of the thoracic spine, its effect will be noted in the lower half of the thoracic spine. With stiffness or excessive recruitment of this muscle, there is the potential for extension and/or rotational asymmetry to develop in the lower and midthoracic region.[81] Imbalance of the latissimus can contribute to excessive flexibility at the midthoracic level because the lower segments are pulled into rotation while the upper segments remain neutral.

The trapezius and rhomboid muscles are also upper extremity muscles with origins on the thoracic spine. The middle and lower trapezius originate on the thoracic vertebrae, first through fifth and sixth through twelfth, respectively.[29] The rhomboid muscles run from the spinous processes of the thoracic vertebrae first to fifth down to the medial border of the scapula. When contracting bilaterally, either the trapezius or the rhomboid muscles can produce an extension moment on the thoracic spine.[96] Clinically, this is can be seen in individuals with a flattened thoracic spine; rhomboid muscle contraction is associated with extension of thoracic spine in the interscapular area. Similar to the latissimus, unilateral contraction of the rhomboid and trapezius muscles can cause contralateral rotation of the thoracic spine.

Anterior Musculature

Generally, abdominal muscles are recognized as having a variety of essential functions: support and protect the internal organs, assist with exhalation, and provide both stabilization and movement of the trunk. Probably less understood is what constitutes ideal abdominal performance. There is often an exaggerated emphasis on abdominal strength, especially the RA, and little attention is paid to motor control. The influence of abdominal muscle length on abdominal muscle function is often underappreciated. Assessment of abdominal muscle length, recruitment patterns, and performance are an important part of a thorough thoracic examination. Furthermore, treating patients with pain syndromes by indiscriminately issuing abdominal exercises may perpetuate their thoracic movement impairments.

Abdominal Muscle Length

Ideal abdominal muscle length promotes ideal trunk alignment. Optimal resting length of each of the abdominal muscles holds the spine, rib cage, and pelvis in the correct position. Because passive tension of the abdominal musculature contributes to postural control, the efficiency of maintaining good trunk alignment is greatly enhanced when the abdominal muscles are at ideal length. Consider the effect that a short RA muscle will have on trunk alignment. Individuals with a short RA muscle appear to have a depressed chest, and the thoracic spine will be kyphotic (Figure 4-23) or swayed posterior because the anterior thorax is pulled down toward the anterior rim of the pelvis. This is because the primary action of the RA muscle, which runs from the pubic rim of the pelvis up to the costal margins of the fifth through seventh ribs and xiphoid process, is to curl the trunk by approximating the sternum to the anterior pelvis.[29] In athletic populations, the RA muscle is often overdeveloped with "sit-up"-type exercises that lead to shortness or an increased stiffness of the muscle. Shortness of the RA muscle can contribute to movement impairments, as well as alignment impairments, by limiting thoracic extension; individuals may perform lumbar extension as a compensation for the lack of thoracic extension. Although the individual appears to have brought the thorax to a more upright position, what has occurred is an exaggeration of the curves in the thoracic and lumbar spines (see Figure 4-28, *B*).

As with the RA muscle, the relationship between standing alignment and length of the oblique abdominal muscles should be considered. An individual who habitually stands in a swayback alignment places the fibers of the external obliques in a lengthened position while the fibers of the internal obliques are slightly shortened.[29] Habitual assumption of a swayback standing posture shifts the center of mass posterior so that the abdominal muscles, RA and internal obliques muscles in particular, play a greater role in holding the upright position, acting as antigravity muscles.

The length of the internal and external oblique muscles is reflected, in part by the subcostal angle. An ideal subcostal angle of approximately 90 degrees is considered to be a reflection of balance between the internal and external obliques.[1] A subcostal angle greater than 90 degrees may indicate shortness of the internal oblique muscles or excessive length of the external oblique muscles, with the latter often the case in individuals who have poor abdominal tone. The individual who routinely has performed abdominal crunches as the main abdominal exercise would be expected to develop shortness or stiffness in the internal oblique (as well as the RA muscle). The result is this individual's subcostal angle may be greater than 90 degrees. Contraction of the internal oblique muscles that

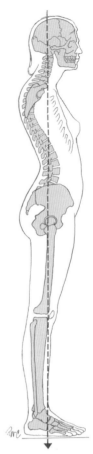

Figure 4-23. Exaggeration of the curves in the thoracic and lumbar spines. (From Kendall FP, McCreary EK, Provance PG: *Muscles: testing and function*, ed 4, Philadelphia, 1993, Lippincott Williams & Wilkins.)

run obliquely in the superomedial direction from the iliac crest to the linea alba and the lower ribs, pulls the thorax toward the pelvis and widens the subcostal angle. Conversely, a narrow subcostal angle could indicate shortness/stiffness of the external oblique muscles. The anterior fibers of the external oblique muscles run inferomedially from the fifth to twelfth ribs toward the linea alba, inguinal ligament, and the anterior pelvic rim. The angle of pull of the external oblique muscles decreases the subcostal angle. The upper fibers of the transversus abdominis muscle may have some ability to narrow the subcostal angle.[29]

Another form of asymmetry commonly found in the abdominal muscles is an alteration in the resting length of the internal and external obliques on one side compared to the other. An individual who has repeatedly rotated the trunk to the right to perform work duties may develop a postural impairment of rib cage rotation to the right and shortness of the left external oblique muscle compared to the right internal oblique muscle. Additionally, the right internal oblique would be expected to be shorter than the left internal oblique. The subcostal margin would be asymmetrical so that the left subcostal margin would be closer to midline than the right (Figure 4-24). The habit of sitting on one's foot or leaning over onto the armrest produces lateral trunk flexion, which can also lead to development of length asymmetries in abdominal muscles. The alteration of length depends on the frequency and constancy of assuming such positions, as well as what other activities or positions the individual performs to reverse the lateral trunk flexion/rotation. An individual with poor abdominal muscle tone is probably more likely to develop this postural scoliosis because they lack the normal muscle stiffness that would help to "derotate" the trunk.

Although the subcostal angle is a useful guide for determining the length of the oblique abdominal muscles, it should not be considered an absolute indicator; variations will occur between individuals because of their body structure, pulmonary dysfunction, or other conditions such as ankylosing spondylitis. The length of the oblique musculature can be assessed further by observing the

movement of the rib cage and subcostal angle with inhalation and with full-arm elevation (Figure 4-25). Average rib cage expansion is 5 to 10 cm[106] going from maximum exhalation to maximum inhalation; with age, rib cage motion does decrease,[106,107] so values on the lower end of normal would be expected in older individuals. Less than 3 cm change in rib cage motion would be considered impaired expansion. Expansion of the rib cage and widening of the subcostal angle during inhalation will be limited by shortness in the abdominal muscles. The limitation in motion will be greater with arms elevated overhead. Failure of the rib cage to expand is a potential sign of shortness in both internal and external oblique muscles. If the subcostal angle does not widen when the subject inhales with the arms overhead, the external oblique muscle is implicated. Limited range of motion and lateral trunk flexion toward the contralateral side may be another indicator of short abdominal muscles. Conclusions about abdominal muscle length should be based on evaluation of the patient's age, body habitus, activity level, and movement tests.

Development of abdominal muscle shortness can occur by overexercising the muscles or continually adopting postures that allow the abdominal muscle to rest at a shortened length. The general public seems to be under the perception that the abdominal muscles cannot be exercised too much. However, excessive abdominal exercise can lead to muscle imbalances as described previously. The imbalance in the abdominal muscle contributes to movement impairments but may have other consequences. Shortness or stiffness of the oblique abdominal muscles can interfere with the ability of the inspiratory muscles to lift and flare the rib cage. Because the oblique muscles assist with exhalation during strenuous breathing, aerobic activity may perpetuate the muscle shortness. Importantly, an increase in the compression forces on the thoracic spine and rib cage may result from oblique abdominal muscle shortness. Some individuals may be creating greater stresses on their thoracic spine by working on abdominal strengthening exercises.

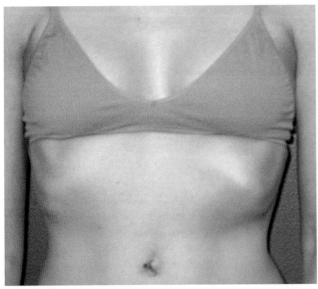

Figure 4-24. Left subcostal margin would be closer to midline than the right.

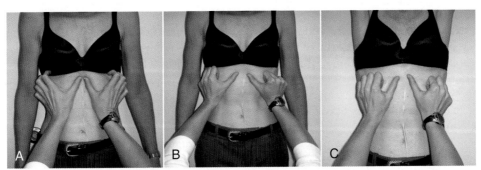

Figure 4-25. Length of the oblique musculature can be assessed further by observing the movement of the rib cage and subcostal angle with inhalation and full-arm elevation. **A,** At rest with narrow subcostal angle. **B,** With inhalation, the angle widens. **C,** Inhalation with arms over the head. The angle does not widen as much as with arms at side.

Muscle Performance

Using the term *muscle performance* to describe the abdominal function encompasses both parameters of strength and recruitment. Defining abdominal muscle function based only on the results of standard manual muscle testing (MMT), such as the leg lowering test, would dismiss the importance of motor control.[108] Stability of the spine and rib cage requires coordinated activation of the abdominal muscles. Modulation of abdominal muscle activity to meet specific functional demands is crucial for appropriate spinal stabilization. Deficits in abdominal muscle motor control have been found in subjects with low back pain[109,110]; however, it is not known if similar motor control impairments exist in the thoracic spine. Furthermore, it is not clear if the alteration in muscle activation patterns is the cause or the effect of the low back pain. Although little attention has been directed at the relationship between thoracic pain syndromes and abdominal muscle performance, some insights may be gleaned from the work examining their affect on the lumbar spine, but caution is advised in attempting to generalize results across spinal segments.

One of the most important functions of the abdominal muscles is to provide isometric support to resist compensatory spinal motions during extremity motion.[1] Porterfield and DeRosa state that ideally the abdominals function as antirotators and antilateral flexors.[104] The anatomical arrangement of the internal and external oblique RA and the transverse abdominus muscles is such that when working optimally, they provide stability of the spine and rib cage. During extremity movements, the trunk should be a stable foundation; the abdominal muscles play a major role by countering the rotational moments placed on the thorax and spine during limb movement.[100,104] Although the oblique muscles are thought of as rotators and lateral flexors of the trunk, their role in providing stability is achieved by resisting those rotational forces. The abdominal muscles continue to be a major source of trunk stability even when the trunk is in flexion, extension, or lateral flexion.[112]

During lower extremity movements, the external oblique muscles help prevent anterior pelvic tilt and work with the internal oblique muscles to prevent rotation of the pelvis. When the pelvis is stabilized, the external and internal oblique muscles should control rotation of the rib cage and thoracic spine. A common movement impairment seen in the thoracic region is rotation of the thorax during extremity motion. This impairment can be found even in individuals who do regular abdominal exercise, usually because their exercise strategies have focused on strength and not control. Treatment of the rotational impairment is accomplished by having the patient practice extremity movements while focusing on maintaining rib cage and spine stability. Often, this exercise must be started at a very low level and then progressed as the patient demonstrates the ability to control the motion.

For example, a patient with pronounced weakness of the abdominal muscles and excessive flexibility in the thorax may need to start exercising by lying supine, contracting abdominals, and easily moving one arm overhead toward flexion. The patient would stop the motion of the arm when rib cage or spinal motion was detected; initially the patient may move through only a limited ROM but with continued practiced should achieve full flexion. Movements of the arm into horizontal abduction would be considered a progression because the abducted position will tend to rotate the thorax. Higher level exercises may use resistance. Exercise movements that target the latissimus dorsi or serratus anterior will require activity of the external oblique to oppose the forces on the rib cage.[1] Lower extremity motions are useful to not only assess abdominal muscle performance and stability of the thorax but also as a method of challenging the muscles.

The TA muscle is often referred to as a *muscular corset*. The activity of the TA muscle has traditionally been considered to be a spinal stabilizer, in part by increasing intraabdominal pressure (IAP). The role of the TA in spinal stabilization has been shown to be minimal.[110a] Increasing IAP does increase spinal stiffness,[111,113] which can help prevent tissue strain.[111] Contraction of the TA muscle does increase IAP via its insertion into the lumbar fascia[111]; however, its contributions to trunk mechanics may be more complex than that of a corset. The TA muscle has been shown to be active with trunk rotation[114] and interestingly, differential activation within portions of the TA.[115] Urquhart and Hodges[115] used a paradigm of pelvic rotation with the thorax fixed and found that the lower and middle regions of the TA muscle were active during contralateral rotation of the pelvis and the upper fibers during ipsilateral rotation. The authors suggested several possible explanations for the apparent contradictory activity of the TA muscle: (1) stabilization of the linea alba and aponeuroses against the pull of the internal oblique or internal obliques, (2) control of the motion of the rib cage and lumbar spine via insertion onto the lumbodorsal fascia, or (3) the contraction served to increase the intraabdominal pressure.[115] These new insights into the function of this muscle correspond to anatomical studies documenting variations in fiber direction within the TA: The upper fibers are oriented horizontally and the middle and lower fibers are angled somewhat inferomedially.[116]

Another example of regional distinction in the TA muscle was noted during arm movements: Recruitment of the upper portion of the TA muscle was delayed in response to arm movement compared to middle and lower regions.[117] Initial investigations into the activity of the TA with extremity movement did not demonstrate differential activity of the muscle dependent on the direction of the arm.[118,119] According to Hodges, the activity of the TA would not depend on the direction of force if it contributes to spinal control through modulation of intraabdominal pressure.[113]

The RA muscle is aligned in such a manner that it does not provide any significant control over rotation.[120,121] Therefore exercise programs that emphasize the RA muscle may lead to a compromise in the control of rotation.[1] Furthermore, RA muscle exercises are often issued with the intent of targeting either the upper or lower portion of the muscle.[122,123] However, in EMG studies, no difference was found between activation of the upper and lower portions of the muscle during common exercise maneuvers.[124] Previous studies that may have demonstrated a difference in activity were flawed because the EMG signals were not normalized.

Treatment of thoracic pain syndromes often involves working on trunk muscle control so that both the abdominals and the posterior trunk muscles work synergistically. Instructing the patient to focus on maintaining stability of the spine, rib cage, and pelvis during extremity movements is a useful strategy aimed at improving motor control. This approach is also ideal when considering the length-tension relationship of the abdominals because performing exercises with the trunk in a neutral alignment works the abdominals at their ideal length. Stabilizing the thorax during movements of the extremities is usually easiest in supine and becomes more difficult when the patient moves into sitting, quadruped, or standing.[117] When lying supine, the compliance of the rib cage is decreased[107]; therefore controlling unwanted rib cage motion should be easier for the patient. Exercises can be adapted to meet the specific needs of the patient. It is worth emphasizing that patients may have the ability to generate sufficient force with their abdominals but still lack the precise control needed. The greater the demands the patient places on his or her body, the greater precision needed from the trunk muscles. For example, a competitive tennis player needs to demonstrate the ability to move the arm against resistance while maintaining spine and rib cage stability in standing. In contrast, a sedentary 65-year-old patient may only be able to move one arm up overhead without allowing the rib cage to move while in the supine position.

With nonstructural alignment impairments, the patient should actively correct the alignment and maintain the correction. This can be done intermittently throughout the day and as the patient gains endurance, the alignment correction can be held for longer periods of time. Holding the corrected position will result in the muscles working at the appropriate length. Eventually, the postural correction can be maintained with mostly passive muscle tension. As discussed earlier, thoracic pain syndromes are frequently associated with alterations in tissue properties and the development of excessive flexibility in specific directions. Although some may consider this to be mostly an arthrokinematic dysfunction, reversal of the dysfunction will best be achieved by teaching the

patient appropriate trunk muscle recruitment, so the patient can limit or stop the undesired motion.

There are those patients, usually very sedentary, who are unable to readily recruit their abdominal muscles. Having these patients practice abdominal contractions in sitting or standing so that they pull in against the abdominal contents will improve their success. They may spend a week between visits practicing the isolation of abdominal contraction versus inhalation or Valsalva maneuver.

Extensive discussion of the mechanics of breathing is beyond this text; however, a review of the basic kinesiology is warranted. Contraction of the diaphragm will widen the subcostal angle and increase the chest volume as it descends toward the abdomen and compresses the viscera. The increase in chest volume is proportional to the rib cage displacement.[125] The resistance of the abdominal muscles, viscera, and the intercostals improves the efficiency of the diaphragm. Optimal performance of the diaphragm relies on a balance between the muscles of ventilation; if the resistance from the intercostals and the oblique abdominal muscles is excessive because of muscle shortness or stiffness, then the diaphragm will be required to work harder during inhalation. Conversely, lack of resistance from abdominal musculature and the intercostals also creates an imbalance that can manifest in two common patterns known as *paradoxical breathing*. In one pattern, when the diaphragm contracts and there is insufficient resistance from the abdominal muscles, the abdomen bulges outward, limiting the need for rib cage expansion. Such is the case with individuals with abdominal muscle paralysis; contraction of their diaphragm will cause abdominal distention rather than chest expansion. The second type of paradoxical breathing occurs when the abdomen is drawn inward during inhalation, which commonly occurs when there is weakness of the diaphragm and is seen in individuals who are ventilator-dependent.

Clinically, what can be observed in a neurologically intact person is inhalation as a substitute for abdominal muscle contraction. A common error when attempting to contract abdominal muscles by "pulling the belly in" is to inhale by contracting the diaphragm or the accessory muscles of inhalation rather than the abdominals, which are muscles of exhalation. Appropriate contraction of the abdominal muscles should flatten the abdomen, change the firmness of the external obliques, and often narrow the infrasternal angle. Treatment should include education and practice to correct the coordination impairment by having the individual gently blow outward as he or she contracts the abdominal muscles.

The traditional view of intercostal muscle function is that the external intercostal muscles elevate the ribs and therefore are considered inspiratory muscles; the internal intercostals, with fibers angled downward and dorsally, pull the ribs closer together assisting with expiration.

Other authors believe that rather than opposing functions, the intercostal muscles work together to stabilize the rib cage against the pull of the diaphragm and the fluctuating pressure in the thorax.[96] This belief is supported by EMG activity of both the internal and external intercostals during both phases of ventilation.[126,127] The anatomical location of the intercostals may explain what appears to be a dichotomy in their function. The expiratory mechanical advantage of the internal intercostals decreases moving from bottom to top of rib cage and the most anterior portion, often as parasternal intercostals, become inspiratory muscles.[128] Although the intercostal muscles are considered primarily ventilatory muscles, EMG studies have demonstrated activity of the intercostals during trunk rotation.[129] Using indwelling electrodes placed in the lateral intercostals, Whitelaw[129] demonstrated that the internal intercostals were active with ipsilateral rotation and the external intercostals were active during contralateral rotation. The activity in muscles was much greater than the activity during breathing. Although the intercostals may assist with trunk rotation, their operating range and their force-generating capacity would be less than that of the abdominals.

MOVEMENT SYSTEM SYNDROMES
of the Thoracic Spine

Movement system syndromes of the thoracic spine are named for the alignment or movement direction that deviates the most from optimal alignment or movement patterns, as follows:

- Thoracic rotation-flexion syndrome
- Thoracic flexion syndrome
- Thoracic rotation-extension syndrome
- Thoracic rotation syndrome
- Thoracic extension syndrome

During an examination, correction of the impaired alignment or movement pattern usually decreases or eliminates the symptoms; however, in many cases of thoracic flexion syndrome, correction of the flexed posture may result in a slight temporary increase in pain. Clinical observation suggests that often even a severe kyphotic posture does not reproduce pain, although the patient may notice some discomfort when modifying the position. Yet, correction of the kyphosis when possible is usually indicated, and even if the patient is unable to fully correct the kyphosis, a partial correction is desirable. In the case of thoracic rotation, modification of the rotation can decrease the symptoms. Correction of excessive thoracic extension can immediately reduce or eliminate the symptoms. In all of the syndromes except the flexion syndromes, alignments or movement impairments that are accompanied by symptoms are weighted more heavily than impairments that do not reproduce pain.

The examination consists of alignment and movement tests of the spine, rib cage, and extremities in a variety of positions. The patient's preferred strategy for assuming an alignment or performing a movement test is termed the *primary test*. Those primary tests that produce or increase the patient's symptoms are followed by a secondary test in which the examiner modifies the movement or alignment and symptom behavior is reported. The location of the patient's pain should be correlated to the region of impaired motion. For example, in a patient with a flat upper thoracic spine and a kyphotic lower thoracic spine and pain in the upper thoracic region, the patient who complains of increased pain when sitting erect is most likely to have a thoracic extension syndrome. Conversely, a patient with the same postural impairments but with pain in the lower thoracic region will most likely have a thoracic flexion syndrome. Although the results of some tests may be more meaningful when determining the diagnosis, the examination is considered combinatorial (rather than algorithmic) so that all of the results of all key tests are used to verify the movement system diagnosis.

Both scapular muscle strain and cervical dysfunction can create pain in the upper thoracic area. For example, pain along the vertebral border of the scapula is characteristic of a cervical spine syndrome[130] (see Chapter 3). Strain of the scapular adductors, consistent with either scapular abduction syndrome or scapular downward rotation syndrome,[1] may mimic a thoracic syndrome because of the overlapping regions of pain. Distinguishing the primary source of pain in patients with midthoracic region pain can be difficult because arm motions stress both the thoracic spine and scapular region. However, if the midthoracic pain is reproduced during lower extremity motions, for example, hip abduction-lateral rotation in supine, then the thoracic spine is implicated as the source of pain. It is possible that more than one area is implicated as a source of a patient's symptoms. A careful systematic examination of the patient will assist in determining the cause of the pain.

Therapists should be aware that the etiology of pain in the thoracic region has a higher likelihood of arising from nonmusculoskeletal sources than other spinal regions.* The therapist must be alert for atypical symptom behavior and other systemic signs or symptoms that the patient may not have associated with the thoracic pain.[135,138,139] Suspicion of visceral or systemic pathology warrants a referral to the patient's physician. Examples of musculoskeletal symptoms suggesting conditions that also warrant a referral to the physician are compression fractures,[140,141] possible disc herniation, or lower extremity neurological complaints that may implicate cord involvement.[87,136,142] Lower extremity neurological complaints may implicate spinal cord involvement, therefore new or unexplained neurological findings should be assessed by a physician. Additional information on screening for pathology is available through other sources.[135]

---

*References 89, 91, 92, 131, 132, 135, and 136.

Conversely, there are several cases in the literature of musculoskeletal problems disguising themselves as visceral pathology.[80,90,134] Therapists working in conjunction with physicians can be instrumental in identifying musculoskeletal causes of visceral, cardiac, or urogenital symptoms.

Compressive forces on the thoracic spine have the potential to contribute to symptoms across all of the different thoracic movement system syndromes. For individuals who report a height loss of 3 to 5 cm or more,[143-145] there is probably a greater likelihood that compression is a contributing factor to their symptoms. Shortness or hypertrophy of the thoracic paraspinals and overdevelopment of the abdominals will add to spinal compression. Compression forces on the spine are greater in unsupported sitting and standing when compared to a recumbent position. Therefore, if compression is a factor, the patient usually has fewer symptoms when lying down. The effect of compression can be assessed by manually lifting the patient's rib cage with the patient in the upright position. The therapist's open hands are placed on each side of the rib cage and while pressing inward, an upward force is applied to the rib cage to help "unload" the spine. If symptoms are reduced with this maneuver, it is likely that compression is contributing to the patient's symptoms. Location of the hands along the rib cage will be dictated by the symptoms, for example, upper thoracic symptoms would require the hands to be placed closer to the axilla. If the patient has radicular symptoms, hand placement directly over the symptomatic region should be avoided. In the patient with osteopenia, manual rib cage elevation should be done very gently. If osteoporosis is present, manual rib cage elevation should be avoided because of the risk of rib fracture.

In all likelihood, pain syndromes develop because of impairments in motor control, muscle generation of force, and changes in tissue stiffness. In other words, the cause of thoracic pain, similar to low back pain, is multifactorial and in certain patients, one component of dysfunction may be a greater contributing factor than another. Rehabilitation of patients will be most successful if treatment is aimed at restoring normal alignment, movement, and muscle recruitment patterns.

THORACIC ROTATION-FLEXION SYNDROME

Thoracic rotation-flexion syndrome is characterized by pain associated with the movement and postures of thoracic flexion and rotation. Asymmetries of the rib cage with a thoracic kyphosis and/or posterior trunk sway are common alignment impairments observed in this syndrome. Common muscle impairments include asymmetry in the length and recruitment of the trunk muscles, including long thoracic paraspinal muscles and scapulothoracic muscles (middle trapezius, rhomboids); short or stiff shoulder girdle muscles (pectoralis minor and major, latissimus dorsi), and the RA muscle; and asymmetrical

length and strength of the oblique abdominal muscles. Motor recruitment dominance of the RA muscle is common in this syndrome. Compression of the spine and asymmetrical approximation of the ribs should be considered contributing factors to pain. There is a paradoxical relationship to the amount of thoracic flexion and the presence of pain; thoracic flexion is easily performed because of the shape of the thoracic facets and the anterior load of the rib cage and upper extremities. Plus, pure thoracic flexion without a rotation component to the motion is commonly not painful. However, excessive posturing or movement into flexion of the thoracic spine is a contributing factor to biomechanical stress that can cause musculoskeletal pain in this region. Creep of the connective tissues of the thoracic spine elongating the posterior elements (posterior longitudinal ligament) while compressing the anterior elements (vertebral bodies and discs) of the spine will occur with prolonged flexion. Thus an individual who spends increased time with the thoracic spine in a flexed position will demonstrate pain when attempting to rapidly improve alignment by straightening the thoracic curve. This individual may be unable to fully correct the posture because the prolonged mechanical stresses have created a structural change at the vertebral bodies, discs, and posterior longitudinal ligament. In addition, rotation occurs early and readily once the thoracic spine is flexed because of the opening of the facets and posterior aspect of intervertebral bodies. Thus flexion with rotation of the thoracic spine would increase not only the anterior forces on the spine but also create asymmetrical compressive forces along the ribs and their attachments into the sternum.

Symptoms and History

Individuals with the thoracic rotation-flexion syndrome complain of pain in the thoracic region, which may radiate into the lateral and anterior rib cage or abdomen. They will note an increase in pain with lying down, reaching, or trunk rotation. Ventilation is affected so that pain occurs with forceful exhalation.[134,146-148] Common recreational activities reported by individuals with a rotation-flexion syndrome include any activity that repeatedly places their trunk into flexion and rotation such as crew, squash, golf, diving, and running (asymmetrical arm swing and trunk rotation). Habitual trunk flexion with rotation during functional activities include arranging the desk so that flexion and/or rotation is required to reach the phone, computer, and files or greet incoming customers/clients. Other habits are sitting shifted to one side (leaning toward the mouse pad side of the desk), sitting on one foot, or leaning on an armrest while working, reading, driving, or watching television. Pain with sitting is reduced or abolished when the individual uses a backrest to keep the spine more erect and to avoid asymmetrical postures such as leg crossing, unilateral armrest use, or sitting on one foot. Individuals with a rotation-flexion syndrome may have a history of loss of motion at the glenohumeral joint because of a frozen shoulder or a rotator cuff injury or a history of chest surgery in which the rib cage or sternum has been surgically manipulated.

Key Tests and Signs

Standing Alignment

Thoracic kyphosis with an asymmetry of the rib cage will be the most common alignment impairment found in this syndrome. Sway of the trunk posterior to the axis of the hip combined with thoracic flexion and asymmetry of the rib cage is also commonly observed in individuals with a thoracic rotation-flexion syndrome. The presence of rib cage asymmetry can be noted from either an anterior or posterior view. The shape of the rib cage and its effect on the position of the scapulae should be noted. A posterior rib cage asymmetry may cause the alignment of the scapulae to appear asymmetrical, because the structural base (rib cage) upon which the scapulae are resting is asymmetrical. An anterior rib cage asymmetry may cause the size or shape of the breast to appear asymmetrical.

Scoliosis may be present, although it is more common for scoliosis to present with a loss of the thoracic curve (as in the thoracic rotation-extension diagnosis). Scoliosis with a thoracic flexion alignment impairment occurs in older individuals who have degenerative changes or who have performed trunk-curl exercises. Passive elevation of the rib cage when pain is present unloads the weight of the upper trunk on the thoracic region and relieves symptoms for individuals with pain from compression.

If a structural kyphosis is suspected, observation of the spinal alignment in supine, prone, and a quadruped position should be done. A structural kyphosis is implicated if there is no reduction in the kyphosis in these alternate positions. The quadruped position is an especially useful position for assessing the amount of extension available in the thoracic spine because it allows unloading of the thoracic spine, and this position often relieves the patient's pain. In this position, it may be helpful to cue the patient to relax the abdominal musculature and lower the apex of the spinal curve. If a structural kyphosis is present, accommodation of the fixed kyphosis is necessary in the treatment planning.

Movement Impairment Analysis

Standing tests. Standing trunk flexion demonstrates excessive flexion and rotation in the thoracic spine; in addition, the presence of a rib hump is more noticeable in a thoracic flexed position compared to standing. The motions of trunk rotation and lateral flexion demonstrate an asymmetry in motion and/or pain with these movements. Either motion may cause a radicular symptom into the chest or abdomen because of neural compromise at either the vertebral foramen or along the length of the ribs. Unilateral shoulder flexion, which is a test for the presence of spine motion during extremity motion,

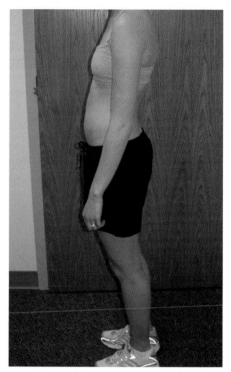

Figure 4-26. Kyphosis-lordosis.

results in variation side to side. Thus, with arm motion there is a resulting motion at the spine and rib cage with or without reproduction of the symptoms. Bilateral shoulder flexion demonstrates an increase in thoracic flexion or sway with unilateral trunk rotation. In the presence of a kyphosis-lordosis alignment impairment (Figure 4-26), rotation may also be present in addition to the increased thoracic and lumbar curves. With both unilateral and bilateral shoulder flexion, pain and motion will be improved if the trunk is supported either by a wall or lying recumbent. The spine will be straighter and aided in the prevention of rotation with the extremity movement. Caution should be used when considering cueing for recruitment of the abdominal musculature for trunk control during this follow-up test, since the increased flexion and spine compression may increase the individual's pain during arm motion. If the individual presents in an early stage of rehabilitation, protection of the thoracic spine and neural tissue can be achieved by performing supported shoulder flexion while facing the wall. Thus the weight of the upper body can be unloaded by the wall, the thoracic spine can be easily extended without overcorrection. The exercises can be progressed once the patient has advanced to a rehabilitation stage to strengthen the thoracic paraspinal muscles in the same position by active shoulder flexion or flexion without support from the wall.

In the presence of a thoracic rotation-flexion impairment, asymmetrical motion of the rib cage will be noted during ventilation (most commonly during bucket-handle assessment of the rib cage). In addition, because of the positional impairment of sternal depression and dominance of the RA muscle, decreased pump-handle motion compared to the relative amount of bucket-handle motion will also be present.

Supine tests. Pain will commonly be reported when assuming the supine position. Accommodation of the thoracic flexion should be done by providing support for both the cervical and thoracic spine into flexion. Padding may be needed unilaterally to accommodate a structural rotation of the rib cage or spine. A follow-up test of removing some of the support after 5 to 10 minutes in the position should be done to determine if the patient can tolerate the straighter position. Examination of the subcostal margin in the supine position will reveal rib cage asymmetries and give insight in muscle length issues related to the internal oblique, external oblique, and the RA muscle. An increased subcostal margin in both standing and supine may indicate a decreased length of the internal oblique muscles and an increase in the length of the external oblique musculature. An asymmetry of the subcostal margin is commonly present in this category. Approximation of the sternum toward the pubis may be present if there is a marked shortness of the RA muscle. During testing of the abdominal musculature, there will be poor control of the oblique abdominal muscles with rotation of the rib cage and/or thoracic spine during upper or lower extremity movement. Use of inhalation to stabilize the rib cage by contraction of the diaphragm and increasing IAP instead of appropriately recruiting the abdominal musculature is commonly observed. In the presence of sway or sternal depression, increased recruitment of the RA muscle over the lateral abdominal musculature can be seen. In younger individuals, the RA muscle will test strong during trunk curling; however, rotation during the trunk curl demonstrates a unilateral weakness of the oblique abdominal musculature. Unilateral shoulder flexion in the supine position will reveal a rib cage motion or thoracic spine motion that will be most pronounced when moving the arm in a diagonal pattern. Pain with arm motion will commonly decrease with cueing to control the rotational movement by increasing abdominal muscle contraction during the motion. If the patient is in Stage 1 for rehabilitation, the recruitment of the abdominal musculature may increase pain from compressive force on the spine and rib cage. Thus caution should be used during abdominal muscle testing by monitoring closely for an increase or worsening of the presenting symptoms. Hip abduction with lateral rotation in the flexed position is commonly assessed if the individual complains of symptoms during functional activities that require leg motions such as driving and walking. Rotation of the thoracic spine and rib cage and pain noted during the leg motion will be reduced by cueing to recruit the trunk musculature during the activity. Both the thoracic spine extensors

(control flexion) and the abdominal musculature (control rotation) may need to be recruited for adequate trunk control during upper and lower extremity motions.

Prone tests. Prone-lying may reduce symptoms in younger more flexible individuals with a thoracic rotation-flexion syndrome. However, older individuals may need increased support in prone to accommodate the amount of thoracic flexion that is present. In the case of a severe kyphosis, prone should not be attempted. Prone lying may also require some lateral trunk support to minimize rotation while in this position. As in the supine position, removal of some of the trunk support can be done after 5 to 10 minutes to see if the individual can tolerate a more extended position of the spine.

Trunk extension in the prone position will test weak in older individuals with a thoracic flexion alignment impairment[149-152]; however, use of this position for testing and exercise should be done with caution because the erector spinae musculature is not isolated to the thoracic region. Recruitment of the erector spinae in the prone position increases both lumbar and thoracic region extension. Because of the high prevalence of osteoporosis and osteoarthritis in older individuals and the mechanical advantage of the lumbar paraspinals to compress the lumbar region, low back pain may occur during prone trunk extension. If not properly positioned into lumbar and thoracic flexion, an imbalance between the strength and control of the upper thoracic paraspinals (weak and decreased recruitment) compared to the lumbar paraspinals (strong and increased recruitment) can worsen the compression forces at the lower rib cage and thoracolumbar junction.

Single arm raises in the prone position in individuals with a thoracic rotation with extension syndrome can reveal thoracic rotation. Cueing to increase paraspinal muscle recruitment aids in the flexion and rotation control that commonly decreases symptoms. In an individual who is unable to tolerate unilateral arm motions, bilateral symmetrical scapular adduction with shoulder abduction (hands on head, elbows flexed, and elbows extended) can be performed in the various degrees of difficulty.

Quadruped tests. When positioned in the quadruped position, there will be a noticeable amount of thoracic flexion with rotation of the rib cage (hump). Quadruped is commonly a pain-relieving position for individuals with thoracic rotation with flexion because the thoracic spine is suspended between the upper and lower extremities, thus providing a position of unloading. Because of upper extremity muscle weakness and rib cage asymmetries, scapular winging or tilting is commonly present. Rocking back in the quadruped position will reveal an increase in thoracic flexion and rotation. Cueing is needed to relax the abdominal musculature during the rocking motion to prevent flexion of the thoracic spine. Shoulder flexion in quadruped can cause rotation of the thoracic spine and rib cage. Instruction to recruit the latissimus dorsi and thoracic back extensors by an isometric contraction (isometric shoulder extension of the weight-bearing arm toward the ipsilateral knee) reduces the rotation. Inability to perform this correctly in the quadruped position should prompt the therapist to downgrade the activity by performing unilateral shoulder flexion in the prone position. In very active populations, crawling can be assessed to create a more unstable activity that requires trunk rotation. Crawling in individuals with thoracic flexion with rotation will reveal an asymmetry in the trunk rotation.

Functional Activities

Observation of the thoracic spine and rib cage should be done during aggravating functional activities. Specific attention should be paid to the amount of abdominal muscle compared to thoracic paraspinal muscle recruitment during the task. If simply cueing to reduce the motion of flexion with rotation does not decrease the symptoms, timing the movement so that the individual is instructed to first relax their abdominals and then perform the task may reduce the tendency to flex the thoracic spine enough to allow the individual to perform with increased thoracic extension reduce rotation and less pain.

Special Consideration of Treatment of Structural Scoliosis

Caution should be used when prescribing abdominal muscle exercises for individuals with a structural scoliosis because of the compressive effects of the abdominal musculature on the thoracic spine and rib cage. Common impairments that can be observed in older individuals with a structural scoliosis include spine compression with an increase in spine and rib cage rotation that occurs because of excessive abdominal muscle contraction. To address spine compression in an older individual with a structural scoliosis, the therapist should prescribe unloading activities and allow relaxation of the abdominal and trunk musculature. Quadruped rocking, back to the wall with supported shoulder flexion, and inhalation to elevate the ribs and elongate the abdominal musculature should be prescribed.

If pain occurs during asymmetrical sitting positions, the patient should be instructed in correcting the alignment. Avoidance of leaning on armrests, equal weight bearing through the pelvis and femurs, and back support should reduce the pain caused by asymmetrical sitting. In contrast to this, if an individual has scoliosis, pain may occur if they attempt to actively sit in a more symmetrical position. If pain occurs with sitting, instruct the individual to sit without attempting to correct the rotation that is structurally present in the spine. Allowing the individual to sit with the thoracic spine in rotation aligns the boney structures and relieves tissue stresses from forcing a "straight position," thus decreasing their

symptoms with sitting. Pads can be used to distribute the pressure on the back of the chair.

CASE PRESENTATION
Thoracic Rotation-Flexion Syndrome
Symptoms and History

A 23-year-old white female graduate student presents with a 1-year history of burning abdominal pain, located just below her umbilicus. The pain is present with sleeping in sidelying, sitting, driving the car, or using the elliptical machine at the gym. The patient is unaware of a position that relieves her symptoms. She denies any gastrointestinal symptoms (nausea, diarrhea, and so on) occurring at the same time of the pain. The severity of abdominal pain caused her to go to the emergency department twice in the past year. She has had upper and lower gastrointestinal examinations to rule out pathology of this system. Radiological studies of her pelvis and spine are negative. She denies a relationship of the symptoms to her menstrual cycle. Her past recreational history includes 12 years of dance with participation on the dance team during her undergraduate studies. Her initial Oswestry disability score was 46%.

Alignment Analysis

The patient is 5 foot 7 inches tall and weighs 130 pounds. She has a long slender trunk and long arms. When standing, the patient demonstrates a lateral trunk shift to the right with T10, T11, and T12 spinous processes rotated right (indicating left rotation of those segments); a posterior sway of the thoracic spine, with the apex of her thoracic kyphosis at the lower thoracic segments; anterior pelvic tilt; and knee hyperextension. No symptoms reported in standing.

Movement Impairment Analysis
Forward bending

The patient demonstrated thoracic motion that was greater than hip motion with forward bending and reproduced her abdominal pain. The secondary test of corrected forward bending abolished her symptoms but required upper extremity support during forward bending to increase her ability to flex her hips and decrease the amount of thoracic flexion. On return from forward bending, the patient reported central lower thoracic pain with no abdominal symptoms. Corrected return from forward bending did not reproduce her pain. (During this point in the examination, the patient noted that she commonly would use trunk extension to attempt to relieve her abdominal pain.)

Sidebending

The patient demonstrated lateral abdominal pain (2/10) with sidebending in both directions. Sidebending left demonstrated greater ROM compared to right sidebending. The secondary test of supported sidebending at the apex of her curve abolished her pain bilaterally.

Single leg stance

During the single leg stance test on the right lower extremity, the patient demonstrated trunk shift right with rotation left, an increase in the posterior sway of the trunk and increased abdominal pain. Correction of these alignment faults abolished her pain. To correct the movement impairments, the patient supported her trunk by using bilateral upper extremity support on the wall, while being cued to keep her trunk still during motion of her leg.

Ventilation in standing

The patient demonstrated less than 3 cm of rib cage expansion with primarily bucket-handle motion. No symptoms were produced during this test.

Sitting position

On assuming the sitting position the patient demonstrated a slumped posture with a trunk shift to the right. Trunk flexion in sitting increased her pain to 2/10, and trunk extension in sitting reduced her pain to 0/10.

Sitting knee extension

From the corrected position, the patient demonstrated thoracic flexion with rotation during terminal knee extension in sitting; however, no symptoms were produced.

Sitting hip flexion

The patient demonstrated a right trunk shift and reproduced her abdominal pain when performing active hip flexion with either leg (2/10) while in the sitting position.

Supine position

The patient reported no symptoms in supine. Shoulder flexion was through full ROM without detectable rib cage changes. During single knee to chest, her upper trunk rotated but not her pelvis nor were her symptoms reproduced.

Sidelying position

In the sidelying position, the patient reported an increase in her symptoms to 4/10. The abdominal pain abolished with support of the rib cage by a thin pillow.

Prone position

The patient noted central 2/10 thoracic pain with initial prone lying. Positioning of the chest and lumbar spine with pillows to decrease lumbar extension and thoracic flexion reduced the symptoms to 0/10. The patient demonstrated left rotation of the thoracic segments T10 to T12 in the prone position. Palpation of the thoracic erector spinae musculature was positive for sensitivity to touch and a hyperemic reaction T10 to T12. Posterior to anterior spring testing of the lower thoracic and upper lumbar segments revealed decreased motion at the (L) facets and spinous process of T10 to T12 compared to the adjacent lumbar segments (L1 to L2). No abdominal pain was produced with spring testing.

Quadruped position

In the quadruped position, the patient reported 1/10 abdominal pain that abolished with correction of the assumed position of thoracic flexion with right trunk shift and left rotation. Arm lift in the quadruped position reproduced her abdominal pain, and the patient's rotation and shift was increased. The patient was unable to correct the thoracic movement in this position.

Functional Activities

The patient consistently sat in thoracic flexion with her legs crossed and tended to lean on the right armrest of the chair. In addition, when observing her driving position, the patient demonstrated the same alignment impairments by consistently shifting toward the center console of the car.

Diagnosis and Staging

The patient's movement system diagnosis was thoracic rotation-flexion syndrome. The tissue impairment was considered Stage 2 because she did not have continuous symptoms and the symptoms could be modified in most positions during the examination. Her prognosis was good to excellent because of the ability to modify her symptom during the examination, her age, and general good health. Negative moderators were her lack of awareness of specific positions that would improve her symptoms and the amount of time that she spends sitting during the day.

Treatment

The patient was seen once a week for 4 weeks, and then decreased to once every other week for an additional 3 more visits. Treatment included instruction in correct performance of functional activities, including bending, sleeping, sitting, driving a car, and aerobic exercise. She was also instructed in a home exercise program to improve the recruitment of her thoracic paraspinal muscles and improve the control of her trunk musculature during the examination items that had produced thoracic flexion, sidebending, and rotation.

During the first visit the patient was instructed to sleep with a support under her rib cage to provide positioning out of trunk sidebending while in the sidelying position. In addition, the use of pillows between her knees aided in control of trunk rotation by placing the pelvis in a neutral position. The patient was also instructed not to cross her legs, to avoid leaning on the armrests of chairs, and to maintain a more erect trunk by keeping her back supported by the back of the chair and her buttocks as far back in the seat as possible.

Initially, to improve the recruitment of her thoracic paraspinal muscles and improve her alignment impairments, she was given bilateral shoulder flexion exercises in standing with her hands and forearms supported on a wall and unilateral shoulder flexion in prone with her upper extremity off the supporting surface. To improve her trunk control during leg motions, she was given supported single leg stance with an emphasis on keeping her trunk still during leg motions. In addition, quadruped rocking and in standing trunk flexion supporting herself with her hands on a counter was given to unload the thoracic spine and improve hip flexion while decreasing the overall amount of thoracic spine flexion.

On subsequent visits, standing alignment was reviewed with a mirror to provide visual feedback of her trunk sway. The home exercise program was progressed to shoulder flexion in quadruped (corrective exercises for both flexion and rotation trunk control problems), shoulder flexion with her back to the wall (to progress load for paraspinal strengthening), and prone trunk extension with positioning to avoid lower lumbar extension (to strengthen thoracic paraspinal muscles without causing a secondary lumbar extension impairment).

At 1 month, the patient reported absence of abdominal pain with sitting and sleeping; however, she would occasionally notice pain during aerobic exercise. At this point the patient was instructed to avoid trunk rotation and bending into the elliptical machine during her workout activities. In addition, during a discussion regarding an appropriate means of abdominal strengthening, the patient reported she had started performing sit-ups after 30 minutes on the elliptical machine. Lower leg and upper extremity motions while keeping her trunk still were performed to demonstrate the abdominal muscle recruitment during these tasks; the patient was given an explanation as to why trunk curling activities were most likely contributing to her pain syndrome. At this stage of her care, light weights were added to the shoulder flexion exercises to increase the demands on the paraspinal and trunk musculature.

Outcome

At the time of her last visit, the patient reported no abdominal pain for the past month; she had been consistently performing her home program 3 times a week with daily implementation of the functional activity changes. She was able to perform 45 minutes on the elliptical trainer and indicated that she understood that she had to avoid trunk curling activities in the future. Spring testing in prone of the lower thoracic vertebral structures was negative. Her Oswestry disability score was 0%.

THORACIC FLEXION SYNDROME

Although the thoracic flexion syndrome is associated with movements and postures of flexion, the movement is not always painful; however, prevention of excessive thoracic flexion is key to preventing other pain syndromes. Excessive flexion predisposes an individual to increased thoracic spine compression, as well as neck and lumbar spine impairments. A thoracic kyphosis and/or posterior trunk sway are common alignment impairments observed in this syndrome. Common muscle impairments include long thoracic paraspinal and scapulothoracic muscles (middle trapezius and rhomboids); short or stiff anterior axioscapular and axiohumeral muscles (pectoralis minor and major and latissimus dorsi, especially in an individual with a kyphosis lordosis), and the RA muscle. Motor recruitment dominance of the RA muscle is common in this syndrome.

If active thoracic flexion and taking a deep breath is painful, compression fracture of the spine should be considered. There is a paradoxical relationship with the amount of thoracic flexion and the presence of pain. An individual may be predisposed to thoracic flexion because of the shape of the thoracic facets and the flexion moment created by the head, shoulders, and rib cage. Usually, thoracic flexion without a rotation component to the motion is not painful. However, excessive flexion of the thoracic spine is a contributing factor to biomechanical stress that can cause musculoskeletal pain in this region. Elongating the posterior elements (posterior longitudinal ligament and other connective tissues) while compressing the anterior elements (vertebral bodies and discs) of the spine is a consequence of the prolonged flexion. An individual who maintains prolonged thoracic flexion may have pain when attempting to decrease the curve and is usually unable to correct his or her alignment because of the structural changes that have developed.

Symptoms and History

In this syndrome, the pain in the thoracic region usually increases when reaching with both arms, lying in the supine position or when trying to straighten the thoracic spine after prolonged flexion. Ventilation will be affected so that pain occurs with forceful exhalation.[134,146-148] Individuals with a flexion syndrome often participate in activities that cause flexion such as bending to garden, prolonged reading, or watching television. Habitual trunk flexion during functional activities is commonly observed in individuals with this syndrome. These individuals sit slouched (leaning toward the mouse pad) or with their hips not fully back into the seat. Pain with sitting is reduced or abolished when the individual is instructed to use the backrest of the chair to keep the spine straight or support the trunk by using the armrests on the chair. Younger individuals with a flexion syndrome report a history of excessive abdominal strengthening exercises. In addition, the current postural trend for students is to sit in thoracic and lumbar flexion.

Key Tests and Signs
Standing Alignment
Thoracic kyphosis with sternal depression is the most common alignment impairment. Sway of the trunk posterior to the axis of the hip combined with thoracic flexion is also common. The patient may have a wide subcostal margin (infrasternal angle). It is important to note the shape of the rib cage and its effect on the position of the scapulae. The scapulae will be more abducted and internally rotated and demonstrate less posterior tilt during shoulder flexion because of the shape of the rib cage. Passive elevation of the rib cage when pain is present

will unload the weight of the upper trunk and relieve symptoms for individuals with a contributing factor of compression.

Movement Impairment Analysis

Standing tests. Standing trunk flexion demonstrates excessive flexion in the thoracic spine. The motions of trunk rotation and lateral flexion do not demonstrate an asymmetry in motion and/or pain with these movements. Unilateral and bilateral shoulder flexion, which is a test for presence of spine motion during extremity motion, demonstrates an increase in thoracic flexion or sway. In the presence of a kyphosis-lordosis alignment impairment, lumbar extension with thoracic flexion may be noted. With both unilateral and bilateral shoulder flexion, pain and motion are improved if the trunk is provided support either from a wall or lying recumbent, thus allowing the spine to be straighter. Caution should be used when considering cueing for recruitment of the abdominal musculature for trunk control during this follow-up test because increased flexion and spine compression may add to the individual's pain during arm motion. If the individual is in an early stage of rehabilitation, protection of the thoracic spine can be achieved by performing supported bilateral shoulder flexion while facing the wall, thus unloading the weight of the upper body by the support of the wall. The thoracic flexion can be decreased by having the patient extend a few degrees and gradually progress the program once the patient has advanced to Stage 2. The program would consist of strengthening the thoracic paraspinal muscles by performing active shoulder flexion from the facing the wall position and then without the wall for support. In the presence of thoracic flexion during ventilation the pump-handle motion of the rib cage is decreased compared to the relative amount of bucket-handle motion.

Supine tests. To avoid pain in the supine position, a support for both the cervical and thoracic spine should be used. Removal of some of the support after 5 to 10 minutes usually indicates that the patient can tolerate the straighter position. The subcostal margin indicates a wide subcostal angle that is consistent with a decrease in the length of the internal oblique muscles and an increase in the length of the external oblique musculature. Approximation of the sternum toward the pubis may be present if there is a marked shortness of the RA muscle. There is poor control of the lateral abdominal musculature. The patient will inhale as an attempt to contract the abdominal muscles instead of appropriate recruitment of the abdominal muscles, which contribute to exhalation. In the presence of trunk sway or sternal depression, increased recruitment of the RA muscle over the lateral abdominal musculature can be observed. In younger individuals, the RA muscle tests strong during trunk curling; however, in the older adult the internal obliques with the RA may test weak during the trunk

curl. The trunk curl is rarely used to assess the performance of the internal oblique muscles in the older individual. Therefore assessment of the relative performance of the abdominals versus the pectoral muscles is best assessed by using arm motions. Unilateral shoulder flexion in the supine position reveals rib cage motion or thoracic spine motion that will be most pronounced when moving the arm in a diagonal pattern. If the patient is in Stage 1 for rehabilitation, as following abdominal surgery or a trauma to the thorax, the recruitment of the abdominal musculature may increase the pain caused by compressive force on the spine and rib cage. Thus caution should be taken during abdominal muscle testing, monitoring closely for an increase or worsening of the presenting symptoms.

Prone tests. The prone position may reduce symptoms in younger more flexible individuals but may increase the symptoms in older less flexible individuals. In the case of a severe kyphosis, prone testing should not be attempted. If the patient is positioned in prone on pillows, removal of some of the trunk support can be done after 5 to 10 minutes to see if the individual can tolerate a more extended position of the spine.

Trunk extension in the prone position tests weak in older individuals with a thoracic flexion alignment impairment[149-152]; however, use of this position for testing and exercise should be done with caution since the erector spinae musculature is not isolated to the thoracic region. These individuals also have excessive cervical extension or an anterior translation of the cervical spine. Recruitment of the erector spinae muscle in the prone position increases both lumbar and thoracic region extension. Because of the high prevalence of osteoporosis, osteoarthritis, and spinal stenosis in older individuals and the mechanical advantage of the lumbar paraspinals to compress the lumbar region, low back pain may occur during this prone trunk extension. If not properly positioned into lumbar and thoracic flexion, an imbalance between the strength and motor control of the upper thoracic paraspinal muscles (weak and decreased recruitment) compared to the lumbar paraspinals (strong and increased recruitment) can worsen the compression forces at the lower rib cage and thoracolumbar junction.

Quadruped tests. When positioned in quadruped, there will be a noticeable amount of thoracic flexion. Quadruped is commonly a pain-relieving position for individuals with thoracic flexion because the thoracic spine is suspended between the upper and lower extremities, thus providing a position of unloading. Because of upper extremity muscle weakness, scapular winging or tilting commonly is present. Rocking back in the quadruped position reveals an increase in thoracic flexion. Cueing is needed to relax the abdominal musculature to prevent activation during motion, which would cause an increase in the flexion moment of the thoracic spine.

Sitting tests. A prolonged slumped or flexed position of the thoracic spine has been related to increased pain in the thoracic, cervical, and lumbar regions.[16,78,153,154] As noted earlier, individuals with long legs may sit with their knees higher than their hips, causing lumbar and thoracic flexion. Reducing the angle so that the knees are not higher than the hip by using a higher chair or a cushion would make it easier to avoid lumbar and thoracic flexion. Correction of the sitting position of thoracic flexion should eliminate any symptoms associated with the alignment fault. The patient may also need to modify the position when working at a desk to avoid thoracic flexion. In addition, the individual's vision should be checked to see if it is partially responsible for the slouching behavior. The habit of leaning forward may be the result of individuals not being able to see what is positioned in front of them. Interestingly, a slouched sitting posture has been reported to be associated with a decrease in shoulder ROM and strength.[155] Therefore it is important to assess reaching by mimicking the typical activities an individual would perform while sitting at the desk. If pain occurs with reaching during sitting in a slouched position, the patient should be instructed to correct the alignment before reaching forward. Individuals with a marked fixed kyphosis usually sit in lumbar extension. Often, a support behind the lumbar spine or not positioning the buttocks against the back of the chair will decrease the symptoms in sitting.

Functional Activities

Observation of the thoracic spine and rib cage should be done during aggravating functional activities. Specific attention should be paid to the pattern of abdominal muscle activity compared to thoracic paraspinal muscle activity during the task. If simply cueing to reduce the motion of flexion does not decrease the symptoms, then the individual should be instructed to first relax the abdominal muscles before performing the task so that the amount of thoracic extension will increase and there will be less thoracic rotation.

Treatment

Treatment of osteoporosis includes load-bearing exercises to stimulate bone growth.[156] Weakness of the back extensors is common in individuals with an osteoporotic kyphosis,[10,12] thus exercise prescription should include strengthening exercises for the thoracic paraspinal musculature. Consideration should be given to the biomechanical stresses applied to the adjacent spinal regions when developing a strengthening program for the thoracic back extensors. Classically, a prone trunk extension exercise is prescribed to improve the strength of the paraspinal musculature in this population[152] (Figure 4-27). Careful observation of the spine during the prone extension exercise is critical for determining the region of the spine that is moving. Commonly, lumbar extension is performed to a greater extent than thoracic extension,

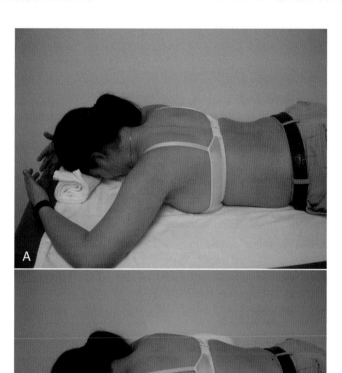

Figure 4-27. Starting position for prine arm lifts. **A,** Insufficient support under thorax allows thoracic extension. **B,** Increased support places thoracic spine in more ideal alignment.

thus increasing the compressive forces at the lumbar spine resulting in pain[152] (Figure 4-28). An alternative to the classic back extensor strengthening exercise is to exercise in a functional position. Sitting and standing with the spine aligned against a wall improves alignment and unloads the weight of the upper trunk. Motions of the upper extremity, shoulder flexion or abduction, can then be used to facilitate contraction of the paraspinal musculature[157] (Figure 4-29). Spine compression and abdominal muscle shortness are contributing factors to the osteoporotic kyphosis, thus deep breathing while appropriately aligned on the wall should be done to increase abdominal muscle length[1,29] and decompress the thoracic spine.[93] Because of the compressive forces on the spine with contraction of the abdominal musculature, care should be taken with strengthening abdominal muscle in individuals with osteoporosis. Generally, patients with a swayback alignment of their trunk are cued to contract their abdominals only enough to hold a corrected alignment of their trunk, while patients with a kyphosis are advised to avoid abdominal muscle contraction in standing.

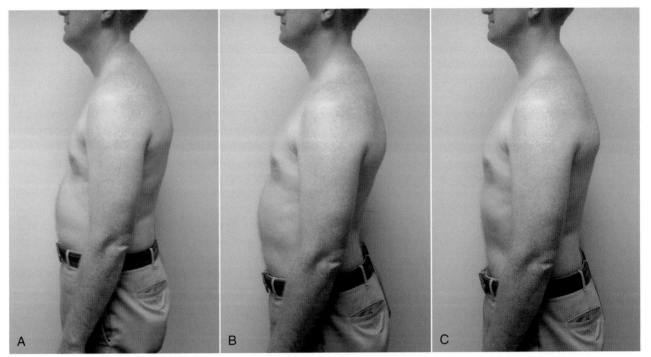

Figure 4-28. A, Kyphosis. **B,** Lumbar extension greater than thoracic extension. **C,** Improved thoracic alignment without lumbar extension.

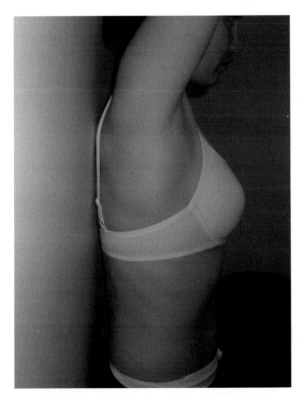

Figure 4-29. Back to wall shoulder flexion.

Older individuals with a total C-curve of both the thoracic and lumbar spines, as well as a flat abdomen, have excessive abdominal muscle activity and markedly diminished back extensor activity. Even in the prone position, while performing shoulder flexion from the overhead position, the abdominal muscles contract rather than the back extensor muscles. Every effort needs to be made to change this recruitment pattern. Therefore these individuals need to avoid any type of abdominal muscle exercise and standing in the swayback position that makes the abdominal muscles the antigravity muscle group.

THORACIC ROTATION-EXTENSION SYNDROME

Symptoms and History

The thoracic rotation-extension syndrome causes pain in the thoracic region that may radiate into the lateral and anterior rib cage or the abdomen. Symptoms may be pain, numbness, or burning. Trunk extension and/or rotation produce symptoms so that motions of unilateral shoulder flexion or reaching are painful because of these associated trunk motions. Similarly, a deep inhalation can cause pain because of associated thoracic rotation-extension.[133,145,158] Positions and alignments that cause rotation or extension forces on the thoracic spine, such as sidelying or sitting up in an exaggerated position of trunk extension, can also cause pain.

Racquet sports, gymnastics, and ballet are activities that may have contributed to the development of the rotation-extension syndrome. Occupations that require working with the arms overhead can also contribute to the development of the syndrome. Patients with the diagnosis of thoracic rotation-extension may report a history of loss of motion at the glenohumeral joint. The loss of glenohumeral motion could cause the patient to substitute thoracic spine motion of extension and/or rotation as a substitute for loss of motion at the shoulder joint.

Key Tests and Signs

Often, patients with this syndrome have asymmetry in the thoracic spine and rib cage. The malalignment may be localized over a few segments or a structural scoliosis. From a posterior view, the spinous processes of the thoracic vertebrae may demonstrate lateral curvature and a rib hump may be present. If the rotation malalignment is in the upper thoracic region, the rib hump may not be obvious because of the scapulae; however, scapular asymmetry is likely. Loss of the normal thoracic sagittal curve is apparent in the posterior view in a few segments or the entire thoracic spine, and often the scapulae appear to wing because of the loss of the normal thoracic curve. Patients who habitually hold their spines in extension can often lessen their symptoms by relaxing thoracic paraspinal muscles and allowing the thoracic spine to flex. Minimal or no change in the thoracic curve will occur when the flat thoracic spine is structural.

From the anterior view, the chest or rib cage may be asymmetrical. The subcostal margin is often flared outward more on one side than the other. The subcostal angle may be wide (>110 degrees), and the rib cage appears to be flared. In such patients, the abdominal muscles will not be stiff or strong enough to counter the pull from the pectoral muscles so overhead movements of the upper extremities cause the rib cage elevation and thoracic spine extension.

Movement Impairment Analysis

The tests described here are considered to be key tests for thoracic rotation-extension syndrome. The tests are listed according to the order they are performed during the examination.

Standing tests. The tests are (1) trunk flexion, (2) trunk rotation, (3) trunk lateral flexion, (4) trunk extension, (5) shoulder flexion, and (6) deep inhalation.

Trunk flexion. The amount of flexion available in the thoracic spine is often less than the expected 30 to 40 degrees of flexion.[2,3] During the return to the upright position, pain may be reported. Cueing the patient to avoid excessive extension and/or rotation during the return from forward bending decreases the symptoms.

Trunk rotation. Asymmetrical rotation is accompanied by complaints of pain. Pain may occur with rotation to either side. The axis of rotation appears to be shifted to one side, producing a twisting motion rather than a motion about a relatively straight line, typically at or close to the painful region.

Trunk or thoracic lateral flexion. Asymmetry and pain can also be noted with lateral flexion to either or both sides. During lateral thoracic flexion, the location and amount of spinal motion is assessed. If pain and a pivot point of motion are observed, the therapist manually stabilizes the segments of increased motion as the patient repeats lateral flexion. Improvement in symptoms while trying to redistribute the motion helps confirm the rotation aspect of the diagnosis.

Thoracic extension. Thoracic extension motion reproduces or increases the patient's pain. Excessive extension range may be observed in a few segments of the thoracic spine.

Shoulder flexion. Unilateral shoulder flexion is considered a positive test if symptoms are reproduced or the thoracic spine is observed to laterally flex, rotate, or extend. If the primary test is positive, during the secondary test the patient is cued to stabilize the thoracic spine or it is manually stabilized during shoulder motion. The accuracy of the diagnosis is further supported if the patient reports a decrease in symptoms with the modified movement.

Ventilation. In some cases, the patient may have pain reproduced with deep inhalation and the thoracic spine is observed to move toward extension.

Supine tests. The tests are (1) shoulder flexion and (2) shoulder diagonal motion. Lying supine may produce a decrease in pain as a result of relaxation of the thoracic paraspinal muscles and decreased compression. If the patient has a large posterior rib hump, there may be an increase in symptoms unless the rotation can be accommodated. A small folded towel placed under the rib cage on the opposite side or manually supporting the rib cage should decrease the pain.

Shoulder flexion. Unilateral shoulder flexion will cause asymmetrical rib cage motion. During bilateral shoulder flexion, the rib cage is often observed to elevate excessively and the motion may be asymmetrical. If the patient reports pain with this test, the same motion should be repeated with contraction of the abdominals or manual stabilization of the rib cage.

Arm diagonal movement. Movement of the arm from a vertical position toward the horizontal on a diagonal line (as if stretching the sternal fibers of pectoralis major) produces rib cage motion. The ribs are observed to deviate toward the side of the moving arm, which is most easily seen by visually monitoring the caudal portion of the sternum and rib angle. Typically, one side is noted to move less than the other or not at all. The secondary test is the same arm motion performed with abdominals contracted to limit the excessive rib cage motion or manual stabilization of the rib cage.

Prone tests. The movement tests are (1) shoulder flexion (arm lift) and (2) trapezius muscle tests. The patient may report a decrease of pain when assuming the prone position because of relaxation of the thoracic paraspinal muscles and a decrease in compressive forces on the spine. A pillow placed under the chest may improve symptoms further.

Shoulder flexion. Unilateral shoulder flexion will cause thoracic rotation. When both arms are lifted off the supporting surface, thoracic extension and pain are produced. The secondary test requires the patient to recruit their abdominal muscles to limit any extension or rotation of the spine. Manual assistance from the therapist may help improve the movement or a pillow can be placed under the thorax and the bilateral shoulder flexion repeated.

Lower and middle trapezius muscle tests. Extension and/or rotation of the thoracic spine may be noted.

Quadruped tests. Movement tests are (1) rocking backward, (2) shoulder flexion, and (3) crawling. Commonly, the patient assumes a position of thoracic extension and rotation or lateral flexion. Correction of extension alignment will reduce symptoms.

Rocking backward. The thoracic spine may extend and/or rotate. As the patient rocks backward, the therapist may need to monitor by palpation the area of the thoracic spine that is believed to be causing the pain to detect the motion.

Shoulder flexion. Movement of the arm into shoulder flexion causes rotation, extension, or lateral flexion of the thoracic spine. This motion may not cause pain because the spine is not subjected to the same compression forces as with standing.

Crawling. The crawling test is generally reserved for higher level patients in whom more demanding activities are required to reveal their movement impairment of thoracic rotation.

Treatment

The treatment emphasis of the rotation-extension syndrome is to prevent extension and/or rotation motions of the thoracic spine in all positions and during motions of the trunk and the extremities. The patient's daily routines and habits, such as sitting positions and body language, should be reviewed and observed to identify contributing factors. Those activities that the patient reports as painful are especially important to simulate in the clinic. For example, if the patient reports pain with running, observation of his or her running pattern will probably reveal asymmetrical arm swing and thoracic extension. The patient should correct this by allowing the thoracic spine to move toward flexion and limiting the arm swing.

Commonly, patients with the diagnosis of thoracic rotation-extension need to be cued to relax their thoracic paraspinal muscles and allow the thoracic spine to slightly flex. This extension posture is usually seen in both standing and sitting, but the position of rotation or lateral flexion occurs more often in sitting than standing. An example is the receptionist who sits erect in her chair and rotates to greet people as they approach her from the side. She should be cued to use the backrest on her chair and allow her trunk to relax into the chair and rotate the chair rather than rotating in her thoracic spine. When sitting, patients also need to refrain from leaning over onto an armrest or sitting on one of their legs that is bent under them.

Exercise Program

The home exercise program should focus on balance of trunk muscle activity, which often necessitates avoiding strengthening the trunk extensors. Frequently, the performance of the abdominal muscles is not optimal, so improving the strength and recruitment of the obliques is indicated. Abdominal activity is beneficial to help control the rotation forces on the rib cage and spine, as well as help balance the paraspinal activity; some patients seem to maintain spinal stability by excessive paraspinal muscle activity. Unilateral arm or leg movements are good exercises for recruiting the abdominal muscles to control the rotation of the trunk and to counter the extension of the thoracic spine.

Prone exercises are also useful for learning to control rotation and extension motions of the thoracic spine. Initially, the patient may need to lay over two pillows to position the thoracic spine in flexion (see Figure 4-27); eventually they can work toward using only one pillow under their chest. Prone unilateral arm movements, such as sliding the arm along a surface toward shoulder flexion or arm lifts, are often more challenging for patients than arm diagonals in supine and therefore should be monitored closely. To effectively stabilize the thorax during the exercise, the patient should be cued to make their trunk stiff and to activate their abdominals.

Quadruped rocking back is also a useful exercise, with the focus on controlling the motion so that the thoracic spine is not rotating or extending as the patient rocks backs. Often, the patient will flex both lumbar and thoracic spines rather than isolating the flexion to thoracic region. It may be helpful to provide manual contact over the posterior lumbar area to promote neutral spine position and gentle pressure at the sternum to promote slight thoracic flexion. A more challenging exercise in the quadruped position than rocking backward is unilateral shoulder flexion. If the patient is unable to control thoracic extension or rotation with the hips at 90 degrees of flexion, increasing the hip flexion angle during the unilateral shoulder flexion makes it easier to perform.

As mentioned earlier, compression may be an underlying source of symptoms with this diagnosis, as well as the others. Positioning strategies taught to the patient include sitting with arms supported on armrests or pillows or a lap board on the patient's lap to help alleviate the compression. The patient may find it helpful to face the wall and rest his/her hands and forearms on the wall at head level, the emphasis is to let the upper extremities help support the weight of trunk and reduce the activity of the posterior thoracic muscles (Figure 4-30, *A*). Additionally, the quadruped and recumbent positions are useful in decreasing the compression of the spine.

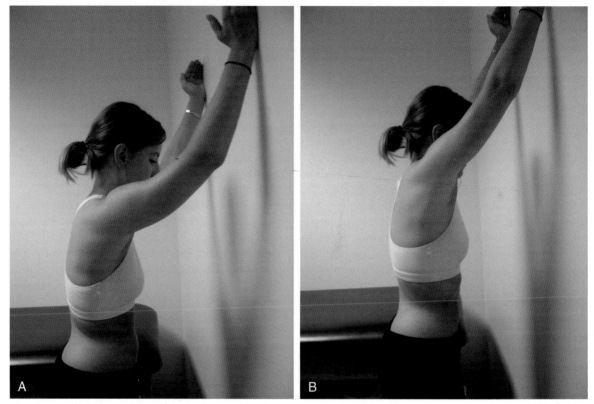

Figure 4-30. **A,** Sliding hands up the wall to perform shoulder flexion. **B,** At maximum flexion, the patient lifts the hand off the wall by posteriorly tilting and externally rotating the scapula.

CASE PRESENTATION
Thoracic Rotation-Extension Syndrome

Symptoms and History

A 34-year-old female was referred to physical therapy for treatment of right shoulder pain. The patient reported a sudden onset of pain in the right scapular region 10 days before her initial visit. Pain progressively worsened over the next few days; she reported breathing was painful at the times when pain was at its worst. She rated her pain as 9/10 at worst and 0 at best using the 0- to 10-point pain scale. Her pain had started to lessen over the 2 days before her initial physical therapy visit so that at the time of initial examination, she reported no pain. The patient attributed the improvement in symptoms to taking time off work and reducing her activity level over the previous week. Her pain was still quite bothersome at night and would interfere with her sleep. During the day, she reported being somewhat guarded with movements and if she twisted or "moved the wrong way," she would get a sharp jab of pain. Lying supine and rolling over onto her side increased pain. Once in a sidelying position, she usually could become more comfortable. Driving was also uncomfortable, and when questioned, the patient admitted to leaning on the console while driving.

The patient was working as a postdoctoral fellow in molecular biology; this work required her to work under a fumigating hood or at a laboratory bench. When sitting at work, she would often have to sit on an elevated stool without back support. Her main computer was a laptop that she carried back and forth with her on a daily basis. She had not been exercising for the past few months, but 3 to 4 months before she had trained for and completed a 5K race. The patient enjoyed knitting as a pastime but even that was painful during the 2 weeks before her visit.

Patient's goals were to resolve pain and return not only to normal work and self-care activities but also to be able to resume some type of exercise. She was concerned that she may need to permanently restrict activities to avoid exacerbating the pain.

Alignment Analysis

Patient was 5 foot 3 inches tall and weighed 142 pounds. She had mild kyphosis in the lower thoracic spine, and the upper thoracic spine was flat. The thorax was rotated and laterally flexed to the right and the right iliac crest was higher than the left. The right scapula was abducted with vertebral border 4 inches from the spine; the left scapula was resting in neutral abduction/adduction. Scapular depression was also noted on the right, corresponding to the right clavicle being aligned horizontally. In the seated position, the patient would assume a slouched posture.

Movement Analysis

Standing

Cervical ROM was pain-free, and the range was considered to be normal. The most significant movement impairment noted during cervical movements was an increase in posterior translation with cervical extension. Trunk forward flexion and lateral flexion were pain-free. Flexion ROM was greater in the lower than in the upper thoracic spine. Rotation to the right was greater in range than rotation to the left, and vague discomfort was present with rotation to the right. Extension of the trunk also produced mild discomfort in the right upper thoracic area, which was the area of her chief complaint. Extension occurred mostly in the upper thoracic spine rather than in the lumbar spine. During trunk rotation and extension, the patient had difficulty isolating motion to the spine, so she moved the scapula while moving the spine. This combination of thoracic and scapular motion made isolating the source of symptoms more difficult.

Assessment of breathing pattern revealed an increase in pump-handle motion, whereas the bucket-handle motion was diminished.

The patient did not note any pain at this time with deep inhalation. Shoulder flexion did not produce symptoms, and range was normal. A movement impairment of scapular depression was noted (right greater than left). A secondary test was not performed because of the lack of symptom reproduction. Palpation of the musculature in the scapular region did not produce pain.

Supine

Active shoulder flexion created rotation in the rib cage. With right shoulder flexion, rib cage rotation occurred almost immediately when she initiated shoulder flexion and caused discomfort; with left shoulder flexion, rotation occurred later in the range and was not as pronounced. During the secondary test, the rib cage was manually stabilized during shoulder flexion and the symptoms were eliminated. Patient was unable to improve the movement pattern using her own abdominal contraction.

Arm diagonal movements were assessed by having the patient move the arm from 90 degrees of humeral flexion outward and down toward horizontal as if stretching the sternal portion of the pectoralis major. Rotation of the rib cage was noted during with arm movement (right greater than left); minimal pain was reported with this movement.

Hip abduction lateral rotation from a hip-flexed position also revealed poor abdominal control because of the pelvic rotation noted with leg movement, however, no pain was reported. The patient did note mild pain moving from supine to sidelying and prone positions. When turning from supine to her side, she moved into a partial sit-up by pushing back with her arm, then as she moved toward her side, she twisted her thoracic spine. Immediate modification of her rolling method resulted in a pain-free motion.

Prone

The patient was positioned over a pillow in the prone position, which did not reproduce any pain. Manual muscle testing of scapular muscles was performed with the patient lying with the pillow under her chest. Strength of the middle trapezius on the right was 4-/5, left 3/5; lower trapezius on the right was 3+/5, on the left 3/5. No pain was produced during tests if the examiner supplied fixation with a hand on opposite side of thorax.[29] Rhomboid strength was 5/5 bilaterally.

The patient was cued to perform bilateral arm lifts with her hands clasped on top of her head. The upper thoracic spine was observed to extend, and the patient was noted to push into cervical flexion so that she pressed her forehead into the supporting towel roll. With cueing to contract her abdominal muscles for stabilization and to avoid extending the upper back, the patient could improve her performance.

Diagnosis and Staging

The patient was diagnosed with a thoracic rotation-extension syndrome. Movements or positions of thoracic rotation reproduced her pain. In particular, rotation moments on the rib cage caused pain. Supporting factors for the extension diagnosis are the flat upper thoracic alignment, extension of upper thoracic spine during trunk extension and prone tests, and pain in the upper thoracic region. The poor abdominal muscle control was a contributing factor to both the rotation and extension movement impairments. The kyphosis in the lower thoracic spine was suspected to contribute to the extension in the upper thoracic spine as compensation. Although strain of the trapezius muscle had been considered as a possible source of the pain, the lack of pain with palpation and during strength testing did not support the hypothesis.

Treatment

Significant time was spent educating the patient on postural corrections. Key corrections included sitting with back support as often as possible, avoiding twisting or rotation of the trunk, and stopping sidebending onto the arm of the chair or the console of the car. The patient found it comfortable to support her arms on pillows while seated, so this was encouraged to help unload the weight of upper extremities off the thoracic region. This support was particularly helpful while knitting.

Bed mobility and transfers were practiced with patient. She was taught to avoid twisting her spine as she moved from one position to another, which helped her avoid symptoms. On her first visit the patient was instructed in (1) wall slides with scapular elevation; (2) prone, with a pillow under her thorax, arm lifts with her hands on her head with instruction to avoid thoracic extension and to contract her abdominal muscles; and (3) hip abduction with lateral rotation in supine.

Her exercise program was designed to improve abdominal muscle performance to help avoid thoracic extension and to control rotation. Improving scapular muscle performance was also to assist in reducing the asymmetrical rotation of her thoracic spine. On the patient's second visit, she was overcorrecting her spinal alignment so that rather than just gently lifting her chest to correct the lower thoracic flexion, she was extending her spine forcefully and causing pain. The overcorrection also occurred during the wall slide exercise and prone arm lifts. Postural correction was practiced with the patient in sitting and standing using a mirror for visual feedback. She was able to reproduce the corrected alignment. Once the patient could distinguish the correct position, she was able to limit the thoracic extension during the wall slides as well. The prone exercise was modified having the patient place two pillows under her thorax so that the upper thoracic spine was placed in slight flexion. Verbal cues for abdominal recruitment were also provided, and the patient could perform the exercise correctly without pain.

Sleeping continued to be disturbed; specifically, the patient awoke with pain when she was changing positions. She remembered pushing her elbow down into the bed while rolling to sidelying from supine. Bed mobility was again practiced with the emphasis on "log rolling" so that her shoulders, trunk, and hips rotated at the same time. Patient was advised to practice rolling a few times each day so that during the night, the correct strategy for rolling would be more automatic.

Over the next month the patient was seen once each week, during which time her exercise program was progressed. Additions to her program included (1) practicing transfers sit to supine to sidelying without allowing lateral flexion or rotation of the trunk, (2) rolling to each side while using hands to hold knees toward chest and keeping head supported, (3) supine bilateral then unilateral shoulder flexion without allowing the rib cage to rotate, and (4) arm diagonals. She also continued with hip abduction lateral rotation from hip flexion with addition of a 2-pound weight at the knee to create a greater load on the obliques, prone arm lifts, and wall slides with scapular elevation.

Shoulder flexion in supine was first given to the patient with instructions to flex both arms at the same time and use abdominal muscles to prevent the rib cage from elevating. Bilateral motion was easier because the patient did not have to prevent rotation. She was eventually progressed to performing the exercise with one arm at a time. Patient was not able to control trunk sufficiently to perform shoulder flexion in the quadruped position.

Outcome

The patient was seen for 5 visits over a 10-week period. At her final visit, she reported resolution of her pain unless she twisted without thinking about how she was moving, but this occurred only occasionally. She had resumed all of her regular responsibilities both at work and at home. She was able to sleep through the night without awakening even with a change of position. Driving was pain-free, although she did have to remind herself to avoid leaning onto the console when she drove the car. The patient also reported that she felt her strength in her arms and trunk had improved.

THORACIC ROTATION SYNDROME

Thoracic rotation syndrome is characterized by pain associated with the movement and postures of thoracic rotation. Asymmetries of the rib cage are the common alignment impairments observed in this syndrome. Common muscle impairments include asymmetry in the length and recruitment of the trunk muscles, including thoracic paraspinal and scapulothoracic muscles (middle trapezius rhomboids), short or stiff anterior scapulohumeral muscles (pectoralis minor and major, latissimus dorsi), and asymmetrical length and strength of the oblique abdominal muscles. Approximation of the ribs resulting from rotation and/or compression from stiffness or shortness of the abdominal muscles should be considered a contributing factor to pain. In addition, thoracic rotation impairments occur in position of both thoracic flexion and extension.

Symptoms and History

Individuals with the rotation syndrome complain of pain in the thoracic region, which may radiate into the lateral and anterior rib cage or abdomen. They note an increase in pain with reaching or trunk rotation. The most common recreational activities reported by individuals with rotation syndrome include any activity that repeatedly places their trunk into rotation, including tennis, softball, sailing, squash, and running (asymmetrical arm swing and trunk rotation). Habitual trunk rotation during functional activities are commonly observed in individuals with this syndrome and include arrangement of their desk so that rotation is required to reach the phone, computer, or files and/or to greet incoming customers/clients; sitting shifted to one side (leaning toward the mouse pad side of desk); sitting on one foot; or leaning on an armrest while working, reading, driving, and watching television. Pain with sitting is reduced or abolished when the individual is instructed to use the backrest to keep the spine straight and to avoid asymmetrical postures, leg crossing, unilateral armrest use, and sitting on one foot. Commonly, individuals with a rotation syndrome report a history of chest surgery in which the rib cage or sternum have been surgically manipulated.

Movement Impairment Analysis

Thoracic rotation with an asymmetry of the rib cage will be the most common alignment impairment found in this diagnosis. The presence of a rib cage asymmetry can be noted from either an anterior or posterior perspective. It is important to note the shape of the rib cage and its effect on the position of the scapulae. A posterior rib cage asymmetry may cause the alignment of the scapulae to appear asymmetrical, when in fact the structural base (rib cage) that the scapulae are resting on is asymmetrical. An anterior rib cage asymmetry may cause the size or shape of the breast to appear asymmetrical. See the preceding Case Presentation, "Thoracic Rotation-Flexion Syndrome" for discussion on the affect of scoliosis on this diagnosis.

Standing tests. Standing trunk flexion demonstrates excessive rotation in the thoracic spine; in addition, the presence of a rib hump is more noticeable in a thoracic-flexed position compared to standing. The motions of trunk rotation and lateral flexion demonstrate an asymmetry or are excessive in a selected group of thoracic segments, with pain with these movements. Either motion may cause a radicular symptom into the chest or abdomen as a result of neural compromise at either the vertebral foramen or along the length of the ribs. Unilateral shoulder flexion, a test for presence of spine motion during extremity motion, results in a side-to-side variation so that arm motion results in a motion at the spine, with or without reproduction of the presenting symptoms. Bilateral shoulder flexion demonstrates unilateral trunk rotation. With both unilateral and bilateral shoulder flexion, pain and motion are improved if the trunk is provided support, either from a wall or lying recumbent, which aids in prevention of rotation with the extremity movement. Recruitment of the abdominal musculature for trunk control during this follow-up test may be needed to control the rotational forces on the spine. In an early stage of rehabilitation, protection of the thoracic spine and neural tissue can be achieved by performing supported shoulder flexion while facing the wall. Thus some of the weight of the upper body is supported by the wall, and the rotation of the thoracic spine can be corrected. Progress can be made once the patient has advanced to Stage 2 to strengthen the thoracic paraspinal muscles in the same position by active shoulder flexion or by lifting the hands off the wall after performing shoulder flexion sliding the hands up the wall. Asymmetrical motion of the rib cage is noted during ventilation (most commonly during bucket-handle assessment of the rib cage).

Supine tests. Pain will commonly be reported when assuming the supine position. Support of the rib cage by appropriate padding can be used unilaterally to accommodate a structural rotation of the rib cage or spine. Examination of the subcostal margin in the supine position reveals rib cage asymmetries and gives insight into muscle length issues related to the internal oblique and external oblique muscles. An increased subcostal margin in standing and supine would indicate a decreased length of the internal oblique and an increased length of the external oblique musculature.

During testing of the abdominal musculature, there is poor control of the oblique abdominal muscles with rotation of the rib cage and/or thoracic spine during lower extremity movement. Unilateral shoulder flexion in the supine position reveals rib cage motion or thoracic spine motion that is most pronounced when moving the arm in a diagonal pattern. Pain with arm motion commonly decreases with cueing to control the rotational movement by increasing abdominal muscle contraction during the motion. If the patient is in Stage 1 of rehabilitation, the recruitment of the abdominal musculature may increase pain because of compressive force on the spine and rib cage. Thus caution should be taken during abdominal muscle testing, monitoring closely for an increase or worsening of the presenting symptoms. Hip abduction with lateral rotation in the flexed position is commonly assessed if the individual complains of symptoms during functional activities that requires lower extremity motions such as running and walking. Rotation of the thoracic spine and rib cage and pain noted during the lower extremity motion is reduced by cueing to recruit the trunk musculature during the activity. Both the thoracic spine extensors and the abdominal musculature may need to be recruited for adequate trunk rotation control during upper and lower extremity motions.

Prone tests. The prone positioning may reduce symptoms in younger more flexible individuals with a thoracic rotation syndrome. However, the spines of older individuals may need increased support in prone to accommodate the amount of thoracic flexion present. Prone lying may also require some lateral trunk support to minimize rotation while in this position.

In individuals with a thoracic rotation diagnosis, unilateral shoulder flexion with scapular posterior tilt starting with the shoulder already in the flexed position while in the prone position will reveal thoracic rotation. Instructing the patient to increase paraspinal muscle recruitment or abdominal muscle recruitment will aid in controlling the rotation and usually decrease the symptoms. In an individual who is not able to tolerate unilateral arm motions, bilateral symmetrical scapular posterior tilt and adduction with shoulder flexion can be performed by increasing the degrees of difficulty such as hands on head, arms bent, or arms straight.

Quadruped tests. When positioned in quadruped, there may not be a noticeable amount rotation of the rib cage (hump); however, rocking backward or shoulder flexion in quadruped may reveal trunk rotation. Quadruped is commonly a pain relieving position for individuals with thoracic rotation because the thoracic spine is suspended between the upper and lower extremities and thus in an unloaded position. Because of upper extremity muscle weakness and rib cage asymmetries, scapular winging or tilting will commonly be present. As initially noted, rocking back in the quadruped position will reveal an increase in rotation, while cueing is needed to relax the abdominal musculature to prevent any contraction of the abdominal muscles during motion, that would cause an increase in the rotation of the thoracic spine. Shoulder flexion in quadruped will cause rotation of the thoracic spine and rib cage, and cueing recruits the latissimus dorsi and thoracic back extensors by an isometric contraction (draw the heel of the weight-bearing hand toward the ipsilateral knee). Shoulder isometric extension will reduce the rotation. Inability to perform this correctly in the quadruped position should prompt the therapist to downgrade the activity by performing unilateral shoulder flexion in the prone position. In very active populations, crawling can be assessed to create a more unstable activity that requires trunk rotation. Crawling in individuals with thoracic rotation will reveal an asymmetry in the trunk rotation during this task.

Functional Activities

Observation of the thoracic spine and rib cage should be done during aggravating functional activities. Specific attention should be paid to the amount of abdominal muscle recruitment compared to thoracic paraspinal muscle recruitment during the task. If simply cueing to reduce the motion of rotation does not decrease the symptoms, timing the movement so that the individual is instructed to first relax the abdominals and then perform the task may reduce the mechanical load enough to allow the individual to perform with decreased compression and reduce rotation and pain.

THORACIC EXTENSION SYNDROME

Symptoms and History

Individuals with thoracic extension syndrome have an altered flexibility of the thoracic spine so that extension occurs too easily. Thoracic extension occurs most often in the interscapular region but can occur in the lower thoracic segments or the thoracolumbar junction. The symptoms associated with thoracic extension syndrome are usually confined to these same areas; however, patients may have a greater distribution of their symptoms. According to Bogduk,[159] pain from the thoracic spine is quasisegmental; the location of pain may be representative of the source of pain with an accuracy of one to two segments.

The habit of holding an erect posture in both sitting and standing is characteristic of individuals with this syndrome, and both positions are associated with pain. The habitual contraction of the spinal extensors contributes to altered flexibility in the thoracic spine so that extension occurs too easily. This syndrome occurs more commonly in younger rather than older people, especially those who participate in dance or gymnastics and who work with their arms overhead.

In some patients, the entire spinal column is flattened so that all of the normal curves of the spine are decreased. The upper thoracic spine, most often between the scapulae, may actually appear to be in some extension. The ability of the thoracic spine to extend may be related to some anomaly of the thoracic vertebrae. Normally, extension is limited by the superior facet impinging onto

the vertebrae below, as well as the contact of the spinous processes. Because this syndrome is often associated with overactivity of both thoracic paraspinals and scapular adductors, an impairment of scapular adduction can be present as well.

Key Tests and Signs

The key tests for thoracic extension syndrome are as follows and are listed in the order they are performed during the examination.

Standing tests. The tests performed in standing are (1) trunk flexion, (2) trunk extension, (3) trunk rotation, (4) lateral flexion, and (5) ventilation.

Trunk flexion. The amount of flexion available in the thoracic spine is often less than the expected 30 to 40 degrees of flexion.[2,3] If the extension impairment involves the upper thoracic spine, the loss of flexion ROM may not be noticeable because normally the upper thoracic spine contributes less than half of the available range[2] (see Figure 4-19). During the return to the upright position, pain may be reported and careful observation may reveal that extension is exaggerated at some segments, usually in the painful area. The distribution of motion between segments is thought to transition gradually, so obvious motion occurring at a few segments would be considered faulty. Cueing the patient to avoid excessive extension during the return from forward bending will improve symptoms.

Trunk extension. Pain will be reproduced with active trunk extension.

Trunk rotation. Rotation ROM may be limited but should not cause pain.

Trunk lateral flexion. Lateral flexion of the trunk should not cause pain or be significantly asymmetrical.

Ventilation. Deep inhalation may reproduce the patient's pain, and in more extreme cases the thoracic spine is observed to move toward extension.

Sitting test. In a sitting test, assessment of a individual's preferred alignment and modification of alignment are performed. The patient will most often sit with the spine held very erect. Cues to relax his or her spine and allow it to slightly flex should decrease the pain. Further relief may be obtained by supporting the spine in the flexed position with the backrest of the chair.

Supine tests. The patient may report a decrease of pain when assuming the supine position as a result of relaxation of the thoracic paraspinals; the reduction of compression on the spine may possibly aid in pain reduction. Assessment of abdominal performance typically reveals weakness.

Shoulder flexion. During bilateral shoulder flexion, the rib cage is often observed to elevate excessively. The patient may be able to feel extension of the involved thoracic segments. If the patient reports pain with this test, the same motion should be repeated with contraction of the abdominals or manual stabilization of the rib cage.

Prone tests. The following movement tests are assessed with the patient in the prone position: (1) shoulder flexion (arm lift) and (2) assessment of trapezius muscle performance. With both movement tests, the impairment and symptoms would be expected to occur more consistently when both arms are lifted off the surface. As with supine, the effect of position on symptoms is assessed. The patient may report a decrease of pain on assuming the prone position caused by relaxation of the thoracic paraspinal muscles and a decrease in compressive forces on the spine. A pillow placed under the chest may improve symptoms further.

Shoulder flexion. Shoulder flexion performed unilaterally might cause thoracic extension; however, when both arms are lifted off the surface, thoracic extension and pain are produced. The secondary test requires the patient to recruit their abdominal muscles to limit extension of the spine. Manual assistance from the therapist may help improve the movement.

Trapezius muscle test. A dominance of the rhomboid muscles may be observed during a middle trapezius test so that the scapula moves toward downward rotation when the patient must support the weight of the arm. With middle and lower trapezius testing, extension of the upper or midthoracic spine may be noted as well. Although the trapezius muscle may test strong during an isolated test, the inability of the patient to control the thoracic spine extension during the test or exercise attempt is the most important finding.

Quadruped tests. In the quadruped position, both alignment and movement tests are performed. Commonly, the patient will assume a position of thoracic extension, and the scapulae will be prominent on the posterior thorax. The patient may appear to be "hanging" on their shoulders and scapulae.

Shoulder flexion. Movement of the arm into shoulder flexion may produce mild extension of the thoracic spine in those individuals whose relative flexibility into thoracic extension is greatly exaggerated. This motion may not cause pain because the spine is not subjected to the same compression forces as with standing.

Treatment

The treatment priority for thoracic extension syndrome is to restrict movement of the spine into extension during the patient's activities. This will be most effective if the patient learns to recognize spinal extension and the extremity movements that induce extension moments on the thoracic region. For example, if the patient routinely has pain associated with styling her hair because arm elevation induces thoracic extension, then it is necessary to teach the patient to hold gentle flexion in the thoracic spine while elevating the arms.

Patients with the diagnosis of thoracic extension syndrome typically exhibit habitual thoracic extension. Instruction to relax the thoracic paraspinals and slightly flex the thoracic spine improves symptoms. Initially, pain will be an indication of faulty positioning; however, long-term management requires that the patient develop an awareness of spinal posture.

If compression is contributing to symptoms, positioning strategies, such as sitting with arms supported, are encouraged. In standing, the patient can help reduce compressive forces by resting the hands and forearms on the wall at head level and relaxing the trunk, so that the upper extremities help support the weight of trunk and reduce the activity of the posterior thoracic muscles. Recumbent positions or quadruped are frequently pain relieving and should be used to help control symptoms.

Exercise Program

The home exercise program should focus on improving the motor control of the thoracic region and reversing the trend of excessive flexibility into thoracic extension or rib cage elevation. Failure to avoid thoracic extension postures and movements will perpetuate the pain problem. Exercises that may be useful when trying to improve the motor control are similar to those listed for treatment of the thoracic rotation-extension syndrome, with the obvious difference being that rotation is not a problem. Often, abdominal muscle activity is emphasized as a means to control or stop the spinal extension. The abdominal muscles may be weak (insufficient contractile elements) or their recruitment pattern is impaired. The corrective exercise is to engage the abdominal muscles to limit thoracic extension or excessive elevation of the rib cage during arm elevation. This exercise can be practiced in standing, sitting, or quadruped.

CONCLUSION

Movement system syndromes of the thoracic spine are most commonly caused by impairments in alignment, stabilization, and movement patterns. Pain syndromes that develop from movement-related tissue injury require consideration of the mechanics that cause tissue injury. This chapter presented key principles for examining alignment, movement, and muscle impairments of the thoracic region. Emphasis was placed on a structured examination, key tests for diagnosis, and treatment for the specific impairments. The emphasis of treatment of movement related syndromes is on education regarding changes in alignment, muscle recruitment, and reduction of thoracic movement by redistribution of motion to other regions. The ultimate goal is to achieve optimal alignment and movement patterns that are consistent with kinesiology. Malalignments and altered movement patterns of the thoracic spine also play a key role in problems of the cervical spine, shoulder, and lumbar spine. Thus optimizing thoracic alignment and trunk control is important in many, if not most, of the musculoskeletal pain syndromes and not just when pain is present in the thoracic spine region.

REFERENCES

1. Sahrmann S: *Diagnosis and treatment of movement impairment syndromes*, St Louis, 2002, Mosby.
2. White AA III, Panjabi M: *Clinical biomechanics of the spine*, ed 2, Philadelphia, 1990, Lippincott-Raven.
3. Neumann DA: *Kinesiology of the musculoskeletal system: foundations of rehabilitation*, St Louis, 2002, Mosby.
4. Harrison DE, Colloca CJ, Harrison DD, et al: Anterior thoracic posture increases thoracolumbar disc loading, *Eur Spine J* 14(3):234-242, 2005.
5. Keller TS, Harrison DE, Colloca CJ, et al: Prediction of osteoporotic spinal deformity, *Spine* 28(5):455-462, 2003.
6. Silverman SL: The clinical consequences of vertebral compression fracture, *Bone* 13(2):S27-S31, 1993.
7. Mueller MJ, Maluf KS: Tissue adaptation to physical stress: a proposed "Physical Stress Theory" to guide physical therapist practice, education, and research, *Phys Ther* 82(4):383-403, 2002.
8. Russek LN: Hypermobility syndrome, *Phys Ther* 79(6):591-599, 1999.
9. Russek LN: Examination and treatment of a patient with hypermobility syndrome, *Phys Ther* 80(4):386-398, 2000.
10. Sinaki M, Itoi E, Rogers JW, et al: Correlation of back extensor strength with thoracic kyphosis and lumbar lordosis in estrogen-deficient women, *Am J Phys Med Rehabil* 75(5):370-374, 1996.
11. Sinaki M, Nwaogwugwu NC, Phillips BE, et al: Effect of gender, age, and anthropometry on axial and appendicular muscle strength, *Am J Phys Med Rehabil* 80(5):330-338, 2001.
12. Sinaki M, Lynn SG: Reducing the risk of falls through proprioceptive dynamic posture training in osteoporotic women with kyphotic posturing: a randomized pilot study, *Am J Phys Med Rehabil* 81(4):241-246, 2002.
13. Willner S: Spinal pantograph: a non-invasive technique for describing kyphosis and lordosis in the thoracolumbar spine, *Acta Orthop Scand* 52(5):525-529, 1981.
14. Mellin G: Measurement of thoracolumbar posture and mobility with a Myrin inclinometer, *Spine* 11(7):759-762, 1986.
15. Gajdosik RL, Albert CR, Mitman JJ: Influence of hamstring length on the standing position and flexion range of motion of the pelvic angle, lumbar angle, and thoracic angle, *J Orthop Sports Phys Ther* 20(4):213-219, 1994.
16. Christie HJ, Kumar S, Warren SA: Postural aberrations in low back pain, *Arch Phys Med Rehabil* 76(3):218-224, 1995.
17. Fon GT, Pitt MJ, Thies AC Jr: Thoracic kyphosis: range in normal subjects, *AJR Am J Roentgenol* 134(5):979-983, 1980.
18. Singer KP, Jones TJ, Breidahl PD: A comparison of radiographic and computer-assisted measurements of thoracic and thoracolumbar sagittal curvature, *Skel Radiol* 19(1):21-26, 1990.
19. Itoi E, Sinaki M: Effect of back-strengthening exercise on posture in healthy women 49 to 65 years of age, *Mayo Clin Proc* 69(11):1054-1059, 1994.
20. Jackson RP, Mcmanus AC: Radiographic analysis of sagittal plane alignment and balance in standing volunteers and patients with low-back-pain matched for age, sex, and size—a prospective controlled clinical-study, *Spine* 19(14):1611-1618, 1994.
21. Korovessis PG, Stamatakis M, Baikousis A: Unrecognized laceration of main bronchus caused by fracture of the T6 vertebra, *Eur Spine J* 7(1):72-75. 1998.
22. Korovessis P, Stamatakis M, Baikousis A: Segmental roentgenographic analysis of vertebral inclination on sagittal plane in asymptomatic versus chronic low back pain patients, *J Spinal Disord* 12(2):131-137, 1999.
23. Tuzun C, Yorulmaz I, Cindas A, et al: Low back pain and posture, *Clin Rheumatol* 18(4):308-312, 1999.
24. Mirza SK, White AA, III: Anatomy of intervertebral disc and pathophysiology of herniated disc disease, *J Clin Laser Med Surg* 13(3):131-142, 1995.
25. Carr AJ, Jefferson RJ, Turner-Smith AR, et al: An analysis of normal back shape measured by ISIS scanning, *Spine* 16(6):656-659, 1991.
26. Crawford MB, Toms AP, Shepstone L: Defining normal vertebral angulation at the thoracolumbar junction, *AJR Am J Roentgenol* 193(1):W33-W37, 2009.
27. Zoeller R, Sahrmann SA, Kuhnline M, et al: Changes in the infrasternal angle with abdominal muscle contractions, *Phys Ther* 73:S104, 1993.
28. Bellemare F, Jeanneret A, Couture J: Sex differences in thoracic dimensions and configuration, *Am J Respir Crit Care Med* 168(3):305-312, 2003.
29. Kendall F: *Muscles: testing and function with posture and pain*, ed 5, Baltimore, 2005, Lippincott Williams & Wilkins.
30. Lowe TG, Line BG: Evidence-based medicine: analysis of Scheuermann kyphosis, *Spine* 32(Suppl 19):S115-S119, 2007.
31. Tribus CB: Scheuermann's kyphosis in adolescents and adults: diagnosis and management, *J Am Acad Orthop Surg* 6(1):36-43, 1998.
32. Poolman RW, Been HD, Ubags LH: Clinical outcome and radiographic results after operative treatment of Scheuermann's disease, *Eur Spine J* 11(6):561-569, 2002.
33. Kanis JA: Diagnosis of osteoporosis and assessment of fracture risk, *Lancet* 359(9321):1929-1936, 2002.
34. Kanis JA, Borgstrom F, De Laet C, et al: Assessment of fracture risk, *Osteoporos Int* 16(6):581-589, 2005.
35. Kotz K, Deleger S, Cohen R, et al: Osteoporosis and health-related quality-of-life outcomes in the Alameda County Study population, *Prev Chronic Dis* 1(1):A05, 2004.
36. Sinaki M, Brey RH, Hughes CA, et al: Significant reduction in risk of falls and back pain in osteoporotic-kyphotic women through a Spinal Proprioceptive Extension Exercise Dynamic (SPEED) program, *Mayo Clin Proc* 80(7):849-855, 2005.
37. Sinaki M, Brey RH, Hughes CA, et al: Balance disorder and increased risk of falls in osteoporosis and kyphosis: significance of kyphotic posture and muscle strength, *Osteoporos Int* 16(8):1004-1010, 2005.
38. O'Sullivan PB, Grahamslaw KM, Kendell M, et al: The effect of different standing and sitting postures on trunk muscle activity in a pain-free population, *Spine* 27(11):1238-1244, 2002.
39. Grieve GP: *Common vertebral joint problems*, London, 1981, Longman Group Limited.

40. Stubgen JP: Rigid spine syndrome: a noninvasive cardiac evaluation, *Pediatr Cardiol* 29(1):45-49, 2008.

41. Omey ML, Micheli LJ, Gerbino PG: Idiopathic scoliosis and spondylolysis in the female athlete. Tips for treatment, *Clin Orthop Relat Res* (372):74-84, 2000.

42. Wynne-Davies R: Familial (idiopathic) scoliosis. A family survey, *J Bone Joint Surg Br* 50(1):24-30, 1968.

43. Burwell RG, Dangerfield PH, Moulton A, et al: Etiologic theories of idiopathic scoliosis: autonomic nervous system and the leptin-sympathetic nervous system concept for the pathogenesis of adolescent idiopathic scoliosis, *Stud Health Technol Inform* 140:197-207, 2008.

44. Bagnall KM, Raso VJ, Hill DL, et al: Melatonin levels in idiopathic scoliosis. Diurnal and nocturnal serum melatonin levels in girls with adolescent idiopathic scoliosis, *Spine* 21(17):1974-1978, 1996.

45. Hilibrand AS, Blakemore LC, Loder RT, et al: The role of melatonin in the pathogenesis of adolescent idiopathic scoliosis, *Spine* 21(10):1140-1146, 1996.

46. Machida M, Dubousset J, Yamada T, et al: Serum melatonin levels in adolescent idiopathic scoliosis prediction and prevention for curve progression—a prospective study, *J Pineal Res* 46(3):344-348, 2009.

47. Smith RM, Pool RD, Butt WP, et al: The transverse plane deformity of structural scoliosis, *Spine* 16(9):1126-1129, 1991.

48. Shohat M, Shohat T, Nitzan M, et al: Growth and ethnicity in scoliosis, *Acta Orthop Scand* 59(3):310-313, 1988.

49. Dickson RA: The etiology and pathogenesis of idiopathic scoliosis, *Acta Orthop Belg* 58 (Suppl 1):21-25, 1992.

50. Cheng S, Sipila S, Taaffe DR, et al: Change in bone mass distribution induced by hormone replacement therapy and high-impact physical exercise in post-menopausal women, *Bone* 31(1):126-135, 2002.

51. Bruyneel AV, Chavet P, Bollini G, et al: Lateral steps reveal adaptive biomechanical strategies in adolescent idiopathic scoliosis, *Ann Readapt Med Phys* 51(8):630-641, 2008.

52. Bruyneel AV, Chavet P, Bollini G, et al: Dynamical asymmetries in idiopathic scoliosis during forward and lateral initiation step, *Eur Spine J* 18(2):188-195, 2009.

53. Lao ML, Chow DH, Guo X, et al: Impaired dynamic balance control in adolescents with idiopathic scoliosis and abnormal somatosensory evoked potentials, *J Pediatr Orthop* 28(8):846-849, 2008.

54. Mallau S, Bollini G, Jouve JL, et al: Locomotor skills and balance strategies in adolescents idiopathic scoliosis, *Spine* 32(1):E14-E22, 2007.

55. Olafsson Y, Odergren T, Persson HE, et al: Somatosensory testing in idiopathic scoliosis, *Dev Med Child Neurol* 44(2):130-132, 2002.

56. Frownfelter D, Dean E: *Cardiovascular and pulmonary physical therapy*, ed 4, St Louis, 2006, Mosby.

57. Santos PS, Resende LA, Fonseca RG, et al: Intercostal nerve mononeuropathy: study of 14 cases, *Arq Neuropsiquiatr* 63(3B):776-778, 2005.

58. Carnett JB: The simulation of gall-bladder disease by intercostal neuralgia of the abdominal wall, *Ann Surg* 86(5):747-757, 1927.

59. Carnett JB, Bates W: The treatment of intercostal neuralgia of the abdominal wall, *Ann Surg* 98(5):820-829, 1933.

60. Hardy PA: Post-thoracotomy intercostal neuralgia, *Lancet* 1(8481):626-627, 1986.

61. Defalque RJ, Bromley JJ: Poststernotomy neuralgia: a new pain syndrome, *Anesth Analg* 69(1):81-82, 1989.

62. Selbst SM: Chest pain in children, *Am Fam Physician* 41(1):179-186, 1990.

63. Gregory PL, Biswas AC, Batt ME: Musculoskeletal problems of the chest wall in athletes, *Sports Med* 32(4):235-250, 2002.

64. Monnin JL, Pierrugues R, Bories P, et al: The slipping rib syndrome: a cause of diagnostic errors in abdominal pain, *La Presse Medicale* 17(1):25-29, 1988.

65. Udermann BE, Cavanaugh DG, Gibson MH, et al: Slipping rib syndrome in a collegiate swimmer: a case report, *J Athl Train* 40(2):120-122, 2005.

66. Coelho MS, Guimaraes PS: Pectus carinatum, *J Bras Pneumol* 33(4):463-474, 2007.

67. Mavanur A, Hight DW: Pectus excavatum and carinatum: new concepts in the correction of congenital chest wall deformities in the pediatric age group, *Conn Med* 72(1):5-11, 2008.

68. Nakaoka T, Uemura S, Yano T, et al: Does overgrowth of costal cartilage cause pectus excavatum? A study on the lengths of ribs and costal cartilages in asymmetric patients, *J Pediatr Surg* 44(7):1333-1336, 2009.

69. Schoenmakers MAGC, Gulmans VAM, Bax NMA, et al: Physiotherapy as an adjuvant to the surgical treatment of anterior chest wall deformities: a necessity? *J Pediatr Surg* 35(10):1440-1443, 2000.

70. Canavan PK, Cahalin L: Integrated physical therapy intervention for a person with pectus excavatum and bilateral shoulder pain: a single-case study, *Arch Phys Med Rehabil* 89(11):2195-2204, 2008.

71. O'Sullivan P, Dankaerts W, Burnett A, et al: Evaluation of the flexion relaxation phenomenon of the trunk muscles in sitting, *Spine* 31(17):2009-2016, 2006.

72. Callaghan JP, Dunk NM: Examination of the flexion relaxation phenomenon in erector spinae muscles during short duration slumped sitting, *Clin Biomech* 17(5):353-360, 2002.

73. Panjabi MM, Krag MH, Dimnet JC, et al: Thoracic spine centers of rotation in the sagittal plane, *J Orthop Res* 1(4):387-394, 1984.

74. Edmondston SJ, Aggerholm M, Elfving S, et al: Influence of posture on the range of axial rotation and coupled lateral flexion of the thoracic spine, *J Manipulative Physiol Ther* 30(3):193-199, 2007.

75. Grice AS: Radiographic, biomechanical and clinical factors in lumbar lateral flexion: part I, *J Manipulative Physiol Ther* 2:26-34, 1979.

76. Panjabi MM, Oxland TR, Yamamoto I, et al: Mechanical behavior of the human lumbar and lumbosacral spine as shown by three-dimensional load-displacement curves, *J Bone Joint Surg Am* 76(3):413-424, 1994.

77. Molnar S, Mano S, Kiss L, et al: Ex vivo and in vitro determination of the axial rotational axis of the human thoracic spine, *Spine* 31(26):E984-E991, 2006.

78. McDonnell MK, Sahrmann S: Movement impairment syndromes of the thoracic and cervical spine. In Grant R,

ed: *Physical therapy of the cervical and thoracic spine*, New York, 2002, Churchill Livingstone.

79. Spitznagle TM: Musculoskeletal chronic pelvic pain. In Carriere B, Feldt C, eds: *The pelvic floor*, Stuttgart, 2010, Georg Thieme Verlag.

80. Lee LJ, Coppieters MW, Hodges PW: Differential activation of the thoracic multifidus and longissimus thoracis during trunk rotation, *Spine* 30(8):870-876, 2005.

81. Oatis CA: *Kinesiology: the mechanics & pathomechanics of human movement*, Philadelphia, 2004, Lippincott Williams & Williams.

82. Sizer PS, Brismee JM, Cook C: Coupling behavior of the thoracic spine: a systematic review of the literature, *J Manipulative Physiol Ther* 30(5):390-399, 2007.

83. McInerney J, Ball PA: The pathophysiology of thoracic disc disease, *Neurosurg Focus* 9(4):e1, 2000.

84. Oppenheim JS, Rothman AS, Sachdev VP: Thoracic herniated discs: review of the literature and 12 cases, *Mount Sinai J Med* 60(4):321-326, 1993.

85. Wilke A, Wolf U, Lageard P, et al: Thoracic disc herniation: a diagnostic challenge, *Man Ther* 5(3):181-184, 2000.

86. Yelland MJ: Back, chest and abdominal pain. How good are spinal signs at identifying musculoskeletal causes of back, chest or abdominal pain? *Aust Fam Physician* 30(9):908-912, 2001.

87. Xiong Y, Lachmann E, Marini S, et al: Thoracic disk herniation presenting as abdominal and pelvic pain: a case report, *Arch Phys Med Rehabil* 82(8):1142-1144, 2001.

88. Rohde RS, Kang JD: Thoracic disc herniation presenting with chronic nausea and abdominal pain. A case report, *J Bone Joint Surg Am* 86(2):379-381, 2004.

89. Jorgensen LS, Fossgreen J: Back pain and spinal pathology in patients with functional upper abdominal pain, *Scand J Gastroenterol* 25(12):1235-1241, 1990.

90. Hamberg J, Lindahl O: Angina pectoris symptoms caused by thoracic spine disorders. Clinical examination and treatment, *Acta Medica Scand Suppl* 644:84-86, 1981.

91. Fruergaard P, Launbjerg J, Hesse B, et al: The diagnoses of patients admitted with acute chest pain but without myocardial infarction, *Eur Heart J* 17(7):1028-1034. 1996.

92. Frobert O, Fossgreen J, Sondergaard-Petersen J, et al: Musculoskeletal pathology in patients with angina pectoris and normal coronary angiograms, *J Intern Med* 245(3):237-246, 1999.

93. Leong JC, Lu WW, Luk KD, et al: Kinematics of the chest cage and spine during breathing in healthy individuals and in patients with adolescent idiopathic scoliosis, *Spine* 24(13):1310-1315, 1999.

94. Massery M: Multi system consequences of impaired breathing mechanics and/or postural control. In Frownfelter D, Dean E, eds.: *Cardiovascular and pulmonary physical therapy evidence and practice*, ed 4, St Louis, 2005, Mosby.

95. Williams PL, Warwick R, Dyson M, et al: *Gray's anatomy*, ed 37, New York, 1989, Churchill Livingstone.

96. From Oatis CA: *Kinesiology: the mechanics & pathomechanics of human movement*, ed 2, Philadelphia, 2009, Lippincott Williams & Williams.

97. Mannion AF, Dumas GA, Cooper RG, et al: Muscle fibre size and type distribution in thoracic and lumbar regions of erector spinae in healthy subjects without low back pain: normal values and sex differences, *J Anat* 190:505-513, 1997.

98. Lee DG: *The thorax: an integrated approach*, ed 2, 2003, Orthopedic Physical Therapy Products.

99. Lee LJ, Coppieters MW, Hodges PW: Anticipatory postural adjustments to arm movement reveal complex control of paraspinal muscles in the thorax: *J Electromyogr Kinesiol* 19(1):46-54, 2009.

100. Hodges PW, Richardson CA: Relationship between limb movement speed and associated contraction of the trunk muscles, *Ergonomics* 40(11):1220-1230, 1997.

101. Briggs AM, Greig AM, Wark JD, et al: A review of anatomical and mechanical factors affecting vertebral body integrity, *Int J Med Sci* 1(3):170-180, 2004.

102. Moseley GL, Hodges PW, Gandevia SC: Deep and superficial fibers of the lumbar multifidus muscle are differentially active during voluntary arm movements, *Spine* 27(2):E29-E36, 2002.

103. Phillips S, Mercer S, Bogduk N: Anatomy and biomechanics of quadratus lumborum. Proceedings of the Institution of Mechanical Engineers. Part H, *J Engineer Med* 222(2):151-159, 2008.

104. Porterfield JA, DeRosa C: *Mechanical low back pain: perspectives in functional anatomy*, Philadelphia, 1991, Saunders.

105. McGill SM: A revised anatomical model of the abdominal musculature for torso flexion efforts, *J Biomech* 29(7):973-977, 1996.

106. Moll JM, Wright V: An objective clinical study of chest expansion, *Ann Rheum Dis* 31(1):1-8, 1972.

107. Estenne M, Yernault JC, De Troyer A: Rib cage and diaphragm-abdomen compliance in humans: effects of age and posture, *J Appl Physiol* 59(6):1842-1848, 1985.

108. Jull GA, Richardson CA: Motor control problems in patients with spinal pain: a new direction for therapeutic exercise, *J Manipulative Physiol Ther* 23(2):115-117, 2000.

109. Hodges PW, Richardson CA: Delayed postural contraction of transversus abdominis in low back pain associated with movement of the lower limb, *J Spinal Disord* 11(1):46-56, 1998.

110. Hodges PW, Richardson CA: Altered trunk muscle recruitment in people with low back pain with upper limb movement at different speeds, *Arch Phys Med Rehabil* 80(9):1005-1012, 1999.

110a. Grenier SC, McGill SM: Quantification of lumbar stability by using two different abdominal activation strategies, *Arch Phys Med Rehabil* 88(1):54-62, 2007.

111. McGill S: *Low back disorders: evidence-based prevention and rehabilitation*, Champaign, IL, 2002, Human Kinetics Publishers.

112. Brown SH, McGill SM: How the inherent stiffness of the in vivo human trunk varies with changing magnitudes of muscular activation, *Clin Biomech* 23(1):15-22, 2008.

113. Hodges PW: Core stability exercise in chronic low back pain, *Orthop Clin North Am* 34(2):245-254, 2003.

114. Cresswell AG, Grundstrom H, Thorstensson A: Observations on intra-abdominal pressure and patterns of abdominal intra-muscular activity in man, *Acta Physiologica Scand* 144(4):409-418, 1992.

115. Urquhart DM, Hodges PW: Differential activity of regions of transverses abdominis during trunk rotation, *Eur Spin J* 14:393-400, 2005.

116. Urquhart DM, Barker PJ, Hodges PW, et al: Regional morphology of the transversus abdominis and obliquus internus and externus abdominis muscles, *Clin Biomech* (20):233-241, 2005.

117. Urquhart DM, Hodges PW, Story IH: Postural activity of the abdominal muscles varies between regions of these muscles and between body positions, *Gait Posture* 22(4):295-301, 2005.

118. Hodges PW, Richardson CA: Transversus abdominis and the superficial abdominal muscles are controlled independently in a postural task, *Neurosci Lett* 265(2):91-94, 1999.

119. Hodges PW, Cresswell AG, Daggfeldt K, et al: Three dimensional preparatory trunk motion precedes asymmetrical upper limb movement, *Gait Posture* 11(2):92-101, 2000.

120. Urquhart DM, Hodges PW, Allen TJ, et al: Abdominal muscle recruitment during a range of voluntary exercises, *Man Ther* 10(2):144-153, 2005.

121. Andersson EA, Grundstrom H, Thorstensson A: Diverging intramuscular activity patterns in back and abdominal muscles during trunk rotation, *Spine* 27(6):E152-E160, 2002.

122. Parfrey KC, Docherty D, Workman RC, et al: The effects of different sit- and curl-up positions on activation of abdominal and hip flexor musculature, *Appl Physiol Nutr Metabol* 33(5):888-895, 2008.

123. Bird M, Fletcher KM, Koch AJ: Electromyographic comparison of the ab-slide and crunch exercises, *J Strength Conditioning Res* (2):436-440, 1920.

124. Lehman GJ, McGill SM: Quantification of the differences in electromyographic activity magnitude between the upper and lower portions of the rectus abdominis muscle during selected trunk exercises, *Phys Ther* 81(5):1096-1101, 2001.

125. Fitting JW: Clinical significance of abnormal rib cage abdominal motion, *Eur Respir J* 1(6):495-497, 1988.

126. Whitelaw MA, Markham DR: Patterns of intercostal muscle activity in humans, *J Appl Physiol* 67(5):2087-2094, 1989.

127. Dimarco AF, Romaniuk JR, Supinski GS: Action of the intercostal muscles on the rib cage, *Respir Physiol* 82(3):295-306, 1990.

128. De Troyer A, Kirkwood PA, Wilson TA: Respiratory action of the intercostal muscles, *Physiol Rev* 85(2):717-756, 2005.

129. Whitelaw WA, Ford GT, Rimmer KP, et al: Intercostal muscles are used during rotation of the thorax in humans, *J Appl Physiol* 72(5):1940-1944, 1992.

130. Cloward RB: Cervical diskography. A contribution to the etiology and mechanism of neck, shoulder and arm pain, *Ann Surg* 150:1052-1064, 1959.

131. Abbott J: Pelvic pain: Lessons from anatomy and physiology, *J Emerg Med* 8(4):441-447, 1990.

132. Howard FM, El-Minawi AM, Sanchez RA: Conscious pain mapping by laparoscopy in women with chronic pelvic pain, *Obstet Gynecol* 96(6):934-939, 2000.

133. Deep K, Bhalaik V: Pain as a presenting feature of acute abdomen in spinal injuries, *Injury* 34(1):33-34, 2003.

134. Lum-Hee N, Abdulla AJ: Slipping rib syndrome: an overlooked cause of chest and abdominal pain, *Int J Clin Pract* 51(4):252-253, 1997.

135. Goodman CC, Snyder TK: *Differential diagnosis for physical therapists: screening for referral*, ed 4, St Louis, 2007, Saunders Elsevier.

136. Bruckner FE, Greco A, Leung AW: 'Benign thoracic pain' syndrome: role of magnetic resonance imaging in the detection and localization of thoracic disc disease, *J Royal Soc Med* 82(2):81-83, 1989.

137. Fruth SJ: Differential diagnosis and treatment in a patient with posterior upper thoracic pain, *Phys Ther* 86(2):254-268, 2006.

138. Nicholas JJ, Christy WC: Spinal pain made worse by recumbency: a clue to spinal cord tumors, *Arch Phys Med Rehabil* 67(9):598-600, 1986.

139. Saha E, Dziadzio M, Irving K, et al: Unusual cause of painful shoulder in an elderly woman with rheumatoid arthritis, *Clin Rheumatol* 26(9):1549-1551, 2007.

140. Cortet B, Roches E, Logier R, et al: Evaluation of spinal curvatures after a recent osteoporotic vertebral fracture, *Joint Bone Spine* 69(2):201-208, 2002.

141. Sutherland CJ, Miller F, Wang GJ: Early progressive kyphosis following compression fractures. Two case reports from a series of "stable" thoracolumbar compression fractures, *Clin Orthop Relat Res* (173):216-220, 1983.

142. Wong-Chung JK, Naseeb SA, Kaneker SG, et al: Anterior disc protrusion as a cause for abdominal symptoms in childhood discitis. A case report, *Spine* 24(9):918-920, 1999.

143. Moayyeri A, Luben RN, Bingham SA, et al: Measured height loss predicts fractures in middle-aged and older men and women: the EPIC-Norfolk prospective population study, *J Bone Miner Res* 23(3):425-432, 2008.

144. Gunnes M, Lehmann EH, Mellstrom D, et al: The relationship between anthropometric measurements and fractures in women, *Bone* 19(4):407-413, 1996.

145. Eggertsen R, Mellstrom D: Height loss in women caused by vertebral fractures and osteoporosis, *Ups J Med Sci* 112(2):213-219, 2007.

146. Arroyo JF, Vine R, Reynaud C, et al: Geriatrics advisor. Slipping rib syndrome: don't be fooled, *Geriatrics* 50(3):46-49, 1995.

147. Meuwly JY, Wicky S, Schnyder P, et al: Slipping rib syndrome: a place for sonography in the diagnosis of a frequently overlooked cause of abdominal or low thoracic pain, *J Ultrasound Med* 21(3):339-343, 2002.

148. Porter GE: Slipping rib syndrome: an infrequently recognized entity in children: a report of three cases and review of the literature, *Pediatrics* 76(5):810-813, 1985.

149. Sinaki M, Grubbs NC: Back strengthening exercises: quantitative evaluation of their efficacy for women aged 40 to 65 years, *Arch Phys Med Rehabil* 70(1):16-20, 1989.

150. Sinaki M, Wahner HW, Bergstralh EJ, et al: Three-year controlled, randomized trial of the effect of dose-specified loading and strengthening exercises on bone mineral density of spine and femur in nonathletic, physically active women, *Bone* 19(3):233-244, 1996.

151. Sinaki M, Itoi E, Wahner HW, et al: Stronger back muscles reduce the incidence of vertebral fractures: a prospective 10 year follow-up of postmenopausal women, *Bone* 30(6):836-841, 2002.

152. Hongo M, Itoi E, Sinaki M, et al: Effect of low-intensity back exercise on quality of life and back extensor strength

in patients with osteoporosis: a randomized controlled trial, *Osteoporos Int* 18(10):1389-1395, 2007.

153. Straker LM, O'Sullivan PB, Smith AJ, et al: Relationships between prolonged neck/shoulder pain and sitting spinal posture in male and female adolescents, *Man Ther* 14(3):321-329, 2008.

154. Straker LM, O'Sullivan PB, Smith AJ, et al: Sitting spinal posture in adolescents differs between genders, but is not clearly related to neck/shoulder pain: an observational study, *Aust J Physiother* 54(2):127-133, 2008.

155. Kebaetse M, McClure P, Pratt NA: Thoracic position effect on shoulder range of motion, strength, and three-dimensional scapular kinematics, *Arch Phys Med Rehabil* 80(8):945-950, 1999.

156. Wolff I, van Croonenborg JJ, Kemper HC, et al: The effect of exercise training programs on bone mass: a meta-analysis of published controlled trials in pre- and postmenopausal women, *Osteoporos Int* 9(1):1-12, 1999.

157. Hodges PW, Richardson CA: Inefficient muscular stabilization of the lumbar spine associated with low back pain. A motor control evaluation of transversus abdominis, *Spine* 21(22):2640-2650, 1996.

158. Ozgocmen S, Cimen OB, Ardicoglu O: Relationship between chest expansion and respiratory muscle strength in patients with primary fibromyalgia, *Clin Rheumatol* 21(1):19-22, 2002.

159. Bogduk N: Innervation and pain patterns of the thoracic spine. In Grant R, editor. *Physical therapy of the cervical and thoracic spine*, ed 3, New York, 2002, Churchill Livingstone.

APPENDIX

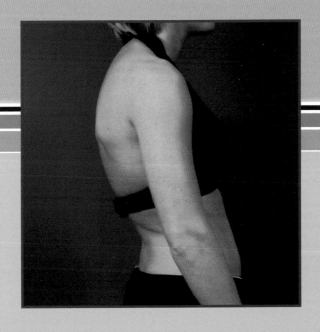

Thoracic Rotation-Flexion Syndrome

Thoracic rotation-flexion syndrome is characterized by pain associated with thoracic flexion and rotation. A posture of thoracic flexion permits rotation to occur readily. There is asymmetry in the length and recruitment of the trunk muscles: Paraspinal, scapulothoracic, and oblique abdominal muscles. Compression should be considered a contributing factor to pain if the individual has loss of height greater than $1\frac{1}{2}$ to 2 inches.[1,2] The source of symptoms in any spinal diagnosis is often difficult to determine; however, the presence of neurological signs or radicular symptoms, in particular the lower extremity, does implicate involvement of neural structures. Pain in the thoracic region has a greater likelihood of arising from nonmusculoskeletal origin; therefore it is important to pay particular attention to the potential diagnoses requiring referral.

Symptoms and History

- Pain location: Thoracic region, may radiate into the lateral and anterior rib cage or abdomen (intercostal nerve)
- Increased pain with lying down, reaching, or trunk rotation
- Pain with forceful exhalation

Activities/Population

- Recreational activities: Crew, squash, golf, running (asymmetrical arm swing and trunk rotation)
- Desk arrangement that requires rotation to reach phone, computer, or files
- Habit of working to one side
- Habit of leaning on armrest
- History of loss of motion at the glenohumeral joint
- History of chest surgery

Common Referring Diagnoses

- Bulging/herniated thoracic disc
- Thoracic pain/strain
- Trapezius strain
- Rhomboid strain
- Costochondritis
- Intercostal neuritis

Key Tests and Signs for Movement Impairment

Alignment Analysis

- Thoracic kyphosis and/or scoliosis
- Asymmetry of the rib cage noted from both posterior and anterior views
- Rib hump noted posteriorly, may cause scapular malpositioning

Unloading Test

- Passive rib cage elevation decreases symptoms

Movement Impairment Analysis

Standing

- Trunk flexion: May see an increase in thoracic rotation or excessive thoracic flexion; asymmetry of rib cage may be more notable during flexion versus standing
- Trunk rotation/lateral flexion: Asymmetrical rotation/lateral flexion of thoracic spine; pain may be reproduced with motion to either or both sides; often rotation will be greater than normal in one direction; may be painful
- Shoulder flexion: Thoracic rotation induced with unilateral > bilateral shoulder flexion; may be painful
  - Pain decreased if trunk stabilized during shoulder flexion
- Ventilation: Asymmetrical motion of rib cage (bucket-handle)

Supine

- Pain increased on assuming the supine position, asymmetry of subcostal margin noted
  - Supporting cervical and upper thoracic spine with pillows for 5 to 10 minutes will alleviate pain
- Lower abdominal muscle testing: Oblique abdominal muscles: poor control
- Shoulder flexion or hip flexion/abdomen/lateral rotation: Rib cage rotation and pain with diagonal movement
  - Pain decreased during extremity movement with stabilization of rib cage by cueing abdominal and spinal extensors to contract

Prone

- Pain increases without support; too difficult to attempt in cases of severe kyphosis (older spine)
  - Supporting with pillow(s) under chest to provide slight flexion and decreased rotation decreases pain initially, after several minutes, remove support to see if patient can tolerate a more extended position
- Pain with single-arm lift, observe or palpate rotation
  - Pain decreases with cue to recruit thoracic paraspinals to assist in rotation control during arm lift

Quadruped

- Increased thoracic flexion and rotation, rib hump may cause scapular winging or tilting
- Rocking back: Thoracic rotation flexion may increase
  - Cue to relax abdominal musculature, allows greater thoracic extension during rocking back
- Shoulder flexion: Causes rotation and/or flexion in thoracic spine
  - Cues to stabilize trunk by recruiting latissimus dorsi/back extensors and/or abdominals for rotation control decreases rotation flexion
- Crawling: Observe thoracic rotation

Aggravating Functional Activity

- Observe thoracic rotation-flexion during activity

Muscle Length Impairments

- Long thoracic paraspinals (based on alignment)
- Rectus abdominis short or stiff
- Asymmetry in length of latissimus dorsi, pectoralis major, and oblique abdominal muscles

Associated Signs or Contributing Factors

- Sternal depression
- Lumbar lordosis
- Generalized hypermobility
- Approximation of rib cage and ilium (older spines)

Structural Variations

- Vertebral wedging noted on x-ray
- Loss of height reported

Muscle Strength/Performance Impairment

- Strain of the scapular muscles because of scapular abduction/internal rotation associated with kyphosis
- Short lumbar paraspinals

Differential Diagnosis

Movement System Diagnoses

- Thoracic extension
- Thoracic rotation-flexion
- Scapular downward rotation
- Scapular abduction
- Cervical syndromes (especially for pain along vertebral border of scapula)

Potential Diagnoses Requiring Referral Suggested by Signs and Symptoms

Neuromusculoskeletal

- Compression fracture
- Scheuermann's disease
- Ankylosing spondylitis
- Disc herniation

Systemic

- Infections (e.g., tuberculosis [TB] or osteomyelitis)
- Rheumatic disease

Visceral

- Neoplasms
- Cardiovascular disease
- Pulmonary disease/pleuritis
- Abdominal organ pathology
- Gynecological dysfunctions
- Renal pathology

Treatment
Patient Education
- Avoid thoracic flexion during functional activities, as follows:
  - *Reaching:* While pain is present, suggest reaching with both arms bent to decrease flexion moment at thoracic spine.
  - *Driving:* Keep hands positioned symmetrically on steering wheel. Education on improved thoracic alignment while driving.
  - *Sports:* Increase motion of hip flexion during sporting activities, reduce amount of trunk flexion during initiation of task (e.g., hip flexion with spine straighter to address golf ball).
- *Positioning:* If tolerating supine, minimize number of pillows under head and shoulders; if initially assuming the position is painful, start with increased flexion/support with pillows and then remove after several minutes.
- *Standing instruction:* Avoid swayed thoracic spine, correct alignment of center of mass over feet so that thoracic paraspinal musculature and gluteals will be required for control of balance. In the presence of severe kyphosis, an assistive device may be needed to improve thoracic extension when standing.
- *Sitting instruction:* Provide trunk support to decrease thoracic flexion of upper thoracic spine; may need to teach unloading with upper extremities if compression is a contributing factor to pain.

Standing
Emphasis on redistribution of motion to increase hip motion and decreasing thoracic flexion with rotation motion.
- *Wall exercises:* Emphasis on improved alignment for flexion, decompression of thoracic spine.
  - *Facing wall shoulder flexion:* Decompression of thoracic spine, relaxation of abdominal musculature, improved postural alignment. Progression to shoulder flexion for strengthening of thoracic paraspinal musculature.
  - *Back to wall:* Decompression of thoracic spine caused by unloading of weight of the upper body. Rib cage elevation manually and with cueing to "hold new position." Emphasis on improved alignment and decompression for symptom relief.
  - *Back to wall shoulder flexion:* Lengthen latissimus dorsi, strengthen thoracic paraspinal musculature, cueing needed to relax abdominal musculature to improve sternal depression. Inhale at top of flexion: Lengthen abdominal musculature; correct ventilation impairment of thoracic flexion with inhalation.
  - *Back to wall shoulder abduction:* Lengthen pectoral major/minor; strengthen thoracic paraspinal musculature. Inhale at top of flexion: Lengthen abdominal musculature; correct ventilation impairment of thoracic flexion with inhalation.
  - *Ventilation:* Emphasis on increasing pump-handle motion during inhalation, with cues to relax abdominal musculature; can be done on the wall or in sitting support for the spine.

Prone
Emphasis on strengthening paraspinal musculature and improving rotation control and alignment of spine.
- *Erector spinae strengthening:* Isometric contraction during middle trap progression.
  - Isometric scapular adduction
  - Bilateral arm lift
  - Single-arm lift arm on table
  - Single-arm lift arm off table
- *Prone trunk extension from a flexed position:* Place trunk in flexion over several pillows; emphasis on upper thoracic paraspinal strengthening with monitoring of lower paraspinal activity.
  - Should not be performed if (1) motion is localized to lumbar paraspinals and do not observe a change in the amount of thoracic flexion or (2) if suspect compression as a component of pain.

Quadruped
Emphasis on improvement of alignment and decompression of thoracic spine.
- *Rocking:* Cueing to relax abdominal musculature; emphasis on reducing thoracic flexion.
- *Arm lifts:* Erector spinae strengthening.

Aggravating Functional Activity
Observe and correct excessive thoracic flexion during functional activities, including reading, eating, tooth brushing, and so on.

NOTES

Thoracic Flexion Syndrome

Thoracic pain is associated with positions or movements of the thoracic spine into flexion. Most often, excessive flexion is noted both in an upright posture and with trunk movements. Movement tests of thoracic flexion are often not painful; however, pain is produced when the patient attempts to rapidly straighten the spine after periods of prolonged flexion. Compression should be considered a contributing factor to pain if the individual has loss of height greater then 1½ to 2 inches.[1,2] The source of symptoms in any spinal diagnosis is often difficult to determine; however, the presence of neurological signs or radicular symptoms, in particular in the lower extremity, does implicate involvement of neural structures. Pain in the thoracic region has a greater likelihood of arising from nonmusculoskeletal origin; therefore it is important to pay particular attention to the potential diagnoses requiring referral.

Symptoms and History

- Pain location: Thoracic region, especially midscapular region (scapular abduction) and lower thoracic region
- Younger spines: Pain worse after sitting in a flexed posture for prolonged periods
- Older spines: More commonly, pain with attempts to straighten the spine from flexed position
- Older spines: Pain associated with walking or standing

Activities/Population

- Sedentary lifestyle (older spine)
- Sits with excessive kyphosis
- Working at low surfaces or with arms extended out in front of body
- Recreational activities: Sit-ups, crew, and bicycling
- Sleeps in sitting position
- Bikers
- Students

Common Referring Diagnoses

- Bulging or herniated thoracic disc
- Thoracic pain/strain
- Trapezius strain
- Rhomboid strain
- Costochondritis
- Intercostal neuritis

Key Tests and Signs for Movement Impairment

Alignment Analysis

- Thoracic kyphosis
- Subcostal margin > 90 degrees
- Swayback
- Scapular abduction
- Increased depth of rib cage
- Pain common with attempt to straighten spine from the flexed position

Unloading Test

- Passive rib cage elevation decreases symptoms

Movement Impairment Analysis

Standing

- Trunk flexion: Excessive thoracic flexion; pain with return to upright position
  - Thoracic flexion: If painful in an older individual, suspect compression fracture
  - Pain decreased with redistributing motion: Increase hip flexion and limit thoracic flexion
- Bilateral shoulder flexion: Increase thoracic flexion/sway; may observe lumbar extension
- Ventilation: Pump-handle motion reduced

Supine

- Pain increased on assuming the supine position
  - Supporting cervical and upper thoracic spine with pillows for 5 to 10 minutes will alleviate pain
- Lower abdominal muscle testing: Poor performance of external oblique and overrecruitment of rectus abdominis (RA) and internal obliques (athletic population)

Prone

- Pain may increase without support; too difficult to achieve in cases of severe kyphosis (older spine)
  - Supporting with pillow(s) under chest to provide slight flexion decreases pain initially; after several minutes, patient can tolerate a more extended position after removal of support
- Manual muscle testing: Weakness of thoracic paraspinals, middle and lower trapezius, and rhomboid muscles

Quadruped

- Increased thoracic flexion, short RA (athletic population)
  - Spinal extension in quadruped often less painful than supine or upright position
- Rocking back: Increases thoracic flexion
  - Cueing to relax abdominal musculature increases thoracic extension during rocking back

Aggravating Functional Activity

- Thoracic extension from a flexed position during activity or excessive thoracic flexion that is painful during activity

Muscle Length Impairments (Based on Alignment)

- Short RA/internal obliques (athletic population)
- Long thoracic paraspinals
- Long scapular adductors

Associated Signs or Contributing Factors

- Sternal depression
- Lumbar lordosis
- Generalized hypermobility
- Approximation of rib cage and ilium (older spines)

Structural Variations

- Vertebral wedging noted on x-ray
- Loss of height reported

Muscle Strength/Performance Impairment

- Strain of the scapular muscles because of scapular abduction associated with kyphosis
- Short lumbar paraspinals

Differential Diagnosis

Movement System Diagnoses

- Thoracic extension
- Thoracic rotation-flexion
- Scapular downward rotation
- Scapular abduction
- Cervical syndromes (especially for pain along vertebral border of scapula)

Potential Diagnoses Requiring Referral Suggested by Signs and Symptoms

Neuromusculoskeletal

- Compression fracture
- Scheuermann's disease
- Ankylosing spondylitis
- Disc herniation

Systemic

- Infections (e.g., TB or osteomyelitis)
- Rheumatic disease

Visceral

- Neoplasms
- Cardiovascular disease
- Pulmonary disease/pleuritis
- Abdominal organ pathology
- Gynecological dysfunctions
- Renal pathology

Treatment

Patient Education

- Avoid thoracic flexion during functional activities, as follows:
  - *Reaching:* While pain is present, reach with both arms bent to decrease flexion moment at thoracic spine.
  - *Driving:* Keep hands positioned symmetrically on steering wheel. Education on improved thoracic alignment driving.
  - *Sports:* Increase motion of hip flexion during sporting activities, reduce amount of trunk flexion during initiation of task (e.g., hip flexion with spine straighter to address golf ball).
- *Positioning:* If tolerating supine, minimize number of pillows under head and shoulders; if initially assuming the position is painful, start with increased flexion/support with pillows and then remove after several minutes.
- *Standing instruction:* Avoid swayed thoracic spine, correct alignment of center of mass over feet so that thoracic paraspinal musculature and gluteals will be required for control of balance. In the presence of severe kyphosis, an assistive device may be needed to improve thoracic extension when standing.
- *Sitting instruction:* Provide trunk support to decrease thoracic flexion of upper thoracic spine; may need to teach unloading with upper extremities if compression is a contributing factor to pain.

Standing

Emphasis on redistribution of motion to increase hip motion and decreasing thoracic flexion with rotation motion.

- *Wall exercises:* Emphasis on improved alignment for flexion, decompression of thoracic spine.
  - *Facing wall shoulder flexion:* Decompression of thoracic spine, relaxation of abdominal musculature, improved postural alignment. Progression to shoulder flexion for strengthening of thoracic paraspinal musculature.
  - *Back to wall:* Decompression of thoracic spine caused by unloading of weight of the upper body. Rib cage elevation manually and with cueing to "hold new position." Emphasis on improved alignment and decompression for symptom relief.

- *Back to wall shoulder flexion:* Lengthen latissimus dorsi, strengthen thoracic paraspinal musculature, cueing needed to relax abdominal musculature to improve sternal depression. Inhale at top of flexion: Lengthen abdominal musculature; correct ventilation impairment of thoracic flexion with inhalation.
- *Back to wall shoulder abduction:* Lengthen pectoral major/minor, strengthen thoracic paraspinal musculature. Inhale at top of flexion: Lengthen abdominal musculature; correct ventilation impairment of thoracic flexion with inhalation.
- *Ventilation:* Emphasis on increasing pump-handle motion during inhalation, with cues to relax abdominal musculature; can be done on the wall or in sitting support for the spine.

Prone

Emphasis on strengthening paraspinal musculature and improving rotation control and alignment of spine.

- *Erector spinae strengthening:* Isometric contraction during middle trap progression.
  - Isometric scapular adduction
  - Bilateral arm lift
  - Single-arm lift arm on table
  - Single-arm lift arm off table
- *Prone trunk extension from a flexed position:* Place trunk in flexion over several pillow; emphasis on upper thoracic paraspinal strengthening with monitoring of lower paraspinal activity.
  - *Should not be performed if (1) motion is localized to lumbar paraspinals and do not observe a change in the amount of thoracic flexion or (2) if suspect compression as a component of pain.*

Quadruped

Emphasis on improvement of alignment and decompression of thoracic spine.

- *Rocking:* Cueing to relax abdominal musculature; emphasis on reducing thoracic flexion.
- *Arm lifts:* Erector spinae strengthening.

Aggravating Functional Activity

Observe and correct excessive thoracic flexion during functional activities, including reading, eating, tooth brushing, and so on.

NOTES

Thoracic Rotation-Extension Syndrome

Thoracic pain is associated with positions or movements of the thoracic spine into extension and rotation. There is an altered distribution of rotation motion across the thoracic spine. Alignment and movement impairments are most often found in a portion of the thoracic spine rather than the entire thoracic spine. The flexibility of the thoracic spine is altered so that extension and rotation occur too easily. Muscle impairments include asymmetry in the length and recruitment of the trunk muscles: paraspinals, scapulothoracic and oblique abdominal muscles. The source of symptoms in any spinal diagnosis is often difficult to determine; however, the presence of neurological sign or radicular symptoms, in particular the lower extremity, does implicate involvement of neural structures. Pain in the thoracic region has a greater likelihood of arising from nonmusculoskeletal origin; therefore it is important to pay particular attention to the potential diagnoses requiring referral.

Symptoms and History

- Pain location: Thoracic region, which may radiate into the lateral and anterior rib cage or abdomen (intercostal nerve)
- Pain increases with sidelying; inhalation; unilateral arm motion, especially overhead; movements of trunk rotation

Activities/Population

- Habitual trunk extension, "good posture"
- Working with arms overhead especially if asymmetrical
- Recreational activities: tennis, ballet, gymnast
- History of glenohumeral joint loss of motion

Common Referring Diagnoses

- Bulging or herniated thoracic disc
- Thoracic pain/strain
- Trapezius strain
- Rhomboid strain
- Slipping rib syndrome
- Rib malpositioned into inhalation

Key Tests and Signs for Movement Impairment

Alignment Analysis

Standing

- Flat or decreased flexion in regions of the thoracic spine
- Decreased A-P depth of rib cage
- Asymmetry of the rib cage noted from both posterior and anterior views:
  - Rib hump noted posteriorly
  - Anterior chest asymmetry
  - Subcostal margin asymmetrical
- Thoracic scoliosis or rotational malalignment in localized area

Unloading Test

- Passive rib cage elevation decreases symptoms

Movement Impairment

Standing

- Trunk flexion: Limited thoracic flexion, thoracic rotation may be more prominent during trunk flexion, and may have pain with return to the upright position at end-range of motion
  - Cueing to avoid excessive extension and/or lateral flexion with return to the upright position at end-range of motion decrease pain
- Trunk rotation/lateral flexion: Asymmetrical rotation/lateral flexion of thoracic spine; pain may be reproduced with motion to either or both sides
  - Supported lateral flexion decreases pain
- Trunk extension is painful
- Shoulder flexion is painful; observe rotation or lateral flexion
  - Cueing to control extension and rotation of thoracic spine decrease symptoms
- Ventilation: May have pain with deep inhalation and may observe thoracic extension and rib cage asymmetry

Supine

- Pain may decrease with supine lying
  - Pain may decrease with correction of rotation of rib cage
- Shoulder flexion: Observe excessive rib cage elevation and asymmetry in rib cage motion
  - Cues to stabilize rib cage achieved by recruiting abdominal musculature

Prone

- Unilateral shoulder flexion: Thoracic extension and rotation noted, overrecruitment of scapular adductors and thoracic paraspinals, may be painful
  - Position in thoracic flexion and/or cueing for abdominal contraction decreases pain and overrecruitment of scapular adductors and thoracic paraspinals

Quadruped

- Preferred position commonly is thoracic extension with lateral flexion
- Shoulder flexion: Causes rotation or lateral flexion in thoracic spine
  - Cues to stabilize trunk by recruiting abdominals and/or latissimus dorsi decreases rotation
- Crawling: Observe thoracic rotation

Aggravating Functional Activity

- Observe thoracic extension rotation during activity

Muscle Length Impairments (Based on Alignment)

- Asymmetrical short/stiff thoracic paraspinals
- Asymmetrical short/stiff scapular adductors
- Asymmetrical oblique abdominals

Associated Signs or Contributing Factors

- Vertebral borders of scapula prominent, one side greater than the other if rib hump present
- Scapular adduction
- Cervical and lumbar spines flat

Muscle Strength/Performance Impairment

- Abdominal muscle weakness

Structural Variations

- Scoliosis

Special Tests

- Positive hooking maneuver

Differential Diagnosis

Movement System Diagnoses

- Thoracic extension
- Thoracic rotation-flexion
- Scapular downward rotation
- Scapular abduction
- Cervical syndromes (especially for pain along vertebral border of scapula)

Potential Diagnoses Requiring Referral Suggested by Signs and Symptoms

Neuromusculoskeletal

- Compression fracture
- Disc herniation

Systemic

- Infections (e.g., TB or osteomyelitis)
- Rheumatic disease

Visceral

- Neoplasms
- Cardiovascular disease
- Pulmonary disease/pleuritis
- Abdominal organ pathology
- Gynecological dysfunctions
- Renal pathology

Treatment
Patient Education
- Avoid thoracic rotation and extension during functional activities, as follows:
  - *Reaching:* While pain is present, reach with both arms to decrease rotational moment at thoracic spine and turn more at hips to avoid thoracic rotation with reach.
  - *Driving:* Avoid leaning on armrest, keep hands positioned symmetrically on steering wheel, assess pain with turning car on or managing car controls. Education on improved thoracic alignment and motion with function.
  - *Racquet sports:* Increase rotation motion at hips to decrease amount of motion across thoracic spine.
- *Positioning:* In sidelying, support thoracic spine out of sidebending and support lower legs to avoid rotation of lumbar region or low thoracic region.
- *Sitting instruction:* Avoid shifting to armrest, crossing legs, or asymmetrical sitting.

Standing
Avoid asymmetrical stance. Emphasis on redistribution of motion to increase hip motion and decrease thoracic rotation and extension with motion. Cueing to avoid excessive extension and/or lateral flexion with return to the upright position at end-range of motion decreases pain.
- *Wall exercises:* Emphasis on improved alignment for rotation control.
  - *Trunk lateral flexion:* Back supported on wall, unilateral lateral flexion with manual support on rib cage.
  - *Back to wall shoulder flexion:* Lengthen latissimus dorsi, strengthen thoracic paraspinal musculature, cueing recruits abdominal musculature to improve rotational motion and control extension.
  - *Back to wall shoulder abduction:* Lengthen pectoral major/minor, strengthen thoracic paraspinal musculature cueing recruit abdominal musculature to improve rotational motion.
  - *Facing wall shoulder flexion:* Decompression of thoracic spine, relaxation of abdominal musculature, improved postural alignment. Progression to shoulder flexion for strengthening of thoracic paraspinal musculature.
  - *Ventilation:* Back on wall to control thoracic extension and manual contact on rib cage to correct asymmetry during ventilation.

Supine
Correct rotation in supine with towel support for positioning.
- *Shoulder flexion:* Cues to stabilize rib cage achieved by recruiting abdominal musculature.

Prone
Emphasis on strengthening paraspinal musculature and improving rotation control and alignment of spine.
- *Position:* Thoracic flexion and/or cueing for abdominal contraction decreases pain and overrecruitment of scapular adductors and thoracic paraspinals.
- *Erector spinae strengthening:* Isometric contraction during middle trap progression.
  - Isometric scapular adduction
  - Bilateral arm lift
  - Single-arm lift arm on table
  - Single-arm lift arm off table

Quadruped
Emphasis on improvement of alignment of thoracic spine.
- *Rocking:* Emphasis on reducing rotation/sidebending with extension during motion.
- *Arm lifts:* Cues to stabilize trunk by recruiting abdominals and/or latissimus dorsi decreases rotation.

NOTES

Thoracic Rotation Syndrome

This syndrome is characterized by pain or symptoms reproduced with thoracic rotation without any obvious bias toward flexion or extension alignment or movement impairments. In this syndrome, there is an imbalance in muscles acting as extrinsic contributors to multiplanar movements rather than principle uniplanar motion. The painful region of the thoracic spine has become the most flexible site for motion. The source of symptoms in any spinal diagnoses is often difficult to determine; however, the presence of neurological signs or radicular symptoms in particular the lower extremity does implicate involvement of neural structures. Pain in the thoracic region has a greater likelihood of arising from nonmusculoskeletal origin; therefore, it is important to pay particular attention to the diagnoses requiring referral.

Symptoms and History

- Pain location: Sharp or pinching pain in the thoracic region, which may radiate into the lateral and anterior rib cage
- Pain provoked with trunk rotation or arm motions

Activities/Population

- Recreational activities: throwing, golf, kayak/canoeing, running
- Desk or work arrangement that requires rotation to reach phone, computer, files
- Habit of working to one side

Common Referring Diagnoses

- Bulging or herniated thoracic disc
- Thoracic pain/strain
- Trapezius strain
- Rhomboid strain
- Costochondritis
- Intercostal neuritis
- Slipping rib syndrome

Key Tests and Signs for Movement Impairment

Alignment Analysis

- Standing: Generally slight malalignment in the area of the painful region, large subcostal angle (>90 degrees)
- Alignment at rest may appear normal
- Unloading: Passive rib cage elevation decreases symptoms

Movement Impairment Analysis

Standing

- Trunk flexion: Observe an increase in thoracic rotation; thoracic rotation and asymmetry of rib cage may be more notable during flexion versus standing
- Both flexion and extension of the thoracic spine can reproduce pain
- Trunk rotation and lateral flexion: Asymmetrical rotation/lateral flexion of thoracic spine; pain may be reproduced with motion to either or both sides
- Shoulder flexion: Thoracic rotation induced with unilateral shoulder flexion; may be painful
  - Pain decreased if trunk stabilized during shoulder flexion

Supine

- Shoulder flexion/hip flexion or abduction/lateral rotation: Rib cage rotation and pain with arm diagonals or hip flexion or abduction/lateral rotation
  - Pain decreased during extremity movement with stabilization of rib cage by cueing abdominal and spinal extensors to contract
- Lower abdominal muscle testing: Oblique abdominal muscles—poor control

Prone

- Pain with single-arm lift, observe rotation

Quadruped

- Position: Rib hump may cause scapular winging or tilting
- Shoulder flexion: Observe rotation in thoracic spine
  - Rotation may be present bilaterally
- Crawling: Observe thoracic rotation

Aggravating Functional Activity

- Observe thoracic rotation during activity

Muscle Length Impairments (Based on Alignment)

- Long thoracic paraspinals
- Long abdominal musculature
- Latissimus dorsi muscle (based on length test)

Associated Signs or Contributing Factors

- Asymmetry of the rib cage
- Asymmetry of scapular position (rib cage rotation)
- Sitting posture: Habitually with lateral flexion

Structural Variation

- Scoliosis

Movement Impairment

Standing

- Ventilation: Asymmetrical expansion of anterior costal margins

Supine

- Pain reproduced with rolling over (twisting)
- Pain eliminated if patient performs log roll

Special Tests

- Positive hooking maneuver

Differential Diagnosis

Movement System Diagnoses

- Thoracic extension
- Thoracic rotation-flexion
- Scapular downward rotation
- Scapular abduction
- Cervical syndromes (especially for pain along vertebral border of scapula)

Potential Diagnoses Requiring Referral Suggested by Signs and Symptoms

Neuromusculoskeletal

- Compression fracture
- Disc herniation
- Ankylosing spondylitis
- Slipping rib syndrome

Systemic

- Infections (e.g., TB or osteomyelitis)
- Rheumatic disease

Visceral

- Neoplasms
- Cardiovascular disease
- Pulmonary disease/pleuritis
- Abdominal organ pathology
- Gynecological dysfunctions
- Renal pathology

Treatment
Patient Education
- Avoid thoracic rotation functional activities, as follows:
  - *Reaching:* While pain is present, reach with both arms to decrease rotational moment at thoracic spine. Turn more at hips to avoid thoracic rotation with reach.
  - *Driving:* Avoid leaning on armrest, keep hands positioned symmetrically on steering wheel, assess pain with turning car on or managing car controls. Education on improved thoracic alignment and motion with function.
  - *Racquet sports:* Increase rotation motion at hips to decrease amount of motion across thoracic spine.
- *Positioning:* In sidelying, support thoracic spine out of sidebending, support lower legs to avoid rotation of lumbar region or low thoracic region.
- *Sitting instruction:* Avoid shifting to armrest, crossing legs, and asymmetrical sitting.

Standing
Avoid asymmetrical stance. Emphasis on redistribution of motion to increase hip motion and decrease thoracic rotation with motion.
- *Wall exercises:* Emphasis on improved alignment for rotation control.
  - *Trunk lateral flexion:* Back supported on wall, unilateral lateral flexion with manual support on rib cage.
  - *Facing wall shoulder flexion:* Decompression of thoracic spine, relaxation of abdominal musculature, improved postural alignment. Progression to shoulder flexion for strengthening of thoracic paraspinal musculature.
  - *Back to wall shoulder flexion:* Lengthen latissimus dorsi, strengthen thoracic paraspinal musculature, cueing recruits abdominal musculature to improve rotational motion.
  - *Back to wall shoulder abduction:* Lengthen pectoral major/minor, strengthen thoracic paraspinal musculature, cueing recruits abdominal musculature to improve rotational motion.
- *Ventilation:* Back on wall with manual contact on rib cage to correct asymmetry during ventilation.

Prone
Emphasis on strengthening paraspinal musculature, improving rotation control and alignment of spine.
- *Erector spinae strengthening:* Isometric contraction during middle trap progression.
  - Isometric scapular adduction
  - Bilateral arm lift
  - Single-arm lift arm on table
  - Single-arm lift arm off table

In some cases, prone trunk extension may be needed for strengthening, and caution should be take to consider the effect of this exercise on the lumbar spine. Isolation of the thoracic paraspinals with this exercise is difficult to achieve in many cases, thus contributing to a lumbar extension movement impairment.

Quadruped
Emphasis on improvement of alignment of thoracic spine.
- *Rocking:* Emphasis on reducing rotation with motion.
- *Arm lifts:* Erector spinae strengthening, rotation control.

NOTES

Thoracic Extension Syndrome

Thoracic pain is associated with positions or movements of the thoracic spine into extension. Typically, these individuals habitually assume a very erect posture to the point of thoracic extension in both sitting and standing. The flexibility of the thoracic spine is altered so that extension occurs too easily. The source of symptoms in any spinal diagnosis is often difficult to determine; however, the presence of neurological signs or radicular symptoms, in particular the lower extremity, does implicate involvement of neural structures. Pain in the thoracic region has a greater likelihood of arising from nonmusculoskeletal origin; therefore it is important to pay particular attention to the potential diagnoses requiring referral.

Symptoms and History

- Pain location: Thoracic region, often interscapular area or thoracolumbar junction
- Pain associated with standing, sitting erect or reaching overhead

Activities/Population

- Habitual "good alignment" such as military personnel
- Dancers, gymnasts
- Working with arms overhead
- Habit of sleeping with arms overhead
- Younger individuals

Common Referring Diagnoses

- Bulging or herniated thoracic disc
- Thoracic pain/strain
- Trapezius strain
- Rhomboid strain

Key Tests and Signs for Movement Impairment

Alignment Analysis

Standing

- Flat or decreased thoracic curve, common at thoracolumbar junction or interscapular region
  - Pain decreased by slightly flexing thoracic spine; cues to relax spine
- Rib cage alignment: Decreased anterior-posterior depth

Unloading Test

- Passive rib cage elevation decreases symptoms

Movement Impairment:

Standing

- Trunk flexion: Limited thoracic flexion during bending, may have pain with return
  - Pain during return to upright is decreased with cues to avoid extending thoracic spine
- Trunk extension: Pain with active extension
- Trunk rotation: Limited but not painful
- Ventilation: May have pain with deep inhalation, may observe thoracic extension

Sitting

- Sits with thoracic spine extended
  - Pain decreased by slightly flexing thoracic spine; cues to relax spine
  - Thoracic spine supported into relaxed flexed position decreases pain

Supine

- Pain may decrease with supine lying
- Bilateral shoulder flexion: Observe elevation of the rib cage

Prone

- Unilateral shoulder flexion: Thoracic extension noted, often upper thoracic; may be painful, excessive recruitment of thoracic paraspinals
  - Position in thoracic flexion and/or cueing for abdominal contraction decreases pain

Quadruped

- Thoracic extension noted, may be painful
  - Pain decreased with flexion of thoracic spine
- Scapulae appear prominent

Aggravating Functional Activity

- Observe thoracic extension during activity

Muscle Length Impairments (Based on Alignment)

- Short/stiff thoracic paraspinals
- Short/stiff scapular adductors

Associated Signs or Contributing Factors

- Vertebral borders of scapula prominent (standing and quadruped)
- Scapular adduction
- Cervical and lumbar spines flat

Muscle Strength/Performance Impairments

- Poor performance in abdominals

Differential Diagnosis

Movement System Diagnoses

- Thoracic extension
- Thoracic rotation-flexion
- Scapular downward rotation
- Scapular abduction
- Cervical syndromes (especially for pain along vertebral border of scapula)

Potential Diagnoses Requiring Referral Suggested by Signs and Symptoms

Neuromusculoskeletal

- Compression fracture
- Metastatic tumor in thoracic spine
- Frank neurological signs

Systemic

- Infections (e.g., TB or osteomyelitis)
- Rheumatic disease
- Shingles

Visceral

- Neoplasms
- Cardiovascular disease
- Pulmonary disease/pleuritis
- Abdominal organ pathology
- Gynecological dysfunctions
- Renal pathology

Treatment
Movement Impairment Exercise
Standing

Patient education regarding relaxing thoracic spinal extensors during standing: Drop chest and allow head / neck to move slightly anterior to plane of shoulders.

- *Forward bending and return:* Correct excessive thoracic extension with return from forward bending.
- *Bilateral shoulder flexion:* Cueing to reduce thoracic extension with end-range of motion.
- *Ventilation:* Correct thoracic extension during inhalation, back to wall to limit trunk motion during ventilation, and cueing manually with hands to increase bucket-handle over pump-handle motion.

Sitting

Patient education to reduce thoracic extension during sitting. Pain decreased by slightly flexing thoracic spine, cues to relax spine.

- *Thoracic spine:* Supported into relaxed flexed position decreases pain, may need to support shoulder girdle with bilateral pillows positioned lengthwise in axilla.

Supine

- *Bilateral shoulder flexion:* In the supine position, cueing to contract abdominal musculature to avoid rib cage elevation, thoracic extension, support cervical spine into flexion to encourage upper thoracic flexion.

Prone

- *Unilateral/bilateral shoulder motions:* Positioning into thoracic flexion, cues to recruit abdominal musculature to control thoracic extension, cueing to recruit scapulothoracic musculature over thoracic paraspinal musculature.

Quadruped

- *Increased thoracic flexion:* May need to accommodate cervical or lumbar position to achieve position of comfort.
- *Rocking backward:* Cueing to increase thoracic flexion at end-range of motion.
- *Arm lifts:* Cues to contract abdominal musculature to maintain "flexed thoracic" position with arm lifts.

Aggravating Functional Activities

Observe and correct thoracic extension during aggravating functional activity.

REFERENCES

1. Keller TS, Harrison DE, Colloca CJ, et al: Prediction of osteoporotic spinal deformity, *Spine* 28(5):455-462, 2003.
2. Silverman SL: The clinical consequences of vertebral compression fracture, *Bone* 13(2):S27-S31, 1992.

Movement System Syndromes of the Hand and Wrist

Cheryl Caldwell, Lynnette Khoo-Summers

INTRODUCTION

Hand dysfunctions may be caused by an acute injury or injury as a result of prolonged or repetitive activities. Effective treatment requires managing the acute tissue injury as well as the underlying movement impairments. Based on years of clinical observations, we have classified the patterns of movement deviations associated with hand dysfunctions. The classifications are labeled as movement system syndromes (Box 5-1). This chapter describes two categories of movement system syndromes: (1) those based on the source or region of the injury, and (2) those based on the principal movement system impairment.

A diagnosis based on the source or pathoanatomy is most commonly used for acute hand dysfunction and is often provided in the referral documentation. In these cases, a complete movement system examination is not possible. The source diagnosis guides physical therapy treatment based on established protocols. These protocols are based on stages of tissue healing because they identify the source (pathoanatomical tissue) that is affected and the degree of the injury.[1] A regional diagnosis, hand impairment is used when the referral documentation does not state the pathoanatomical or source diagnosis for an acute injury (see Box 5-1). After resolution of this early or severe stage of tissue injury, a complete movement system examination should be performed to establish a diagnosis of the principal movement impairment.

A diagnosis based on the principal movement system impairment should also be used for hand dysfunction caused by prolonged or repetitive activities. These types of slowly developing conditions do not have a protocol for treatment or even an established standardized examination, particularly one that assesses movement. The repetitive movements that induce the pain conditions result in slight deviations from precise movement and thus an examination to assess movement characteristics is essential.[2]

In addition to the movement system impairment, or source or regional diagnosis (see Box 5-1), assignment of a stage helps guide the development of the treatment plan. The staging system is described in Chapter 2.

Movement system impairments are influenced by a variety of factors, including age, structural variations, and body type. For example, a patient who is obese may have a resting alignment of shoulder abduction. This shoulder alignment results in increased wrist ulnar deviation (UD) when typing on a keyboard. Repetitive wrist ulnar and radial deviation may cause tissue injury at the wrist such as is found in de Quervain's disease. Another example of the influence of structural variation is the musician whose anthropometrics may influence choices made regarding an instrument. A musician with short arms and fingers may compensate by using a slightly different movement pattern compared to a musician with longer extremities playing the same instrument.

For any of the movement system syndromes, the most important movement pattern to address in treatment may be the result of either hypomobility (physiological and accessory motion), hypermobility (excessive motion), force production deficit (decreased strength), or movement pattern coordination deficit (impaired motor control: timing, magnitude, or duration).[3]

The movement system syndromes of insufficient finger or thumb flexion, insufficient finger or thumb extension, and insufficient thumb abduction and/or opposition are used to teach the principles of examination and treatment of the hand to physical therapy students and therapists who have not specialized in hand therapy. The content within these three syndromes is not new to the experienced hand therapist, but it is organized in a unique way to facilitate teaching therapists who do not specialize in the hand how to determine the cause of the dysfunction (referred to as the *source of signs and symptoms* in the Chapter 5 Appendix). A major objective of the systematic examination of the hand for these syndromes is to identify the cause of the dysfunction instead of only identifying isolated impairments, such as decreased active

BOX 5-1

Movement System Syndromes of the Hand

- Insufficient finger and/or thumb flexion syndrome
- Insufficient finger and/or thumb extension syndrome (not discussed in text but is included in the Chapter 5 Appendix)
- Insufficient thumb palmar abduction and/or opposition syndrome
- Thumb carpometacarpal (CMC) accessory hypermobility syndrome
- Finger (or thumb) flexion syndrome with and without rotation syndrome
- Source or regional impairment diagnosis of the hand
  Conditions that may fall under the regional impairment diagnosis of the hand when the pathoanatomical source diagnosis is not provided on the referral documentation are as follows:

INJURIES

- Injuries that may be treated initially conservatively or surgically include but are not limited to gamekeeper's thumb, ligament injuries, fractures, de Quervain's disease, boutonnière, mallet, osteoarthritis (OA) of CMC of thumb (depending on the stage), tendinopathy, and carpal tunnel syndrome (CTS).

POSTOPERATIVE

- Stabilization: Indications are fractures, ligament injuries, pain, instability, deformity, avascular necrosis (AVN), bony tumors).
  - Open reduction internal fixation (ORIF), external fixation, fusion, limited intercarpal arthrodesis, percutaneous pins, or cast
- Arthroplasty: Indications are joint destruction or deformity secondary to rheumatoid arthritis (RA), OA, degenerative joint disease (DJD).

- Metacarpophalangeal (MP): Most common
- Ligament reconstruction tendon interposition (LRTI)
- Proximal interphalangeal (PIP) joint
- Total wrist
- Nerve decompression: Indications are median, radial. or ulnar nerve compression resulting in pain, loss of sensation or motor function.
- Replantation and/or amputation.
- Compartment decompression: Indication is crush injury with secondary loss of arterial blood flow.
- Repair: Indications are tear, avulsion, laceration, and rupture.
  - Ligament, tendon, triangular fibrocartilage complex (TFCC), nerve (grafts and repair), and artery
- Incision and drainage: Indication is infection.
- Tendon and nerve transfers: Indication is paralysis of a muscle, with resultant loss of function.
- Soft tissue release and/or resection: Indications are Dupuytren's disease, adhered tendon resulting in loss of active functional use of hand. Synovectomy indicated with prolonged swelling, pain, and dysfunction, no evidence of joint destruction.
  - Compartment or pulley release: Indications are de Quervain's disease or trigger finger/tenosynovitis), fasciotomy = compartment release, tenolysis, synovectomy, aspiration or excision (indicated with ganglion), excision of palmar fascia (indicated with Dupuytren's), surgical decompression (indicated with intersection syndrome), and skin graft or skin with significant loss of soft tissue.

range of motion (AROM). For example, for the movement system syndrome, insufficient finger or thumb flexion, there are several potential causes of the limitation of movement, including flexor or extensor tendon adhesion (hypomobility), extensor muscle shortness (hypomobility), weakness or rupture of the finger flexors (force production deficit), shortened ligaments (hypomobility), and so on. Treatment should address the cause of dysfunction instead of the isolated impairments. If treatment is based on goniometric measurement of AROM without taking into account the cause of the limitation, the treatment may not be the most effective or efficient.

The movement system syndromes, thumb carpometacarpal (CMC) accessory hypermobility and finger flexion with and without rotation, are unique and have not been previously described this way. CMC accessory hypermobility syndrome is based on information available in the literature, as well as clinical experience observing and treating the movement impairments associated with thumb pain. Young patients with hypermobile joints and patients with early osteoarthritis (OA) or degenerative

joint disease (DJD) of the CMC of the thumb are often assigned this syndrome.

Knowledge of normal alignment, movement, and muscle function guides the therapist in identifying alignment and movement impairments and prescribing treatment to correct those impairments. Unique to the movement system examination of the hand is the emphasis on first evaluating the patient's preferred pattern of movement and correlating this with the onset of symptoms (referred to as the *primary test*). The examiner focuses on identifying the joint that is relatively most flexible and is the cause of the patient's chief complaint. The primary test is immediately followed by a secondary test in which the symptom-provoking preferred pattern of movement is modified to determine the effect on the symptoms. This sequence of testing is performed throughout the examination, as well as during the observation of functional activities. Identifying and modifying the functional activities is a critical aspect in the physical therapy management of the patient's pain.

Key elements in the examination and treatment of the hand for all diagnostic groups presented in this chapter that may be unique are as follows:

- Identify the joint that is relatively most flexible (this is the concept of relative flexibility or the body taking the path of least resistance to movement) and train the patient to move less at the flexible joint and more at the stiffer joint. Identify the repeated or prolonged functional activity that has caused the adaptations in joint flexibility.[2]
  - Examination of patients with the movement system syndrome insufficient finger or thumb flexion caused by metacarpophalangeal (MP) collateral ligament shortness shows that the MP joint is the stiffest and the least likely to move. Therefore, for treatment to be most effective, the proximal interphalangeal (PIP) and distal interphalangeal (DIP) joints must be stabilized or made stiffer. The goal is the normal balance of stiffness around the joints and between the joints.
- Identify the specific muscle impairments contributing to the movement dysfunction of the affected joints. Muscle impairments include recruitment, stiffness, or changes in length or weakness.
  - Stiffness throughout the range of motion (ROM) should be assessed at the time muscle length is assessed instead of solely making a determination of length at the end-range. Stiffness is assessed by comparing muscles on opposite sides of the body, as well as on opposing sides of a joint. A balance of stiffness around the joint is a prerequisite for precise motion at that joint.[2,4]
  - Each muscle has an ideal length. Excessive length is as bad as or worse than decreased length (shortness).
  - Increased muscle stiffness or muscle shortness may cause joint compression contributing to the patient's symptoms.
- Identify alignment and movement impairments in the proximal upper extremity and relate these impairments to the symptomatic hand. Proximal impairments may result in increased muscle exertion distally and may place distal nerves at increased risk for injury.[5]
- Restore the precise pattern of movement. This principle can be applied to patients with degenerating painful joints to decrease their symptoms and the rate of degeneration.[2] Restoring the precise pattern of movement is most effective in the early stages of degeneration. The inevitable process of degeneration progresses through stages from hypermobility to eventual hypomobility. Degeneration occurs because of both intrinsic (genetic) and extrinsic (mechanical) factors. Although it is not possible to stop the process of aging and degeneration, it may be possible to slow or delay the effects of degeneration by changing the extrinsic factors. For example, in the early stages of OA

at the CMC joint of the thumb, the CMC joint becomes relatively too flexible and other structures, such as the adductor pollicis, become too stiff.[6] These impairments result in imprecise movement of the thumb, particularly at the CMC joint.

- For example, a young hairdresser with thumb CMC pain performed repeated thumb adduction when using scissors to cut hair. The excessive adductor stiffness contributed to imprecise movement of her thumb CMC joint and pain while cutting hair. The patient was educated to modify the movement pattern to decrease CMC adduction and increase flexion of the distal joints. Changing to scissors of a different design that deemphasized thumb adduction during hair cutting was helpful. When not cutting hair, the patient was instructed to maintain the arc of the thumb as much as possible during functional activities. Exercises to increase the extensibility of the thumb adductor and increase the performance of the thumb abductors were prescribed. The patient's symptoms resolved within a few treatments.
  - Imprecise movement at the CMC joint rarely occurs in isolation but is also associated with movement impairments at the MP and interphalangeal (IP) joints.[7]
- Modification of the movement pattern during habits, functional activities, and specific exercises (motor performance) is practiced during treatment.[2]
- Train muscles to stabilize the joint that is relatively too flexible.[2]
  - Increasing or decreasing muscle stiffness restores the balance of stiffness around a joint.
  - Modify patterns of muscle recruitment (timing, duration, and magnitude).
- If necessary, use splints to prevent the site that is relatively most flexible from moving and encouraging movement at the less flexible site.
- Use the physical stress theory to guide gradual progression of stresses to the tissues, resulting in tissue adaptations.[8]
- Emphasize maintaining the corrected movement pattern during practice of exercises, habits, and functional activities[2] as the stresses are increased on the tissues (i.e., after immobilization as with de Quervain's disease, initiating exercises to gradually stress the tissues versus just discontinuing the splint and returning to full activity).

Symptoms in the hand may be referred from the neck, thoracic outlet,[5] elbow, forearm, or wrist.[9-11] Therefore the examination of the hand should include differentiating whether the source of the symptoms is from the hand or referred from one of these regions.

Edema and scar are impairments that may exist in any of the syndromes and must be addressed for treatment to be effective, but identification of the edema and scar is not critical for assigning the movement system diagnosis.

EXAMINATION AND KEY TESTS

Subjective Examination

During the history, particular attention is paid to questioning the patient regarding the daily activities that are performed repeatedly and which of those are associated with increasing and decreasing the symptoms.

Objective Examination

I. Screening[12]
II. Posture and/or alignment
III. Palpation and/or appearance: Skin, scar, circulation, edema, sympathetic, atrophy, or nodules
IV. Functional activities: Work, activities of daily living, sports, and leisure
V. Movement analysis
  A. AROM
    1. Arc of motion
    2. Orientation of fingers toward scaphoid
    3. Onset of pain
    4. Sequence of PIP and DIP motion (flexion usually occurs together and extension always occurs together)
    5. Quality of motion: Flexibility, timing, and sequencing of movement at one joint relative to another
    6. Metacarpal arch
    7. Total AROM: Note excessive, as well as limited, ROM
  B. Passive ROM (PROM)
    1. Ligament integrity
    2. Limited ROM as the result of shortness of joint structures (MP collateral ligaments, IP volar plate and accessory collateral ligaments, and oblique retinacular ligament [ORL])
    3. Joint accessory motion
    4. Muscle length tests: When assessing muscle length, particular attention is paid to stiffness throughout the ROM, as well as the end-feel and quantity of motion. Comparison of stiffness and length is made to the same muscle on the uninvolved side and to synergists and antagonists on the involved side.
      a. Intrinsic muscle length (interossei)
      b. Extrinsic finger flexor muscle length and adhesion
      c. Extrinsic finger extensor muscle length and adhesion
      d. Wrist flexor and extensor length
      e. Thumb extrinsic and intrinsic length and adhesion
  C. Strength
    1. Manual muscle testing (MMT)[13]
    2. Resisted tests for soft tissue differential diagnosis[14]
    3. Grip test with dynamometer
    4. Pinch test with pinch gauge
    5. Quick tests of strength:
      a. Ulnar: Froment's sign and crossing fingers
      b. Median: Opposition
      c. Radial: Finger and wrist extension

Synthesize the findings from the movement testing (AROM, PROM, and resistive tests) to determine the reason for the loss of motion (source of signs). For example, insufficient finger flexion may be because of the following:

- Flexor tendon adhesions
- Extensor tendon adhesions
- Weakness of finger or thumb flexors
- Rupture of finger or thumb flexors
- MP collateral ligament shortness or adhesion
- Shortness of extrinsic finger or thumb extensors
- Shortness of interossei and lumbricals
- IP joint dorsal capsule shortness or adhesions
- Shortness of ORL
- Ligament sprain
- Swan neck deformity

See the description of the movement system syndromes in the Chapter 5 Appendix for specific test findings.

VI. Sensory testing[5]
  A. Threshold
    1. Pinprick
    2. Temperature
    3. Light touch (Semmes-Weinstein monofilaments)
    4. Vibration
  B. Functional
    1. Static and moving 2-point discrimination
    2. Localization
    3. Moberg's pick-up test
  C. Quantification
  D. Objective
    1. Ninhydrin
    2. Wrinkle test
  E. Provocative sensory testing
  F. Tinel's test
VII. Other special tests, including but not limited to the following:
  A. Finkelstein's test[15,16]
  B. Crank and grind test[17]
  C. Phalen's test[18]

ALIGNMENT OF THE HAND AND WRIST

Prolonged postures or repeated movements performed by the patient result in adaptations in the tissues (tissue impairments). These tissue impairments (i.e., short, stiff, long, overused, or weak muscles) result in imprecise movement patterns that eventually result in tissue injury.[2] The identification of impairments in alignment provides insight into possible existing impairments in the tissues that will be verified later in the examination.

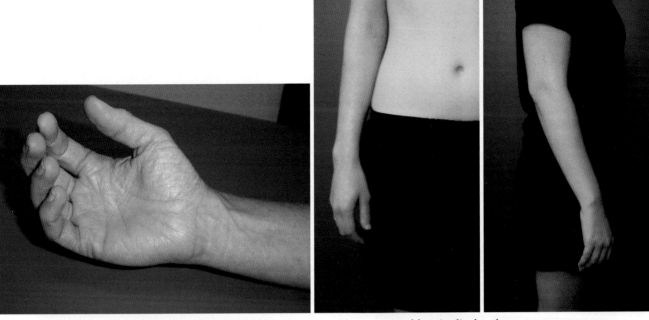

Figure 5-1. Normal resting alignment: Transverse and longitudinal arches.

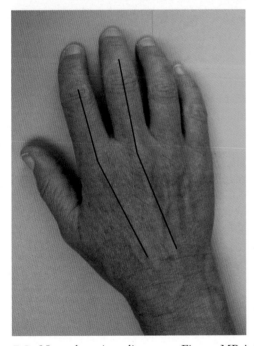

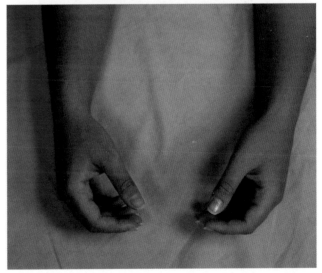

Figure 5-3. Normal resting alignment: Thumb in abduction.

Figure 5-2. Normal resting alignment: Finger MP joints in slight ulnar deviation.

Normal Standing Alignment

Normal alignment gives an indication of the preferred patterns of muscle use and resting muscle lengths. Normal alignment of the hand at rest includes the following:

1. Transverse arch at the carpal tunnel and at the heads of the metacarpals[4]
2. Fingers and thumb resting in slight flexion, forming the longitudinal arches of the hand, fingers, and thumb (Figure 5-1)[4,19]

3. Finger MP joints in slight UD[20,21] (Figure 5-2)
4. Neutral rotation of the PIP and DIP joints of the fingers
5. Rotation of the MP joints of the fingers[4]
6. Thumb in slight palmar abduction (Figure 5-3)[7]
7. Wrist in neutral to slight extension and UD (Figure 5-4)[22]
8. Radial styloid process extends distally farther than the ulnar styloid process[23]
9. Cascade of the metacarpals, decreasing in length from radial to ulnar sides[20] (Figure 5-5)

Examining the alignment of the forearm, elbow, and shoulder girdle is an important component of evaluation

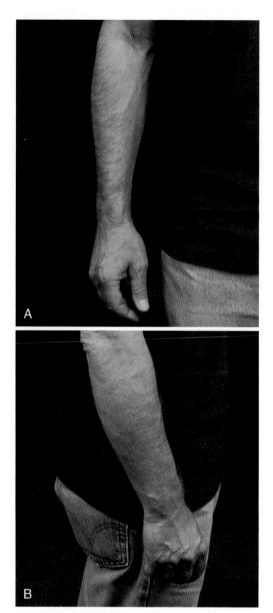

Figure 5-4. **A,** Normal resting alignment of wrist in slight extension, front view. **B,** Normal resting alignment of wrist in slight ulnar deviation, side view.

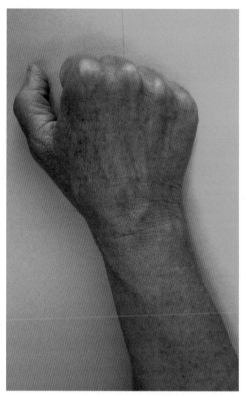

Figure 5-5. Normal decreasing length of metacarpals from radial to ulnar side of hand.

of hand dysfunction. Visual appraisal of muscle and tendon development should also be examined when assessing alignment. Muscles should be equally defined between muscles on the same side or symmetrical when compared to the same muscle on the opposite side.

Impaired Alignment

Impaired alignment provides important clues regarding the source of the signs or symptoms and indicates the preferred patterns of muscle use and resting muscle stiffness or lengths. However, assessment of alignment is only the first step in the objective examination and any clues obtained need to be confirmed via the rest of the tests.

Impaired alignment of the hand includes clawing (Figure 5-6), stiff hand position (wrist flexion, finger MP extension, IP flexion, and thumb adduction); rotation of the fingers (Figure 5-7); boutonnière (Figure 5-8) or swan neck alignment of the thumb or fingers (Figure 5-9); mallet, radial deviation (RD), or UD of the IP joints of the fingers or thumb (Figure 5-10); flexion of the DIP joints of the fingers (Figure 5-11); deviations in the longitudinal arch of increased flexion (Figure 5-12) or extension (Figure 5-13) as a whole or at individual joints (arch no longer smooth); deviations of the transverse arch (increased or decreased) (see Figure 5-13, *B*); increased UD of the MP joints (see Figure 5-8, *C*); and adduction and/or flexion (Figure 5-14; see Figure 5-10, *B*) or abduction of the CMC joint of the thumb.[24]

Many of these impaired alignments are classically thought of as a result of an acute injury or a chronic disease process. Some impaired alignments may be due to prolonged position of immobilization required for tissue healing after an injury or surgery. However, people that have not had an injury or a chronic disease may have a mild version of these impairments in alignment. These may be due to genetics, as well as the repeated movement patterns used during daily activities. Theoretically, modification of these impaired alignments may help to prevent tissue injury or alleviate pain in the presence of tissue injury.

Clawing, a resting position of flexion of the IP joints of the fingers with MP joint hyperextension (see Figure

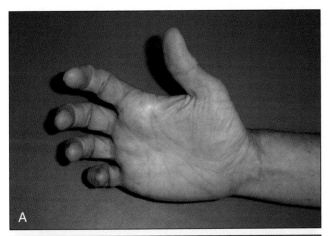

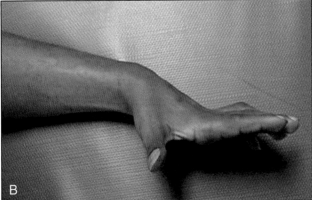

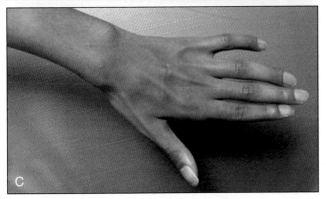

Figure 5-6. Impaired alignment. **A,** Decreased arches. **B** and **C,** Clawing.

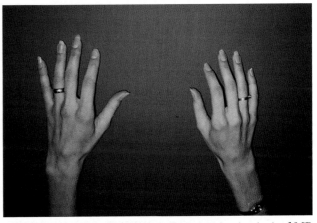

Figure 5-7. Impaired alignment: Rotation (supination) of MP joints of index fingers right greater than left.

the flattening of the transverse arches.[25,26] The static alignment of the posttraumatic stiff hand is similar to the claw hand position: wrist flexion, finger MP extension, IP flexion, and thumb adduction.[24]

A classic boutonnière deformity (see Figure 5-8, *A*), PIP flexion with DIP hyperextension, is a sign of injury to the central slip of the extensor mechanism. With rupture to the central slip, the extensor mechanism retracts increasing the tension on the terminal tendon, thus contributing to hyperextension of the DIP joint. Over time, the lateral bands migrate anteriorly and thus become PIP joint flexors instead of extensors. However, this same alignment can be seen with a PIP flexion contracture without injury to the extensors (pseudoboutonnière). Prolonged positioning in this alignment may also result in shortening of the oblique retinacular ligament. Shortness of the ORL then contributes further to the deformity.[27-29]

A swan neck deformity (see Figure 5-9, *A*) is described as PIP hyperextension with MP and DIP flexion. This can be due to anything that increases tension on the central slip of the extensor mechanism (ED, intrinsics) but most often may be caused by shortness or increased activity of the finger intrinsics. A prerequisite for the PIP hyperextension to occur is laxity of the volar plate at the PIP joint. As the PIP hyperextends, the lateral bands migrate farther from the axis of rotation in a posterior direction, increasing their efficiency as PIP extensors. PIP hyperextension places increased passive tension on the FDP resulting in DIP flexion. A nonfunctional FDS may also contribute to PIP hyperextension. A swan neck deformity may also result secondary to a mallet finger injury. When the terminal tendon of the extensor mechanism is ruptured in a mallet finger injury, the extensor mechanism retracts, increasing the tension on the central slip that is still attached. This results in PIP hyperextension if the PIP volar plate is lax.[30-33]

RD or UD of the IP joints of the fingers or thumb (see Figure 5-10) is usually either an indication of an injury to the collateral ligaments or of degeneration as a

5-6, *B* and *C*), is classically a sign of ulnar or combined ulnar and median nerve injury and is due to loss of function of the interossei and lumbricals (intrinsics). Insufficient function of the intrinsics results in an imbalance at the MP joint where the extensors (extensor digitorum [ED]) predominate over the flexors (intrinsics, flexor digitorum profundus [FDP], and flexor digitorum superficialis [FDS]) because the intrinsics are no longer functioning. The predominance of the ED at the MP joint results in increased passive tension on the FDP further contributing to the flexion of the IP joints. Clawing also results in flattening of the transverse arches of the hand. Ulnar nerve injury affects the hypothenar muscles and median nerve injury the thenar muscles, contributing to

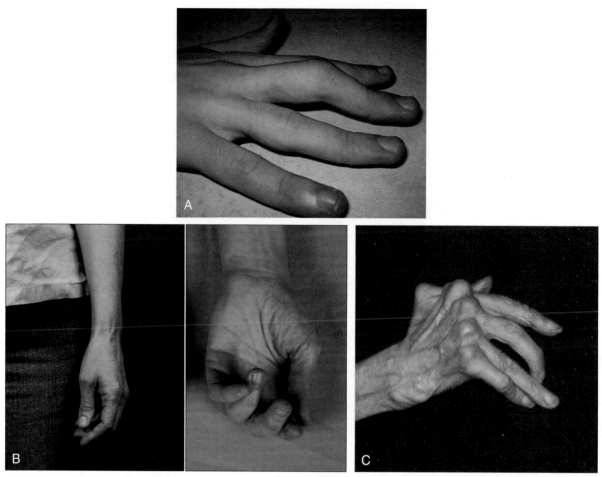

Figure 5-8. **A,** Classic boutonnière posture of proximal interphalangeal (PIP) joint flexion and distal interphalangeal (DIP) joint hyperextension. **B,** Impaired alignment: Tendency toward boutonnière of thumb (MP flexion with IP extension). **C,** Impaired alignment: Subluxation and ulnar deviation of MP joints and intrinsic plus (increased flexion of MP joints and extension of IP joints); boutonnière of thumb (MP flexion with IP extension). (**A,** From DeLee JC, Drez D, Miller MD: *DeLee and Drez's orthopaedic sports medicine,* Philadelphia, 2010, Saunders.)

result of OA.[17,34,35] Abnormal UD of the MP joints of the fingers is usually an indicator of inflammatory arthritis (e.g., rheumatoid or lupus). As the fingers deviate, muscle function changes. With UD of the fingers at the MP joints, the FDP and FDS may become ulnar deviators of the joint if the pulleys no longer hold the tendons centrally on the bone.[36-38] Likewise, the ED may become a deviator of the joint if it slips in a radial or ulnar direction off the head of the metacarpal.

UD of the MP joints of the fingers (see Figure 5-8, *C*) may be suggestive of inflammatory arthritis. However, some people that have laxity of the joints and little muscle stiffness may also have increased UD of the MP joints[21] that is associated with their symptoms and can be modified with patient education.

Flexion of the DIP joints of the fingers is usually either an indicator of a mallet finger injury or the result of OA of the DIP joints (see Figure 5-11).[17]

Adduction (see Figure 5-10, *B*) or abduction of the CMC joint of the thumb is usually associated with degeneration of the CMC joint of the thumb. Adduction of the

CMC is usually associated with flexion[26] and may indicate shortness or relative stiffness of the adductor pollicis and the flexor pollicis brevis (FPB) and insufficient function or excessive length of the abductor pollicis longus (APL), abductor pollicis brevis (APB), opponens pollicis (OP), and first dorsal interossei (DI) muscles. Abduction of the CMC indicates shortness, relative stiffness, or excessive recruitment of the APL, and if associated with MP flexion, shortness or stiffness of the FPB, and lengthened or insufficient recruitment of the extensor pollicis brevis (EPB). The adducted or abducted positions of the CMC joint of the thumb are also associated with compensatory impairments in alignment of the MP[39] and IP joints of the thumb, either a boutonnière (MP flexion with IP hyperextension) (Figure 5-8, *B* and *C*) or swan neck (MP hyperextension with IP flexion) deformity (see Figure 5-9, *B*).[6,40,41]

Rotation of the fingers at the MP or PIP joints (see Figure 5-7), deviations in the longitudinal arch of increased flexion (see Figure 5-12) or extension (see Figure 5-13, *A* and *B*) as a whole or at individual joints

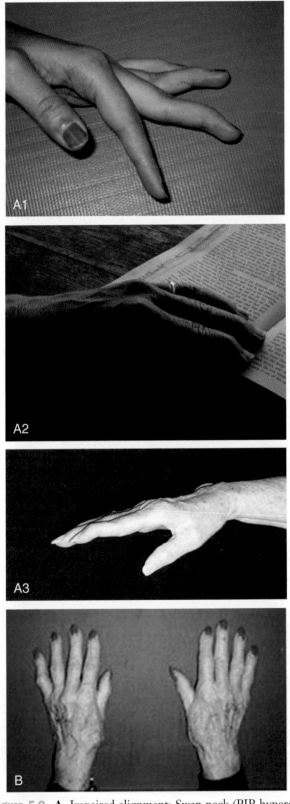

Figure 5-9. A, Impaired alignment: Swan neck (PIP hyperextension with MP and DIP flexion) of fingers. **B,** Impaired alignment: Swan neck of thumbs left greater than right.

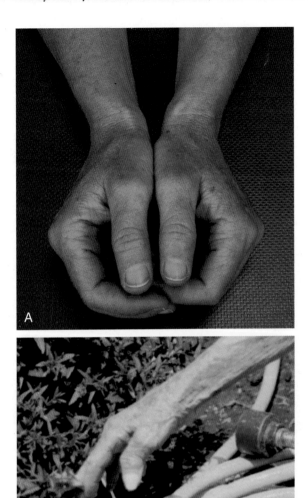

Figure 5-10. A, Impaired alignment: Radial deviation of IP of thumb and adduction of CMC of thumb early stages of degeneration. **B,** Impaired alignment: Radial deviation of IP of thumb and adduction of CMC of thumb late stages of degeneration.

(arch no longer smooth), or deviations of the transverse arch (increased or decreased) may indicate an imbalance of the muscular forces on opposing sides of the joints (in the absence of a structural change or nerve injury from trauma). Rotation may be the result of overuse or increased stiffness of the interossei on one side of the finger and underuse or use in a lengthened position of the interossei on the opposite side of the finger. The FDP, FDS, and ED may be underused and the intrinsics overused (intrinsic plus position of MP flexion and IP extension). Alteration of the longitudinal arch of increased finger MP flexion and decreased IP flexion may be the result of overuse of the finger intrinsics and underuse of the FDP, FDS, and ED (see Figure 5-9, *A2*). Clawing, boutonnière, swan neck, and mallet are all disruptions in the longitudinal arch. These are usually attributed to a nerve injury or injury to the extensor mechanism. However, when similar alignments are identified in the

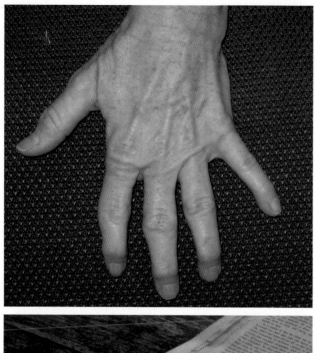

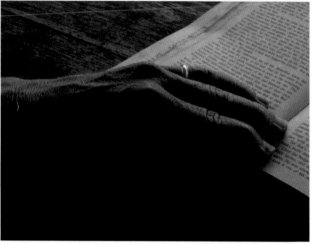

Figure 5-11. Impaired alignment: DIP flexion and osteo-arthritis.

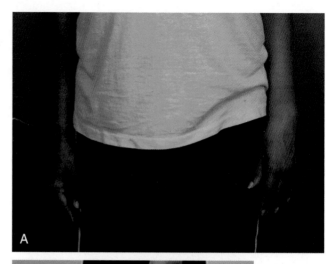

A

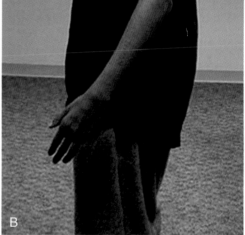

B

Figure 5-13. A, Impaired alignment: Alteration of longitudinal arch of fingers of decreased flexion (left elbow injury). **B,** Impaired alignment: Alteration of longitudinal arch of fingers of decreased flexion and decreased transverse arch (ulnar nerve injury).

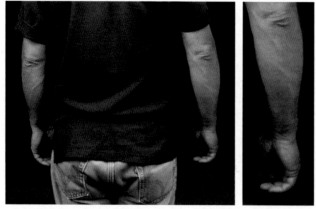

Figure 5-12. Impaired alignment: Alteration of longitudinal arch of fingers of increased flexion.

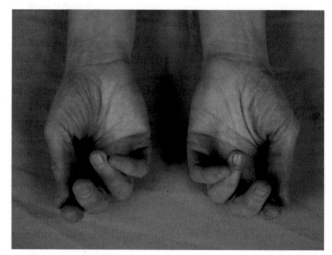

Figure 5-14. Impaired resting alignment: Thumb CMC flexion right greater than left.

absence of a specific nerve or extensor mechanism injury, the therapist should identify the muscles that may be under or overused, contributing to the impaired alignment. Similarly, muscles that contribute to increasing the transverse arch are the opponens pollicis and digiti minimi, APB, abductor digiti minimi (ADM), flexor digiti minimi (FDM), FPB, and the interossei. The transverse arch is decreased when the ED, extensor pollicis longus (EPL), is dominant compared to the interossei.

An increase in the longitudinal arch of the fingers and thumb is indicative of overuse or relative stiffness of the FDS, FDP, and FPL (see Figure 5-12). A decrease in the longitudinal arch is associated with relative decreased muscle stiffness of the FDS, FDP, and flexor pollicis longus (FPL) (see Figure 5-13, *A*).

The most common wrist alignment impairment is wrist flexion (Figure 5-15, *A* and *B*), but RD or UD may also be present. Wrist flexion may be due to obesity and secondary abduction of the shoulder. The effect of gravity then is to flex the wrist. A resting alignment of wrist flexion may also be the result of repeated use of the finger or wrist flexors with the wrist in a flexed position. The finger or wrist flexors may be relatively

stiff, short, or overused compared to the wrist extensors. A resting alignment of wrist RD with extension is indicative of stiffness, shortness or overuse of the extensor carpi radialis longus (ECRL) or extensor carpi radialis brevis (ECRB) relative to the extensor carpi ulnaris (ECU). Wrist radial deviation with wrist flexion is indicative of overuse of the flexor carpi radialis (FCR) relative to the flexor carpi ulnaris (FCU). Overuse of the FCU may result in wrist UD with wrist flexion and overuse of the ECU, wrist UD with extension. Prolonged alignment with the wrist in UD may contribute to injury of the tissues on the ulnar side of the wrist such as the triangular fibrocartilage complex (TFCC) (Figure 5-15, *C*).

Shoulder alignment must be considered in making the determination of elbow, forearm, wrist, and hand alignment impairments. If distal impairments are noted, then scapular and humeral alignment should be corrected to determine if the origin of this malalignment is distal or proximal. Impairments in shoulder girdle alignment may affect patterns of muscle use in the hand or cause proximal or distal nerve compression with symptoms radiating into the hand.[5,42]

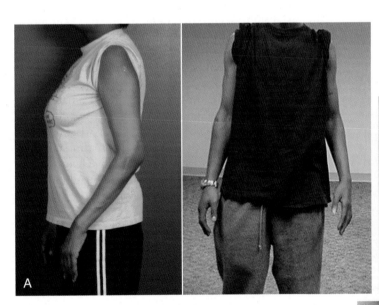

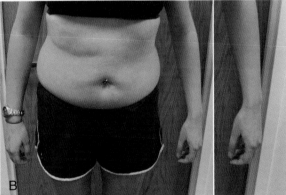

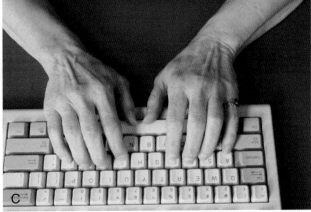

Figure 5-15. A, Impaired alignment: Wrist flexion secondary to elbow hypomobility and lack of elbow extension. **B,** Impaired resting alignment of wrist flexion secondary to wide thorax and shoulder abduction (without pain or injury). **C,** Impaired alignment of wrist in ulnar deviation resulting in left ulnar-sided wrist pain.

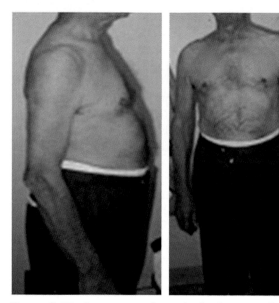

Figure 5-16. Asymmetry of muscle development: Decreased biceps and increased wrist extensors.

Visual appraisal of muscle and tendon development should also be examined when assessing alignment. Asymmetry of muscle bulk between muscles on the same side or compared to the same muscle on the opposite side is another indicator of impaired patterns of muscle use or of nerve injury (Figure 5-16).

An important component of examination of the hand is assessment of appearance, including skin, creases, web spaces, scar, circulation, temperature, edema, sympathetic changes, and nodules. These are not described in detail in this chapter because they are covered well in other texts. However, a brief description of the examination of edema and scar is provided in Box 5-2.

NORMAL MOTIONS OF THE HAND AND WRIST

Wrist Motions

Normally, the wrist extends with slight radial deviation and flexes with slight UD during functional wrist motion.[26]

Wrist flexion occurs in the sagittal plane around a medial to lateral axis through the capitate.[20] Full range is approximately 65 to 80 degrees.[43] During wrist flexion if the fingers and thumb are relaxed, finger and thumb extension will occur secondary to tenodesis[43] or passive tension on the finger and thumb extensors. During wrist flexion, the proximal carpal row glides posteriorly on the distal radius[43,44] and articular disc, the scaphoid and lunate volarflex, and the triquetrum dorsiflexes.[45] Relative volarflexion of the scaphoid "unlocks" the midcarpal joint so most of the motion during wrist flexion occurs at the midcarpal joint.[45] The articular surface of the distal end

of the radius has an inclination anteriorly that allows for greater wrist flexion than extension ROM.[43]

Wrist extension occurs in the sagittal plane around a medial to lateral axis through the capitate.[20] Full range is approximately 55 to 70 degrees.[43] During wrist extension if the fingers and thumb are relaxed, finger and thumb flexion will occur secondary to tenodesis of the finger and thumb flexors.[43] During wrist extension, the proximal carpal row glides anteriorly on the distal radius[43,44] and on the articular disc, the scaphoid and lunate dorsiflex, and the triquetrum volarflexes.[45] Relative dorsiflexion of the scaphoid "locks" the midcarpal joint so most of the motion during wrist extension occurs at the radiocarpal joint.[45]

Radial deviation occurs in the coronal plane around an anterior-to-posterior axis through the capitate. Full range is approximately 15 degrees,[43] and maximum range is achieved with the wrist in neutral with respect to flexion and extension. During wrist radial deviation, the proximal carpal row glides ulnarly[44] and the scaphoid and lunate volarflex.[43,45]

Ulnar deviation occurs in the coronal plane around a anterior-to-posterior axis through the capitate. Full range is approximately 30 degrees,[43] and maximum range is achieved with the wrist in neutral with respect to flexion and extension. Ulnar deviation is greater than radial deviation because of the medial inclination of the articular surfaces of the distal radius and ulna.[43] The radial styloid process extends distally farther than the ulnar styloid process. During wrist UD , the proximal carpal row glides radially[44] and the scaphoid and lunate dorsiflex.[45] Normally there are greater compressive forces on tissues of the ulnar side of the wrist during wrist UD with the forearm pronated than with the forearm supinated because of a dynamic change in the relative length of the radius and ulna.[46] During pronation, the ulna moves slightly distally, whereas during supination it moves slightly proximally.[47]

Finger Motions

Finger Flexion

MP, PIP, and DIP flexion occurs in the sagittal plane around a medial-to-lateral axis. Full range is approximately 90 degrees for the MP joint. The range increases progressively toward the ulnar side of the hand to about 110 degrees.[43] Manual workers with fingers that have a greater circumference tend to have less ROM compared to nonmanual workers.[4] Normal range for the PIP is 100 to 120 degrees and 70 to 90 degrees for the DIP.[43] Rotation of the MP joints contributes to the fingers being oriented toward the scaphoid at the end of the range of finger flexion (Figure 5-17).[20] Normally, the fingers adduct as they flex. Although movement at the CMC and gliding of the intermetacarpal joints are not usually measured clinically, normal finger flexion range and deepening of the arches of the hand require slight flexion at the

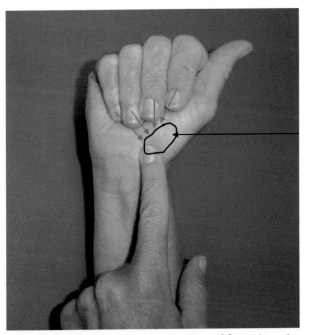

Figure 5-17. Normal movement pattern of fingertips oriented toward scaphoid during finger flexion.

CMC and gliding at the intermetacarpal joints. There is increased movement at the CMC and intercarpal joints on the ulnar side of the hand compared to the second and third CMC and intercarpal joints. Usually the PIP and DIP joints flex simultaneously.[48] The normal total active motion (TAM) of the fingers is 270 degrees. Normally, the fingertips make a large arc of motion[20,49] with the PIPs flexing first, followed by MP, and last by DIP flexion[20] (Figure 5-18, *A*). During active finger flexion, the wrist should extend slightly.[20,43] During finger flexion at the MP, PIP, and DIP joints, the direction of the glide of the distal articular surface on the proximal articular surface is anterior.[44]

Finger Rotation

Finger MP and IP rotation occurs in a transverse plane about a longitudinal axis. Average range of passive MP rotation is 30 to 40 degrees and is greatest for the ring and little fingers.[20,43] Rotation during active finger MP flexion varies from 1 to 13 degrees of supination.[50] The direction of MP rotation of the index finger is variable.[50,51] Rotation during active finger PIP flexion varies from 1 to 6 degrees of pronation for the index and middle fingers and 8 to 9 degrees of supination for the ring and small

Text continued on p. 184

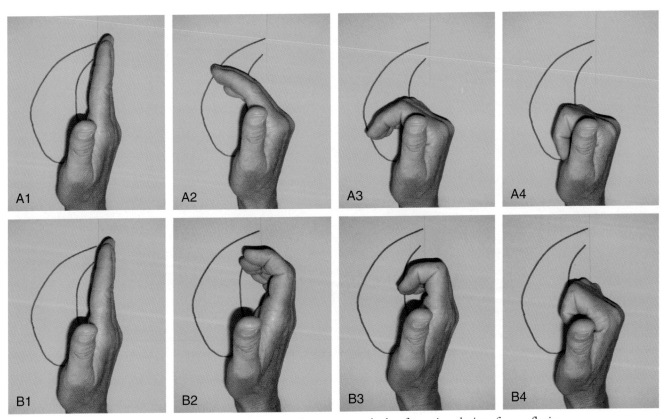

Figure 5-18. A, Normal large arc of motion made by fingertips during finger flexion. **B,** Decreased arc of motion made by fingertips during finger flexion with decreased intrinsic function.

BOX 5-2

Examination and Treatment of Scar and Edema

EXAMINATION OF SCAR
- Location gives clues to future potential loss of motion.

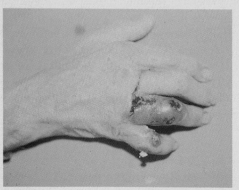

Appearance of scar. Dorsal scar on proximal phalanx and over PIP joint may result in limited MP and PIP range of motion and adherence of extensor mechanism. (Used with permission from Ann Kammien, PT, CHT, St Louis, Mo.)

- Note color and size (i.e., raised, length).[1]

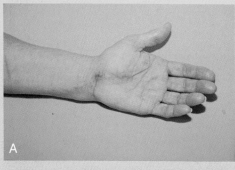

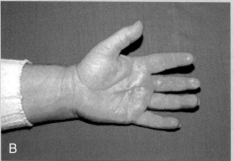

Appearance of scar. **A,** red; **B,** raised. (Used with permission from Ann Kammien, PT, CHT, St Louis, Mo.)

- Assess mobility: Muscles and tendons in hand *must* be free to glide.[1]

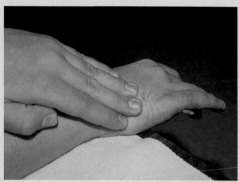

Assessment of mobility of scar. Scar adhered to extensor tendon with limited extensor tendon glide resulting in decreased active PIP extension. (Used with permission from Ann Kammien, PT, CHT, St Louis, Mo.)

- Assess for hypersensitivity: By palpation.

SCAR CLASSIFICATION[2]
- Mature scar: As a scar matures, it gets whiter in color and flattens. It may take a scar up to 2 years to mature.
- Immature scar is red and slightly elevated and can be painful.
- Linear hypertrophic immature scar is confined to border of the original surgical incision.
- Widespread hypertrophic scar (example: burn).
- Keloid: Raised scar that does not flatten as it matures and extends over normal tissue.

TREATMENT OF SCAR[2]
- Prevention is the key: Avoid shearing forces to area (tape placed longitudinally along the scar can help decrease shearing forces).
- Best evidence is treatment with silicone gel sheeting, which should begin early and continue for at least 1 month (for linear scars).
- Limited evidence for pressure, but it is still recommended in combination with silicone sheeting for widespread scars.
- Further research is needed regarding the efficacy of massage.

General treatment guidelines for superficial scar
- If hypersensitive:
  - Desensitization[3,4]
- If firm and raised, use the following:
  - TopiGel sheeting (chemical reaction)[5]
  - Compression/pressure[5]

AROM, Active range of motion; *DIP,* distal interphalangeal; *IP,* interphalangeal; *MP,* metacarpophalangeal; *PIP,* proximal interphalangeal; *PROM,* passive range of motion.

1. Schneider LH, Feldscher SB: Tenolysis: dynamic approach to surgery and therapy. In Mackin EJ, Callahan AD, Osterman AL, et al, eds: *Rehabilitation of the hand and upper extremity,* ed 5, St Louis, 2002, Mosby.
2. Mustoe TA, Cooter RD, Gold MH, et al: International clinical recommendations on scar management, *Plast Reconstr Surg* 1102:560-571, 2002.
3. Skirven TM, Callahan AD: Therapist's management of peripheral nerve injuries. In Mackin EJ, Callahan AD, Osterman AL, et al, eds: *Rehabilitation of the hand and upper extremity,* ed 5, St Louis, 2002, Mosby.
4. Walsh MT, Muntzer E: Therapist's management of complex regional pain syndrome reflex sympathetic dystrophy. In Mackin EJ, Callahan AD, Osterman AL et al, eds: *Rehabilitation of the hand and upper extremity,* ed 5, St Louis, 2002, Mosby.

BOX 5-2

Examination and Treatment of Scar and Edema—cont'd

- If immobile, do the following:
  - Gradually applying stress to scar helps the scar remodel in such a way that it allows gliding between structures.
  - AROM and PROM
  - Splinting[5]
  - Modalities

Treatment of hypersensitive scar

- Desensitization should include the following five categories as tolerated[3,4]:
  - Massage
  - Tapping
  - Vibration
  - Textures
  - Functional use of the involved finger

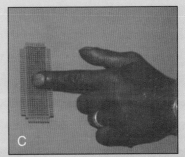

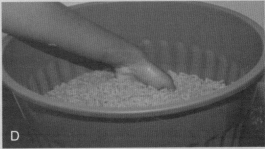

C and **D,** Textures. Treatment of hypersensitive scar using desensitization. Use of textures to bombard sensory receptors and raise their threshold of firing. (Used with permission from Ann Kammien, PT, CHT, St Louis, Mo.)

- Parameters for desensitization
  - Textures, particles, vibration, tapping, scar massage, functional use, 30 seconds each texture for total of 5 to 10 minutes, 5 to 6 times/day.
  - Begin with texture that is challenging for the patient but tolerable. Progress to more noxious stimuli as tolerated.[3]

Treatment of immobile or adhered scar

- Massage
  - Circular and retrograde[1]
  - Minimum 5 to 6 times/day, 5 minutes each time
  - Dycem or wearing a latex glove on uninvolved hand may be helpful to increase friction.
- Vibration
- AROM and resistive exercises as tolerated
- Compression[5]
  - Elastomer or Otoform K secured with Coban, ace wrap, Tubigrip, or compression glove to provide compression on the scar.
  - Use as much of the day as possible without limiting functional use of the involved region.

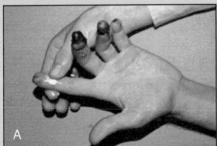

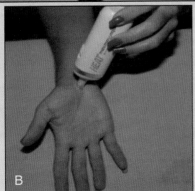

A, Massage. Treatment of desensitization using massage.
B, Vibration. Treatment of desensitization using vibration.

5. Grigsby DE, Linde L, Knothe B: Therapist's management of the burned hand. In Mackin EJ, Callahan AD, Osterman AL, et al, eds: *Rehabilitation of the hand and upper extremity,* ed 5, St Louis, 2002, Mosby.

Continued

BOX 5-2

Examination and Treatment of Scar and Edema—cont'd

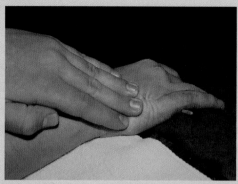

Treatment of immobile scar using massage combined with exercise. Scar is moved distally as tendon glides proximally during active finger extension. (Used with permission from Ann Kammien, PT, CHT, St Louis, Mo.)

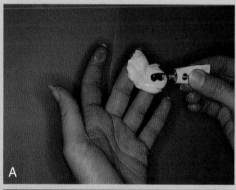

A

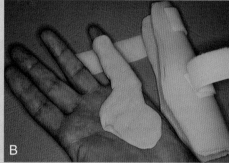

B

Treatment of raised scar using compression and/or pressure. **A,** Mixing red enzyme (catalyst) with Otoform K putty. **B,** Completed otoform mold with splint to hold fingers in extension in patient that had Dupuytren's release.

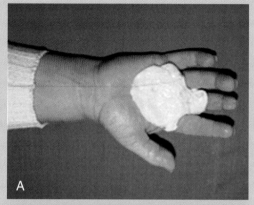

A

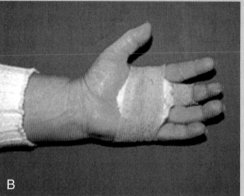

B

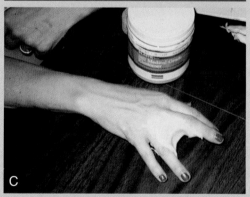

C

Treatment of raised scar using compression. **A,** Otoform K. **B,** Otoform K held on with Coban. **C,** Elastomer used for serial molds to stretch scar in web space for pianist that had limited range of finger spread after injury.

BOX 5-2

Examination and Treatment of Scar and Edema—cont'd

- Silopad finger caps contain mineral oil that helps moistens scar; does not contain silicone.
- TopiGel and/or silicone gel: Acting mechanism is a chemical reaction, so it requires no pressure.[5]

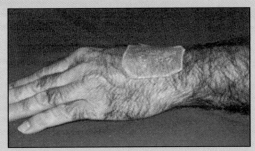

Treatment of raised scar using TopiGel sheeting.

- Wear for a minimum of 12 hours and wash 1 to 2 times/day[2] and dry flat.
- Usually worn at night.
- Each piece of silicone can last about 2 to 3 weeks.
- Watch for allergic reaction.
- Scar pump: Option not commonly used.

Treatment of raised scar[1]
- Compression and/or pressure: Refer to previous section for specifics.
- TopiGel and/or silicone gel: Refer to previous section for specifics.

Treatment of scar with splinting[5]
- Purpose: To provide gentle and prolonged tension to the maturing scar to lengthen the tissue and add compression to the scar.
- Methods
  - Static progressive: Night use with scar at end-range length
  - Dynamic: 4 to 6 times/day, 20 to 30 minutes, with tissues at end-range length

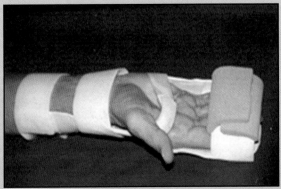

Treatment of scar using static progressive splinting to provide a prolonged stretch. (Used with permission from Ann Kammien, PT, CHT, St Louis, Mo.)

Treatment of scar with modalities
- Purpose
  - Increase extensibility of scar
  - Best if administered with scar on stretch
- Examples

- Paraffin[5]
- Moist heat
- Ultrasound[5]
- Fluidotherapy: Superficial heat plus a desensitizing effect and AROM during treatment
- Heat massager

EXAMINATION OF EDEMA
- Appearance[6]
  - Most common on dorsum of hand[7]
  - Shiny skin
  - Decreased skin creases

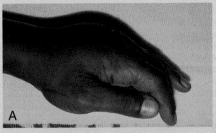

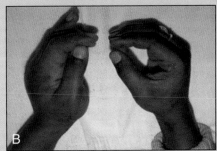

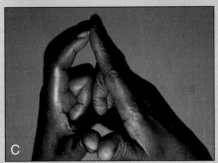

Appearance. **A** and **B,** Dorsal hand edema. **C,** Shiny skin, decreased skin creases, and decreased passive PIP extension left index finger. (Used with permission from Ann Kammien, PT, CHT, St Louis, Mo.)

- Resting posture
  - Joints rest in loose-packed position (finger MP extension, IP flexion, thumb adduction).
  - Decreased longitudinal and transverse arches of hand.
- Objective signs of edema
  - Increased circumference and/or volume measures.[7]
  - Loss of AROM and PROM (A = P) with a soft end-feel.[6]
  - Palpation may be pitting or brawny.[6]

Continued

BOX 5-2

Examination and Treatment of Scar and Edema—cont'd

PROCEDURES FOR MEASUREMENT OF EDEMA
Circumferential gauge or measuring tape
- Procedure
  - Measure at proximal phalanx, PIP joint, middle phalanx, and DIP joint
  - Try to use consistent amount of tension on tape
- Results
  - Compare to uninvolved side
- Indications
  - When swelling is limited to a finger compared to the whole hand

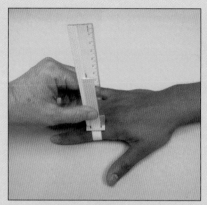

Circumferential gauge.

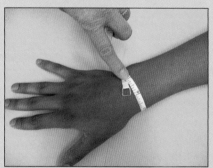

Using measuring tape to measure wrist circumference.

Volumeter[7,8]

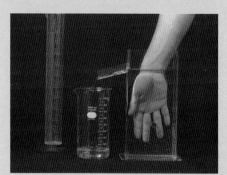

Volumeter. (From Fess EE: Documentation: essential elements of an upper extremity assessment battery. In Mackin EJ, Callahan AD, Osterman AL, et al, eds: *Rehabilitation of the hand and upper extremity,* ed 5, St Louis, 2002, Mosby.)

- Procedure
  - Calibrate volumeter by filling with water until it overflows and stops dripping.
  - Sit back in chair, place palm in anatomical position, and lower one-third of forearm slowly into volumeter, positioning web space between long and ring fingers over horizontal rod. Hold hand there until water no longer flows from spout.
- Results
  - Compare to uninvolved side.
  - Nondominant hand may be slightly smaller (3.43%) than dominant hand.[9]
- Indications
  - When the whole hand and/or forearm are swollen.

TREATMENT OF EDEMA
Early intervention is the key.
Elevation[6,7]
- Hand above heart.[6,7]
- Best with elbow extended.
- The level of the hand must be lowered if arterial occlusion is suspected or raised if venous occlusion is suspected.

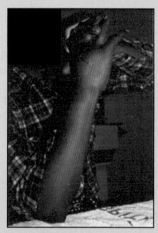

Treatment of edema. Massage with hand elevated.

Compression
- Massage[7]
  - Distal to proximal massage
    - Effective for low plasma protein edema
    - Utilizes venous system
  - Manual edema mobilization[10]
    - Effective for high plasma protein edema
    - Utilizes lymphatic system
    - Light massage done in segments
    - Proximal to distal, then distal to proximal

BOX 5-2

Examination and Treatment of Scar and Edema—cont'd

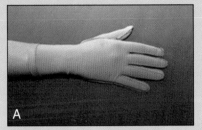

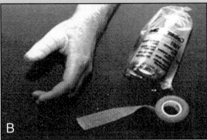

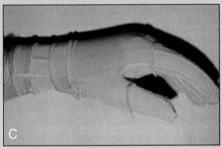

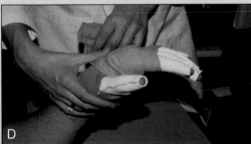

Treatment of edema. Compression: **A,** Isotoner glove. **B,** Coban. **C,** Jobst garment. **D,** Ace wrap and finger sleeves. (Used with permission from Ann Kammien, PT, CHT, St Louis, Mo.)

- Ace wrap, Coban, Isotoner glove, or Jobst glove[7]
  - Caution with donning compressive garments when motion restrictions are present

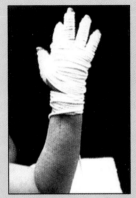

Treatment of edema with string wrapping. (From Villeco JP: Edema: therapist's management. In Mackin EJ, Callahan AD, Osterman AL, et al, eds: *Rehabilitation of the hand and upper extremity,* ed 5, St Louis, 2002, Mosby.)

- String wrapping[7]: Used less commonly
  - Wrap distal to proximal for 5 minutes, followed by gripping exercise
- Intermittent compression pumps[7,11]: Used less commonly

Modalities
- Cold[7]
- Heat
  - Hand must be elevated but only in the later phases of healing
- Electrical galvanic stimulation (EGS)[7]

GENERAL PRINCIPLES OF POSITIONING THE SWOLLEN HAND[7]
- Fingers: Intrinsic-plus or closed-packed position
- Thumb: Abducted
- Wrist: Slight extension

Exercise
- Usually elevated
- AROM stimulates venous and lymphatic drainage.[6,7]
- Avoid the following:
  - Exercise that is overly aggressive or complete immobilization: A delicate balance exists between the appropriate amount of rest and exercise.
  - Whirlpool: If a whirlpool treatment must be used with a patient with edema, decrease water temperature to 96° F to avoid increasing edema with dependent position.
  - Exercising with hand dependent.
  - Compression to wrist and hand without compression on the fingers.
  - Use of a sling because the hand is not elevated sufficiently.

6. Colditz JC: Anatomic considerations for splinting the thumb. In Mackin EJ, Callahan AD, Osterman AL, et al, eds: *Rehabilitation of the hand and upper extremity,* ed 5, St Louis, 2002, Mosby.

7. Villeco JP, Mackin EJ, Hunter JM: Edema: therapist's management. In Mackin EJ, Callahan AD, Osterman AL, et al, eds: *Rehabilitation of the hand and upper extremity,* ed 5, St Louis, 2002, Mosby.

8. Brand PW, Hollister AM: *Clinical mechanics of the hand,* ed 3, St Louis, 1999, Mosby.

9. van Velze CA, Kluever I, van der Merwe CA, et al: The difference in volume of dominant and nondominant hands, *J Hand Ther* 46:6-9, 1991.

10. Artzberger SM: Manual edema mobilization: treatment for edema in subacute hand. In Mackin EJ, Callahan AD, Osterman AL, et al, eds: *Rehabilitation of the hand and upper extremity,* ed 5, St Louis 2002, Mosby.

11. Innis PC: Surgical management of the stiff hand. In Mackin EJ, Callahan AD, Osterman AL, et al, eds: *Rehabilitation of the hand and upper extremity,* ed 5, St Louis 2002, Mosby.

fingers. Rotation of the DIP joints of all fingers vary from 1 to 5 degrees of pronation.[50]

Finger Extension

MP, PIP, and DIP extension occurs in the sagittal plane around a medial to lateral axis. Full range is approximately 0 to 45 degrees for the MP joint.[52] Normal range for the PIP and DIP joints is 0 degrees.[52] Although movement at the CMC and gliding of the intermetacarpal joints are not usually measured clinically, normal finger extension range and a decrease of the arches of the hand require extension at the CMC and gliding at the intermetacarpal joints. The sequence of finger extension occurs first at the MP followed by PIP and DIP.[4] Normally, the PIP and DIP always extend together.[43,48] During finger extension, the wrist should not flex excessively but should stay relatively stable, the IP joints of the fingers should extend through full ROM, and the MP joints should extend at least to neutral (0 degrees). During finger extension at the MP, PIP, and DIP joints, the direction of the glide of the distal articular surface on the proximal articular surface is posterior.[44]

Finger Abduction

Finger MP abduction occurs in the coronal plane about an anterior-to-posterior axis. To our knowledge, there are no normal values for AROM for MP abduction. Normal passive range is 9 to 19 degrees of radial deviation and 20 to 43 degrees of UD.[21] Normal finger abduction should occur without MP extension beyond neutral (0 degrees).[43] The direction of the glide of the proximal phalanx on the metacarpal during finger abduction at the MP joints is radial for the index, radial and ulnar for the middle, and ulnar for the ring and small fingers.[44] Pronation (medial rotation) occurs at the MP joints during finger radial deviation, and supination occurs during finger UD.[21]

Thumb Motions

During isolated movements of the thumb, the wrist and fingers should stay stable.

Thumb Flexion

Normal motion occurs around an anterior-to-posterior axis in the coronal plane. Normal range of thumb MP flexion is highly variable but normally about 50 degrees.[43] IP flexion is 70 degrees.[43] The thumb CMC also flexes 15 degrees[52] but is usually not measured clinically. Our observation is that the sequence of movements of the joints of the thumb during flexion from a resting alignment are CMC flexion first followed by MP and IP flexion. During thumb flexion, the thumb medially rotates slightly (pronates).[20] The IP joint pronates and adducts during pinch.[53] The glide of the distal articular surface on the proximal articular surface at the MP and CMC joints is in an anteroulnar direction.[44]

Thumb Extension

Normal motion occurs around an anterior-to-posterior axis in the coronal plane. Normal range of thumb MP and IP extension is 0 degrees. The IP has varying degrees of hyperextension and should be compared with the opposite thumb. The CMC joint extends to 10 to 15 degrees from anatomical position.[43] Our observation is that the sequence of movements of the joints of the thumb during extension from a resting alignment are CMC extension first followed by MP and IP extension. Thumb extension (also known as *radial abduction*) should occur without excessive adduction or abduction. During thumb extension, the thumb laterally rotates slightly (supinates). The glide of the distal articular surface on the proximal articular surface at the MP and CMC joints is in a posteroradial direction.[44]

Thumb Palmar Abduction

Normal motion occurs around a medial to lateral axis in the sagittal plane. A slight amount of abduction occurs at the MP joint, but the primary movement occurs at the CMC joint and is about 45 degrees.[43,48] During thumb abduction the MP and IP joints should stay in a fairly neutral position.[54] During thumb abduction, the wrist should stay stable and the CMC joint should not extend.[4,20] The direction of the glide of the distal articular surface on the proximal articular surface at the MP joint is radial and at the CMC joint is dorsal.[43] The CMC joint is most stable in abduction and extension.[7,20] It is in abduction and extension that most of the supporting ligaments of the CMC joint are taut.[7]

Thumb Adduction

Thumb adduction occurs around a medial-to-lateral axis in the sagittal plane. A slight amount of adduction occurs at the MP joint, but the primary movement occurs at the CMC joint.[43,48] Normal movement is to be able to adduct the thumb against the radial side of the second metacarpal and index finger.[43] The direction of the glide of the distal articular surface on the proximal articular surface at the MP joint is ulnar and at the CMC joint is volar.[43,44]

Thumb Opposition

Thumb opposition consists of thumb flexion, abduction, and medial rotation (pronation) bringing the tip of the thumb toward the tip of the small finger to line up the fingernails.[7,43] During opposition, the CMC and MP joints flex simultaneously throughout the motion. The CMC and MP abduct simultaneously only at the beginning of the movement.[54] Often, opposition is not measured goniometrically in the clinic but instead is assessed qualitatively.

Assessment of Range of Motion

AROM assesses the contractile and noncontractile structures.[14] When assessing movement of the hand, the patient's preferred pattern of active ROM is assessed first and correlated with the timing and onset of symptoms. If symptoms are produced and impairments are noted, the movement is immediately modified (when possible) to determine the effect on symptoms. During AROM, the timing of onset of muscle activity and increases and decreases relative to the normal ROM should be noted. A joint that moves relatively too much can be just as or more problematic than a joint with limited motion.

Besides noting the quantity of motion at each joint (increased or decreased), particular emphasis is placed on noting the quality of motion during the composite motion. Impairments to be noted during the assessment of the quality of active finger and thumb flexion and extension include the following:

1. A decrease (Figure 5-18, *B*) or increase in the arc of the motion that the tips of the digits make during flexion and extension
2. Flexing the MPs more than the IPs
3. Keeping the MPs extended and flexing primarily the IP joints (see Figure 5-18, *B*)
4. Increased rotation at the MP joints
5. Rotation at the IP joints
6. A relative increase or decrease in the flexion or extension of one joint relative to the other joints (Figure 5-19)
7. PIP flexion with DIP extension
8. PIP extension with DIP flexion
9. A change in the normal orientation of the fingers toward the scaphoid during finger flexion with the DIPs extended
10. A decrease in the range of flexion of the ulnar fingers versus the middle and index (Figure 5-20)
11. Lack of deepening of the transverse arches of the hand during finger and thumb flexion

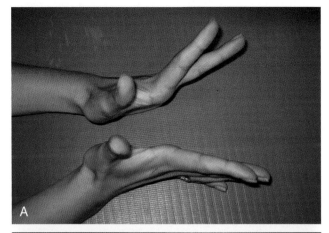
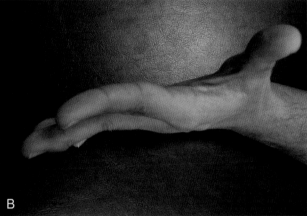

Figure 5-19. **A,** Excessive MP extension during active finger extension; left worse than the right. **B,** Insufficient MP extension with excessive IP extension during active finger extension (increased used of intrinsic).

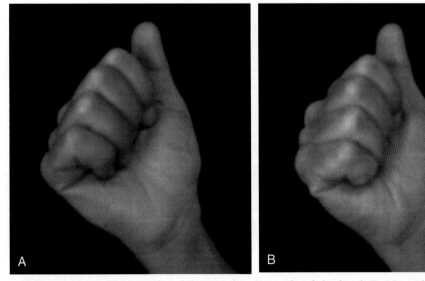

Figure 5-20. **A,** Decreased mobility on the ulnar side of the hand. **B,** Normal mobility on ulnar side of hand noted during strong grip.

12. Lack of flattening of the transverse arches during finger and thumb extension
13. RD or UD of the PIP or DIP joints
14. Excessive UD of the finger MP joints
15. Excessive MP extension instead of PIP joint extension (Figure 5-21).

In addition, impairments during AROM of the thumb include (1) insufficient or excessive thumb CMC, MP or IP extension or flexion relative to the other joints of the thumb; (2) insufficient or excessive CMC or MP abduction relative to the other joint (CMC or MP); (3) flexion of one joint of the thumb with extension of another or vice versa; and (4) wrist movement during active thumb motion (Figures 5-22 to 5-28).

When observing active finger flexion and extension, the alignment and movement of the wrist should also be

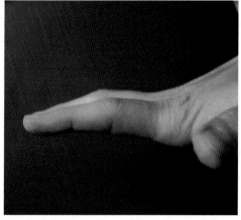

Figure 5-21. Excessive MP extension instead of IP extension (clawing with finger extension without nerve injury).

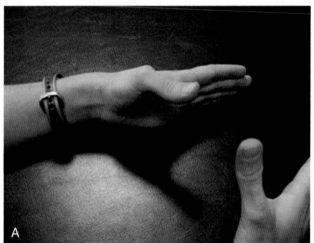

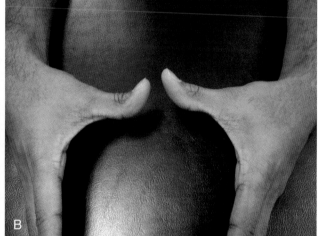

Figure 5-22. A, Insufficient thumb MP extension and excessive IP and CMC extension. **B,** Insufficient thumb MP extension and excessive IP and CMC extension.

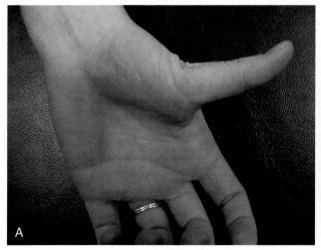

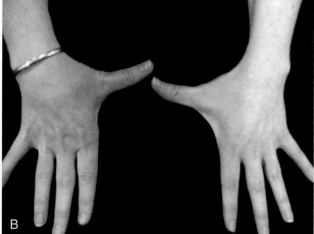

Figure 5-23. A, Insufficient thumb CMC extension with excessive thumb MP extension. **B,** Insufficient CMC extension and too much MP extension on right hand.

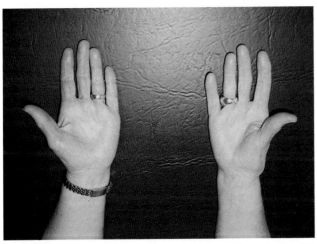

Figure 5-24. Insufficient CMC extension with excessive IP extension, right greater than left.

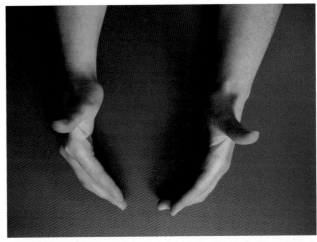

Figure 5-25. Excessive thumb adduction during thumb extension.

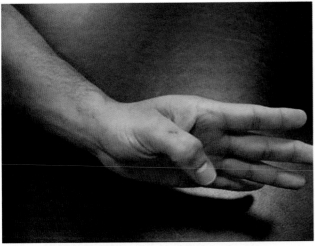

Figure 5-26. Insufficient thumb MP flexion with increased CMC and IP flexion.

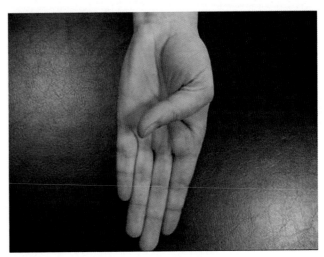

Figure 5-27. Insufficient thumb IP flexion with increased MP flexion.

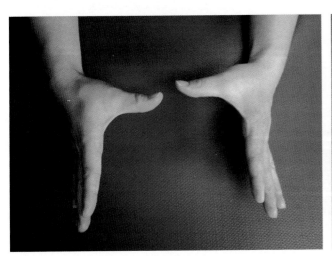
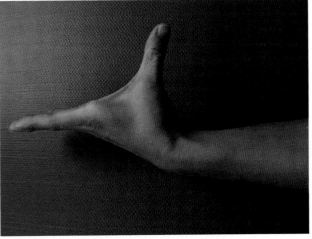

Figure 5-28. Wrist flexes instead of maintaining neutral wrist position during active thumb palmar abduction.

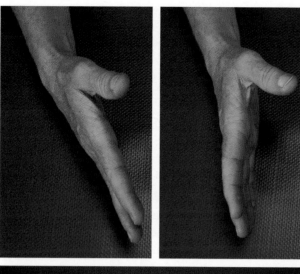

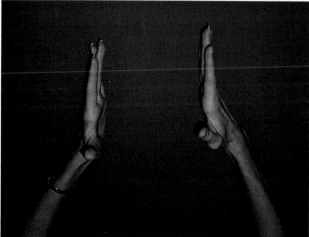

Figure 5-29. Wrist flexion during active finger extension: wrist not stable.

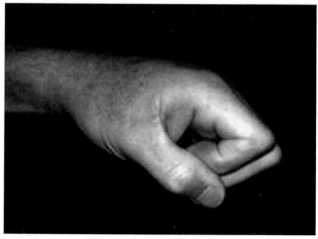

Figure 5-30. Wrist flexion instead of slight wrist extension during active finger flexion. (Used with permission from Ann Kammien, PT, CHT, St Louis, Mo.)

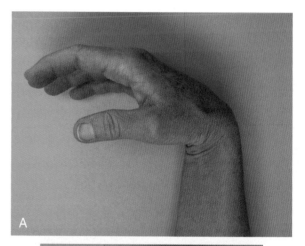

Figure 5-31. Tenodesis.

noted. During active finger extension, the wrist should not flex excessively (Figure 5-29). During active finger flexion, the wrist should not flex but instead should extend slightly (Figure 5-30). During active wrist extension and flexion, the fingers should flex and extend, respectively, as the result of tenodesis[4,20,55] (Figure 5-31). For example, during active wrist extension, the fingers should stay relaxed in a relatively flexed position instead of extending.

Resistance may provoke movement impairments when AROM is normal or may exaggerate the impairment noted during AROM (Figures 5-32 to 5-39).

Finally, during AROM or resistive ROM of the fingers or thumb, the examiner should also note the alignment and movement of the proximal upper extremity (forearm, elbow, and shoulder). The source of symptoms in the hand may come from the cervical spine, the thoracic outlet,[5] elbow, forearm, wrist, or the hand.[9-11] When the shoulder girdle is impaired, the distal muscles may generate excessive force to compensate for the proximal impairments.[4,42,56,57] Decreased strength of the scapular muscles

and poor scapular alignment may result in compression of nerves proximally causing symptoms in the hand or predisposing injury to the nerves distally (double crush).[5] Ideal alignment and strength of the shoulder girdle provides a stable base on which the distal upper extremity can function.

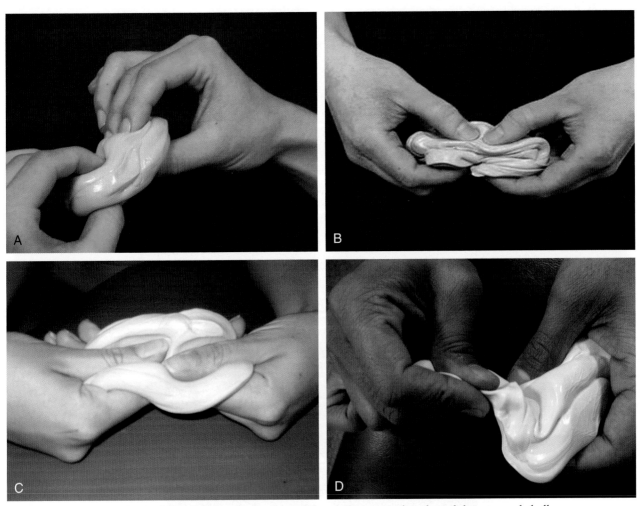

Figure 5-32. **A,** Normal longitudinal arc of thumb during pinch and good thenar muscle bulk. **B,** Collapse of first MC into flexion and adduction during pinch (left worse than right). **C,** Excessive thumb CMC adduction and flexion with wrist flexion during pinch. **D,** Excessive thumb IP extension and MP flexion during pinch (boutonnière).

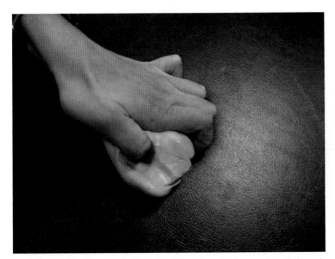

Figure 5-33. Excessive thumb adduction during resisted thumb flexion.

Following AROM, PROM should be assessed, paying particular attention to identifying the cause of the impairments. For example, what is the reason for the limited AROM?

Of particular interest during assessment of PROM is the resistance felt to passive motion (stiffness). Passive tests should include tests of muscle length, ligament integrity, joint capsular pattern, joint accessory motion, and ligament length. When assessing muscle length, particular attention is paid to relative flexibility and stiffness not just absolute length. Stiffness is compared between one muscle or group relative to another and between muscles on one side compared to the same muscles on the opposite side. The onset of pain should also be noted during PROM and compared to the pain behavior during AROM. This helps determine whether the contractile or noncontractile structures are involved.[14]

PROM can then be followed by resistive testing to identify involvement of the contractile structures and to

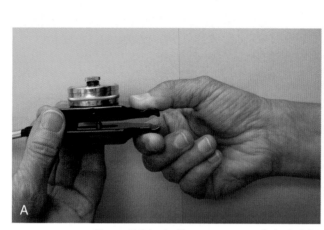

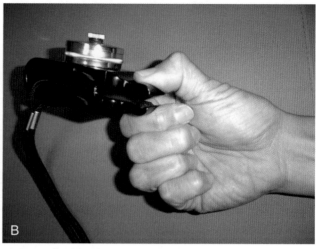

Figure 5-34. **A,** Correct pattern of pinch: Maintaining arch of the first metacarpal. **B,** Collapse of first MC into flexion and adduction (swan neck) during pinch.

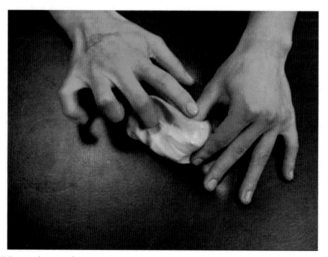

Figure 5-35. Normal arc of movement during resisted finger flexion on right middle finger.

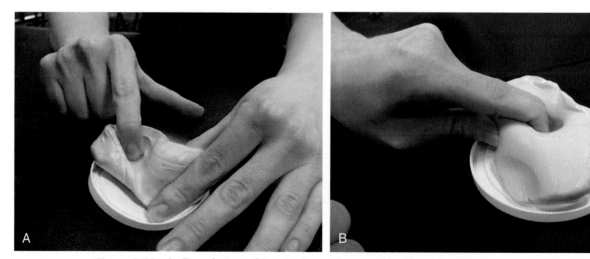

Figure 5-36. **A,** Dorsal view of impaired arc of movement: Excessive MP flexion and PIP extension (swan neck) index finger during resisted finger flexion. **B,** Radial or lateral view.

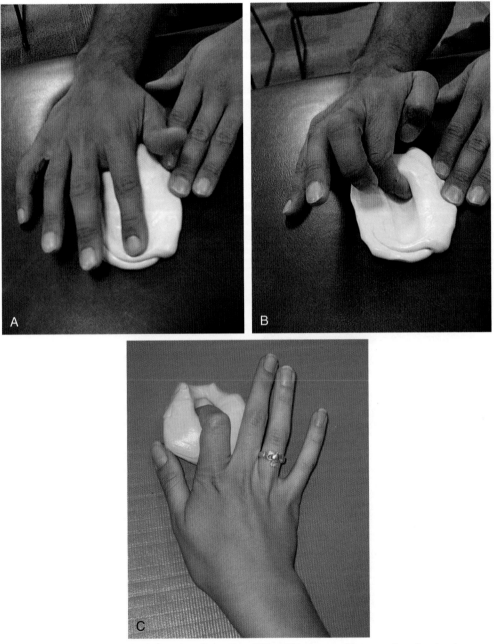

Figure 5-37. Impaired movement: Excessive MP adduction and/or rotation (supination = lateral rotation) of the index finger during resisted finger flexion. **A,** Starting position. **B** and **C,** MP adduction with rotation.

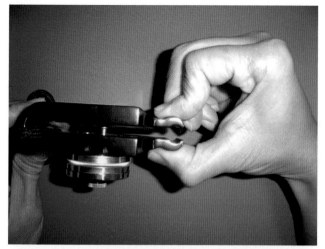

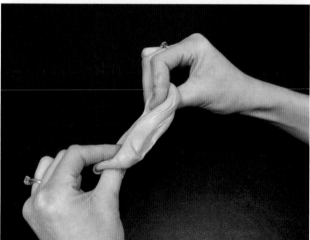

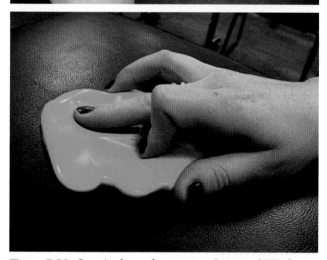

Figure 5-38. Impaired arc of movement: Increased PIP flexion and DIP hyperextension (boutonnière) of index finger during resisted finger flexion.

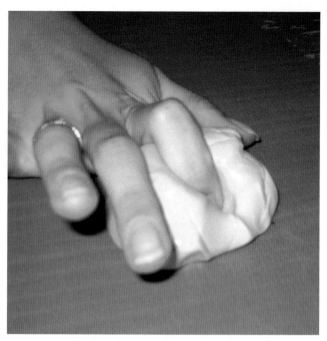

Figure 5-39. Impaired arc of movement: Excessive MP extension during resisted finger flexion indicating insufficient use of interossei.

FUNCTIONAL ACTIVITIES OF THE HAND AND WRIST

Subjective Examination

During the history, the patient should be questioned about those daily activities that are performed repeatedly and which of those are associated with either increasing and decreasing the symptoms. These activities include work, leisure, and activities of daily living (ADLs).

The patient must be asked to describe and demonstrate the preferred alignment and movement patterns they use repeatedly during their daily activities. Attention is given to the entire upper quarter and trunk and the potential effect of those areas on the distal symptoms. Any impairments that are identified are immediately modified to determine the effect the modification has on the patient's symptoms.

Assessment of the person's preferred pattern of performance of functional activities is a crucial part of examining the patient with symptoms in the hand. Activities or postures that are used frequently during the day or during sleep are assessed. Simulation of the posture or movement should be performed during the examination. Attention should be paid to onset of symptoms, alignment and movement patterns of the entire upper extremity. If symptoms are present and impairments are noted in the posture or movement pattern, the posture or movement pattern should be immediately modified to determine if the modification alleviates the symptoms. The patient should then be educated regarding the

determine strength of individual or groups of muscles. Although a muscle may test strong in the midrange, it might test weak in the shortened range. The findings from the AROM, PROM, and resisted tests are evaluated to determine the cause of the movement impairments. This evaluation helps focus the treatment.

impaired posture or movement pattern, and practice of the modified movement pattern should be done during the therapy session until the patient is able to adequately perform the modification independently. The modification must be easy enough for the patient to perform so that he or she can perform it correctly. If the patient is having difficulty, the examiner should prescribe a different modification that is easier. Symptoms should not be produced or increased during the modification of the movement or posture. Frequently, patients with symptoms in the hand also need modifications to the alignment or movement of the shoulder to alleviate the symptoms.[5] Taking breaks frequently to improve the performance of the opposing muscles from those used repeatedly is often beneficial.

Examples of modifications in functional activities that may be necessary are detailed in the next sections.

Writing

Modifications in writing focus on restoring the normal arch of the thumb and fingers used in grip, and correcting the alignment of the wrist, trunk, and shoulder girdle. The thumb CMC should be in relatively more abduction and pronation instead of adduction, flexion, and supination. Avoiding prolonged positioning with the joints at end-ranges may decrease stresses on the joint structures. At times, compensatory techniques may be useful such as using a writing utensil with a larger diameter or taping or splinting to facilitate correct alignment. Writing using a prehensile pattern of a 3-point grip with the DIP joint of the index finger in hyperextension and the PIP joint flexed may increase the compressive forces on the dorsal surfaces of the DIP joint and increase the tensile forces on the volar structures. With this type of grip the FDP is underused and the FDS may be overused. The ORL may become shortened and may need stretching. Writing with the thumb CMC positioned in adduction places the CMC joint in a less stable position and may result in stiffness or shortness of the adductor pollicis and insufficient use of the APB and the OP (Figures 5-40 to 5-44).

Using a Computer Mouse and Typing

The computer mouse and keyboard should be positioned on the desk so they can be reached while maintaining good alignment of the proximal upper extremity. The upper extremity should be supported to maintain the trunk and shoulder girdle in ideal alignment, the elbow flexed slightly less than 90 degrees, the forearms supported, and the wrists in very slight extension. The fingers should rest in the normal longitudinal arch (Figure 5-45) and in a relatively neutral position regarding ulnar or radial deviation (Figures 5-46 to 5-48).[58] Consideration of alternate keyboard or mouse styles, adjustable chair armrests, and adjusting chair and monitor height are often helpful to achieve the ideal alignment. In our experience, in most cases the preferred alignment of the

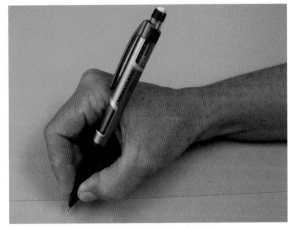

Figure 5-40. Writing: Ideal alignment.

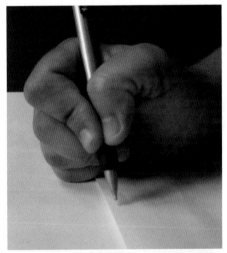

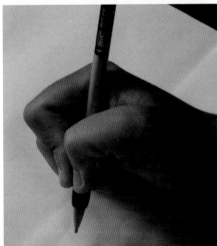

Figure 5-41. Writing: Impaired alignment. Excessive CMC adduction, thumb IP flexion, and index DIP extension.

shoulder girdle is in scapular depression. Adjustments need to be made to the arm support to elevate the shoulder girdle to ideal alignment. At times, placing the keyboard on the desk instead of using the computer tray is optimal. This positioning may require moving the

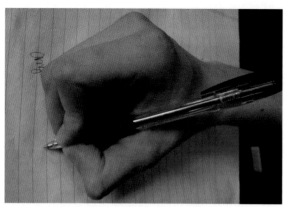

Figure 5-42. Writing: Impaired alignment. Normal CMC alignment with excessive thumb IP flexion and index DIP extension.

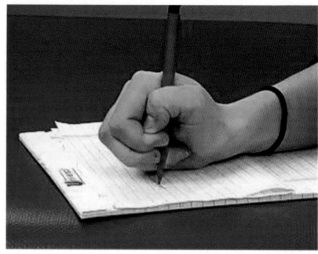

Figure 5-44. Writing: Impaired alignment. Excessive CMC adduction, thumb IP, and index DIP flexion.

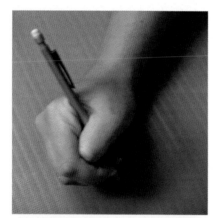

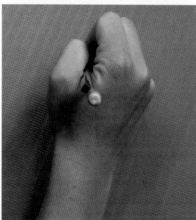

Figure 5-43. Writing: Impaired alignment. Excessive CMC adduction and thumb IP flexion.

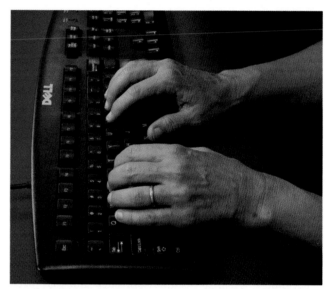

Figure 5-45. Typing: Normal longitudinal arc of index.

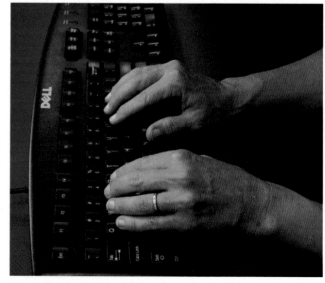

Figure 5-46. Typing: Impaired longitudinal arc. Increased MP flexion and IP extension of index.

monitor back on the desk so the keyboard can be placed a few inches away from the edge of the desk, allowing the distal one-half to two-thirds of the forearms to be supported by the desk. A preferred alignment of some shoulder abduction can result in increased wrist UD and extension contributing to symptoms on the ulnar side of the wrist. Taking breaks to stand with the back against the wall and performing shoulder flexion, as well

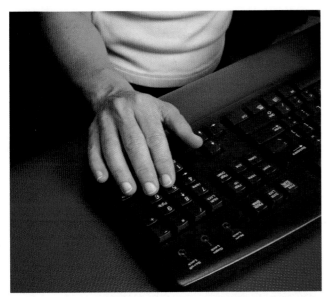

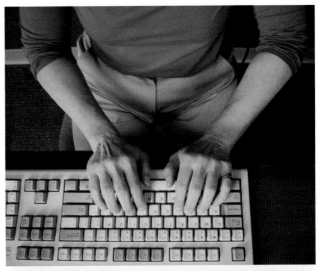

Figure 5-47. Typing: Repeated use of index MP in ulnar deviation contributing to an imbalance between the antagonistic interossei and MP joint pain.

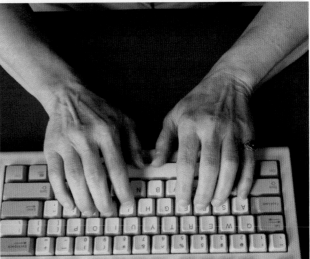

Figure 5-48. Typing: Ulnar-sided left wrist pain caused by keyboard/typing position; increased shoulder abduction and wrist ulnar deviation on left.

as stretching the finger flexors and extensors can be helpful.

Lifting
Lifting with the elbow flexed and the forearm supinated instead of pronated often helps decrease symptoms for patients with lateral epicondylitis (wrist extension with forearm pronation syndrome).

Sleeping
Particular attention should be paid to sleeping position when the alignment of the shoulder girdle is a factor contributing to the patient's symptoms in the distal upper extremity. At times, a wrist or hand splint may be necessary to maintain the proper alignment of those joints. For example, in patients who have carpal tunnel syndrome (CTS), the wrist should be kept in a neutral position. Splinting the wrist is used to maintain the wrist position in patients with CTS, but proper support of the arm may also be helpful (Figure 5-49).

Reading
The pattern of grip used to hold the book while reading and the alignment of the proximal upper extremity, neck, and trunk should be noted. Resting and propping the reading material up on pillows and tilting it helps maintain the correct alignment of the head and decreases the need for prolonged gripping of the reading material (Figure 5-50).

Gripping Objects
Identification of repeated use of a particular preferred pattern of grip or pinch directs treatment. The pattern is modified either by varying the pattern or by alternating

the pattern with one that uses a different set of muscles. For example, if a person tends to grip using an intrinsic plus type grip (MP flexion with IP extension; see Figure 5-50, *A* and *B*), instruction to use a style of grip that uses the extrinsic finger flexors more (hook- or power-type grip[48]; see Figure 5-50, *C*) may be beneficial. If an intrinsic plus grip must be used repeatedly, then taking breaks to stretch those muscles is necessary. Gripping objects so that a prolonged force is placed on the joints into ulnar or radial deviation should be avoided (Figure 5-51).

Playing an Instrument
Maintaining the ideal alignment of the trunk, neck, shoulder girdle, and distal upper extremity while playing an instrument is important. Particular attention is paid to subtle deviations in the alignment of the fingers (rotation, UD, or loss of the arch) and wrist, especially

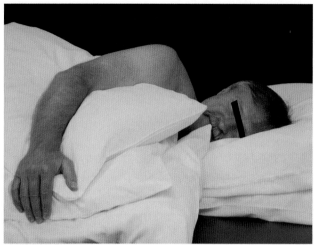

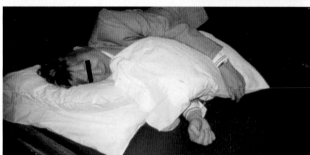

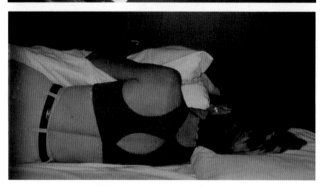

Figure 5-49. Sleeping position with good arm support.

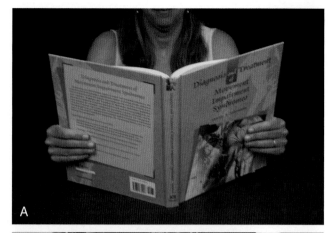

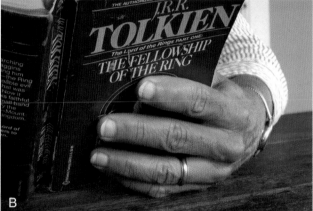

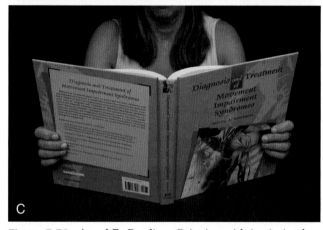

Figure 5-50. **A** and **B,** Reading: Gripping with intrinsic-plus-type pattern of grip (MP flexion and IP extension). **C,** Reading: Gripping without intrinsic-plus–type pattern of grip (increased PIP flexion and MP extension).

during functional use as force is increased. Small changes in the alignment of the shoulder girdle and elbow can result in beneficial decreases in the stresses on the hand.[4,56] For example, while playing the harp with the scapula aligned in excessive abduction, the musician may excessively flex the elbow or extend the wrist to reach the close strings. Adducting the scapula slightly results in less extension of the wrist and less elbow flexion.

Manual Therapy

When the therapist applies force using the fingers or thumbs during joint mobilization techniques or massage, repeated or prolonged positioning of the therapist's joints at end-ranges should be avoided. A common impairment noted with the thumb position is collapse of the CMC

into adduction and flexion and the MP and IP into excessive flexion or excessive extension. Modification of this alignment to a more neutral position may help reduce stresses on the tissues (Figure 5-52).

Many other functional activities may need to be addressed depending on those used by the patient. Examples may be eating, cooking, driving, other work activities, fitness, and hygiene.

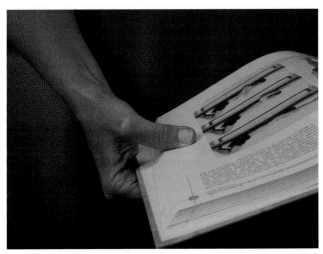

Figure 5-51. Reading: Functional pattern of use contributing to stress on ulnar collateral ligament of the MP of the thumb.

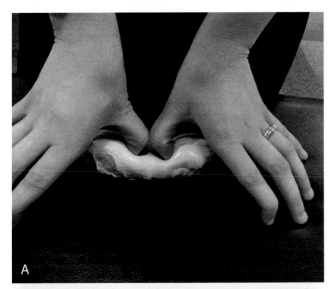

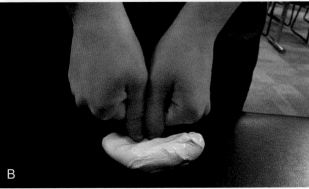

Figure 5-52. **A,** Preferred pattern of motion of physical therapy student performing simulated functional activity of joint mobilization. **B,** Modified pattern of motion of physical therapy student performing simulated functional activity of joint mobilization intended to decrease stresses on thumb joints.

MUSCULAR ACTIONS OF THE HAND AND WRIST

Muscles of the Wrist

The ECRL and ECRB are wrist extensors and radial deviators.[13] They are in the second extensor compartment.[59] The ECRL is a better radial deviator than the ECRB. The ECRL may also help flex the elbow[13] and supinate the forearm.[26]

During finger flexion, gripping, or pinching, it is critical that the ECRL and ECRB are active to ensure the correct length tension capabilities of the finger flexors.[20,43,60] During contraction of the finger flexors as with attempted gripping or pinching, weakness of the wrist extensors will result in the wrist flexing. Wrist flexion decreases the mechanical advantage of the finger flexors, limiting the ability to grip or pinch.[20] Another example of compensatory wrist flexion occurring during active finger flexion is when finger flexion is limited by stiffness, shortness, or adhesions. Maximizing active finger flexion ROM requires that the wrist be maintained in 20 to 30 degrees of extension.[20]

During active wrist extension, if the wrist extensors are weak, the fingers may extend, indicating substitution by the ED. This is common after a wrist fracture. To strengthen the wrist extensors, it is critical to keep the fingers relaxed in flexion to avoid substitution by the ED.

The ECRL may often become overused, stiff, short, or painful. The ECRL has a good moment arm for elbow flexion[49] in any forearm position but is the greatest with the forearm pronated.[61] Repeated flexion of the elbow with the forearm pronated contributes to overuse of the ECRL. This is often the case with patients with lateral epicondylosis. During forearm pronation, compensatory humeral medial rotation will allow the ECRL to remain stiff or short. Humeral medial rotation should be avoided during exercises designed to increase the extensibility of the ECRL. If the ECRL is overused because the elbow is repeatedly flexed with the forearm in pronation, an important part of treatment is educating the patient to increase the use of the biceps by flexing the elbow with the forearm supinated instead of pronated. In addition, the ECRL also tends to be overused because it is active as a synergist during any gripping or pinching activities, which includes most daily functional activities.[43]

When performing resisted tests to differentiate between the ECRL or ECRB as the source of the symptoms, modification of elbow position can be helpful.[13] Symptomatic resisted wrist extension with the elbow flexed implicates the ECRB, whereas the elbow extended implicates the ECRL.

Flexibility and strengthening exercises are often beneficial for patients with lateral elbow pain associated with overuse of the wrist extensors. Combined wrist flexion, forearm pronation, and elbow extension[11] with the humerus stabilized places maximal stretch on the ECRL and ECRB. Shortness of the ECRL and ECRB results in a resting alignment of wrist extension and radial deviation.[13] Stiffness of the ECRL and ECRB is identified by increased resistance to stretch during wrist flexion and ulnar deviation when the forearm is pronated with the elbow extended and the humerus stabilized. Progression of exercises should take into consideration the multiple joints that the muscle crosses when the goal is to avoid excessive stresses on the ECRL and ECRB.[62] For example, performing wrist extension and flexion exercises with the forearm in neutral rotation and the elbow flexed places less tensile stress on the ECRL than with the forearm pronated and elbow extended.

The ECU extends and ulnarly deviates the wrist.[13] The ECU is in the sixth extensor compartment.[59] It is a better wrist extensor with the forearm supinated than with the forearm pronated because the tendon slips anteriorly during forearm pronation.[48,49] The ECU is active as an antagonist during wrist flexion[63] and stabilizes the wrist during thumb abduction.[20] The ECU works along with the ECRL and ED during wrist extension. Through the attachments of its sheath to the TFCC,[45] the ECU contributes to the stability of the distal radioulnar joint (DRUJ)[43] and the ulnar carpals. Repeated use of the wrist in UD[47] and wrist extension causes increased compression on the TFCC potentially resulting in tissue injury and symptoms. A resting alignment of slight shoulder abduction while typing on a standard computer keyboard has been observed to contribute to increased wrist extension and UD, with symptoms on the ulnar side of the wrist. Shortness of the ECU results in a resting alignment of UD with slight wrist extension.[13] Stiffness of the ECU is identified by increased resistance to stretch during wrist flexion and radial deviation with the forearm pronated, elbow extended, and humerus stabilized.

The FCR flexes and radially deviates the wrist. The FCR may also assist in pronation of the forearm and elbow flexion.[13,26] The FCR contracts during RD to counterbalance the extensor component of the ECRL.[43] During movements of the wrist, the FCR also plays a role in stabilizing the distal pole of the scaphoid.[64] Shortness of the FCR results in a resting alignment of wrist flexion and RD.[13] Stiffness of the FCR is identified by increased resistance to stretch during wrist extension and ulnar deviation with the forearm supinated, elbow extended and humerus stabilized.

The FCU flexes and ulnarly deviates the wrist. It also assists with elbow flexion.[13] The FCU is a very strong muscle with a large cross-sectional area.[43,49] The FCU is less active as an ulnar deviator than the ECU.[49] The FCU stabilizes the pisiform during contraction of the ADM.[65] An imbalance between the forces of the FCU and ADM caused by repeated abduction of the small finger with the wrist in excessive extension may result in pain in the region of the pisiform or pisotriquetral joint. Overuse, stiffness, or shortness of the FCU may contribute to ulnar nerve compression at the elbow.[11] Shortness of the FCU results in a resting alignment of wrist flexion with UD.[13] Stiffness of the FCU is identified by increased

resistance to stretch during wrist extension and radial deviation with the forearm supinated, elbow extended, and humerus stabilized.

The palmaris longus is a pure wrist flexor. It is absent in about 10% of people.[43] It tenses the palmar fascia and assists with elbow flexion.[13]

Extrinsic Muscles of the Fingers

Finger Extensors

The extensor digitorum communis (EDC), extensor indicis (EI), and extensor digiti minimi (EDM) extend the MP joints of the fingers via their attachment into the sagittal bands.[20] No other muscles can extend the MP joints of the fingers.[19,20] All three muscles assist with IP extension if the MPs are not fully extended. The ED assists with abduction of the index, middle, and ring fingers, and both the ED and the EDM assist with abduction of the small finger.[13] If the DI are weak, the ED and EDM may substitute for finger abduction. The EI assists with adduction of the index finger.[13] The EI also allows independent extension of the index finger with the other fingers flexed.[19] The juncturae between the tendons of the ED and sharing of the muscle bellies of the ED in the forearm contribute to limited independence of finger motion.[20,66] The ED also assists with wrist extension and RD.[13,43,63] The ED and EI are in the fourth extensor compartment, whereas the EDM is in the fifth.[59,66]

Normally, the finger extensor tendons should remain centered over the dorsum of the head of the metacarpal if the sagittal bands are intact.[66] Normally during finger flexion, the ED tendons move ulnarly slightly because of the increased mobility on the ulnar side of the hand.[20] Laxity of the sagittal bands allows the extensor tendons to sublux, usually to the ulnar side of the joint, during finger flexion.[49,66]

During normal active finger extension when the forces of the MP flexors (FDP, FDS interossei and lumbricals) and MP extensors (ED) are balanced, the ED extends the MP but does not cause MP hyperextension. If some of the MP flexors (interossei and lumbricals) are weak, the ED causes increased MP hyperextension, which prevents the ED from being able to extend the IP joints fully.[24,26] This pattern of movement (mild "clawing") is often observed in musicians such as pianists.

During finger flexion, when applying pressure to a surface (i.e., piano keys), or any type of pinch, the PIP joint should not hyperextend, but the finger should maintain its normal longitudinal arch. Maintenance of the arch requires the balanced action between the intrinsic long finger flexors and the ED. Overuse of the intrinsics results in a swan neck–type posture.[30,31]

During active finger extension, if the forces between the intrinsics and long finger extensors are balanced, the fingertips should move through a wide arc of motion. If the extensors (ED) dominate, the arc of motion is smaller.[67]

During active finger extension, the wrist flexors should stabilize the wrist to prevent excessive wrist extension by the ED.[65] If the wrist flexors are overused during active finger extension, the wrist flexes because the wrist flexors are no longer just stabilizing but are overactive, flexing the wrist.

An example of the finger extensors (ED) dominating is displayed when the ECRL and/or ECRB is weak (i.e., after a Colles' fracture). As the patient attempts wrist extension, the fingers extend instead of remaining relaxed in a flexed position.

During cylindrical grip, such as in holding a hammer, the ED helps stabilize the MP joint. Acting with MP flexors, the ED increases joint stability and compression. During spherical grip, such as in holding a baseball, the role of the finger extensors is to balance the finger flexors. The finger extensors also function to open the hand and release objects.[48]

During the passive length test for the ED, shortness or stiffness of the ED results in the MP and IP joints of the fingers extending if the wrist is flexed, or if the MP and IP joints are flexed, the wrist will extend. Shortness[13] or stiffness of the finger extensors may also contribute to subluxation of the tendon over the head of the metacarpal during finger flexion.

Finger Flexors

The primary action of the FDS is to flex the PIP joints of the fingers. However, the FDS also assists with flexion of the CMC, MP, and wrist joints.[13] The FDS powers most individual finger motion[49] and crosses the elbow joint, whereas the FDP does not. The primary action of the FDP is flexion of the distal interphalangeal joints of the fingers. However, the FDP also assists with wrist, CMC, MP, and PIP flexion.[13] In the normal hand, the flexor tendons cross the MP joint slightly from the ulnar side. However, the flexor tendons do not ulnarly deviate the MP joint unless the annular ligaments are lax or damaged, allowing the flexors to become ulnar deviators.[49] During finger flexion, the FDP assists adduction of the index, ring, and small MP joints of the fingers. Interconnections of the muscle fibers of the FDP in the forearm inhibit the independent function of the individual tendons of the FDP.[49] Therefore, to prevent the FDP from working on the finger being tested during MMT of the FDS, the other fingers are stabilized.[68] After surgical repair of the FDP, uninvolved fingers adjacent to the involved finger may need to be immobilized to prevent forces from the adjacent fingers being transferred to the repaired tendon.

Good gliding of the FDS and FDP tendons relative to each other and to the bone is critical to good hand function. Restoring normal gliding of these tendons is often a focus of therapy in patients with traumatic hand injuries.[69] Good hand function also requires normal length of the FDS and FDP. Shortness,[13] stiffness, or adhesion of the FDS will result in flexion of the MP and PIP joints of the fingers if the wrist is extended or flexion of the wrist if the fingers are maintained in extension. Shortness,[13] stiffness, or adhesion of the FDP will result in MP, PIP,

and DIP flexion if the wrist is extended or wrist flexion if the finger is maintained in extension. Findings from flexor muscle length testing in patients with overuse syndromes often reveal that the absolute length of the muscles is normal, but the involved side is noticeably stiffer through the range than the uninvolved side. Caution should be used when stretching the FDS and FDP to prevent the MP and IP joints from flexing. Overstretching should also be avoided. Combined stretching of the wrist and fingers should not exceed 80 degrees of wrist extension and zero degrees of finger extension.

During cylindrical gripping, the FDP is more active during the dynamic phase of flexion movements of the fingers, whereas the FDS is more active during the static phase.[48] During types of prehension that require DIP flexion, such as picking up a pin, the FDP is active.[48] The FDS is active when the DIP is extended during PIP flexion.

There is a decrease in tension of the FDS and FDP at the more distal joints of the fingers when the wrist flexes.[65] Thus when the focus of treatment is regaining finger flexion, the wrist should be maintained in at least 20 to 30 degrees of extension. The benefit of wrist extension for the length-tension properties of the flexor tendons has been discussed previously in the "Muscles of the Wrist" section.

CTS may be aggravated during gripping or prehension when using the finger flexors with the wrist flexed because this movement pattern results in anterior movement of the flexor tendons. The anterior movement of the flexor tendons decreases the distance between the finger flexor tendons and the flexor retinaculum relative to using the finger flexors with the wrist in extension, thus increasing the pressure on the median nerve at the wrist.[70] Maintaining the wrist in neutral-to-slight extension during contraction of the finger flexors prevents the anterior movement of the flexor tendons.[70] A movement impairment of wrist flexion during active finger extension has also been observed in patients with CTS (see Figure 5-29). Repeated use of the wrist flexors with the wrist in flexion may result in an impairment of the wrist flexors noted during active finger extension. Normally during active finger extension, the wrist flexors should stabilize the wrist against the wrist extensor force provided by the finger extensors. However, if the wrist flexors have been used repeatedly in a position of wrist flexion, the wrist flexors may flex the wrist during finger extension instead of stabilizing the wrist. Patients with this movement pattern should be instructed to practice active finger extension, maintaining the wrist in slight extension.

During finger flexion while applying pressure to a surface (such as playing the piano or any type of pinch), the fingers maintain a longitudinal arch when the actions of the FDS and FDP are balanced by the actions of the ED and the finger intrinsics.[4] During open-chain active finger flexion, the fingertips should move through a wide arc of motion if there is balanced action between the intrinsics and long finger flexors. If the long finger flexors dominate, the arc of motion is decreases[20,49] (see Figure 5-18). More details regarding specific movement impairments related to imbalances between these muscles are described later in this chapter in the discussion on the movement system syndromes.

The median nerve may become compressed as it travels under the proximal edge of the FDS producing symptoms in the anterior forearm and hand. Contraction of the FDS to the middle finger increases the compression, aggravating the symptoms.[71]

During active finger flexion in end-range power gripping, we have observed a movement impairment of an excessive increase in the ulnar side of the distal transverse arch and UD of the fingers at the MP joint in some patients. This movement impairment may also contribute to subluxation of the finger extensors over the head of the metacarpals and is more likely to be observed in the patient with hypermobile joints. Manually supporting the MP heads to prevent the excessive increase in the transverse arch abolishes the popping of the finger extensors over the heads of the metacarpals. Treatment may include limiting the finger flexion ROM, using splinting to assist avoiding excessive UD and increase in the transverse arch, exercising to increase the stiffness of the radial deviators of the MP joints of the fingers, and actively practicing the corrected movement pattern.

Intrinsic Muscles of the Fingers

The intrinsic muscles of the fingers include the DI and palmar interossei (PI) and the lumbricals.[19] The DIs abduct the fingers away from the midline of the hand, which is through the middle finger and third metacarpal.[72] The first DI assists with adduction of the thumb[13] and may assist with stabilizing the first CMC joint.[49] The three palmar interossei adduct the fingers.[13] All of the interossei and the four lumbricals flex the MP and extend the IP joints of the fingers.[19] The lumbricals are good extensors of the IP joints, regardless of the position of the MP joint.[20] Because both of the lumbrical attachments are into tendons and the lumbricals have many sensory organs, the lumbricals balance the tension between the finger extensor mechanism and the finger flexors (FDP).[20] When the lumbricals contract, the FDP tension is released and tension on the extensor mechanism is increased, facilitating finger IP extension.[20] The lumbricals are relatively silent during cylindrical grip (gripping a tennis racket), whereas the interossei are very active.[48] The interossei become more efficient as MP flexors as the fingers move farther into flexion.[49] The role of the interossei during cylindrical grip and pad-to-pad prehension is to help flex, abduct, and adduct the MP joints of the fingers.[48] The interossei contribute to ulnarly deviating all of the MP joints during gripping.[48] The function of the interossei is critical for normal active finger flexion and extension. Weakness results in "clawing," which has already been described (see sections on ED and impaired alignment). Absence of interossei

function for the small finger results in a resting alignment of MP abduction and extension as a result of the unopposed action of the ED, which is referred to as Wartenberg's sign.[12,73]

Shortness or stiffness of the intrinsics may result from overuse or immobilization at a shortened length. Shortness may not be evident when making a fist, but PIP and DIP flexion may be severely limited with the MP joint maintained in extension.[19,20] Subtle differences in the length of the interossei may be identified only by abduction or adduction of the finger while maintaining the MP joint in extension and the IP joints in flexion. Shortness, stiffness, or overuse of the interossei on one side of the finger relative to the interossei on the opposite side of the finger may result in a rotation impairment of the MP or PIP joint of the finger. For example, if the first DI is underused and the first palmar interosseous is overused, the patient may present with the index finger resting in increased supination compared to the opposite side. The patient might present with pain in the area of the MP joint or PIP joint, depending on which joint is most affected by the rotation. A repeated activity that might contribute to this impairment is using the number keys on the right side of the computer keyboard instead of using the keys at the top of the keyboard. This movement impairment is described further in the "Movement System Syndromes" section.

Some patients that have normal ulnar nerve function demonstrate a movement impairment of mild clawing of the fingers only during functional use. MP hyperextension is noted presumably because the ED (MP extensor) is no longer counterbalanced by intrinsics (MP flexors) at the MP joint even though the intrinsics may test normal during strength testing. The ED cannot effectively extend IP joints because it is actively insufficient because of MP hyperextension. MP hyperextension puts passive tension on long finger flexors pulling the IPs into flexion. Teaching these patients to modify their preferred movement pattern may help prevent or relieve symptoms.

Weakness of the finger intrinsics has been described as common in patients who are performing artists, so strengthening the intrinsics is recommended.[57] However, we find the muscles do not necessarily test weak when testing the strength of the intrinsics with MMT. We have observed instead that the preferred pattern of movement used by the patient is not ideal, and modification of that movement pattern results in relieving the patient's symptoms. The focus of the modification is to maintain the longitudinal arch of the hand and fingers and neutral rotation of the fingers while playing an instrument, balancing the use of the long finger flexors and intrinsics.[4] Changing the movement pattern is required to achieve a reduction of symptoms and strengthening alone is not as effective. To learn the correct movement pattern, patients need to perform the motion with decreased resistance and difficulty. If resistance is added before learning the new movement pattern, patients will resort to using the preferred impaired pattern of movement.

Thenar Muscles

The thenar muscles are crucial for positioning the thumb during functional grasping and manipulating objects.[4,48] Contraction of the APB and the OP deepen the concavity or transverse arches of the hand facilitating grasp. The activity of these muscles varies, depending on whether the thumb is being opposed to the radial or ulnar fingers and on the force applied.[48]

The APB palmarly abducts the CMC and MP joints of the thumb[13] and assists thumb IP joint extension through its attachments to the extensor mechanism. Most of the thumb abduction occurs at the CMC joint. The APB may assist flexion and medial rotation of the MP joint and assists with opposition of the CMC joint.[13] The APB is often underused compared to the adductor pollicis and FPB, but in the absence of a nerve injury, the APB rarely tests weak during MMT. The APB is active during pinch of thumb with any finger and increases to equal the activity of the adductor pollicis during firm pinch with the small finger.[48] Shortness or stiffness of this muscle is rare.

The OP flexes, abducts and medially rotates the CMC joint of the thumb. Cupping the hand, the APB and OP deepen the transverse arch at the carpal tunnel. Opposition of the thumb also results in deepening the proximal transverse arch of the hand. The OP and the APB originate on the flexor retinaculum.[13] Weakness of the opponens results in the inability to oppose the tip of the thumb to the tip of the small finger, lining up the fingernails and making prehensile types of grip difficult if not impossible.[13] Substitution using the FPB may allow the patient to touch the tip of the small finger to the thumb, but the patient will be unable to rotate the first metacarpal to line up the fingernails.[74] During pinch, the activity of the opponens increases as the pinch with the thumb moves from the index to the small finger.[48] The OP is often underused compared to the adductor pollicis and FPB, but in the absence of a nerve injury, rarely tests weak with MMT. Shortness or stiffness of this muscle is rare.

The FPB flexes the MP and CMC joints of the thumb. The FPB assists in opposition of the thumb and helps extend the IP joint via the extensor mechanism.[13] The FPB has increased activity with increased force of pinch.[48] The FPB is often overused along with the adductor pollicis. Shortness or stiffness of the FBP results in MP flexion of the thumb.

The adductor pollicis adducts the CMC and MP joints of the thumb and assists with MP flexion. It also assists with IP extension through its attachments to the extensor mechanism.[13] The adductor pollicis has the largest torque potential of any muscle affecting the CMC joint of the thumb[7] This muscle is active during all types of strong pinch but especially active during key or lateral pinch.[48] During key pinch, if the adductor is weak, the FPL will

substitute for the adductor pollicis, resulting in thumb IP flexion (positive Froment's sign).[49] If the adductor pollicis is nonfunctional, by using tenodesis,[43] the thumb can be positioned for key pinch by extending the wrist. Because the adductor is used in all types of strong pinch and grip and the thumb is usually flexed and adducted during functional use,[75] the adductor pollicis is frequently overused, stiff, or short. Overuse, stiffness, or shortness of the adductor contributes to alignment impairments, imprecise movement, and symptoms at the CMC joint of the thumb. An extreme example is OA with subluxation of the CMC joint of the thumb. During prehensile gripping, because of the distal attachment of the adductor pollicis on the first metacarpal, the adductor pollicis contributes to adduction, flexion, and lateral rotation (supination) of the thumb instead of helping maintain the longitudinal arch of the thumb.

Extrinsic Muscles of the Thumb

The APL abducts and extends the CMC joint of the thumb. Although it is named as an abductor, the movement it performs is really more extension of the thumb.[49] The APL assists with radial deviation and flexion of the wrist.[13] The APL is in the first extensor compartment with the EPB.[66] The APL is the key muscle to maintain the arch of the pinch in the absence of deformity[49] and thereby provides stability to the CMC joint.[7] It is opposed by the adductor pollicis.[49] The APL will substitute for the APB when the APB is weak, resulting in thumb extension with abduction instead of pure thumb palmar abduction. Increased stresses are placed on the tendons in the first extensor compartment with repeated RD of the wrist with the thumb stabilized, forceful wrist RD with abduction and extension of thumb, rapid rotational movements of forearm, and forceful UD of the wrist.[76]

The APL and the EPB can be the source of symptoms in two different locations: at the wrist over the first extensor compartment (deQuervain's disease) and more proximally where the muscle crosses the ECRL and ECRB (intersection syndrome).[77] The APL and the EPB must glide freely through the retinacular compartment to be symptom-free and function well. Shortness or stiffness results in wrist RD when the thumb is flexed or thumb extension when the wrist is ulnarly deviated. The length test for this muscle (similar to Finkelstein's test) may provoke symptoms at the first extensor compartment if the APL or EPB is the source of the symptoms.

The EPL extends the IP joint of the thumb and assists with MP and CMC extension.[13] The EPL assists with adducting the thumb CMC joint[49] and extending and radially deviating the wrist.[13] The EPL is in the third extensor compartment.[66] Although the EPL is the primary thumb IP extensor, the deep head of the FPB, adductor pollicis, and the APB may assist in extending the IP joint of the thumb via their attachments into the extensor mechanism on the thumb.[13] During thumb extension, if adduction occurs during extension, the EPL may be overused compared to the EPB and APL (see Figure 5-25). The APL, EPL, and EPB are synergists during thumb extension. Excessive thumb adduction during thumb extension indicates overuse of the EPL relative to the APL and EPB. Shortness of the EPL results in thumb extension when the wrist is ulnarly deviated with flexion or wrist extension and RD when the thumb is flexed. The ability to extend and adduct the thumb off the table when the hand is resting on the table with the palm down verifies that the EPL is intact.[19]

The EPB extends the MP joint of the thumb, extends and abducts the CMC, and assists with wrist RD.[13] The EPB tendon is in the first extensor compartment of the wrist with the APL[66] but is generally weaker than the APL. Weakness of the EPB is common. During thumb extension, if adduction occurs with extension, the EPB and APL may be underused compared to the EPL. Modifying the extension so the patient extends with more abduction will increase the use of the EPB and APL versus the EPL. During active thumb extension, other movement impairments involving the EPB can occur and are described in detail in the treatment section of the Chapter 5 Appendix for the thumb CMC accessory hypermobility syndrome. Shortness, stiffness, or adhesion of the EPB results in thumb MP extension when the thumb is flexed and the wrist is ulnarly deviated.

The FPL flexes the IP joint of the thumb, assists with MP and CMC flexion, and may assist with wrist flexion.[13] The FPL is active during cylindrical grip along with the thenar muscles.[48] During pad-to-pad and tip-to-tip prehension, the FPL is important to control IP flexion.[48] The function of the FPL along with the APL is essential to maintain the longitudinal arch of the thumb. The patient is unable to form a circle with tip-to-tip pinch between the thumb and the index finger with severe weakness of the FPL. This is referred to as a positive *circle sign*.[78] Shortness, stiffness, or adhesion of the FPL results in flexion of the thumb IP joint when the thumb and wrist are extended.

Hypothenar Muscles

During cylindrical grip, the muscles of hypothenar eminence are active.[48] When working with patients that have limited flexion of the ulnar fingers caused by stiffness of the joints, there is often insufficient recruitment of the hypothenar muscles. Specific cues to contract these muscles, especially the FDM, help the patient recruit these muscles. We have not observed shortness of these muscles. All of the hypothenar muscles help cup or deepen the concavity of the palm,[13,19] which is required for grasping objects and normal functional use of the hand.

The ADM abducts the MP joint of the small finger and assists in opposition and flexion of the small finger. The ADM also assists in extension of the IP joints through its attachment into the extensor expansion.[13] The FCU stabilizes the pisiform during contraction of the ADM.[65] An imbalance between the forces of the FCU and ADM caused by repeated abduction of the small

finger with the wrist in excessive extension may result in pain in the region of the pisiform or pisotriquetral joint.

The opponens digiti minimi (ODM) opposes the small finger (flexion with slight rotation of the CMC joint) so it is possible to perform tip-to-tip prehension between the little finger and the thumb. The ODM also helps deepen the transverse arch or "cup" the palm.[13]

The FDM flexes the MP joint of the small finger and assists in opposing the little finger to the thumb.[13]

MOVEMENT SYSTEM SYNDROMES
of the Hand

The proposed movement system syndromes of the hand have been developed based on clinical experience and examination of the literature but are still a "work-in-progress" and need testing and refining based on feedback from other clinicians with expertise in treating patients with hand problems.

To our knowledge, no other classification systems have been described to guide physical therapy management of the patient with hand dysfunction. Commonly, it is the physician's diagnoses related to the pathoanatomical source of pain, established protocols, and isolated impairments that guide treatment. The premise of this chapter is that syndromes are composed of clusters of impairments and when identified, more effectively guide physical therapy management of patients with hand problems than if no movement system diagnosis has been made. The physician's diagnosis, while important and helpful, is not sufficient to guide the physical therapy management of the patient with hand problems. For patients whose treatment is guided by protocols, it is still important for the therapist to identify the cause (source) of the symptoms and signs. Thus the diagnoses presented here have two parts: one that identifies the principal movement that is impaired and the second that identifies the tissue that is the source of the impaired movement.

Some patients with hand symptoms have problems that are not guided by established protocols. Based on the premise that the physical therapist has primary expertise in analysis of the movement system, we have developed a set of movement system–based syndromes for the hand to guide physical therapy treatment of these patients. The syndromes are named either for the alignments and movements that appear to be related to the patient's symptom behavior or for the primary cause of the patient's impairments. The focus of the diagnoses is on the movement that produces the symptoms rather than the pathoanatomical source of the symptoms. In many cases, the symptom is associated with movement, thus we believe that alterations in the precision of movement are the cause of the tissue irritation and need to be corrected to achieve optimal outcomes. A patient might be assigned more than one syndrome, but usually, one syndrome is primary.

This section of the chapter focuses on the overall description of each syndrome and on symptoms and history, key tests and signs, and source of signs and symptoms (the first three columns of the Chapter 5 Appendix). The Chapter 5 Appendix includes a complete description of each syndrome, as well as associated signs or contributing factors and differential diagnosis for each syndrome.

INSUFFICIENT FINGER AND/OR THUMB FLEXION SYNDROME

The principal impairment of insufficient finger and/or thumb flexion syndrome is limited finger or thumb flexion AROM, but the key to prescribing the appropriate treatment is differentiating between the sources causing the limited flexion. The sources of the limited flexion can be broadly classified into two main categories: hypomobility (physiological and accessory motion) and force production deficit (decreased strength). Insufficient finger and/or thumb flexion syndrome is most commonly secondary to a trauma or injury or after a period of immobilization to allow for tissue healing. In the acute stage, these patients may be assigned a hand impairment diagnosis Stage 1, but an underlying movement system diagnosis of insufficient finger or thumb flexion may help guide treatment. As the tissues heal, the diagnosis may change from pathoanatomical source or regional hand impairment to another movement system diagnosis. Items 1 to 11 in the following list are the potential causes (source of signs and symptoms) of insufficient finger or thumb flexion. The identified cause of insufficient finger and/or thumb flexion is the second part of the name of the syndrome. Insufficient finger or thumb flexion may be caused by the following:

1. Flexor tendon adhesion[69,79]
2. Extensor tendon adhesion[66,79]
3. Shortness extrinsic extensors[19,79]
4. MP collateral ligament shortness and/or adhesion[20,79]
5. IP joint dorsal capsule shortness and/or adhesion[79]
6. Shortness of oblique retinacular ligament[19]
7. Shortness of interossei and lumbricals[19,20]
8. Swan neck deformity[33] (A swan neck deformity is usually not a problem until it progresses so that the PIP joint of the involved finger hyperextends and "locks," preventing flexion. At that point the swan neck deformity would be classified under this syndrome.)
9. Ligament sprain[34,79]
10. Weakness of finger or thumb flexors[13]
11. Rupture of the finger or thumb flexors[80]

Symptoms and History

Patients with insufficient finger and/or thumb flexion may complain of (1) the inability to make a fist, (2) difficulty gripping objects, and (3) difficulty using the involved hand for functional activities such as feeding, dressing, and writing. They usually report symptoms in the hand or forearm and may report swelling in the hand, wrist or forearm. They may also report numbness and tingling. Patients that have insufficient finger and/or thumb flexion may be referred to physical therapy with the following common referring diagnoses: status/postsynovectomy for arthritis, extensor or flexor tendon repair, tendon adhesion, ligament sprain (grade I or II), stiffness after fracture, or nerve injury. Patients with insufficient finger and/or thumb flexion may also be in the later healing stages after any of the surgical procedures listed for the hand impairment diagnosis in Box 5-1.

Key Tests and Signs

Alignment Analysis

Impairments in alignment and appearance for patients with this syndrome include joints that are red and swollen compared to the opposite hand, scar on flexor or extensor surface, resting alignment of decreased flexion of one or more joints of the involved finger, resting alignment of MPs in extension with increased IP flexion, and adducted thumb (typical stiff-hand posture). See Box 5-2 for examination and treatment for scar and edema.

Movement Impairment Analysis

Movement impairments noted in this syndrome include (1) the joint adjacent to the joint with the limited flexion flexes more readily than the joint that is limited; (2) during finger flexion; the wrist or fingers move into extension if the finger extensors are short[13] or adhered; and (3) during finger flexion the wrist flexes if the finger joint structures are the source of the limited finger flexion and the wrist is relatively less stiff or the wrist extensors are weak.

Joint Integrity

Active and passive finger and/or thumb ROM should be assessed; and active flexion will be limited at one or more joints. Passive flexion and extension of the fingers and/or thumb may or may not be limited; depending on the cause of the limitation. The onset of pain is often at the end-range of the flexion ROM (see the "Source of Signs and Symptoms" section for further explanation). Table 5-1 includes the procedure for restricted joint motion testing.

Ligament integrity and/or length. One of the sources of limitation of finger and/or thumb flexion can be the joint structures, including the MP collateral ligaments, the ORL, and the dorsal capsule.[19,79] Examination of the hand should include testing for integrity and length of the ligaments and differentiating whether the limitation of flexion ROM is the result of the joint structures or other causes. See Table 5-1 for specific procedures for these tests.

Joint accessory motion. Assessing joint accessory motion should also be performed to clarify whether the source of the signs is the result of the joint or other structures.

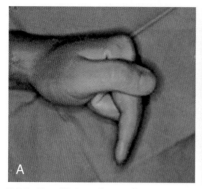 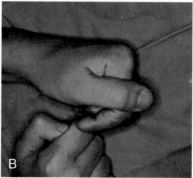

Figure 5-53. Insufficient finger flexion caused by flexor tendon adhesions: AROM less than PROM. **A,** AROM. **B,** PROM greater than AROM. (Used with permission from Ann Kammien, PT, CHT, St Louis, Mo.)

Muscle Length Tests

Tests of muscle length must be performed passively. Particular attention is paid to the amount of resistance to stretch (stiffness) throughout the ROM during the test and to which joint moves most easily. The length tests provide information regarding whether the limitation of flexion ROM is due to shortness or adhesion of the respective muscle and/or tendon. The tests of muscle length that should be performed are extrinsic finger or thumb flexors, extrinsic finger or thumb extensors, and the interossei muscles (see Table 5-1 for specific procedures).

Muscle Strength/Performance Impairments

Assessing strength is important to determine the source of the signs assuming there are no precautions regarding risk of injury to the tissues. Tests of strength include: grip and pinch strength using a grip dynamometer and a pinch gauge and MMT of the finger and/or thumb flexors.[13,19] Strength may be decreased as the result of weakness of the extrinsic finger and/or thumb flexors or intrinsics or decreased gliding of the tendons.[13,68,79] When performing these tests, the examiner should note the preferred pattern of movement and any impairments compared to normal. Impairments include limited ROM or an alteration in the sequencing and timing of joint movement.

Source of Signs and Symptoms

Based on the findings from a comprehensive examination, impairments are identified. Determination of the source of the signs and symptoms requires knowledge of and recognition of the cluster of impairments that are characteristic of each source. Identifying the source will guide management of the patient more effectively and efficiently than treating isolated impairments. For example, if treatment is focused on isolated impairments one could conclude that weakness is the cause of AROM into flexion being less than PROM (when PROM into flexion is normal). The appropriate treatment for weakness would be to overload the muscle to build strength. However, if the source of the limitation of AROM into flexion is flexor tendon adhesion, the initial focus of

treatment would instead be restoring gliding of the flexor tendons. The clusters of impairments for each potential source and/or cause of insufficient finger or thumb flexion are as follows.

Hypomobility

Flexor Tendon Adhesion (Figure 5-53)
- Active finger and/or thumb flexion ROM is less than PROM; passive flexion ROM is normal.[68]
- Extrinsic finger and/or thumb flexor length test findings are positive for shortness or adhesion (PROM and AROM into composite finger and/or thumb extension are equally decreased).[68]
- Adherence of the flexor muscle or tendon may be palpated and visually observed especially during active flexion.[68]
- During the MMT of the extrinsic flexors, a strong contraction of the muscle is palpable and the muscle can hold against resistance within a limited ROM; however, there is an abrupt stop to the active ROM into flexion.

Extensor Tendon Adhesions (Figure 5-54, p. 213)
- Active finger and/or thumb extension ROM is less than PROM ("extensor lag").
- Extrinsic finger and/or thumb extensor length test findings are positive for shortness or adherence (PROM and AROM into composite finger and/or thumb flexion are equally decreased).[66]
- Adherence of the extensor muscle or tendon may be palpated or observed visually, especially during active extension.[66]
- During the MMT of the extrinsic extensors, a strong contraction of the muscle is palpable and the muscle can hold against resistance within a limited ROM; however, there is an abrupt stop to the active ROM into extension.

Extensor Muscle Shortness (Figure 5-55, p. 213)
- Normal active and passive finger and/or thumb extension ROM.

Text continued on p. 214

TABLE **5-1**
Procedures for Testing Restricted Joint Motion and Muscle Length

Tests	Procedure	Results	Indications
PASSIVE RANGE OF MOTION			
Test for limited joint ROM caused by the joint capsule/ligaments[1,2]	If checking for finger flexion ROM, compare passive flexion of the distal joint (i.e., PIP) with the proximal joint (i.e., MP or wrist) extended versus with the proximal joint (i.e., MP or wrist) flexed. If checking for finger extension ROM, compare passive extension of the distal joint with the proximal joint extended versus with the proximal joint flexed.	Limitation of PROM of involved joint remains consistent regardless of proximal joint's position. Short collateral ligament at MP joints: Limited passive MP flexion, regardless of the position of the wrist and/or IP joints. Short accessory collateral ligaments and volar plate at IP joints: Limited passive IP extension, regardless of the position of the MP joints and/or wrist.	Limited active or passive flexion or extension ROM of the digits.
Ligament Integrity/Length Oblique retinacular ligament length test[3,4]	Compare passive DIP flexion with the PIP joint extended versus with the PIP joint flexed.	If the ORL is short, DIP flexion will be less with the PIP joint extended than with the PIP joint flexed. Compare to uninvolved side to see if decrease in DIP flexion with PIP extended is significant. Should be >5 degree difference.	If DIP flexion is limited. With boutonnière deformity.

Continued

TABLE **5-1**
Procedures for Testing Restricted Joint Motion and Muscle Length—cont'd

Tests	Procedure	Results	Indications
Test for integrity of collateral ligaments at MP and PIP joints of fingers 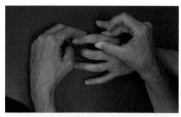 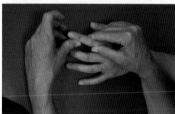 PIP joint varus and valgus stress testing. 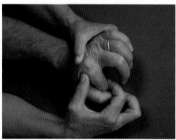 Tests for MP joint ulnar collateral ligament integrity.	Apply an adduction or abduction force to the joint with the IP joints extended to test the PIP collateral ligament integrity. (May test IP joint collateral ligaments with the joint in full extension as well, as with the joint in slight flexion to test different fibers of the ligament. The end-feel should be firm and ligament taut in both positions.) Apply an adduction or abduction force to the joint with the MP joints flexed to test the integrity of the MP joint collateral ligaments.	Normal should be a firm end-feel without pain and little motion. Compare to the uninvolved side.	Traumatic joint injury. Complains of insidious onset of joint pain with history of repetitive forces applied to that joint.

TABLE **5-1**
Procedures for Testing Restricted Joint Motion and Muscle Length—cont'd

Tests	Procedure	Results	Indications

Muscle Length Tests
Muscle length tests should be performed passively. During testing, identify sites that are relatively most flexible and feel for relative differences in stiffness.

Interossei muscle length test[1,5,6] Does not test lumbricals because it is a passive test—no contraction of FDP so lumbricals are not taut.	*Procedure 1* 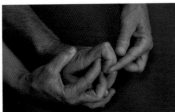 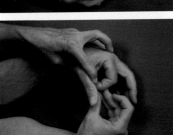 Compare passive flexion of the PIP joint with the MP joint in full extension versus with the MP joint flexed. (The DIP joint is also flexed with the PIP joint, but usually the PIP joint is the one that is measured.) Best to position the wrist in 20 to 30 degrees of extension during this test.	The intrinsic muscles are short if the PIP flexion is less with the MP joint extended than with the MP joint flexed.	Swan neck deformity. Hand has been immobilized in an intrinsic plus position. Limited active or passive flexion ROM of the fingers.
	Procedure 2 A more aggressive interossei muscle length test. (Lumbricals do not abduct and adduct.) 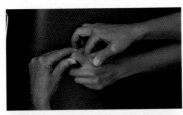 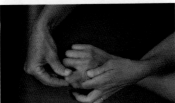 Compare how much MP abduction or add there is with the PIP and DIP joints in full flexion and the MP joint extended (compared to the opposite hand).[7]	Compare to the opposite hand.	Signs of intrinsic shortness, such as supination or pronation of the finger at the MP or IP joints, are present, but the intrinsic muscles do not test short using Procedure 1. Patient complains of pain of unknown origin in the area of the MP or IP joints or between the metacarpals.

Continued

TABLE **5-1**
Procedures for Testing Restricted Joint Motion and Muscle Length—cont'd

Tests	Procedure	Results	Indications
Extrinsic Muscle Length			

If the amount of limitation of movement in one joint depends on the position of another joint, the restricting tissue lies outside the joint.

Tests	Procedure	Results	Indications
Extrinsic flexor length/adhesion test (FDS and FDP). 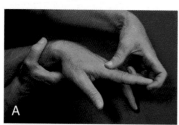 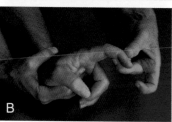 **A** and **B,** Passive finger extension with wrist flexed versus extended. This procedure is used if there is significant shortness. 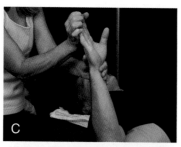 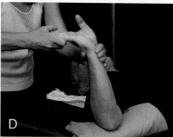 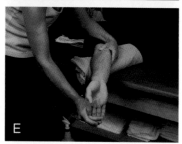 **C** to **E,** This procedure is used when the shortness is not as significant.	Compare passive extension of the distal joint (PIP) with the proximal joint (MP or wrist) flexed versus with the proximal joint extended.	Composite wrist and finger extension are limited. Positive if there is more extension of the distal joint (PIP) into extension with the proximal joint (MP or wrist) flexed than with it extended.	Limited active or passive extension ROM of the digits.

TABLE 5-1

Procedures for Testing Restricted Joint Motion and Muscle Length—cont'd

Tests	Procedure	Results	Indications

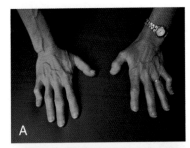

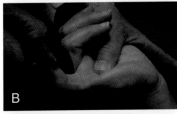

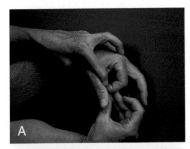

Example of short or hypoplastic flexor digitorum superficialis. **A** and **B**, Limitation of PIP extension with wrist extended. **C**, Normal range of PIP extension with wrist flexed.

Extrinsic extensor length/adhesion test[1,5] (ED, EI, EDM)

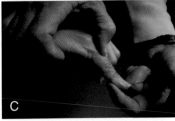

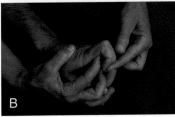

Passive finger PIP flexion with wrist flexed **(A)** versus extended **(B)**. This procedure is used if there is significant shortness.

Extrinsic extensor length/adhesion test (ED, EI, EDM)	Compare passive flexion of the distal joint (PIP) with the proximal joint (MP or wrist) extended versus with the proximal joint flexed.	Composite wrist and finger flexion are limited. Positive if there is more flexion of the distal joint (i.e., PIP) into flexion with the proximal joint (i.e., MP or wrist) extended than with it flexed.	Limited active or passive flexion ROM of the digits. Determining which joint to use to place the muscle on slack to see if there's a change in ROM at the limited joint depends on the exact problem or area of involvement of the muscle. For now, use an *adjacent joint* where there is a significant amount of tendon glide. (i.e., there is generally more tendon glide across the wrist than across the IP joints).

Continued

TABLE **5-1**
Procedures for Testing Restricted Joint Motion and Muscle Length—cont'd

Tests	Procedure	Results	Indications
Extrinsic extensor length/adhesion test *(Continued)* 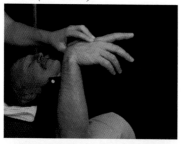 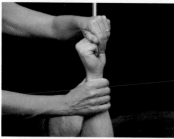 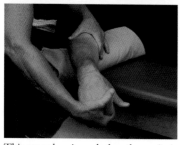 This procedure is used when the extrinsic extensor shortness is not as significant.			
Flexor pollicis brevis length test 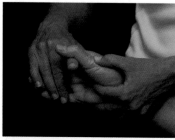 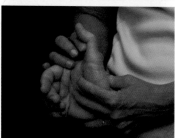 Thumb MP extension with the CMC flexed versus extended.	Compare the passive extension of the thumb MP joint with the CMC joint flexed to the CMC joint extended.	Positive if the thumb MP extension is more limited with the CMC joint extended than with CMC joint flexed.	Limited active or passive thumb extension.

TABLE **5-1**

Procedures for Testing Restricted Joint Motion and Muscle Length—cont'd

Tests	Procedure	Results	Indications
Extensor pollicis brevis length test 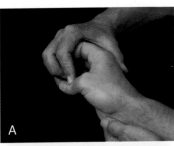 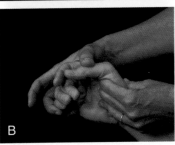 **A,** MP flexion with CMC flexed and wrist in slight extension and ulnar deviation. **B,** MP flexion with CMC extended and wrist in slight flexion and radial deviation.	Compare the range and stiffness of passive flexion the MP joint with the CMC joint extended and wrist flexed and radially deviated to range of MP flexion with the CMC joint flexed and the wrist extended and ulnarly deviated.	Positive if there is less MP flexion with the CMC joint flexed and the wrist extended and ulnarly deviated than with the CMC joint extended and the wrist flexed and radially deviated.	Limited active or passive thumb flexion or wrist ulnar deviation.

Length Test of APB and OP

No procedure is described because clinically there is rarely an issue of shortness. In most clinical problems, the issue is loss of the first web space not an increased web space.

Length Test of Adductor Pollicis

Normal ROM of palmar abduction is 45 degrees.[8] It is difficult to differentiate between the joint versus the muscle limiting the movement.

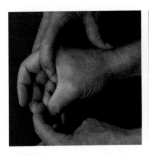 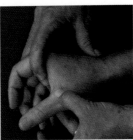

Continued

Tests	Procedure	Results	Indications
Extensor pollicis longus length test 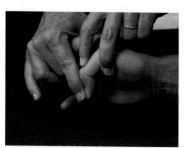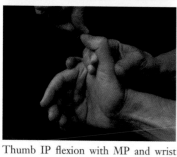 Thumb IP flexion with MP and wrist flexed versus extended.	Compare flexion the thumb IP, MP, and CMC with the wrist in radial deviation and slight extension to flexion of the thumb IP with the MP and CMC in flexion and the wrist flexed and in ulnar deviation.	Positive if there is less thumb IP flexion with the MP and CMC joints flexed and wrist flexed and in ulnar deviation than with the MP and CMC joints in extension and wrist extended and in radial deviation.	Limited active or passive thumb flexion or wrist ulnar deviation.
Flexor pollicis longus length test 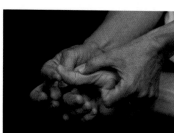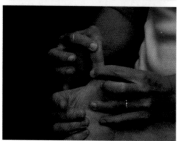 Thumb IP extension with CMC and wrist flexed versus extended.	Compare passive thumb IP extension with MP, CMC, and wrist joints flexed to thumb IP extension with the MP, CMC, and wrist joints extended.	Positive if thumb IP extension is less or relatively stiffer with the MP, CMC, and wrist joints extended than flexed.	Limited active or passive thumb or wrist extension.

APB, Abductor pollicis brevis; *CMC,* carpometacarpal; *DIP,* distal interphalangeal; *ED,* extensor digitorum; *EDM,* extensor digitorum minimi; *EI,* extensor indicis; *FDP,* flexor digitorum profundus; *FDS,* flexor digitorum superficialis; *FPL,* flexor pollicis longus; *IP,* interphalangeal; *MP,* metacarpophalangeal; *OP,* opponens pollicis; *ORL,* oblique retinacular ligament; *PIP,* proximal interphalangeal; *PROM,* passive range of motion; *ROM,* range of motion.

1. Aulicino PL: Clinical examination of the hand. In Mackin EJ, Callahan AD, Osterman AL, et al, eds: *Rehabilitation of the hand and upper extremity,* ed 5, St Louis, 2002, Mosby.
2. Cambridge-Keeling CA: Range-of-motion measurement of the hand. In Mackin EJ, Callahan AD, Osterman AL, et al, eds: *Rehabilitation of the hand and upper extremity,* ed 5, St Louis, 2002, Mosby.
3. Landsmeer JM: The anatomy of the dorsal aponeurosis of the human finger and its functional significance, *Anat Rec* 104(1):31-44, 1949.
4. Shrewsbury MM, Johnson RK: A systematic study of the oblique retinacular ligament of the human finger: its structure and function, *J Hand Surg Am* 2(3):194-199, 1977.
5. Dell PC, Sforzo CR: Ulnar intrinsic anatomy and dysfunction, *J Hand Ther* 18(2):198-207, 2005.
6. Bunnell S: Ischaemic contracture, local, in the hand, *J Bone Joint Surg Am* 351:88-101, 1953.
7. Rosenthal EA: The extensor tendons: anatomy and management. In Mackin EJ, Callahan AD, Osterman AL, et al, eds: *Rehabilitation of the hand and upper extremity,* ed 5, St Louis, 2002, Mosby.
8. Neumann DA: *Kinesiology of the musculoskeletal system: foundations for physical rehabilitation,* St Louis, 2002, Mosby.

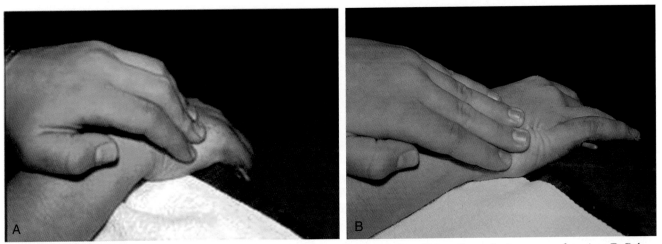

Figure 5-54. Insufficient finger flexion caused by extensor tendon adhesion. **A,** Insufficient finger flexion range of motion. **B,** Palpation of adherence of extensor tendon and extensor lag at PIP joint. (Used with permission from Ann Kammien, PT, CHT, St Louis, Mo.)

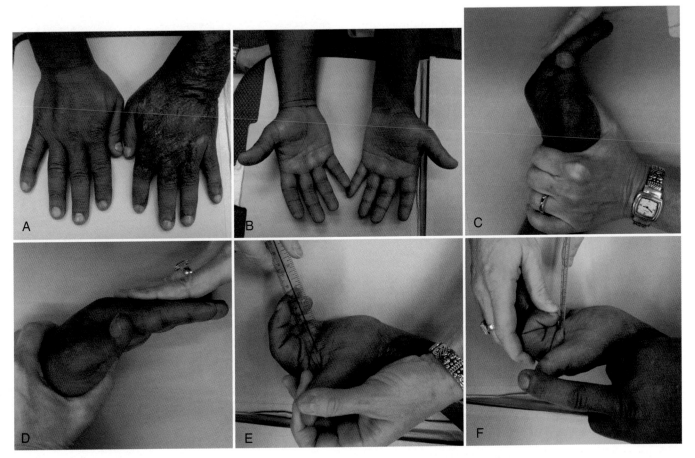

Figure 5-55. Insufficient finger flexion caused by extrinsic extensor shortness and dorsal scar. **A,** Appearance of dorsal scar. **B,** Appearance of anterior surface of hands and forearms. **C to D,** Passive range of MP flexion with wrist extended greater than passive MP flexion with wrist flexed. **E,** Active range of composite finger flexion. **F,** Passive range of composite finger flexion.

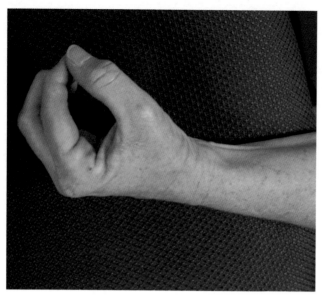

Figure 5-56. Insufficient finger flexion caused by joint structures and osteoarthritis.

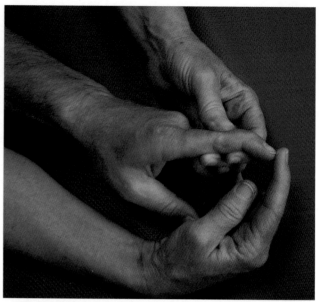

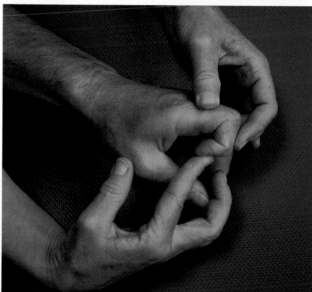

Figure 5-57. Oblique retinacular ligament length test. Limitation of passive DIP joint flexion with PIP joint in extension but not with PIP joint flexed indicates shortness of ORL.

- Extrinsic extensor muscle length test findings are positive for shortness (equally decreased passive and active composite wrist, finger, and/or thumb flexion).[19]

Metacarpophalangeal Collateral Ligament Shortness or Adhesion (Figure 5-56)
- Findings during passive finger and/or thumb MP joint flexion ROM include equal limitation of passive and active MP flexion regardless of the position of adjacent joints.[52] There is a firm end-feel to the PROM into flexion.
- Assessment of accessory joint motion findings are decreased posterior to anterior glide of the proximal phalanx on the metacarpal.[43]

Interphalangeal Joint Dorsal Capsule Shortness or Adhesion (see Figure 5-56)
- IP joint active and passive flexion ROM is equally limited, regardless of the position of the adjacent joints.[19,52]
- There is a firm end-feel to the PROM into flexion.
- Assessment of accessory joint motion findings are decreased posterior to anterior glide of the proximal or middle phalanx on the middle or distal phalanges, respectively.[43]

Shortness of Oblique Retinacular Ligament (Figure 5-57)
- ORL ligament length test findings are positive for shortness (DIP joint flexion limited with PIP joint in extension but not limited with PIP joint flexed).[19]
- Patient may have resting alignment of PIP flexion and DIP hyperextension (boutonnière deformity).[27-29]

Shortness of Interossei and Lumbricals (Figure 5-58)
- Interossei muscle length test findings are positive for shortness.[19] Passive composite finger flexion can be normal with shortness of interossei because the interossei are not stretched across the MP joint when the MP joints are flexed.
- Composite finger extension can be normal with short interossei because the interossei are not stretched across the IP joints when the IP joints are extended.
- PROM should be equal to AROM when the ROM is tested in the exact same position for active and passive.
- Palpation findings may reveal tenderness over the muscle bellies or tendons of the interossei.

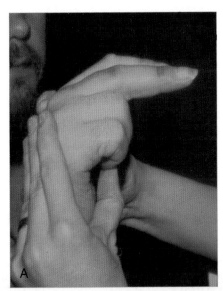

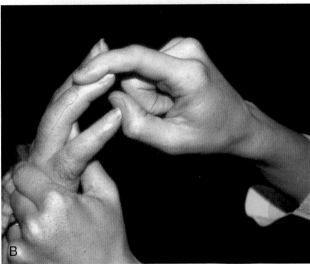

Figure 5-58. Insufficient finger flexion caused by shortness of interossei: Passive PIP and DIP flexion less with MP extended than with MP flexed. **A,** IP flexion with MP flexed. **B,** IP flexion with MP extended. (Used with permission from Ann Kammien, PT, CHT, St Louis, Mo.)

Swan Neck Deformity[33] (see Figure 5-9)
- Resting alignment of PIP hyperextension with MP and DIP flexion.
  - Hypermobility of the PIP (laxity of volar plate)
  - Intrinsic muscle shortness
  - Mallet finger (increases tension on central slip).
  - Fracture of middle phalanx with shortening (decreases tension on the terminal tendon).
  - Extensor tendon adhesion over dorsum of hand.
  - Extensor tendon shortness.
  - Nonfunctional FDS
  - Volar subluxation of the MP joint (increases tension on EDC)

Ligament Sprain[34,79]
- Ligament integrity test findings are positive.

Force Production Deficit
Insufficient finger flexion caused by force production deficit is likely the result of either weakness caused by ulnar or median nerve injury or rupture of the extrinsic flexor tendons.

Weakness of Finger and/or Thumb Flexors
- Active finger and/or thumb flexion ROM is less than passive ROM.
  - Strength determined by MMT is graded 2/5 or less.[13]
  - Weakness is noted throughout ROM of finger and/or thumb flexion.
- Passive finger and/or thumb ROM is normal.

Rupture of Finger and/or Thumb Flexors
(see Figure 5-59)
- Absent active function of the involved tendon; passive flexion ROM of finger and/or thumb is normal.
- Absent tenodesis (involved finger and/or thumb does not flex with wrist extension)[68]
- History of sudden onset with report of audible "pop."

Associated Signs or Contributing Factors
Patients with insufficient finger flexion usually present with associated edema and scarring of the hand or forearm and less frequently loss of sensation. Although these impairments are important to identify and treat, they are not key findings that help differentiate between diagnoses. For this reason, edema, scar, and sensation are listed as "associated signs or contributing factors." See the Chapter 5 Appendix and Box 5-2 for the tests and treatment used to manage edema and scar. The Chapter 5 Appendix includes the complete listing of associated signs or contributing factors for this syndrome.

Differential Diagnosis
The movement system diagnoses, finger flexion with or without rotation syndrome and hand impairment, are those syndromes that most closely overlap with insufficient finger and/or thumb flexion and should therefore be ruled out during the examination of the patient. Source or regional impairment of the hand is discussed briefly in this chapter as it relates to patients with hand injuries, but Chapter 2 describes those diagnoses in more detail. Finger rotation with or without rotation syndrome is discussed in more detail later in this chapter, as well as the Chapter 5 Appendix.

Potential diagnoses requiring referral, as suggested by the patient's signs and symptoms, are diagnoses of neuromusculoskeletal, visceral, or systemic origin that indicate that the patient should be referred to the physician for further evaluation. Refer to the Chapter 5 Appendix for the listing of these conditions.

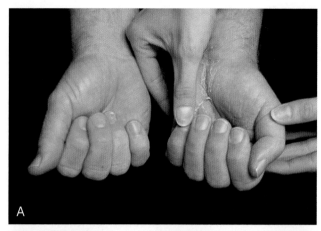

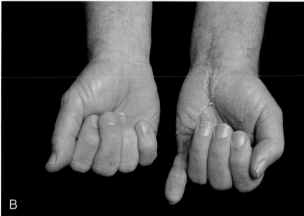

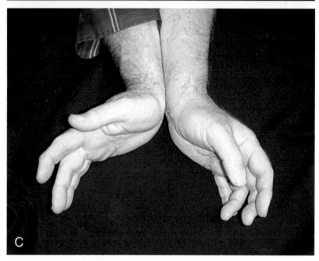

Figure 5-59. Insufficient finger flexion caused by flexor tendon rupture. **A,** Small finger passive flexion range normal. **B,** Small finger active flexion limited. **C,** Lack of normal tenodesis causing finger flexion during wrist extension on left small finger.

Treatment

The Chapter 5 Appendix includes a description of treatment for each of the causes of insufficient finger and/or thumb flexion. Box 5-2 includes description of the treatment of scar and edema. Treatment for sensory deficits is not be covered here because it is covered well in other texts.[74]

The usual expectation is that AROM should increase by a minimum of 10 degrees per week except when the cause of the limitation is due to profound weakness or rupture. If ROM is not improving by at least 10 degrees per week, then more aggressive treatment, such as passive stretching or splinting, should be considered. However, pain and edema should be decreasing gradually over the course of treatment. If pain and edema are not decreasing, one reason could be that the treatment is too aggressive, resulting in the lack of progress with ROM (see Box 5-2).

INSUFFICIENT FINGER AND/OR THUMB EXTENSION SYNDROME

The principal impairment of insufficient finger and/or thumb extension syndrome is limited finger or thumb extension AROM, but the key to prescribing the appropriate intervention is differentiating between the sources causing the limited extension. The identified cause of insufficient finger and/or thumb extension is the second part of the name of the syndrome. Insufficient finger or thumb extension may be caused by the following:

1. Flexor tendon adhesion[69,79] (Figure 5-60)
2. Extensor tendon adhesion[66] (Figure 5-61)
3. Flexor shortness[79] (Figure 5-62)
4. MP, PIP, or DIP volar plate and accessory collateral ligament shortness or adhesion[79] (Figure 5-63)
5. Shortness of ORL[19,80]
6. Shortness of interossei and lumbricals[13]
7. Ligament sprain[34]
8. Weakness of EDC or thumb extensors[13]
9. Weak interossei and lumbricals (finger intrinsics)[13] (see Figure 5-6, *B* and *C*)
10. Rupture of finger or thumb extensors

Insufficient finger and/or thumb extension syndrome is not be described further here because the principles for understanding it are the same as for insufficient finger and/or thumb flexion syndrome. See the Chapter 5 Appendix for additional details related to examination and treatment for this syndrome.

INSUFFICIENT THUMB PALMAR ABDUCTION AND/OR OPPOSITION SYNDROME

The principal impairment of insufficient thumb palmar abduction and/or opposition syndrome is limited thumb AROM into thumb palmar abduction and/or opposition, but the key to prescribing the appropriate intervention is differentiating between the sources causing the limited opposition and/or abduction. The sources of the limited thumb palmar abduction and/or opposition can be broadly classified into two main categories: hypomobility (physiological and accessory motion) or force production deficit (decreased strength). Pain may or may not be

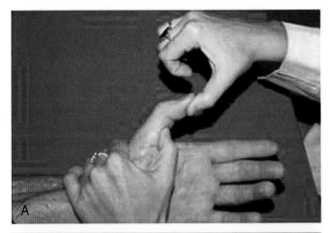

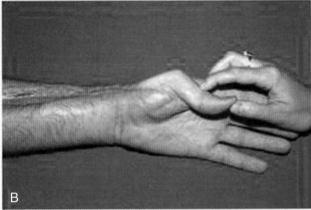

Figure 5-60. Insufficient thumb extension caused by adhered flexor pollicis longus. **A,** Limited passive range of thumb IP extension with MP extended. **B,** Normal IP extension with thumb MP flexed. (Used with permission from Ann Kammien, PT, CHT, St Louis, Mo.)

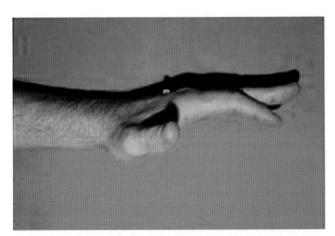

Figure 5-61. Insufficient finger extension caused by extensor adhesion (PIP extensor lag). (Used with permission from Ann Kammien, PT, CHT, St Louis, Mo.)

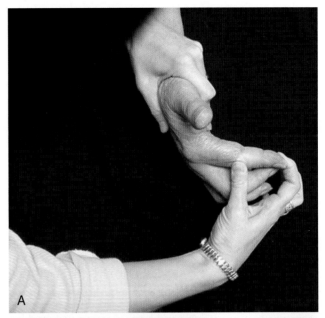

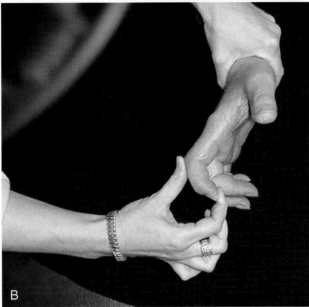

Figure 5-62. Insufficient finger extension caused by extrinsic flexor shortness. **A,** Normal range of PIP and DIP extension with MP and wrist flexed. **B,** Limited PIP extension with MP and wrist extended.

associated with the limited movement. Contracture resulting in insufficient thumb palmar abduction and/or opposition (hypomobility) is most commonly secondary to a trauma or injury or after a period of immobilization to allow for tissue healing.[81] Acutely, these patients may

be assigned a pathoanatomical source diagnosis or hand impairment Stage 1, but the underlying movement system diagnosis of insufficient thumb palmar abduction and/or opposition syndrome may help guide treatment. As the tissues heal, the diagnosis may change from a pathoanatomical source or regional hand impairment to insufficient thumb palmar abduction and/or opposition syndrome. Contracture resulting in insufficient thumb palmar abduction and/or opposition (hypomobility) may also be secondary to paralysis caused by a median nerve injury.[81] However, if there is any active function of the median nerve innervated muscles, then the diagnosis

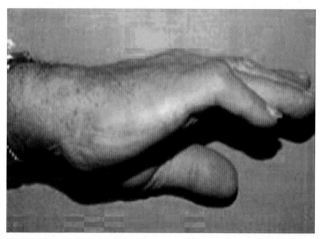

Figure 5-63. Insufficient finger extension caused by contracture of volar plate and accessory collateral ligaments. (Used with permission from Ann Kammien, PT, CHT, St Louis, Mo.)

force production deficit would guide treatment. A third reason for insufficient thumb palmar abduction and/or opposition (hypomobility) is joint subluxation and deformity secondary to the later stages OA of the CMC joint of the thumb.[7,82] The "Source of Signs and Symptoms" section provides key information regarding the cluster of findings identifying the cause of the insufficient thumb palmar abduction and/or opposition for this syndrome.

Symptoms and History

The patient with insufficient thumb palmar abduction and/or opposition may complain of difficulty gripping objects, pain in the hand and/or the forearm, and a history of median nerve injury or trauma.[81] If patients have had a nerve injury, they may also report a loss of sensation. Patients with DJD of the CMC of the thumb may report slowly developing joint pain, stiffness and limitation of motion, and difficulty with functional activities caused by pain. Activities related to DJD of the CMC joint of the thumb include needlework or repetitive use of scissors (e.g., a hairdresser). DJD of the CMC of the thumb is more common in women than men, and the onset is usually in the fifth to seventh decades of life.[83] Common referring diagnoses may include status/postfracture after immobilization, median nerve injury, crush injury, spinal cord injury, brachial plexus injury, hand pain, or DJD of the CMC joint of the thumb.

Key Tests and Signs

Alignment Analysis

Impairments in alignment and appearance for patients with this syndrome include decreased first web space (thumb resting in more adduction than normal), scar, and muscle atrophy. In addition, patients in the later stages of DJD of the CMC joint of the thumb may have swelling at the CMC joint of thumb, prominence, and subluxation and an adduction deformity of the thumb CMC joint (see

Figures 5-9, B, and 5-10, B). Associated alignment impairments of flexion or hyperextension at the thumb MP joint may also be noted.[7,82]

Movement Impairment Analysis

Movement impairments noted in this syndrome include decreased thumb CMC joint abduction during functional activities requiring opening of the hand in preparation for pinch or grip, inability maintaining the normal longitudinal arch of the thumb, and in some cases the MP joint may abduct excessively to compensate for the lack of CMC joint abduction.

Joint Integrity

Active and passive thumb ROM should be assessed. Findings will be limited active CMC palmar abduction, opposition, or extension. The onset of pain will likely be at the end of the ROM. If there is paralysis caused by a median nerve injury, there will be no active thumb palmar abduction or opposition. Passive thumb abduction and opposition ROM may or may not be limited. Crepitus may be palpable during PROM in patients with DJD of the CMC of thumb.[82] See the "Source of Signs and Symptoms" section for further details.

Joint accessory motion. Assessing joint accessory motion should be performed to clarify whether the source of signs is due to the joint or other structures.

Muscle Length Tests

Tests of muscle length should be performed for the adductor pollicis and FPB (see Table 5-1). These tests should be performed passively with particular attention paid to the amount of resistance to passive stretch (stiffness) throughout the ROM during the test and to which joint moves most easily. The purpose of the test is to identify whether decreased muscle length is contributing to the limitation of the thumb abduction and/or opposition ROM. Differentiating whether the limitation of motion is due to the adductor pollicis muscle length versus joint structures may not be possible.

Other special tests. Two special tests have been described to help determine if the source of the signs and symptoms is degeneration at the CMC joint of the thumb. The first test, Swanson's crank and grind test,[84] will be positive as articular degeneration advances, and pain, crepitus, or instability will be present.[82] The second test, the shoulder sign,[85] will also be positive.

Muscle Strength/Performance Impairments

Assessing muscle strength is important to determine whether the insufficient thumb abduction and/or opposition is caused by decreased muscle strength. A quick test of strength[72] can be done by having the patient oppose the tip of the thumb to the tip of the small finger. If weakness of the thenar muscles is suspected, follow-up testing should be done using MMT. Three-point or lateral pinch strength can be assessed with a pinch gauge and compared to the uninvolved side. When performing these tests, the examiner should note the preferred pattern of movement and any impairments compared to normal. Impairments include limited ROM or an alteration in the sequencing and timing of joint movement. Patients with DJD of CMC of thumb may have decreased pinch strength with collapse of the first metacarpal and weakness of the OP, APL, and APB.

Palpation. Tenderness of the CMC joint along the entire joint line is characteristic of patients that are having pain caused by DJD of the CMC of the thumb.[82]

Source of Signs and Symptoms

The clusters of impairments for each potential source or cause of insufficient thumb abduction and/or opposition follow.

Force Production Deficit

If the patient has insufficient thumb abduction and/or opposition because of a median nerve injury, the following signs may be seen:

- Passive thumb abduction and/or opposition ROM will be greater than AROM but some AROM will be present.
- Strength of the APB and OP will be 2/5.[13]
- If pain is associated with the limited PROM, it will be at the end-ROM.

Hypomobility

Contracture caused by thumb adductor muscles, CMC joint structures, or scar may have the following signs:

- Active thumb abduction and/or opposition ROM will be limited and equal to PROM.
- There may be palpable superficial firm and immobile scar in the first web space.
- Thumb CMC joint accessory motions will be decreased for abduction.
- If pain is associated with the limited PROM, it will be at the end ROM.

Median nerve injury:

- Passive thumb abduction and/or opposition ROM will be normal and greater than AROM, and no AROM is possible without substitution.
- The strength grade of the APB and OP based on MMT will be equal to or less than 1/5.
- Treatment is required to prevent loss of PROM and contracture as described in the previous section.

CMC subluxation and/or deformity (see Figure 5-9, *B*, and Figure 5-10, *B*):

- Active thumb abduction and/or opposition ROM will be equal to PROM.
- Swelling may be present at the thumb CMC joint.[82]
- The thumb CMC joint will be prominent.[82]

- There will be an adduction deformity of the thumb CMC joint.[82]
- Thumb CMC joint accessory motion impairments are variable but will likely be decreased in some direction.[86]
- Pain will occur during ROM in multiple directions.

Associated Signs or Contributing Factors

Patients with insufficient thumb abduction and/or opposition caused by contracture secondary to soft tissue injury will often present with associated edema and scarring of the hand. See the Chapter 5 Appendix for the complete listing of associated signs or contributing factors, differential diagnoses, and treatment for this syndrome, as well as Box 5-2 for tests and treatment used to manage edema and scar.

CASE PRESENTATION
Insufficient Thumb Abduction and/or Opposition Syndrome

Symptoms and History

Patient is a retired 60-year-old overweight female with a medical history of juvenile rheumatoid arthritis (JRA). She was referred to physical therapy 1 month after bilateral thumb CMC arthroplasties with carpal tunnel releases. Her past medical history includes attention deficit hyperactivity disorder (ADHD), multiple surgeries to her cervical (fusion) and lumbar spine, bilateral total knee arthroplasties, and vasculitic neuropathy. The patient had multiple deformities, especially in her hands, and atrophy of the muscles in all extremities, greater on the right side compared to the left.

The patient reported difficulty using her hands for daily activities and complained of clumsiness in her hands. She reported dropping things frequently. She also complained of decreased strength and the inability to use her hands functionally because of decreased thumb motion. She reported requiring assistance from her husband for opening jars and other functional activities. At the time of the initial visit, the patient did not report much pain in her hands.

Alignment Analysis

The patient had significant deformity of thumbs with prominence of the CMC joint and MP joint hyperextension. Both thumb CMC joints were adducted with atrophy of the thenar muscles.

Movement Analysis

The patient had insufficient thumb abduction and opposition for gripping objects such as a large coffee cup. Also noted was decreased thumb CMC abduction and extension resulting in compensatory excessive thumb MP and IP extension (they were in hyperextension) when trying to grasp objects, as well as occasional excessive wrist flexion during grasping activities.

Muscle Length and Strength Analysis

The patient had stiffness and shortness in the thumb CMC adductors and joint structures and excessive laxity of the volar plate at both MP and IP joints of the thumbs. Strength of specific muscles, grip, or pinch were not tested at the initial examination due to the recent thumb surgery. Generalized weakness of bilateral hands was noted when examining the patient performing functional activities.

Diagnosis

Insufficient thumb opposition and/or palmar abduction syndrome, Stage 2 for rehabilitation was assigned because the patient did not have any pain but was more limited in the functional use of her hands as a result of weakness and deformity.

Treatment

A static hand-based splint was fabricated for the patient for both hands to be used at night to attempt to increase thumb CMC abduction and opposition ROM without increasing MP and IP hyperextension. The patient was also instructed to use the splint when using her hands for most functional activities to protect the structures of the CMC joint from injurious stresses.

In the later stages of rehabilitation, attempts were made using resistive putty to strengthen her thumb MP and IP flexors without increasing the deformity. General grip strengthening was also added to her home exercise program.

Correcting postural habits

Patient education was provided that focused on extending the CMC joint and avoiding MP and IP extension during grasping activities throughout the day.

Outcome

The patient was seen for a total of 8 visits over 3 months for ROM, strengthening, and correction of movement impairments during functional activities. She was able to increase the functional use of her hands through gentle ROM and strengthening of hand muscles and mostly with patient education to decrease the stresses on the thumb CMC joints. She reported decreased frequency of dropping objects; however, she was still unable to perform activities, such as opening jars, that require more strength.

THUMB CARPOMETACARPAL ACCESSORY HYPERMOBILITY SYNDROME

Patients with thumb CMC accessory hypermobility syndrome have pain at the CMC joint, but the alignment and movement impairments occur at all joints of the thumb. The CMC joint may be either extended/abducted or adducted/flexed. The impairments at the CMC joint are associated with either (1) MP flexion with IP extension or (2) MP hyperextension with IP flexion and result in loss of the normal longitudinal arch of the thumb. This movement pattern is due to an inability to coordinate the

timing and sequencing of the movements between the IP, MP, and CMC joints of the thumb and adaptive changes in the tissues. Correction of the impairments during the secondary test decreases the symptoms. The adductor pollicis and FPB are frequently overused relative to the APL, APB, opponens pollicis, EPB, and FPL. Patients assigned to this diagnosis must have a modifiable movement pattern. This diagnosis is not intended for patients with neurological injury or later stages of arthritis.

Symptoms and History

Patients with thumb CMC accessory hypermobility syndrome may complain of pain in the area of the CMC joint of thumb that is exacerbated by pinching activities. They may also complain of weakness secondary to the pain that occurs with use of the thumb. Populations in which this is seen include patients who perform activities requiring repetitive pinch or gripping with the thumb adducted such as those who write by hand, hairdressers using scissors, and surgeons. Patients with this syndrome are often young with hypermobile joints or middle aged with early stages of DJD of the CMC of the thumb. DJD of the CMC of the thumb is more common in women than in men.[7,87] Common referring diagnoses include thumb pain, wrist pain, DJD of CMC of the thumb (Eaton's stages I or II[82]), thumb arthritis, and basal joint arthritis or pain. Others have classified and described thumb deformities and the progression through the stages of degeneration.[6,88]

Key Tests and Signs

Alignment Analysis

The impairments in alignment and appearance that have been observed for patients with this syndrome include a CMC joint resting alignment of: extension/abduction or adduction/flexion. The impairments at the CMC joint are associated with either (1) MP flexion with IP extension or (2) MP hyperextension with IP flexion.[6,39-41]

Movement Impairment Analysis

A common movement impairment noted in this syndrome is the inability to maintain the arc of pinch during functional activities that produces symptoms (see Figures 5-32, *B* to *D*; 5-34, *B*; 5-41 to 44; and 5-52). The CMC joint remains in an extended/abducted position with associated MP joint flexion and IP joint hyperextension (see Figure 5-32, *D*) or the CMC joint collapses into adduction/flexion with associated MP flexion with IP extension or MP hyperextension with IP flexion (see Figure 5-32, *B*). Correction of arc of pinch decreases or abolishes the symptoms at the CMC joint.

Two different preferred patterns of movement may be noted during active thumb extension: (1) the CMC joint extending relatively more (amount and timing) than the MP joint (boutonnière = MP flexion with IP extension)[6] (see Figure 5-22, *A* and *B*), or (2) the MP joint extending relatively more than the CMC joint (swan neck = MP hyperextension with IP flexion)[6] (see Figure 5-23). During active thumb flexion, the impaired patterns of movement include the CMC joint flexing more readily than the MP joint (see Figure 5-26), or the CMC remains in a relatively abducted and extended position while the MP joint flexes excessively and the IP joint remains extended or hyperextends (see Figure 5-27). During thumb palmar abduction, the MP joint abducts relatively more than the CMC joint. Correction of these movement impairments during the secondary test decreases or abolishes the symptoms at the CMC joint for the patient with thumb CMC accessory hypermobility syndrome. Correction of the alignment or movement pattern at the CMC joint may not be optimal without simultaneous correction at adjacent joints such as the MP and IP.

Joint Integrity

Range of motion/muscle length. Although active and passive thumb ROM should be assessed, in this syndrome, limitation of ROM is generally not a problem. More commonly, excessive ROM is noted. However, if the ROM is limited, the limitation is slight. Active ROM is usually equal to PROM. During PROM, particular attention is paid to differences in stiffness compared to the opposite side. Thumb active and passive abduction[14] and extension may be slightly limited and painful at CMC joint. The limitation in PROM indicates a relatively stiff or short adductor pollicis and/or FPB. In some cases, MP extension may be stiff or limited and IP extension excessive. In other cases, MP flexion may be stiff or limited and IP flexion excessive.

Joint Accessory Mobility

The CMC joint of the thumb may be hypermobile in a variety of directions but commonly in the dorsoradial direction.[49]

Ligament Integrity

Ligament laxity may be noted at the CMC joint.

Other Special Tests

Swanson's crank and grind test[17,84] (Figure 5-64) involving compression of the CMC joint has been described to help determine if the source of the signs and symptoms is degeneration at the CMC joint of the thumb. Swanson's test will be positive as articular degeneration advances, and pain, crepitus, or instability are present. However, in the early stages of DJD of the CMC joint of the thumb, as seen in thumb CMC accessory hypermobility syndrome, distraction instead of the compression and rotation of the MC on the trapezium may reproduce pain.[82]

Muscle Strength/Performance Impairments

The main impairment in muscle strength and performance in thumb CMC accessory hypermobility syndrome is insufficient muscle performance of the OP,

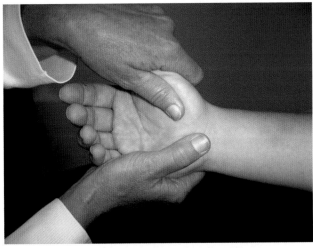

Figure 5-64. Swanson's crank and grind test.

APL, and APB relative to the adductor pollicis and the FPB. The first dorsal interosseous muscle may also help stabilize the base of the first metacarpal at the CMC joint when there is excessive motion of the base of the metacarpal dorsally and radially.[49] Impairments in muscle performance may not be detectable on MMT but identified based on the functional pattern of use. Pinch strength may be decreased and painful.

Source of Signs and Symptoms

The structures of the CMC joint of the thumb are the source of the signs and symptoms for thumb CMC accessory hypermobility syndrome. The cluster of impairments identifying the CMC joint as the source are listed in the following.

CMC Joint

- Preferred pattern of movement of thumb CMC adduction/flexion or CMC extension/abduction reproduces pain.
  - Correction during secondary test by restoring the normal arc of the thumb decreases symptoms.
- The thumb CMC joint may be slightly prominent and swollen.
- The thumb CMC joint accessory motion impairments are variable but will likely be decreased in some direction.[86]
- There may be tenderness to palpation of the CMC joint along the entire joint margin but especially over the radiovolar margin of the CMC joint.[82]
- Crepitus may also be palpable with ROM.[82]
- Pinch strength is decreased and painful.[89]

See the Chapter 5 Appendix for the complete listing of associated signs or contributing factors, differential diagnoses, and treatment for this syndrome.

Treatment

The primary focus of treatment is to educate the patient to maintain the arc of the thumb during active, functional, and resisted isometric thumb movements (see Figures 5-32, *A*; 5-34, *A*; 5-40; and 5-52, *B*). During therapy, the therapist must work with the patient correcting and practicing the movement pattern used during the functional activity that is causing the symptoms. The symptoms should not be reproduced with correct alignment and movement patterns.

In addition, specific exercises are prescribed to increase the performance (motor recruitment and strength) of the muscles required to correct the movement pattern (often the APB, APL, and OP). Others have recommended specific exercises with a focus on thumb abduction because abduction contributes to the stability of the CMC joint.[7,88,89] However, in addition to strengthening of the abductors, we emphasize the precision of movement with the exercise. Working on thumb abduction simultaneously increases the extensibility (stretching) of the antagonistic muscle. The exercises are performed with particular attention to the relative amount and timing of movement between joints. For example, during abduction of the thumb, most of the motion should occur at the CMC joint with the MP and IP joints in a fairly neutral position. Resistive exercises are not performed until the patient is first able to move the thumb actively with the correct pattern of movement. As resistance is added, special care is taken to maintain the correct pattern of movement. The patient is instructed to take frequent breaks to stretch throughout the day to help increase the extensibility of stiff muscles, especially during the functional activity that is contributing to the impairment. The focus is on stretching the muscles that are used the most, usually the adductors and flexors. Stretching helps to relax the muscles in addition to increasing muscle extensibility.

Modification of tools used at work or adaptive equipment is often helpful to facilitate use of the correct alignment and movement pattern[17] (Figure 5-65).

Although not the mainstay of treatment, use of splinting or taping part of the time may be helpful for increasing the extensibility or length of tissues such as the adductor pollicis. See the Chapter 5 Appendix for the specific treatment for this syndrome.

CASE PRESENTATION
Thumb Metacarpophalangeal Flexion with Carpometacarpal Accessory Hypermobility Syndrome

Symptoms and History

A 50-year-old female violin teacher, who is right-hand dominant, presented to her initial physical therapy visit with bilateral thumb pain and a referring diagnosis of hyperflexible joints. She reported the symptoms had been present for the past 10 years. Previous treatment consisted of two types of neoprene splints. One splint had a strap holding the CMC in abduction and the other provided some support to the MP and wrapped around the hand. The patient's goal was to play an orchestral concert and a "gig" on the same day without increasing her symptoms.

The location of symptoms was the MP joint area of bilateral thumbs. Her symptoms were aggravated by playing the piano, prolonged playing of the violin, and lifting. The initial onset of her symptoms followed lifting a container of hand bells. She had to discontinue playing the viola because of her thumb pain. The patient also reported that her thumb pain was aggravated by pulling files, twisting, lifting cases containing hand bells, typing, and playing the piano. The patient reported having obtained an ergonomic keyboard before the initial visit to physical therapy. At the time of the initial examination, she rated the intensity of her resting pain on a verbal numeric scale with 0 being no pain and 10 being severe pain, at 1/10 on the right and 0.5/10 on the left.

Alignment Analysis

Visual appraisal revealed no obvious swelling, scars, or discoloration of either thumb. Bilateral thumb resting alignment was CMC flexion/adduction (right > left), MP flexion, and IP extension (left > right) increased relative to normal. Bilateral ring finger alignment was increased flexion compared to normal. In general, her muscles were not bulky or well defined. There was no obvious atrophy (Figure 5-66).

Movement Analysis

Active ROM into flexion of the right thumb MP/IP was decreased slightly compared to the left (Figure 5-67).

During active thumb extension, the patient's preferred pattern of movement was insufficient thumb MP extension and excessive IP extension. In addition, the CMC joint adducted during thumb extension (Figure 5-68). During functional activities, the thumbs assumed a supinated/adducted position rather than an abducted/pronated position. Modification of the preferred movement pattern by instructing the patient to maintain the arch of

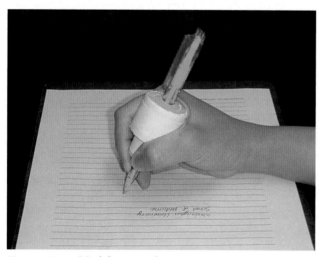

Figure 5-65. Modification of pencil to help maintain arc of thumb during writing.

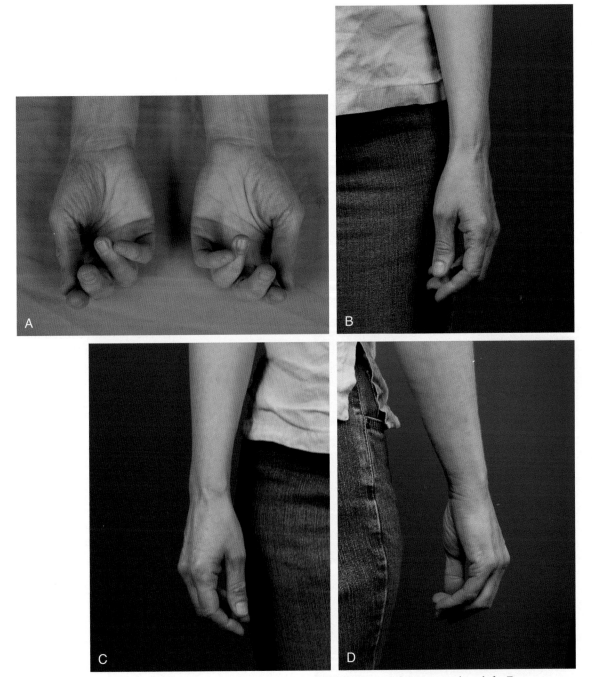

Figure 5-66. Resting alignment. **A,** Increased CMC flexion, right greater than left. **B** to **C,** Thumb MP flexion and IP extension. **D,** Increased flexion of ring finger.

the thumb during functional use decreased her thumb symptoms.

When playing the violin, the patient's preferred pattern of use was the right hand holding the bow with the thumb CMC adducted, the MP joint extended, and IP joint flexed instead of maintaining the arch of the thumb (Figure 5-69, *A* and *C*). Her left hand held the neck of the violin with slight pressure into thumb CMC adduction (Figure 5-69, *D*). In addition, when playing the violin, the left scapula anteriorly tilted and abducted more than the right scapula (Figure 5-69, *E* and *F*).

With ligament integrity testing, there was a firm end-feel but increased laxity of the collateral ligaments of the thumb MP joint with symptoms reproduced with stress to the ulnar collateral ligament.

Muscle Length and Strength Analysis

MMT was performed as described by Kendall et al.[13] Findings were as follows:

- APB 3/5 (tended to substitute with APL)
- EPB 2/5 (tended to adduct during extension)
- First DI 5/5

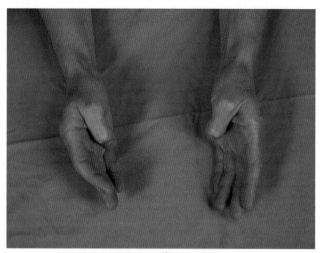

Figure 5-67. Active thumb flexion: Slight decreased range right thumb MP and IP joints compared to left.

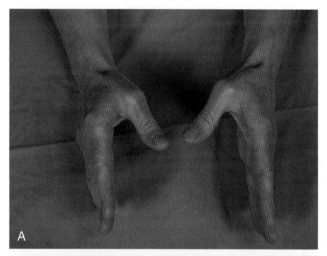

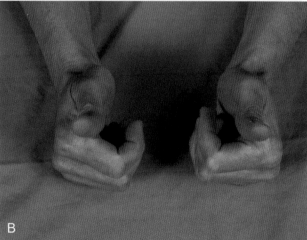

Figure 5-68. Active thumb extension. **A,** Insufficient MP extension and excessive IP extension. **B,** CMC adduction.

The finger flexors and extensors and the thumb MP flexors were relatively stiffer than the patient's other muscles as determined during the length tests. No muscle shortness was found except possibly the finger extensors (ED). As the thumb was passively extended during the length test of the thumb flexors, stiffness was felt throughout the range and wrist RD occurred more readily than thumb extension, indicating possible increased stiffness of the FPB.

Initial Disabilities of the Arm, Shoulder, and Head (DASH) score: 17.24% overall, 18.75% on work, and 0% performing arts for violin.

Diagnosis

The movement system diagnosis was thumb MP flexion with CMC accessory hypermobility syndrome, Stage 2.

Treatment

The primary focus of the treatment was correction of the patient's alignment and movement impairments. The initial treatment included patient education, splinting, and exercises. The patient was educated to maintain the arch of the thumb during functional use (e.g., typing, writing, and playing the violin (Figure 5-69, *B*). She was also educated about correct scapulae alignment while playing the violin (Figure 5-69, *G* and *H*).

Hand-based, custom-made static thumb splints designed to stabilize the thumb MP joints in extension and prevent UD or RD of the MP joints were fabricated (Figure 5-70). The purpose of the splints was to provide added stability to the thumb MP joint during functional use, including playing the violin. Other splint options were discussed with the patient such as silver ring or a more supportive thermoplastic thumb splint immobilizing the CMC and MP joints. The patient was not interested in other splint options. On the patient's last visit, the patient requested neoprene splints, in addition to the thermoplastic splints, because of the possible impact of the thermoplastic splints on her violin while playing. After discussing various splint options, the patient chose the Comfort Cool thumb CMC restriction splint (North Coast Medical, Inc., Morgan Hill, Calif.) (Figure 5-71).

In addition to patient education and splinting, the patient was instructed in home exercises for improving the performance of the EPB, opponens, and APB. During the exercise for the EPB, the patient was instructed to focus on moving at the MP joint instead of the IP joint and to avoid thumb CMC adduction during active thumb extension (avoiding overuse of EPL). When exercising the opponens and the APB, the patient was educated to focus on moving at the CMC joint instead of the MP joint of the thumb during active opposition and abduction. The patient used the lid of a jar as a guide for proper movement into thumb opposition. Once the patient was able to perform the exercise actively with the correct movement pattern, the exercise was progressed by adding rubber band resistance.

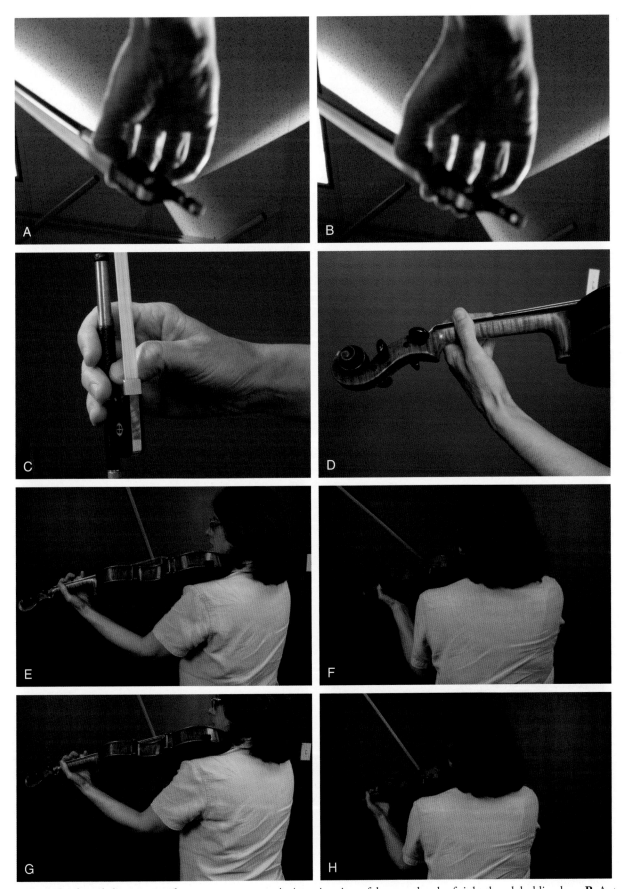

Figure 5-69. Preferred alignment and movement pattern. **A,** Anterior view of decreased arch of right thumb holding bow. **B,** Anterior view of corrected alignment of right thumb holding bow. **C,** Anterolateral view of decreased arch of right thumb holding bow. **D,** Left thumb CMC adduction during holding neck of violin. **E,** Posterolateral view of left scapular anterior tilt and abduction. **F,** Posterior view of left scapular anterior tilt and abduction. **G,** Posterolateral view of corrected scapular alignment. **H,** Posterior view of corrected scapular alignment.

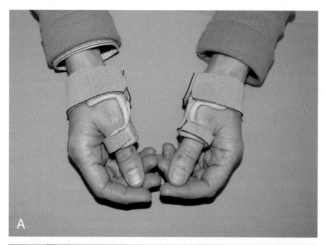

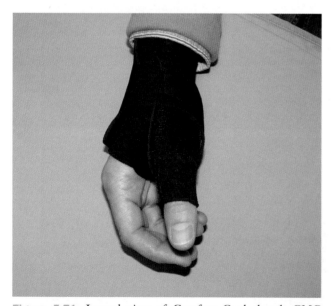

Figure 5-70. Hand-based, custom-made thumb splints designed to stabilize the thumb MP joints in more extension and prevent ulnar or radial deviation of the MP joints. **A,** Lateral view. **B,** Anterior view.

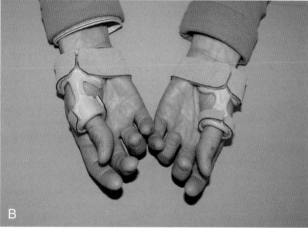

Figure 5-71. Lateral view of Comfort Cool thumb CMC restriction splint.

Outcome

The patient was seen for a total of 4 visits over a 7-week period. At the last visit, the patient reported that she was playing her violin for 45 minutes at a time and wearing the Comfort Cool splints most of the time to control her symptoms. Playing the viola continued to aggravate her symptoms.

Final DASH score: 13.79% overall, 0% work, and performing arts (violin) modules.

Overall, the patient reported being very pleased with her outcomes from physical therapy. She reported an overall 75% improvement in her symptoms when using the splints, which she was doing most of the time. She also reported being pain-free most of the time, as long as she complied with correcting her movement impairments during functional activities such as while playing her instruments. After several months of using the thermoplastic and neoprene splints, the patient decided to be measured for thumb silver ring splints. She has continued performing the exercises prescribed in physical therapy and uses the thumb splints regularly. She reports no longer having thumb pain.

FINGER (OR THUMB) FLEXION SYNDROME

The movement system syndrome finger (or thumb) flexion is a preferred pattern of movement in which the normal alignment of the finger is not maintained during finger flexion. This includes one or more of the following: the longitudinal arch, neutral rotation, or neutral abduction/adduction of the finger (see Figures 5-36 to 5-39, 5-41, 5-42, and 5-46). The movement impairment occurs during the pain-provoking functional or occupational activity involving grip or resisted isometric finger flexion. The movement pattern may be due to an inability to coordinate the timing and sequencing of the movements, an alteration of the relative amount of motion between the IP and MP joints of the finger, or overuse during a repetitive activity. Finger MP or PIP joint pain associated with rotation is due to insufficient performance of one interossei muscle and overuse of the antagonistic interossei muscle at the same joint.[90] The overused muscle is relatively stiffer than its antagonist. This results in the principal impairment of rotation at the painful joint and results from a repetitive activity. Finger AROM and strength are usually normal. Correction of the movement impairments does not always immediately modify symptoms but instead symptoms modify over time. Patients assigned to this diagnosis must have a modifiable movement pattern. This diagnosis is not intended for patients with neurological injury or later stages of arthritis. This syndrome can be associated with a scapular movement syndrome, but the symptoms are not referred from the shoulder or neck structures. Restoration of normal scapular alignment is believed to provide proximal stability, allowing distal segments to work optimally by decreasing excessive stresses on distal tissues.

FINGER (OR THUMB) FLEXION SYNDROME WITH ROTATION

Symptoms and History

Patients with finger (or thumb) flexion syndrome with rotation may have a history of repetitive activity involving use of the finger intrinsic muscles. They may complain of pain at the MP or PIP joints of the finger. This has been observed most commonly in the index and small fingers.

Patients with finger (or thumb) flexion syndrome with rotation may report performance of repetitive activities such as typing on a computer, carrying a bag by the handle with the finger in UD, grasping a golf club, cutting hair (hairdresser), and playing a musical instrument.

Finger MP or PIP joint pain is a common referring diagnosis for patients with finger flexion syndrome with rotation.

Key Tests and Signs

Alignment/Appearance Analysis

The key impairment in alignment/appearance is a relative increase in the amount of rotation (supination or pronation) of the joint compared to the same finger or another uninvolved finger on the uninvolved side (see Figure 5-7).

Movement Impairment Analysis

The key movement impairment is noted during the pain-provoking functional or occupational activities involving grip or resisted isometric finger flexion and the patient does not maintain the finger in neutral rotation and in the normal longitudinal arc. Correction of the rotation and restoration of the normal longitudinal arc of the finger decreases or abolishes the symptoms. Three different impairments may be noted, as follows:

1. A pattern of MP flexion with IP extension (loss of normal longitudinal arc of finger) and UD of the MP joint during finger flexion. This pattern of use indicates that the interossei on one side of finger are being overused relative to the interossei on the opposite side of the same finger and the interossei are being overused relative to the ED (at the MP joint), the FDP, and the FDS (at the IP joints) (see Figures 5-46 and 5-47).
2. Rotation of the finger (most commonly into supination) at the MP joint noted during resisted isometric finger flexion (e.g., string player) (Figure 5-72; see Figure 5-37, *C*).
3. The index finger MP tends to adduct and supinate versus staying in neutral rotation during index finger flexion with abduction (e.g., string player).

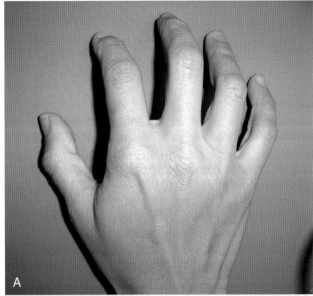

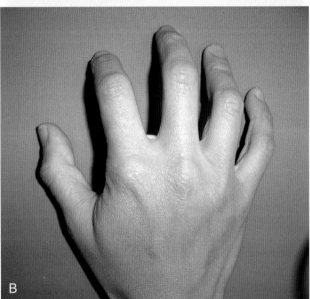

Figure 5-72. Finger flexion syndrome with rotation. **A,** Increased supination of index MP. **B,** Corrected alignment of MP to neutral rotation.

This pattern of use indicates overuse of the first PI relative to the first DI (see Figure 5-37, *B*).

Joint Integrity

Range of motion. Active finger flexion, extension, abduction, and adduction ROM should be assessed to identify any movement impairments. Active and passive finger ROM will usually be normal, but the pattern of movement may be impaired.

Ligament Integrity

Patients with finger (or thumb) flexion syndrome with rotation may have laxity of the collateral ligament on one side of the joint compared to the same finger on the uninvolved side (see Table 5-1).

Muscle Length Tests

The length of the interossei, extrinsic finger flexors, and extensors should be assessed. Table 5-1 lists the specific procedures for these length tests. Findings on the interossei muscle length test include shortness or relative increased stiffness of the interossei on one side of the involved finger and a long or relatively less stiff interossei on the opposite side of the involved finger. Stretch of the overused interossei may produce or aggravate symptoms.

Muscle Strength/Performance Impairments

Resisted tests for soft tissue differential diagnosis should be performed on the contractile structures in the symptomatic area. Contraction of the overused interossei may produce or aggravate symptoms (painful and weak or strong and painful). Pinch strength may be normal, but the movement impairments noted in the section on movement impairments previously may be evident during the test.

MMT of the extrinsic finger flexors, extensors, and interossei should also be performed. Often, no weakness will be detected with MMT. The relative performance between muscle groups is usually the impairment versus weakness detected on MMT. Findings from MMT of the interossei are relative strength or recruitment differences (timing and amount) for the interossei on opposite sides of involved finger. The ED, FDS, and FDP are usually strong but may be recruited relatively less than the interossei (depending on the pattern of impaired movement) as determined by the preferred pattern of movement used during the test.

Palpation. The overused finger muscle may be tender to palpation.

Source of Signs and Symptoms

The source of the symptoms in finger flexion syndrome with rotation is usually the joint structures of the symptomatic joint, but the overused contractile tissues directly affecting the alignment and movement of that joint, such as the interossei, may also be a source of symptoms, as well as a source of the signs.

CASE PRESENTATION
Finger Flexion with Rotation Syndrome, Wrist Flexion Syndrome, and Scapular Depression

History and Symptoms

A 13-year-old female reported left wrist pain that started after increasing practice time on her cello for an audition. She reported that she was right-hand dominant and a serious cellist with auditions to join junior orchestras in the near future. Her symptoms started a few months before her initial physical therapy evaluation. She had seen an occupational therapist for this problem previously, but the progress had plateaued so she was referred to a therapist trained to treat musicians. The patient reported practicing at least 4 hours per day, but she experienced pain during practice, which required taking breaks from playing. The diagnosis provided by an orthopedic surgeon was flexor tendonitis.

The patient reported pain in the area of the left anterior wrist crease only when playing her cello. The production of the pain depended on the position of her wrist and hand when reaching for different notes, and the patient reported that the pain persisted after playing, depending on the number of hours spent practicing.

Alignment Analysis

The patient is a very slender, thin (including her fingers) teenager with little muscle definition. Her preferred sitting alignment when not playing the cello is extreme lumbar and thoracic flexion.

Movement Impairment Analysis

The principal movement impairments noted with her preferred pattern of playing the cello included the following:

- Left wrist in excessive flexion and UD (string arm).
  - Symptoms decreased with modification of her playing alignment so her wrist was in a more neutral alignment.
- Excessive rotation at the finger MP joints (string arm).
- Difficulty maintaining the longitudinal arch of the fingers during application of force to the strings.
- Pain increased with performance of a trill or sustained or prolonged positions during playing.
- Movement was primarily produced distally instead of proximally. For example, she moved her fingers up and down the neck of the cello by abducting/rotating with her fingers and flexing and ulnarly deviating at the wrist without moving the elbow or shoulder.
- Proximal movement impairments of bilateral scapular depression and abduction (right side greater than the left in the degree of movement impairment).
  - Decreased proximal stability of the shoulder girdle to support distal force production.

Muscle Length and Strength Analysis
Muscle strength

Muscle	Result
Interossei	4/5
FDS and FDP	5/5
EDC, ECRL, and ECRB	5/5
FCU and FCR	5/5 (Patient reported resistance to these muscles would have been painful previously.)
Trapezii: Middle and lower	3/5

Diagnosis

- Finger flexion with rotation syndrome
- Wrist flexion syndrome
- Scapular depression

Stage 3 for rehabilitation was assigned because the patient had symptoms only with playing the cello and not with functional activities. Her symptoms increased with increased practice time on the cello.

Treatment

The primary focus of treatment was the redistribution of motion during function (playing the cello) by minimizing the amount of wrist flexion, UD, and finger abduction by increasing the movement of the hand up or down the neck of the cello and moving more at the elbow and shoulder. To achieve this correction, a cue was given to decrease wrist flexion by abducting the glenohumeral joint, which resulted in an immediate decrease in pain. In addition, the therapist worked with the patient to maintain the longitudinal arch of the finger and neutral rotation while maintaining correct scapular alignment. Strategies for treatment included correcting proximal impairments to facilitate better distal function and correcting distal impairments. Correcting the proximal impairments included patient education regarding avoiding scapular depression and abduction during playing the cello and exercises for the trapezius.

Exercises to improve the performance of the trapezius were as follows:

- Standing shoulder flexion facing the wall with cues to increase scapular elevation using the upper trapezius.
- Prone scapular adduction and elevation (middle and upper trapezius), progressing from resting the hands on the head to lifting the arms off the surface with the elbows flexed.

Exercises to correct distal impairments were as follows:

- Putty exercises used for facilitating proper recruitment of muscles rather than for strengthening: Simulating application of force to the strings by focusing on using the long finger flexors (FDS and FDP) to help maintain the longitudinal arch of the fingers. Simulating application of force to the strings, avoiding excessive rotation of the MP joints of the fingers.
- Rubber band exercises for strengthening the interossei: Focus on finger MP joint abduction/adduction.

Correcting postural habits

Patient education to correct sitting alignment while at school and while doing homework was as follows:

- Sitting with good back support and close to work surface.
- Sitting with scapulae in neutral alignment was achieved by focusing on adducting and elevating the scapulae slightly.

Outcome

The patient was seen for total of 4 visits over 3 months, and at the final visit, she reported that she was able to play her cello for any length of time without any symptoms.

FINGER (OR THUMB) FLEXION SYNDROME WITHOUT ROTATION

Symptoms and History

Patients with finger flexion syndrome without rotation may report symptoms that are poorly localized in the hand, wrist, or forearm. Patients also may report symptoms while performing repetitive activities such as playing string instruments or the piano, writing, or any kind of grip or pinch activity.

Key Tests and Signs

Alignment Analysis

The patient with finger flexion syndrome without rotation may have impairments with use of the finger, but the resting finger alignment is often normal. However, associated impairments in scapular alignment may be noted such as scapular depression, abduction, anterior tilt, internal rotation, or downward rotation.

Movement Impairment

The key movement impairment is noted during the pain-provoking functional or occupational activity involving grip or resisted isometric finger flexion, and the patient does not maintain the normal longitudinal arc of finger, transverse arch of hand, and scapular alignment. Correction by restoration of the normal longitudinal arc of the finger and scapular alignment decreases symptoms over time. Movement impairments of the scapula include depression, abduction, internal rotation, downward rotation, or tilt. Restoration of normal scapular alignment is believed to provide proximal stability, allowing the distal segments to work optimally by decreasing excessive stresses on distal tissues.[42]

In addition to the scapular impairments, the following three different finger movement impairments may be noted:

1. Flexion of the finger MP joints with the IP joints in relative extension. This pattern of use indicate overuse of the interossei relative to the FDS, FDP, and ED (see Figure 5-50, *A* and *B*).
2. Flexion of the MP joints with PIP joint hyperextension and DIP joint flexion (swan neck).[30-33] A prerequisite for this pattern of movement to occur is laxity of the volar plate at the PIP joint. This pattern of movement also indicates overuse of the interossei relative to the FDS, FDP, and ED (see Figure 5-36).
3. Flexion of the PIP joint with DIP joint hyperextension (boutonnière).[27-29] This pattern of use is indicative of overuse of the FDS relative to the FDP and laxity of the volar plate of the DIP joint (see Figure 5-38).

Joint Integrity

Range of motion. Active finger flexion, extension, abduction, and adduction ROM should be assessed to identify any movement impairments. Active and passive finger ROM will usually be normal, but the pattern of movement may be impaired.

Ligament Integrity

Patients with finger flexion syndrome without rotation that have a boutonnière type pattern of movement may have shortness of the ORL or laxity of the PIP or DIP volar plates, so the length of these structures should be assessed (see Table 5-1).

Muscle Length Tests

The length of the interossei, extrinsic finger flexors, and extensors should be assessed. Table 5-1 has the specific procedures for these length tests. Muscle length may be normal, but the muscle may be relatively stiffer than on the unaffected side.

Muscle Strength/Performance Impairments

Pinch strength should be assessed and may be normal, but the impairments noted in the section on movement impairments may be evident during the test. MMT of the extrinsic finger flexors, extensors, and interossei should be performed. However, often no weakness is detected. The relative recruitment (timing and amount) between muscle groups is usually the impairment rather than weakness detected on a MMT.

Source of Signs and Symptoms

The source of the symptoms is usually the joint and soft tissue structures of the symptomatic region. However, it is often difficult to reproduce the symptoms with any test during the examination. The impaired pattern of movement is believed to contribute to increased stresses on the tissues in the symptomatic area and correction of the pattern of movement decreases these stresses, thereby reducing the symptoms over time. See the Chapter 5 Appendix for the complete listing of associated signs or contributing factors, differential diagnoses, and treatment for this syndrome.

Treatment

The primary focus of treatment is to educate the patient to maintain the arc and neutral rotation of the fingers during functional activities and active and resisted isometric finger movements. The therapist must work with the patient during the therapy visits on correcting and practicing the movement pattern during the functional activity that is causing the problem. The symptoms should not be reproduced with correct alignment and movement patterns.

In addition, specific exercises are prescribed to increase the performance (motor recruitment and strength) of the muscles required to correct the movement pattern. Thus the extensibility of the antagonistic muscle is simultaneously increased (stretched). The exercises are performed with particular attention paid to the relative amount and timing of movement between joints. Resistive exercises are not performed until the patient is first able to move the fingers actively with the correct pattern of movement. As resistance is added, special care is taken to maintain the correct pattern of movement. The patient is instructed to take frequent breaks to stretch throughout the day to help increase the extensibility of stiff muscles, especially during the functional activity that is contributing to the impairment. The focus on stretching is on the muscles that are used the most. Besides increasing extensibility, stretching helps with relaxation of the muscle.

Modification of tools used at work, musical instruments, or adaptive equipment is often helpful to facilitate use of the correct alignment and movement pattern.

Although not the mainstay of treatment, use of splinting or taping part of the time may be helpful for increasing extensibility or length of tissues and facilitating recruitment of underused tissues. See the Chapter 5 Appendix for specific treatment for this syndrome.

CASE PRESENTATION
Finger Flexion without Rotation Syndrome with a Secondary Diagnosis of Scapular Depression and Shoulder Medial Rotation

History and Symptoms

The patient is a 17-year-old female high school student who plays the bassoon (primarily), violin, and trombone, and loves drawing, writing, and typing. She plays in the youth symphony, and also reports working occasionally on ceramics. She has no history of other medical or musculoskeletal problems. At the time of the initial physical therapy examination, the patient was on summer break so she had not practiced or typed as much as during the school year. Initial movement system examination occurred 6 months after onset of symptoms.

The patient reported generalized bilateral dorsal and volar wrist and hand pain (right more than left). She also reported occasional pain in her right elbow antecubital crease area and upper back pain. She reported her pain was aggravated with playing the bassoon and typing for school but did subside within a few minutes after cessation of those activities. The quality of the pain was described as aching. She reported no problems with sleeping and stated she awakened without any symptoms.

Alignment Analysis
Standing

- Swayback: Increased thoracic kyphosis, lumbar flexion and trunk swayed posteriorly relative to pelvis
- Cervical: Forward head with prominence of paraspinals (right > left)

- Downwardly rotated, abducted, and depressed scapulae
- Medially rotated humeri
- Forearm pronation
- Flat thoracic spine with slight left rotation

Movement Analysis

Standing
Cervical ROM was normal without symptom reproduction. Shoulder ROM was also normal but movement impairments of insufficient scapular elevation, downward rotation, and slight scapular abduction bilaterally were noted. Arm elevation did not reproduce the patient's symptoms at the time of the initial physical therapy examination.

Quadruped
Rocking back had noted movement impairments of cervical extension with insufficient elevation of scapulae. While playing the bassoon, the preferred pattern of playing was with the wrist flexed and the ring and small fingers in the intrinsic plus position (MP flexion with IPs extended). When instructions were provided to correct the movement impairments, the patient's fingers assumed the "boutonnière" position (PIP flexion with DIP hyperextension). The scapulae were depressed while playing.

Muscle Length and Strength Analysis

Supine
- Length tests:
  - Latissimus was stiff and slightly short on the right; normal on the left.
  - Pectoralis major was stiff bilaterally but not short.
  - Teres major was short and stiff bilaterally.
  - Pectoris minor was bilaterally stiff.
  - Shoulder AROM: Medial and lateral rotation ranges were normal.

Prone

Shoulder	Right	Left
Lateral rotation	3/5	3+/5
Medial rotation	3/5	3+/5
Middle and lower trapezii	3/5	3+/5

Movement impairments noted during the MMT of the trapezii included humeral medial rotation, scapular depression, and anterior tilt.

Wrist and hand
MMT of the wrist and hand did not reproduce the patient's symptoms. The right hand was generally weaker than left by one muscle grade. The long finger flexors (FDP and FDS) of the right index and middle fingers were stronger than the long finger flexors of the ring and small fingers.

Diagnosis
Scapular depression, shoulder medial rotation, wrist flexion, finger flexion without rotation syndrome.

Treatment
Exercises were provided to correct the movement impairments noted during the movement system examination. The patient was instructed to do the following:
- Elevate and slightly adduct the scapulae.
- Maintain neutral or lateral rotation of the shoulder during the following home exercises:
  - Shoulder flexion facing the wall
  - Prone exercise for the trapezii
  - Shoulder abduction with lateral rotation performed standing with the back against the wall (reverse T).
- Wrist and hand: The patient was instructed in general strengthening of the long finger flexors using resistive putty and rubber bands, with particular attention paid to maintaining the arc of motion of each finger, especially the ring and small fingers on right side.
- Correcting postural habits: During playing of bassoon the patient was instructed to use mirrors to provide feedback when correcting the alignment of her scapula, wrist, and fingers.

Outcome
The patient was seen in physical therapy for a total of 3 visits. She reported decreased symptoms in her wrist and hand, and she was able to practice close to 2 hours without any symptoms.

SOURCE OR REGIONAL IMPAIRMENT OF THE HAND

Patients in the regional impairment of the hand category usually have a history of acute trauma or injury to the hand or the patient is in the early postoperative phase. When known, the pathoanatomical or source diagnosis assigned by the physician, followed by the name of the operative procedure provided on the referral, is used as the diagnosis that will guide the physical therapy treatment. For example, flexor tendon laceration, flexor tendon repair, Stage 1. If the referral does not state the pathoanatomical or source diagnosis or the procedure that was performed by the physician, the regional diagnosis, hand impairment, will be used.

The focus of treatment is protecting the injured tissues. Usually, there is a history of acute trauma or injury to the hand or it is early in the postoperative phase. Medical precautions have often been issued. Because of the acuity of the condition, the patient's typical movement pattern cannot be assessed at this time. The prognosis of tissue healing and normal movement is expected. The determination of the use of component versus compensatory treatment methods depends on the expectations of the final outcome. Initially, while precautions are required, compensatory methods may be necessary. The guidelines provided in the Chapter 5 Appendix are intended to be general, therefore the consulting physician's protocols for specific precautions and progressions are necessary. Appropriate application of the protocols, however, requires that the therapist be familiar with the tissues that are affected by the surgical procedure, the specific surgical approach, and the variables that need to be considered while applying stresses to the healing tissues. This knowledge, as well as communication with the physician, allows the therapist to make appropriate adjustments in the protocol as needed.

See the source or regional impairment of the hand diagnosis in the Chapter 5 Appendix and Box 5-3 for more specific information regarding common referring diagnoses, examination, and general treatment guidelines for this diagnosis. Underlying movement system syndromes that should be considered are insufficient finger or thumb flexion, insufficient finger or thumb extension, insufficient thumb abduction and/or opposition, thumb CMC accessory hypermobility, or finger (or thumb) flexion syndrome with or without rotation.

MOVEMENT SYSTEM DIAGNOSES FOR THE WRIST

To date, movement system diagnoses for the wrist have not been described in the detail presented here for the hand. However, suggested names for wrist diagnoses would follow the principles for naming the diagnoses in other regions. Suggested names are wrist flexion, wrist extension, a combination of wrist flexion or extension with RD or UD, wrist hypomobility, and wrist accessory hypermobility. For example, a patient with CTS who has symptoms that are provoked by repeated activity performed with the wrist in flexion might be assigned the diagnosis of wrist flexion syndrome.

CONCLUSION

Effective physical therapy treatment of hand dysfunction requires managing the acute tissue injury as well as the underlying movement impairments. In this chapter, we have described movement system diagnoses for hand dysfunctions in detail, and we have proposed the names for some movement system diagnoses for the wrist. These diagnoses need further testing in the clinic and by well-designed studies.

BOX 5-3

General Treatment Guidelines

PATIENT EDUCATION
- Educate the patient regarding precautions and maintaining the precautions during hygiene, the tissues involved, and the differences between *AROM, AAROM,* and *PROM.*
- Specific instructions for splint use, care, precautions, wearing schedule, and donning and doffing the splint should be provided to the patient.

PAIN
- Some pain is expected after surgery. Pain is an indicator of the status of tissue healing and should be used as a guide in clinical decision making regarding tissue tolerance to loads. The pain should not be severe nor last more than 1 hour after exercise.
- Increasing pain, pain that is not decreasing over the course of treatment, or burning pain may indicate that treatment is too aggressive or there is a disruption in the usual course of healing.
- After tenolysis, the patient must be encouraged to work through pain, thus the coordination of analgesics with therapy is critical.

EDEMA
- Early management is the key to good outcome.
- Increasing edema or edema that is not decreasing over the course of treatment may indicate that treatment is too aggressive, exercises are being performed too frequently, or there is a disruption in the usual course of healing.

SCAR
- Early management contributes to good outcome.
- Factors that contribute to increased scar include overly aggressive exercise, prolonged edema, and infection.
- Individuals vary in the amount of scar that is laid down during healing. Treatment must be adjusted appropriately based on these individual differences. After a tendon repair, an individual that heals with less scar will be progressed more slowly compared with the individual that heals with a lot of scar.

RANGE OF MOTION
- Early motion is the key to successful outcomes and avoiding a stiff hand.
- The length of time the hand is immobilized and the number of joints immobilized should be minimized. Whenever possible, the hand should be immobilized in the closed-packed position to maintain the length of the ligaments: flexion of the finger MP joints, extension of the finger IP joints, and abduction of the thumb.
- Maintaining the ROM of all uninvolved joints of the upper extremities is important.
- Indicators for progression of exercise include decreasing pain and edema and improved ROM. The usual expectation is that AROM should increase by a minimum of 10 degrees per week, except when the cause of the limitation is due to profound weakness or rupture.
- Since the body takes the path of least resistance, braced or blocking exercises are used to prevent the joint that is

BOX 5-3

General Treatment Guidelines—cont'd

relatively most flexible from moving and encouraging the stiffer segment to move.

STRENGTH

- Indicators for progression of exercise from active to resistive include the ability to perform AROM with the ideal movement pattern and resistive exercise without a significant increase in pain relative to the intensity of pain produced during AROM.
- Progression of exercise is guided by normal timeframes for tissue healing, moderating factors such as age and medications, and precautions prescribed by the surgeon.
- Use of light resistance can be helpful to increase muscle recruitment before the tissue will tolerate enough resistance for true overload.
- Vital signs should be monitored when initiating an upper extremity resistive exercise program using equipment like the Baltimore Therapeutic Equipment (BTE) work simulator.

FUNCTION

Using the hand in functional activities throughout the course of treatment is critical. The ideal pattern of movement should be encouraged as the patient is able. Examples of functional activities include writing, driving, work, eating, sleeping, and hygiene.

TISSUE FACTORS

Bone

- Early motion is the key to good outcome.
- Indicators for progression to PROM and static progressive or dynamic splinting are determined by the status of fracture healing, often determined by radiographic tests.
- Indicators for progression to strengthening exercises are ROM is acceptable and the fracture is healed (generally about 6 to 8 weeks).
- Crepitus, persistent pain at the site of the fracture, or point tenderness over the fracture site are signs that the fracture is not healed.

Ligament

- Prevention of ligament shortness is the key.
- Whenever possible, the hand should be immobilized in the closed-packed position to maintain the length of the ligaments: flexion of the finger MP joints, extension of the finger IP joints, and abduction of the thumb.
- If the hand has been immobilized in the close-packed position, intrinsic muscle stretching exercises may be indicated.

NERVE

- Early motion is imperative while avoiding excessive tension on the repair site.

- The return of sensibility and motor function is tested periodically to document progress.

Cartilage

- Grinding or crepitus may be sign of joint cartilage loss or damage.

Skin

- Edema contributes to decreased ROM and pain.
- Dressings for wounds should be minimized to maximize ROM.
- Skin maceration from straps, splints, or wound dressings should be avoided.

Muscle

- The position of immobilization may result in muscle shortness.
- The function after muscle repair is generally restored more easily than the function after laceration and repair of a tendon.

Tendon

- The key to good outcome is preserving tendon gliding.
- The zone of the tendon that was injured, type and extent of injury, the type and number of sutures, and the condition of tendon at time of repair determines the amount of tension that can be placed on the repaired tendon during treatment.
- During the healing phase, the goal is to maintain ROM of the joints and the tendon gliding without placing excessive stresses on the repaired tendon.
- Judgments regarding the progression of the treatment protocol depend on the general timeframes for tendon healing but may need to be modified, depending on the individual patient's pattern of scarring.
- The patient who has poor tendon gliding and appears to have a lot of scarring may need to be progressed faster than the patient who has excellent tendon gliding and little scarring.

GUIDELINES FOR TREATMENT OF HYPERSENSITIVITY

Desensitization

- The purpose of desensitization is to decrease pain or hypersensitivity by gradually bombarding the sensory nervous system with a variety of stimuli, resulting in a rise in pain threshold.
- Desensitization is indicated for painful or hypersensitive areas secondary to nerve injury or scar or for areas that have been overprotected.
- Procedures for desensitization consist of bombarding the affected area with stimuli, including: massage, tapping, vibration, graded textures, functional use, and eventual progression to weight-bearing activities
- Desensitization should be done at least 6 times/day, 30 seconds each item.

AAROM, Active assistive range of motion; *AROM,* active range of motion; *IP,* interphalangeal; *MP,* metacarpophalangeal; *PROM,* passive range of motion.

REFERENCES

1. Cannon NM, Beal BG, Walters KJ, et al: *Diagnosis and treatment manual for physicians and therapists: upper extremity rehabilitation*, ed 4, Indianapolis, 2001, The Hand Rehabilitation Center of Indiana.

2. Sahrmann SA: *Diagnosis and treatment of movement impairment syndromes*, St Louis, 2002, Mosby.

3. Scheets PK, Sahrmann SA, Norton BJ: Diagnosis for physical therapy for patients with neuromuscular conditions, *Neurol Rep* 23(4):158-169, 1999.

4. Tubiana R, Chamagne P, Brockman R: Functional anatomy of the hand/movements of the fingers/fundamental positions for instrumental musicians [anniversary article], *Sci Medicine* 20(4):183-194, 2005.

5. Novak CB, Mackinnon SE: Evaluation of nerve injury and nerve compression in the upper quadrant, *J Hand Ther* 18(2):230-240, 2005.

6. Nalebuff EA: Diagnosis, classification and management of rheumatoid thumb deformities, *Bull Hosp Joint Dis* 29(2):119-137, 1968.

7. Neumann DA, Bielefeld T: The carpometacarpal joint of the thumb: stability, deformity, and therapeutic intervention, *J Orthop Sports Phys Ther* 33(7):386-399, 2003.

8. Mueller MJ, Maluf KS: Tissue adaptation to physical stress: a proposed "Physical Stress Theory" to guide physical therapist practice, education, and research, *Phys Ther* 82(4):383-403, 2002.

9. Pratt N: Anatomy of nerve entrapment sites in the upper quarter, *J Hand Ther* 18(2):216-229, 2005.

10. Forman TA, Forman SK, Rose NE: A clinical approach to diagnosing wrist pain, *Am Fam Physician* 72(9):1753-1758, 2005.

11. Dutton M: *Orthopaedic examination, evaluation, and intervention*, New York, 2004, McGraw-Hill.

12. Magee DJ: *Orthopedic physical assessment*, ed 3, Philadelphia, 1997, Saunders.

13. Kendall FP, McCreary EK, Provance PG, et al: *Muscles: testing and function with posture and pain*, 5 ed, Baltimore, 2005, Lippincott Williams & Wilkins.

14. Cyriax J: *Textbook of orthopaedic medicine*, ed 7, London, 1978, Bailliere Tindall.

15. Finkelstein H: Stenosing tendovaginitis at the radial styloid process, *J Bone Joint Surg Am* 12(3):509-540, 1930.

16. Ahuja NK, Chung KC: Fritz de Quervain, MD (1868-1940): stenosing tendovaginitis at the radial styloid process, *J Hand Surg Am* 29(6):1164-1170, 2004.

17. Melvin JL: Therapists' management of osteoarthritis in the hand. In Mackin EJ, Callahan AD, Osterman AL, et al, eds: *Rehabilitation of the hand and upper extremity*, ed 5, St Louis, 2002, Mosby.

18. Phalen GS: The carpal-tunnel syndrome. Seventeen years' experience in diagnosis and treatment of six hundred fifty-four hands, *J Bone Joint Surg Am* 48(2):211-228, 1966.

19. Aulicino PL: Clinical examination of the hand. In Mackin EJ, Callahan AD, Osterman AL, et al, eds: *Rehabilitation of the hand and upper extremity*, ed 5, St Louis, 2002, Mosby.

20. Tubiana R, Thomine J, Mackin E: *Examination of the hand and wrist*, ed 2, London, 1996, Informa Healthcare.

21. Hakstian RW, Tubiana R: Ulnar deviation of the fingers: the role of joint structure and function, *J Bone Joint Surg Am* 49(2):299-316, 1967.

22. Pahle JA, Raunio P: The influence of wrist position on finger deviation in the rheumatoid hand. A clinical and radiological study, *J Bone Joint Surg Br* 51(4):664-676, 1969.

23. Katolik LI, Trumble T: Distal radioulnar joint dysfunction, *J Am Soc Surg Hand* 5(1):8-29, 2005.

24. Bunnell S: The early treatment of hand injuries, *J Bone Joint Surg Am* 33(3):807-811, 1951.

25. Bunnell S: Ischaemic contracture, local, in the hand, *J Bone Joint Surg Am* 35(1):88-101, 1953.

26. Steindler A: Arthritic deformities of the wrist and fingers, *J Bone Joint Surg Am* 133-A(4):849-862, 1951.

27. Littler JW, Eaton RG: Redistribution of forces in the correction of boutonniere deformity, *J Bone Joint Surg Am* 49(7):1267-1274, 1967.

28. Matev I: The boutonnière deformity, *Hand* 11(2):90-95, 1969.

29. Stanley J: Boutonniere deformity, *J Bone Joint Surg Br* 86(Supp 3):216-221a, 2004.

30. Welsh RP, Hastings DE: Swan neck deformity in rheumatoid arthritis of the hand, *Hand* 9(2):109-116, 1977.

31. Dell PC, Sforzo CR: Ulnar intrinsic anatomy and dysfunction, *J Hand Ther* 18(2):198-207, 2005.

32. Nalebuff EA: The rheumatoid swan-neck deformity *Hand Clin* 5(2):203-214, 1989.

33. Knight SL: Assessment and management of swan neck deformity, *Int Congr Ser* 1295:154-157. 2006.

34. Campbell PJ, Wilson RL: Management of joint injuries and intraarticular fractures. In Mackin EJ, Callahan AD, Osterman AL, et al, eds: *Rehabilitation of the hand and upper extremity*, ed 5, St Louis, 2002, Mosby.

35. Swanson AB, de Groot SG: Osteoarthritis in the hand, *Clin Rheum Dis* 11(2):393-420, 1985.

36. Smith EM, Juvinall RC, Bender LF, et al: Role of the finger flexors in rheumatoid deformities of the metacarpophalangeal joints, *Arthritis Rheum* 7:467-480, 1964.

37. Smith RJ, Kaplan EB: Rheumatoid deformities at the metacarpophalangeal joints of the fingers, *J Bone Joint Surg Am* 49(1):31-47, 1967.

38. Ellison MR, Flatt AE, Kelly KJ: Ulnar drift of the fingers in rheumatoid disease. Treatment by crossed intrinsic tendon transfer, *J Bone Joint Surg Am* 53(6):1061-1082, 1971.

39. Moulton MJ, Parentis MA, Kelly MJ, et al: Influence of metacarpophalangeal joint position on basal joint-loading in the thumb, *J Bone Joint Surg Am* 83(5):709-716, 2001.

40. Terrono AL: The rheumatoid thumb, *J Am Soc Surg Hand* 1(2):81-92, 2001.

41. Tomaino MM: Classification and treatment of the rheumatoid thumb, *Int Congr Ser* 1295:162-168, 2006.

42. Pascarelli EF, Hsu YP: Understanding work-related upper extremity disorders: clinical findings in 485 computer users, musicians, and others, *J Occup Rehabil* 11(1):1-21, 2001.

43. Neumann DA: *Kinesiology of the musculoskeletal system: foundations for physical rehabilitation*, St Louis, 2002, Mosby.

44. Kisner C, Colby LA: *Therapeutic exercises: foundations and techniques*, ed 5, Philadelphia, 2007, FA Davis.

45. Taleisnik J: *The wrist*, New York, 1985, Churchill Livingstone.

46. LaStayo PC, Lee MJ: The forearm complex: anatomy, biomechanics and clinical considerations, *J Hand Ther* 19(2):137-144, 2006.

47. LaStayo PC: Ulnar wrist pain and impairment: a therapist's algorithmic approach to the triangular fibrocartilage complex. In Mackin EJ, Callahan AD, Osterman AL, et al, eds: *Rehabilitation of the hand and upper extremity*, ed 5, St Louis, 2002, Mosby.

48. Levangie PK, Norkin CC: *Joint structure & function: a comprehensive analysis*, ed 3, Philadelphia, 2001, FA Davis.

49. Brand PW, Hollister AM: *Clinical mechanics of the hand*, ed 3, St Louis, 1999, Mosby.

50. Degeorges R, Parasie J, Mitton D, et al: Three-dimensional rotations of human three-joint fingers: an optoelectronic measurement. Preliminary results, *Surg Radiol Anat* 27(1):43-50, 2005.

51. Williams PL, Barnester LH, Berry MM, et al: *Gray's Anatomy*, ed 38, New York, 1995, Churchill Livingstone.

52. Cambridge-Keeling CA: Range-of-motion measurement of the hand. In Mackin EJ, Callahan AD, Osterman AL, et al, eds: *Rehabilitation of the hand and upper extremity*, ed 5, St Louis, 2002, Mosby.

53. Hollister A, Giurintano DJ: Thumb movements, motions, and moments, *J Hand Ther* 8(2):106-114, 1995.

54. Li ZM, Tang J: Coordination of thumb joints during opposition, *J Biomech* 40(3):502-510, 2007.

55. Su FC, Chou YL, Yang CS, et al: Movement of finger joints induced by synergistic wrist motion, *Clin Biomech* 20(5):491-497, 2005.

56. Brandfonbrener AG: Musculoskeletal problems of instrumental musicians, *Hand Clinics* 19(2):231-239, 2003.

57. Hochberg FH: Upper extremity difficulties of musicians. In Mackin EJ, Callahan AD, Osterman AL, et al, eds: *Rehabilitation of the hand and upper extremity*, ed 4, St Louis, 1995, Mosby.

58. Baker NA, Cham R, Cidboy EH, et al: Kinematics of the fingers and hands during computer keyboard use, *Clin Biomech* 22(1):34-43, 2007.

59. Netter FH: *Atlas of human anatomy*, ed 4, Philadelphia, 2006, Saunders.

60. Hazelton FT, Smidt GL, Flatt AE, et al: The influence of wrist position on the force produced by the finger flexors, *J Biomech* 8(5):301-306, 1975.

61. An KN, Hui FC, Morrey BF, et al: Muscles across the elbow joint: a biomechanical analysis. *J Biomech* 14(10):659-669, 1981.

62. Cannon NM: Lecture at Indiana Hand Care Course, 2004.

63. Basmagian JV, DeLuca CJ: *Muscles alive: their functions revealed by electromyography*, ed 5, Baltimore, 1985, Williams and Wilkins.

64. Maas M, Dijkstra PF, Bos KE, et al: *Kinematics of the painful wrist: a videofluoroscopic approach*, Amsterdam, 1996, Academie Medical Centre, Department of Radiology and Plastic Reconstructive and Hand Surgery.

65. Smith LK, Weiss EL, Lehmkuhl LD: *Brunnstrom's clinical kinesiology*, ed 5, Philadelphia, 1996, FA Davis.

66. Rosenthal EA: The extensor tendons: anatomy and management. In Mackin EJ, Callahan AD, Osterman AL, et al, eds: *Rehabilitation of the hand and upper extremity*, ed 5, St Louis, 2002, Mosby.

67. Chase RA, White WL, Kravitt S, et al: *Functional anatomy of the hand video*, 1978, Yale University School of Medicine and University of Pittsburg School of Medicine.

68. Culp RW, Taras JS: Primary care of flexor tendon injuries. In Mackin EJ, Callahan AD, Osterman AL, et al, eds: *Rehabilitation of the hand and upper extremity*, ed 5, St Louis, 2002, Mosby.

69. Stewart Pettengill KM, van Strien G: Postoperative management of flexor tendon injuries. In Mackin EJ, Callahan AD, Osterman AL, et al, eds: *Rehabilitation of the hand and upper extremity*, ed 5, St Louis, 2002, Mosby.

70. Skie M, Zeiss J, Ebraheim NA, Jackson WT: Carpal tunnel changes and median nerve compression during wrist flexion and extension seen by magnetic resonance imaging, *J Hand Surg* 15(6):934-939, 1990.

71. Lee MJ, LaStayo PC: Pronator syndrome and other nerve compressions that mimic carpal tunnel syndrome, *J Orthop Sports Phys Ther* 34(10):601-609, 2004.

72. American Society for Surgery of the Hand: *The hand: examination and diagnosis*, ed 3, Aurora, CO, 1978, The Society.

73. Eyler DL, Markee JE: The anatomy and function of the intrinsic musculature of the fingers, *J Bone Joint Surg Am* 36(1):1-9, 1954.

74. Skirven TM, Callahan AD: Therapist's management of peripheral-nerve injuries. In Mackin EJ, Callahan AD, Osterman AL, et al, eds: *Rehabilitation of the hand and upper extremity*, ed 5, St Louis, 2002, Mosby.

75. Cooney WP III, Lucca MJ, Chao EY, et al: The kinesiology of the thumb trapeziometacarpal joint, *J Bone Joint Surg Am* 63(9):1371-1381, 1981.

76. Piligian G, Herbert R, Hearns M, et al: Evaluation and management of chronic work-related musculoskeletal disorders of the distal upper extremity, *Am J Ind Med* 37(1):75-93, 2000.

77. Skirven TM, Osterman AL: Clinical examination of the wrist. In Mackin EJ, Callahan AD, Osterman AL, et al, eds: *Rehabilitation of the hand and upper extremity*, ed 5, St Louis, 2002, Mosby.

78. Andreisek G, Crook DW, Burg D, et al: Peripheral neuropathies of the median, radial, and ulnar nerves: MR imaging features, *Radiographics* 26(5):1267-1287, 2006.

79. Innis PC: Surgical management of the stiff hand. In Mackin EJ, Callahan AD, Osterman AL, et al, eds: *Rehabilitation of the hand and upper extremity*, ed 5, St Louis, 2002, Mosby.

80. Alter S, Feldon P, Terrono AL: Pathomechanics of deformities in the arthritic hand and wrist. In Mackin EJ, Callahan AD, Osterman AL, et al, eds: *Rehabilitation of the hand and upper extremity*, ed 5, St Louis, 2002, Mosby.

81. Colditz JC: Anatomic considerations for splinting the thumb. In Mackin EJ, Callahan AD, Osterman AL, et al, eds: *Rehabilitation of the hand and upper extremity*, ed 5, St Louis, 2002, Mosby.

82. Eaton RG, Glickel SZ: Trapeziometacarpal osteoarthritis. Staging as a rationale for treatment, *Hand Clin* 3(4):455-471, 1987.

83. Wajon A, Ada L, Edmunds I: Surgery for thumb (trapeziometacarpal joint) osteoarthritis. *Cochrane Database Syst Rev* (4):CD004631, 2005.

84. Swanson AB: Disabling arthritis at the base of the thumb: treatment by resection of the trapezium and flexible (silicone) implant arthroplasty, *J Bone Joint Surg Am* 54(3):456-471. 1972.

85. Tomaino MM, Pellegrini VD, Jr, Burton RI: Arthroplasty of the basal joint of the thumb. Long-term follow-up after

ligament reconstruction with tendon interposition, *J Bone Joint Surg Am* 77(3):346-355, 1995.

86. Kovler M, Lundon K, McKee N, et al: The human first carpometacarpal joint: osteoarthritic degeneration and 3-dimensional modeling, *J Hand Ther* 17(4):393-400, 2004.

87. Pellegrini VD Jr: Pathomechanics of the thumb trapezio-metacarpal joint, *Hand Clin* 17(2):175-viii, 2001.

88. Pellegrini VD Jr: Osteoarthritis at the base of the thumb, *Orthop Clin North Am* 23(1):83-102, 1992.

89. Poole JU, Pellegrini VD Jr: Arthritis of the thumb basal joint complex, *J Hand Ther* 13(2):91-107, 2000.

90. Schreuders TAR, Brandsma JW, Stam HJ: The intrinsic muscles of the hand: function, assessment and principles for therapeutic intervention, *Phys Med Rehab Kuror* 17:20-27, 2007.

APPENDIX

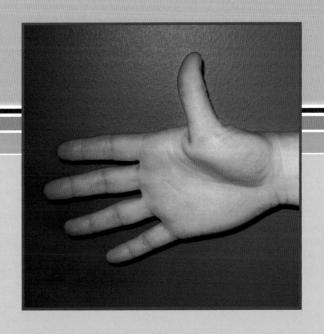

Insufficient Finger and/or Thumb Flexion Syndrome

The principal impairment in insufficient finger and/or thumb flexion syndrome is limited finger or thumb flexion AROM, but the key to prescribing the appropriate interventions is differentiating between the sources causing the limited flexion. The sources of the limited flexion can be broadly classified into two main categories: hypomobility (physiological and accessory motion) or force production deficit (decreased strength). Insufficient finger and/or thumb flexion syndrome is most commonly secondary to a trauma or injury or after a period of immobilization to allow for tissue healing. Initially, these patients may be assigned a movement system diagnosis of hand impairment Stage 1, but an underlying movement system diagnosis of insufficient finger and/or thumb flexion syndrome may help guide treatment. As the tissues heal, the diagnosis may change from hand impairment to another movement system diagnosis such as insufficient finger and/or thumb flexion syndrome. The "Source of Signs and Symptoms" column provides key information regarding the cluster of findings identifying the source of the limited flexion. The identified source or cause of insufficient finger and/or thumb flexion comprises the second part of the name of the syndrome.

Symptoms and History

- Inability to make a fist; difficulty gripping objects and using hand for functional activities such as feeding, dressing, or writing
- Pain in hand and/or forearm
- Swelling in hand, wrist, and/or forearm. If significant swelling is present, may also complain of numbness and tingling
- If swan neck deformity, PIP joint of finger hyperextending can "lock," preventing flexion. May have eventual inability to flex PIP joint

Common Referring Diagnoses

- S/p synovectomy for arthritis
- Extensor or flexor tendon repair
- Tendon adhesion
- Ligament sprain (grade I or II)
- Stiffness after fracture
- Nerve injury

Key Tests and Signs for Movement Impairment

Alignment Analysis and Appearance

- Joint may be painful, red, and swollen compared to opposite hand
- May have scar on flexor or extensor surface
- Absence of normal resting position of some flexion secondary to lack of tenodesis on affected finger (ruptured flexors)
- May observe rotation of finger if isolated shortness of one intrinsic (see finger rotation)

Movement Impairment Analysis

- The joint that is not stiff flexes more readily than the stiff joint
  - During finger/thumb flexion, the wrist may flex more readily than the fingers/thumb
  - During finger/thumb flexion, the wrist or fingers move into extension (short[1] or adhered finger extensors)

Source of Signs and Symptoms

Hypomobility

Flexor Tendon Adhesions[4,5]

- Active flexion ROM is less than PROM; passive flexion ROM is normal.[3]
- Extrinsic finger/thumb flexor length test findings are positive for shortness or adhesion (PROM and AROM into composite finger/thumb extension are equally decreased).[3]
- Adherence of flexor muscle or tendon may be palpated and visually observed, especially during active flexion.[6]
- During MMT of extrinsic flexors, a strong contraction of muscle is palpable and the muscle can hold against resistance within a limited ROM; however, there is an abrupt stop to AROM into flexion.

Extensor Tendon Adhesions[5,6]

- Active extension ROM is less than PROM ("extensor lag").
- Extrinsic finger/thumb extensor length test findings positive for shortness or adherence (PROM and AROM into composite finger/thumb flexion are equally decreased).[6]
- Adherence of extensor muscle or tendon may be palpated or observed visually, especially during active extension.[2]
- During MMT of extrinsic extensors, a strong contraction of the muscle is palpable and the muscle can hold against resistance within a limited ROM; however, there is an abrupt stop to the AROM into extension.

Extrinsic Finger/Thumb Extensor Muscle Shortness[2,5]

- Normal active and passive extension ROM.
- Extrinsic extensor muscle length test findings positive for shortness (equally decreased passive and active composite finger/thumb flexion).[7]

MP Collateral Ligament Shortness or Adhesion[5,8]

- Findings during passive finger/thumb MP joint flexion ROM include equal limitation of passive and active MP flexion, regardless of the position of adjacent joints.[9]
- Firm end-feel to PROM into flexion.
- Accessory joint motion finding is decreased posterior-to-anterior glide of the proximal phalanx on the metacarpal.[2,7]

IP Joint Dorsal Capsule Shortness or Adhesion[5]

- IP joint active and passive flexion ROM is equally limited, regardless of the position of the adjacent joints.[9]
- Firm end-feel to the PROM into flexion.
- Accessory joint motion finding is decreased posterior-to-anterior glide of the proximal or middle phalanx on the middle or distal phalanges, respectively.[2]

Associated Signs or Contributing Factors

Alignment Analysis and Appearance
Posture
- Stiff hand posture (MP joints extended, IP joints flexed, and thumb adducted)

Edema[16,17]
Alignment and Appearance
- Skin: Shiny with decreased creases
- Size: Enlarged locally or diffuse
- Tends to accumulate on dorsal hand
- Loss of arches with dorsal hand edema; tends to position joints in their "loose-packed" position

Range of Motion
- Soft end-feel to PROM

Measurement
- Circumference increased when compared to uninvolved side
- Volumeter increased when compared to opposite side[17,18]

Palpation
- Edema can be pitting or brawny[16]

Scar
Appearance/Palpation
- Visible superficial scar adheres to tendon when pushed in opposite direction of active tendon glide
- Scar may be red, raised, supple, mature, immature, keloid, hypertrophic, or adherent[19]
- Scar should be assessed for hypersensitivity, whether it is raised, and mobility

Sensation
- Decreased if associated with nerve injury

Palpation
- With intrinsic muscle shortness, may have tenderness over the intrinsic muscle bellies

Differential Diagnosis

Movement System Diagnosis
- Insufficient finger/thumb extension
- Finger rotation syndrome
- Hand impairment

Potential Diagnoses Requiring Referral Suggested by Signs and Symptoms
*Neuromusculoskeletal**
- Rupture of flexor tendon
- Radial, median, or ulnar nerve injury
- CRPS
- Fracture
- Subluxation/dislocation
- Ligament sprain (grade III) or volar plate injury
- Tenosynovitis
- Trigger finger or thumb
- Muscle disease
- Spasticity/other neurological disorders
- OA[20]
- Brachial plexus injury
- Cervical radiculopathy

Edema[20]
- Hemiplegia
- Cervical rib
- TOS

Visceral
Edema
- Neoplasms
- Cardiovascular disease
- Renal disease
- Hepatic disease
- Aneurysm
- Raynaud's phenomenon

Systemic
- Gout[21]
- RA[21]
- Scleroderma[21]
- Diabetes[21]

Symptoms and History	Key Tests and Signs for Movement Impairment	Source of Signs and Symptoms
	Joint Integrity	**Shortness of ORL**[2]
	Range of Motion	• ORL length test findings are positive for shortness (DIP joint passive flexion limited with PIP joint in extension but not limited with PIP joint flexed).[10-12]
	• Often have pain at end-range flexion	• May have resting alignment of PIP flexion and DIP hyperextension (boutonnière deformity).[10]
	• Active finger/thumb flexion:	**Shortness of Interossei and Lumbricals**[2,8]
	• Limited at one or more joints	• Interossei muscle length test findings are positive for shortness[2] (see Table 5-1).
	• Absent active flexion (ruptured flexor tendon)	• Passive composite finger flexion can be normal with shortness of interossei because interossei are not stretched across MP joint when MP joints are flexed.
	• If associated with swan neck, finger may snap into flexion with effort or PIP may lock in hyperextension	• Composite finger extension can be normal with short interossei because interossei are not stretched across IP joints when IP joints are extended.
	• Passive ROM	• PROM should be equal to AROM when ROM is tested in the exact same position for both.
	• Flexion ROM may or may not be limited	• Palpation findings may reveal tenderness over the muscle bellies or tendons of the interossei.
	• Extension ROM may or may not be normal	**Swan Neck Deformity**[3,5,13]
	Ligament Integrity/ Length	• Swan neck deformity progression that limits finger flexion is usually associated with RA. For patients with swan neck deformity in this syndrome, PIP flexion would be available but not normal.
	• ORL length	• Alignment of MP flexion with PIP hyperextension and DIP flexion. This alignment may be due to hypermobility of PIP (laxity of volar plate) and one or more of the following:
	• Ligament integrity	• Intrinsic muscle shortness
	Joint Accessory Motion **Muscle Length Tests**	• Mallet finger increases tension on central slip
	• Extrinsic finger/thumb flexor length test	• Fracture of middle phalanx with shortening decreases tension on the terminal tendon
	• Extrinsic finger/thumb extensor length test[2]	• Extensor tendon adhesion over dorsum of hand
	• Interossei muscle length test[2]	• Extensor tendon shortness
	Muscle Strength/ Performance Impairments[3]	• Nonfunctional FDS
		• Volar subluxation of the MP joint increases tension on EDC
	• Strength of grip and pinch may be decreased as a result of decreased gliding of extrinsic flexor (FDP, FDS, FPL) tendons or weakness of interossei	**Ligament Sprain**[5,13,14]
		• Ligament integrity test findings are positive.
		Force Production Deficit
		Weakness of Finger or Thumb Flexors[15]
		• Active finger/thumb flexion ROM is less than PROM
	• MMT of finger/thumb flexors	• Strength determined by MMT is graded 2/5 or less[13]
		• Weakness is noted throughout ROM of finger/thumb flexion
		• Passive finger/thumb ROM is normal
		Rupture of Finger or Thumb Flexors[13]
		• Absent active finger/thumb flexion; passive flexion ROM of finger/thumb is normal
		• Absent tenodesis (involved finger/thumb does not flex with wrist extension)[3]
		• History of sudden onset with report of audible "pop"

*Refer to Magee[20] or Goodman[21] for a comprehensive list of other potential differential diagnoses that might present with neuromuscular changes or edema of the hand.

APB, Abductor pollicis brevis; *APL*, abductor pollicis longus; *AROM*, active range of motion; *AVN*, avascular necrosis; *CMC*, carpometacarpal; *CPM*, continuous passive motion; *CRPS*, complex regional pain syndrome; *CTS*, carpal tunnel syndrome; *DIP*, distal interphalangeal; *DJD*, degenerative joint disease; *ED*, extensor digitorum; *EDC*, extensor digitorum communis; *EPB*, extensor pollicis brevis; *FDP*, flexor digitorum profundus; *FDS*, flexor digitorum superficialis; *FPB*, flexor pollicis brevis; *FPL*, flexor pollicis longus; *IP*, interphalangeal; *LRTI*, ligament reconstruction tendon interposition; *MMT*, manual muscle testing; *MP*, metacarpophalangeal; *OA*, osteoarthritis; *OP*, opponens pollicis; *ORIF*, Open reduction internal fixation; *ORL*, oblique retinacular ligament; *PIP*, proximal interphalangeal; *PROM*, passive range of motion; *RA*, rheumatoid arthritis; *ROM*, range of motion; *RSD*, reflex sympathetic dystrophy; *s/p*, status/post; *SCI*, spinal cord injury; *TFCC*, triangular fibrocartilage complex; *TOS*, thoracic outlet syndrome.

NOTES

Treatment

See Box 5-2 for treatment of scar and edema. The usual expectation is that AROM should increase by a minimum of 10 degrees per week except when the cause of the limitation is due to profound weakness or rupture. Pain and edema should decrease gradually over the course of treatment. The therapist must avoid applying excessive force when performing passive stretching exercises on patients that have hand injuries. Overly aggressive exercise increases swelling and may result in increased fibrosis and limitation of ROM.

Treatment for Insufficient Finger and/or Thumb Flexion Syndrome Caused by Flexor Tendon Adhesion

Treatment of adhesions requires active and resistive contraction of flexors and stretching into composite extension (see Box 5A-1 for General Guidelines for Treatment Progression).

A. *Soft tissue massage*[4,22]
   1. Adhesions: Retrograde massage over flexors pushes skin distally while actively flexing fingers and pulls skin proximally while extending wrist and fingers.
B. *Passive stretches*[4,16] (flexor tendon gliding distally; Figures 5A-1 and 5A-2)
   1. Composite finger extension: Progression is accomplished by sequentially adding wrist extension, forearm supination, and elbow extension as tolerated (Figure 5A-2, *A*).
   2. A static splint stabilizing fingers in extension may be helpful during passive wrist extension[4] (Figure 5A-2, *B*).

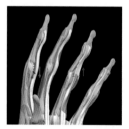

Figure 5A-1. Direction of tendon glide. Flexor tendon glides proximally with active flexion. Flexor tendon glides distally with active or passive finger extension. (From Interactive Hand 2000, Copyright 2001.)

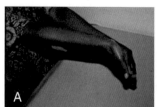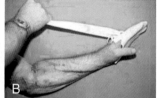

Figure 5A-2. Composite stretching fingers and wrist into extension for distal gliding of adhered finger flexor tendons or lengthening the finger flexors. **A,** Manual stretching using opposite hand. **B,** Stretching with assist of splint to maintain finger extension. (Used with permission from Ann Kammien, PT CHT, St Louis, Mo.)

C. *Active flexion* (flexor tendon gliding proximally) (Figure 5A-3)
   1. Composite, blocked flexion and isolated flexor tendon exercise[4,22] (Figure 5A-4).
   2. Differential tendon gliding[22] (see Figure 5A-3).

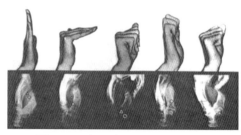

Figure 5A-3. Flexor tendon gliding exercises. Straight fist: FDS glides maximally with respect to sheath and bone. Hook fist: Maximum gliding between FDS and FDP. Fist: FDP glides maximally with respect to sheath and bone. (Reprinted from Wehbe MA, Hunter JM: Flexor tendon gliding in the hand. II. Differential gliding, *J Hand Surg* 10A:575-579, 1985.)

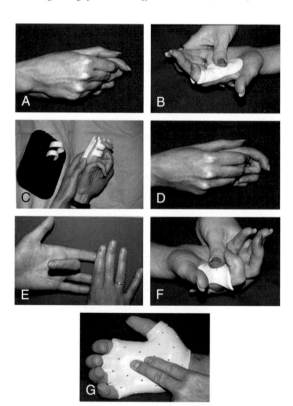

Figure 5A-4. Active finger flexion exercises to increase flexor tendon gliding proximally. **A,** Active braced or blocked DIP flexion to increase gliding of flexor digitorum profundus. **B,** Use of thermoplastic splint to isolate movement to DIP joint and block PIP and MP joint motion. **C,** Use of Bunnell block to isolate DIP flexion. **D,** Active braced or blocked PIP flexion to increase gliding of flexor digitorum superficialis. **E,** Exercising flexor digitorum superficialis by actively flexing middle finger PIP joint, preventing flexor digitorum profundus from working by stabilizing other fingers in extension. **F** and **G,** Use of thermoplastic splints to isolate movement to PIP joint and block MP joint motion. (Used with permission from Ann Kammien, PT CHT, St Louis, Mo.)

D. *Resisted flexion* (proximal flexor tendon gliding with additional force)
   1. Resistive putty, hand grippers (adjust grip size to maximize effectiveness), elastic band[4,22] (Figure 5A-5)

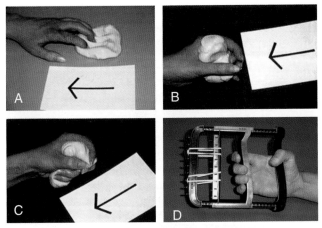

Figure 5A-5. Resistive finger flexion exercises to increase proximal tendon gliding of the finger flexors. **A,** Finger flexion into putty resting on table. **B,** Composite finger flexion done incorrectly: Involved index finger is not touching putty. **C** and **D,** Composite finger flexion done correctly with putty and hand gripper, respectively, resisting involved index finger. (**A** to **C,** Used with permission from Ann Kammien, PT CHT, St Louis, Mo.)

E. *Static progressive/dynamic splinting into extension*[16]
   1. Composite wrist and finger extension splint positioned in slightly better extension than when the patient presents. Straps are adjusted to tolerance for a gradual stretch of the flexors and the splint is used at night[4] (Figure 5A-6, *A*).
   2. Dorsal forearm splint with a tolerable force from fishing line, rubber band, or spring, holding the digits in extension. Static progressive splint should be worn 30 minutes 3 times/day. Dynamic splint may be worn 20 to 30 minutes 3 to 5 times/day. The patient may need to start with 10 minutes and gradually increase the time to 30 minutes[4] (Figure 5A-6, *B*).

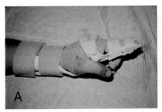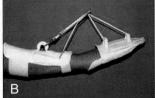

Figure 5A-6. Splinting for insufficient finger flexion caused by flexor shortness or adhesions. **A,** Static splint to maintain wrist and fingers at end-range extension used at night. **B,** Static progressive or dynamic splint to increase composite wrist and finger extension. (Used with permission from Ann Kammien, PT CHT, St Louis, Mo.)

F. *Modalities* (used when other treatment options are not effective)
   1. Electrical stimulation (Russian) to flexors to assist active contraction[4]
   2. Ultrasound over adherent tendon[4]
G. *Progression of resistance for return to function*
   1. Upper extremity ergometer, isokinetic, and Baltimore Therapeutic Equipment (BTE) machines[23]

BOX 5A-1

General Guidelines for Treatment Progression

General guidelines for progression of treatment from easiest or least aggressive to most aggressive for an adhered tendon:
1. Circular massage and active exercise
2. Retrograde massage with active exercise
3. Composite stretching passively into limited ROM
4. Static progressive or dynamic composite splinting into limited ROM
5. Resistive exercises

Treatment for Insufficient Finger and/or Thumb Flexion Syndrome Caused by Extensor Tendon Adhesions/Extrinsic Extensor Muscle Shortness

Treatment of both shortness and adhesion requires stretching into composite flexion. Treatment of adhesions only requires active and resistive contraction of extensors.

A. *Soft tissue massage*[22] (Figure 5A-7)
   1. Adhesions: Retrograde massage over extensors pushes skin distally while actively extending fingers and pulls skin proximally while flexing wrist and fingers.

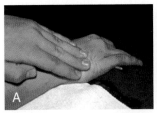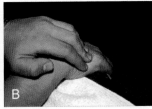

Figure 5A-7. Massage for Insufficient finger flexion caused by extensor tendon adhesions. **A,** Pushing scar distally the opposite direction of the tendon glide during active finger extension. **B,** Pushing scar proximally during active finger flexion. (Used with permission from Ann Kammien, PT CHT, St Louis, Mo.)

B. *Passive or active stretches* (provides extensor tendon gliding distally)[16] (Figure 5A-8, *A, B,* and *D* to *F*)
   1. Composite finger flexion: Progression is accomplished by sequentially adding wrist flexion, forearm pronation, and elbow extension as tolerated.
   2. A flexion glove stabilizing fingers in flexion may be helpful during passive wrist flexion.
   3. Holding a dumbbell weight and working on wrist flexion is another method of stretching the extensors.

C. *Active extension* (proximal extensor tendon glide) (Figure 5A-8, *C*)
  1. Composite and isolated: Differential tendon gliding (claw position for EDC)[22,24]

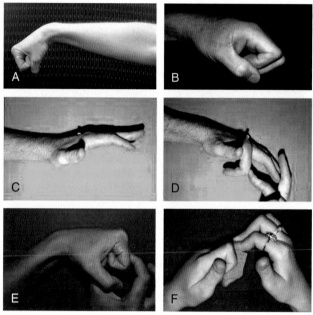

Figure 5A-8. Exercises for insufficient finger flexion caused by extensor tendon adhesions or shortness. **A** and **B,** Active composite finger flexion for shortness or adhesions. **C,** Active composite extension for adhesions to increase extensor tendon gliding proximally. **D,** Passive finger flexion for adhesions to increase extensor tendon gliding distally. **E** and **F,** Composite passive finger flexion for adhesions to increase extensor tendon gliding distally or lengthen short extensors. (**B** to **F,** Used with permission from Ann Kammien, PT CHT, St Louis, Mo.)

D. *Resisted extension* (proximal tendon glide with additional force)[24] (Figure 5A-9)
  1. Resistive putty, rubber bands, elastic band

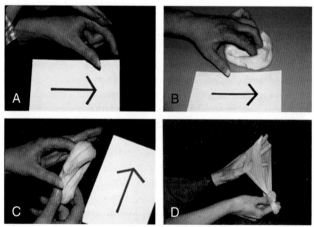

Figure 5A-9. Insufficient finger flexion caused by extensor tendon adhesions. Resisted finger extension exercises to increase extensor tendon gliding. **A,** Manually resisted MP extension. **B** and **C,** Resistive putty. **D,** Elastic band. (Used with permission from Ann Kammien, PT CHT, St Louis, Mo.)

E. *Static progressive/dynamic splinting into flexion*[16] (Figure 5A-10)
  1. Wrist cock-up splint in slight wrist flexion with flexion glove[5] can be worn, if tolerated, at night or periodically through the day (minimum of 20 minutes).
  2. Dorsal splint with outrigger for MP and IP flexion (wrist positioned in neutral or slight flexion) can be worn 20 to 30 minutes 4 to 6 times/day.

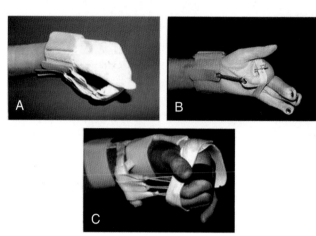

Figure 5A-10. Insufficient finger flexion caused by extensor tendon shortness or adhesions. **A,** Flexion glove for gentle composite stretch to fingers into flexion. **B,** Addition of elastic band around hand and middle phalanges to flexion glove to increase MP and PIP flexion. **C,** Dynamic MP and IP flexion splint. (Used with permission from Ann Kammien, PT CHT, St Louis, Mo.)

F. *Modalities*
  1. Moist heat[25] over dorsal surface with extensors on a stretch (wrist or fingers flexed)
  2. Electrical stimulation (Russian) to extensors to assist active contraction[24]
  3. Ultrasound[25] over adherent tendon or shortened muscle while on a stretch
G. *Progression of resistance for return to function*
  1. Upper extremity ergometer, isokinetic, and BTE machines[23,24]
  See guidelines for progression of treatment in section on flexor tendon adhesions (see Box 5A-1).

Treatment for Insufficient Finger and/or Thumb Flexion Syndrome Caused by MP Collateral Ligament and/or IP Dorsal Capsule Shortness or Adhesion[5,16]

Treatment isolates motion to the joint that is stiff so that the joint that is relatively most flexible does not move. Often, decreasing the amount of effort is helpful to obtain precise movement at the involved joint.

A. *AROM and PROM specific to short structure* (Figures 5A-11 and 5A-12)
  1. Passive or active blocking exercises for MP joint flexion to stretch collateral ligaments

2. Passive or active blocking exercises for PIP or DIP flexion to stretch the dorsal capsule
3. Joint mobilization techniques (e.g., volar glide and distraction to increase MP or IP flexion).
4. Most patients with limited PIP flexion also have limited PIP extension so the following exercises would also be appropriate:
   a. Passive or active blocking exercises for PIP or DIP extension to stretch volar plate
   b. Joint mobilization gliding distal joint surface dorsally to increase IP extension

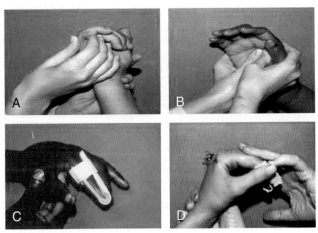

Figure 5A-11. Exercises for insufficient finger flexion caused by joint structures. **A,** Active braced or blocked PIP flexion. **B,** Active braced or blocked MP flexion. **C,** Active MP flexion with uninvolved IP joints immobilized in extension. **D,** Passive MP flexion with wrist stabilized. (Used with permission from Ann Kammien, PT CHT, St Louis, Mo.)

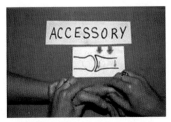

Figure 5A-12. Insufficient finger flexion caused by joint structures. Treatment using joint mobilization. (Used with permission from Ann Kammien, PT CHT, St Louis, Mo.)

B. *Static splints*
1. To increase PIP extension, static splints can be worn at night or periodically throughout the day (e.g., a volar gutter splint in 0 degrees extension with dorsal strap over PIP joint).
2. Splints maintain gentle stretch on short structure.
C. *Static progressive/dynamic splints*
1. Specific to short structure (20 to 30 minutes/4 to 6 times/day).

2. Flexion glove, often worn at night, is best for increasing MP flexion unless an additional strap is added to increase PIP flexion[5] (see Figure 5A-10, *A* and *B*).
3. Static progressive/dynamic MP[5] or IP flexion splint (Figures 5A-13 and 5A-14).
4. Static progressive/dynamic PIP extension splint.

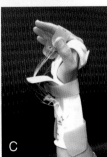

Figure 5A-13. Insufficient finger flexion caused by shortness of PIP or DIP dorsal capsule. Elastic flexion splint to increase PIP and DIP flexion (best for DIP). (Used with permission from Ann Kammien, PT CHT, St Louis, Mo.)

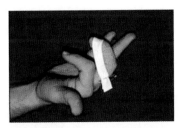
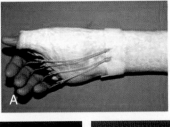
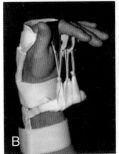

Figure 5A-14. Insufficient finger flexion caused by MP collateral ligament shortness or adhesions. **A,** Treatment initiated early while still casted by adding slings to pull MP joints into flexion. **B,** Dynamic MP flexion splint. **C,** Static progressive MP flexion splint. (Used with permission from Ann Kammien, PT CHT, St Louis, Mo.)

D. *CPM*[26]
1. For isolated or composite motions, CPM is most helpful acutely while in hand impairment Stage 1 or after tenolysis.
E. *Modalities*[25]: Not usually the priority for treatment but used when exercise, splinting, edema, and scar management techniques alone are not effective
1. Hot/cold packs/paraffin
2. Electrical stimulation to assist active contraction and provide feedback
3. Ultrasound for increased tissue extensibility
   a. Underwater

b. Continuous at 0.5 to 1.0 W/cm² (using 3 mHz frequency)
c. Always with restricted tendon/muscle on a stretch

Treatment for Insufficient Finger and/or Thumb Flexion Syndrome Caused by ORL Shortness[24] (Figure 5A-15)

Treatment is simultaneous DIP flexion with PIP extension exercises performed actively, passively, or with resistance. In some cases, splinting to hold the PIP joint in extension may be helpful.

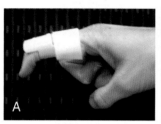
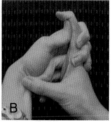

Figure 5A-15. **A** and **B**, Exercises for insufficient finger flexion caused by short ORL.

Treatment for Insufficient Finger and/or Thumb Flexion Syndrome Caused by Intrinsic Muscle Shortness[16]

A. *Passive stretches:* MP joint positioned in full extension while passively flexing the IP joints (Figure 5A-16, *A*)
B. *Active "hook grip" position:* MP joint extension and IP joint flexion (Figure 5A-16, *B*)
C. *Active and passive MP joint abduction or adduction:* IP joints held in flexion with the MP joint in full extension for unilateral finger intrinsic shortness or stiffness (Figure 5A-16, *C*)
D. *Resistive hook grip* with resistive putty (Figure 5A-16, *D*)
E. *Static progressive/dynamic splinting:* Dorsal hand or forearm-based splint extending to the PIP joint level (MP joints extended) with adjustable straps positioning the IP joints in end-range flexion
F. *Patient education*
1. Modify grip to avoid prolonged or repeated intrinsic-plus position as possible.
2. If intrinsic plus position is required for daily activities, performance of active and passive stretches is recommended frequently during day.

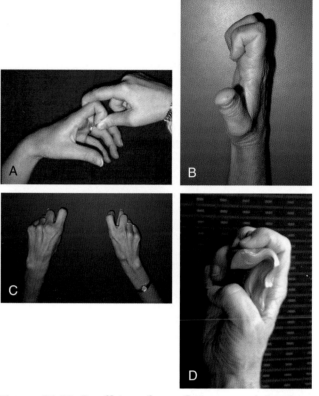

Figure 5A-16. Insufficient finger flexion caused by short intrinsic muscles. **A,** Passive IP flexion with MP in extension to stretch interossei. **B,** Active IP flexion with MP's in extension. **C,** Index MP abduction with IPs flexed and MP in extension to stretch first palmar interossei. **D,** Resistive hook fist with resistive putty.

Treatment for Insufficient Finger and/or Thumb Flexion Syndrome Caused by Swan Neck Deformity

Treatment is controversial; some experts say no improvement occurs with conservative treatment or splinting. Others recommend splinting and exercises to correct joint contractures and intrinsic shortness in the early stages.[27] Surgery is usually necessary for lasting correction.
A. *Exercise*
1. Active and passive intrinsic muscle stretching exercises (see Figure 5A-16, *A* and *B*)
2. Active and passive composite finger and wrist flexion to maintain appropriate length of EDC if needed (see Figure 5A-8, *A* and *B*)
3. Patient education to correct faulty movement patterns (intrinsic plus position) during functional activities by increasing use of FDP, FDS, and extensor digitorum
B. *Splinting*[28]
1. Night splint hand with MPs in extension and IPs flexed.
2. Daytime constant use of button-hole splint to prevent PIP hyperextension but allow PIP flexion. (Use 6 weeks and then as needed.) (Figure 5A-17, *A* and *B*)

3. If splints are needed long term, silver ring splints may be preferable to thermoplastic splints[27]

4. Patient education regarding splint use, skin precautions (e.g., redness of skin, avoid leaving splint in hot place, instructions regarding how to don and doff splint)

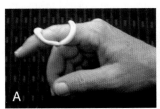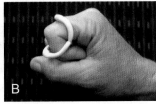

Figure 5A-17. Insufficient finger flexion due to swan neck. **A,** Static buttonhole splint preventing PIP hyperextension. **B,** Static buttonhole splint allows PIP flexion.

Treatment for Insufficient Finger and/or Thumb Flexion Syndrome caused by Weakness of Flexors

Overload the muscle progressively as appropriate for the specific strength of the muscle. Exercises should be done every other day, 3 sets of 10 to 15 repetitions each time, once strength is greater than 3+/5. Exercises can be performed more often at the weaker grades. May need to use tenodesis action with the wrist to achieve finger flexion if no finger flexion available actively.

Treatment for Insufficient Finger and/or Thumb Flexion Syndrome Caused by Rupture of Flexor Tendon

Contact physician same day and schedule appointment for patient to see physician.

Insufficient Finger and/or Thumb Extension Syndrome

The principal impairment in insufficient finger and/or thumb syndrome is limited finger and/or thumb extension AROM, but the key to prescribing the appropriate intervention is differentiating between the sources causing the limited extension. The sources of the limited extension can be broadly classified into two main categories: hypomobility (physiological and accessory motion) or force production deficit (decreased strength). Insufficient finger and/or thumb extension syndrome is most commonly secondary to a trauma or injury or after a period of immobilization to allow for tissue healing. Initially, these patients may be assigned a movement system diagnosis of hand impairment Stage 1, but an underlying movement system diagnosis of insufficient finger and/or thumb extension syndrome may help guide treatment. As the tissues heal, the diagnosis may change from hand impairment to another movement system diagnosis such as insufficient finger and/or thumb extension syndrome. The "Source of Signs and Symptoms" column provides key information regarding the cluster of findings identifying the source of the limited extension. The identified source or cause of insufficient finger and/or thumb extension comprises the second part of the name of the syndrome.

Symptoms and History

- Difficulty gripping objects
- Pain in hand and/or forearm
- Swelling in hand, wrist, and/or forearm
- If significant swelling is present, may also complain of numbness and tingling

Common Referring Diagnoses

- S/p synovectomy for arthritis
- Extensor or flexor tendon repair
- Tendon adhesion
- Ligament sprain (grade I or II)
- Stiffness after fracture

Key Tests and Signs for Movement Impairment

Alignment Analysis and Appearance

- Joint may be painful, red, and swollen compared to opposite hand
- May have scar on flexor or extensor surface
- Absence of normal resting posture of fingers secondary to lack of tenodesis on affected finger (ruptured extensors)

Movement Impairment Analysis

- The joint that is not stiff extends more readily than the stiff joint
  - During finger/thumb extension, wrist or uninvolved finger joints may extend more readily than involved joint(s) of the fingers/thumb
  - During finger/thumb extension, wrist or fingers move into flexion (short or adhered finger flexors)

Joint Integrity

Range of Motion

- Often have pain at end-range extension
- Active finger/thumb extension ROM:
  - Limited at one or more joints
  - Absent active MP extension (ruptured EDC, EI, and/or EDM tendon)
- Passive ROM
  - Extension ROM may or may not be limited.
  - Flexion ROM may or may not be normal.

Ligament Integrity/Length

- ORL length
- Ligament integrity

Source of Signs and Symptoms

Hypomobility

Flexor Tendon Adhesions[4,5]

- Active flexion ROM is less than PROM; passive flexion ROM is normal.
- Extrinsic finger/thumb flexor length test findings are positive for shortness or adhesion (PROM and AROM into composite finger/thumb extension are equally decreased).
- Adherence of the flexor muscle or tendon may be palpated and visually observed, especially during active flexion.
- During MMT of extrinsic flexors, a strong contraction of the muscle is palpable and the muscle can hold against resistance within a limited ROM; however, there is an abrupt stop to the active ROM into flexion.

Extensor Tendon Adhesions[6]

- Active extension ROM is less than PROM ("extensor lag").
- Extrinsic finger/thumb extensor length test findings positive for shortness or adherence (PROM and AROM into composite finger/thumb flexion are equally decreased).
- Adherence of extensor muscle or tendon may be palpated or observed visually, especially during active extension.
- During the MMT of the extrinsic extensors, a strong contraction of the muscle is palpable and the muscle can hold against resistance within a limited ROM; however, there is an abrupt stop to the AROM into extension.

Flexor Muscle Shortness[5]

- Normal active and passive flexion ROM
- Extrinsic flexor muscle length test findings positive for shortness (equally decreased passive and active composite finger/thumb extension)

MP, PIP, or DIP Volar Plate and Accessory Collateral Ligament Shortness or Adhesion[5]

- Extension ROM
  - Equally limited active and passive extension of joint and limited regardless of position of adjacent joints
  - Firm end-feel to passive extension ROM
- Accessory joint motion findings
  - Decreased AP glide of MP, PIP, or DIP joints
- Chronic boutonnière
- Ligament sprain
  - Ligament integrity test is positive

Associated Signs or Contributing Factors

Alignment Analysis
Posture
- Stiff hand posture (MP joints extended, IP joints flexed, and thumb adducted)

Edema[16,17]
Alignment Analysis and Appearance
- Skin: Shiny with decreased creases
- Size: Enlarged locally or diffuse
- Tends to accumulate on dorsal hand
- Loss of arches with dorsal hand edema tends to position joints in their "loose-packed" position

Range of Motion
- Soft end-feel to PROM

Measurement
- Circumference: increased when compared to uninvolved side
- Volumeter increased when compared to opposite side[17,18]

Palpation
- Edema can be pitting or brawny[16]

Scar
Appearance/Palpation
- Visible superficial scar, adheres to tendon when pushed in opposite direction of active tendon glide
- Scar is described as red, raised, supple, mature, immature, keloid, hypertrophic, and adherent[19]
- Scar should be assessed for hypersensitivity, whether it is raised, and mobility

Sensation
- Decreased if associated with nerve injury

Palpation
- With intrinsic muscle shortness, may have tenderness over the intrinsic muscle bellies

Differential Diagnosis

Movement System Diagnosis
- Insufficient finger flexion
- Hand impairment

Potential Diagnosis Requiring Referral Suggested by Signs and Symptoms

*Neuromusculoskeletal**
- Joint dislocation
- Fracture
- Extensor tendon injuries[24]
  - Zone 1: Mallet (DIP)
  - Zone 2: Middle phalanx
  - Zone 3: Boutonnière (PIP)
  - Zone 4: EDC (proximal phalanx)
  - Zones 5-7: MP to wrist
- Tenosynovitis
- Trigger finger or thumb
- Ligament sprain (grade III)
- Radial nerve injury
- Brachial plexus injury
- Cervical radiculopathy
- OA
- Dupuytren's contracture[21]

Edema Caused by Neuromusculoskeletal Problems[20]
- Hemiplegia
- Cervical rib
- TOS

Visceral
Edema Caused by Visceral Problems[20]
- Neoplasms
- Cardiovascular disease
- Renal disease
- Hepatic disease
- Aneurysm
- Raynaud's phenomenon

Systemic
- Gout[21]
- RA[21]
- Scleroderma[21]
- Diabetes[21]

Symptoms and History	Key Tests and Signs for Movement Impairment	Source of Signs and Symptoms
	Joint Accessory Motion Muscle Length Tests • Extrinsic finger/thumb flexor length test • Extrinsic finger/thumb extensor length test[2] • Interossei muscle length test[2] **Muscle Strength/ Performance Impairments** • Strength of grip and pinch may be decreased as a result of decreased gliding of extrinsic extensors, weakness of interossei, or in presence of weakness of wrist extensors caused by radial nerve injury • MMT of finger and thumb extensors[13]	***Shortness of ORL***[2,15] • ORL length test findings are positive for shortness (DIP joint passive flexion limited with PIP joint in extension but not limited with PIP joint flexed). • May have resting alignment of PIP flexion and DIP hyperextension (boutonnière deformity). ***Shortness of Interossei and Lumbricals***[13] • Interossei muscle length test findings are positive for shortness. • Passive composite finger flexion can be normal with shortness of interossei because interossei are not stretched across the MP joint when MP joints are flexed. • Composite finger extension can be normal with short interossei because interossei are not stretched across IP joints when IP joints are extended. • PROM should be equal to AROM when ROM is tested in exact same position for active and passive. • Palpation findings may reveal tenderness over muscle bellies or tendons of interossei. ***Ligament Sprain***[14] • Ligament integrity tests are positive. **Force Production Deficit** ***Weakness of ED or Thumb Extensors***[13] • Active finger or thumb MP extension ROM is less than PROM. • PROM of MP into extension is normal. • MMT: Strength is 2/5 or less. • Weakness is noted throughout ROM of finger/thumb extension. ***Weakness of Intrinsics***[13]***: "Clawing"*** • Decreased IP extension actively • PROM IP extension full • MMT interossei <3/5 ***Injury to or Rupture of Finger or Thumb Extensors (Chronic)*** • Absent active extension • Absent tenodesis • Chronic boutonnière

*Refer to Magee[20] or Goodman[21] for a comprehensive list of other potential differential diagnoses that might present with neuromuscular changes or edema of the hand.

NOTES

Treatment for Insufficient Finger and Thumb Extension

See Box 5-2 for treatment of scar and edema. The therapist must avoid applying excessive force when performing passive stretching exercises on patients that have hand injuries. Overly aggressive exercise increases swelling and may result in increased fibrosis and limitation of ROM.

Treatment for Insufficient Finger and/or Thumb Extension Syndrome Caused by Flexor Tendon Adhesions/Shortness

Treatment of adhesions requires active and resistive contraction of flexors. Treatment of both adhesions and shortness require stretching into composite extension (see Box 5A-2).

A. *Soft tissue massage*[4,22]
   1. Adhesions: Retrograde massage over flexors pulls skin proximally while actively extending wrist and fingers and pushes skin distally while actively flexing fingers.
   2. Muscle shortness: Soft tissue massage techniques can be helpful before stretching.
B. *Passive stretches* (flexor tendon glides distally)[4,16]
   1. Composite elbow extension, forearm supination, wrist, and finger extension (modify to tolerance by adding one joint at a time) (see Figure 5A-2, *A*).
   2. A static splint stabilizing fingers in extension may be helpful during passive wrist extension[4] (see Figure 5A-2, *B*).
C. *Active flexion* (flexor tendon glides proximally) (see Figure 5A-4)
   1. Composite and blocked flexion[4,22]
   2. Differential tendon gliding[22] (Figure 5A-3)
D. *Resisted flexion* (flexor tendon glides proximally with increased force)
   Resistive putty, hand grippers (adjust grip size to maximize effectiveness), elastic band[4,22] (see Figure 5A-5)
E. *Static progressive/dynamic splinting into extension*[16] (see Figure 5A-6)
   1. Composite wrist and finger splint positioned in slightly better extension than that with which patient presents. Straps are used to apply gentle tension for a gradual stretch of the flexors (to be used at night).[4]
   2. Dorsal forearm splint with attached rubber band, spring, or elastic Velcro applying a gentle force to the wrist, MP, and IP joints into extension. Worn 20 to 30 minutes 4 to 6 times/day.[4]
G. *Modalities*[25]
   1. Moist heat over volar surface with flexors on a stretch
   2. Electrical stimulation (Russian) to flexors to assist active contraction[4]
   3. Ultrasound[25] over adherent tendon or shortened muscle while on a stretch[4]
H. *Progression of resistance for return to function*
   1. Upper extremity ergonometer, isokinetic, and BTE[23] machines

---

BOX 5A-2

General Guidelines for Treatment Program

General guidelines for progression of treatment from easiest or least aggressive to most aggressive for an adhered tendon:
1. Circular massage and active exercise
2. Retrograde massage with active exercise
3. Composite stretching passively into limited ROM
4. Dynamic or static progressive composite splinting into limited ROM
5. Resistive exercises

Treatment for Insufficient Finger and/or Thumb Extension Syndrome Caused by Extensor Tendon Adhesion

A. *Soft tissue massage*[22] (see Figure 5A-7)
   1. Adhesions: Retrograde massage over extensors pushes skin distally while actively extending fingers and pulls skin proximally while flexing wrist and fingers.
B. *Passive and active stretches* (provides extensor tendon gliding distally[16] (see Figure 5A-8, *A*, *B*, and *D* to *F*)
   1. Composite elbow extension, forearm pronation, wrist and finger flexion (modify to tolerance by adding one joint at a time).
   2. Flexion glove stabilizing fingers in flexion may be helpful during passive wrist flexion.
C. *Active extension* (proximal extensor tendon glide) (see Figure 5A-8, *C*)
   1. Composite and isolated
   2. Differential tendon gliding (claw position for EDC, MP blocked in flexion with active IP extension for intrinsics)[22,24]
D. *Resisted extension* (proximal extensor tendon glide with additional force)[24] (see Figure 5A-9)
   1. Resistive putty, rubber bands, elastic band
E. *Static progressive/dynamic splinting into flexion*[16] (see Figure 5A-10)
   1. Wrist cock-up splint in slight wrist flexion with flexion glove can be worn, if tolerated, at night or periodically through the day (minimum of 20 minutes).[5]
   2. Dorsal splint with outrigger for MP and IP flexion (wrist positioned in neutral or slight flexion). Worn 20 to 30 minutes 6 to 8 times/day.
F. *Modalities*[25]
   1. Moist heat over dorsal surface with extensors on a stretch (wrist or fingers flexed)
   2. Electrical stimulation (Russian) to extensors to assist active contraction[24]
   3. Ultrasound over adherent tendon or shortened muscle while on a stretch
G. *Progression of resistance for return to function*
   1. Upper extremity ergonometer, isokinetic, and BTE machines[23,24]

General guidelines for progression of treatment as with flexor adhesions (Box 5A-2).

Treatment for Insufficient Finger and/or Thumb Extension Syndrome Caused by MP, PIP, or DIP Volar Plate and Accessory Collateral Ligament Shortness or Adhesion[5,16]

A. *AROM and PROM specific to tight structure*
1. Passive or active PIP extension to stretch volar plate (Figure 5A-18)
2. Joint mobilization techniques (e.g., dorsal glide to increase IP extension)

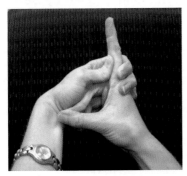

Figure 5A-18. Exercises for insufficient finger extension caused by shortness of PIP volar plate and accessory collateral ligaments. Active PIP extension while preventing MP extension.

B. *Static progressive splints* (Figure 5A-19, *A* and *B*)
1. Can be worn at night or periodically throughout the day (e.g., a volar gutter splint in 0 degrees extension with dorsal strap over PIP joint)
2. Maintains gentle stretch on tight structure

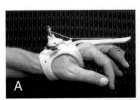
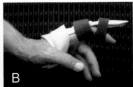
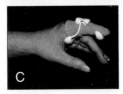
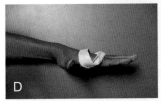
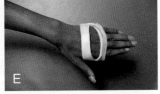

Figure 5A-19. Insufficient finger extension caused by shortness of PIP volar plate and accessory collateral ligaments. **A** and **B,** Static progressive PIP extension splint to increase PIP extension. **C,** Dynamic PIP extension splint (DeRoyal LMB Spring Finger extension assist [DeRoyal Industries, Powell, Tenn.]) used during the day to increase PIP extension ROM. **D** and **E,** Anti-claw splint can be used as an aide to exercise, preventing MP extension while working to increase PIP extension.

C. *Dynamic splints specific to tight structure* (20 to 30 minutes/6 to 8 times/day)
1. Dynamic PIP extension splint (Figure 5A-19, *C*)
2. Anti-claw splint to encourage PIP extension with MP extension blocked by splint (Figure 5A-19, *D* and *E*)
D. *CPM*
1. For isolated or composite motions, CPM is most helpful acutely while in hand impairment Stage 1 or after tenolysis.
E. *Modalities*[25]
1. Hot/cold packs/paraffin
2. Electrical stimulation to assist active contraction and give feedback
3. Ultrasound for increased tissue extensibility
a. Underwater
b. Continuous at 0.5 to 1.0 W/cm^2 (using 3-mHz frequency)
c. Always with restricted tendon/muscle on a stretch

Treatment for Insufficient Finger and/or Thumb Extension Syndrome Caused by Shortness of ORL[24]

Treatment is active, passive, or resistive exercises into simultaneous PIP extension with DIP flexion. In some cases, splinting to hold the PIP joint in extension may be helpful (see Figure 5A-15).

Treatment for Insufficient Finger and/or Thumb Extension Syndrome caused by Intrinsic Muscle Shortness[16] (see Figure 5A-16)

A. *Passive stretches:* MP joint positioned in full extension while passively flexing the IP joint
B. *Active "hook fist" position:* MP joint extension and IP joint flexion
C. *Active and passive MP joint abduction or adduction:* IP joints held in flexion with the MP joint in full extension (for unilateral finger intrinsic shortness or stiffness)
D. *Resistive hook grip* with resistive putty
E. *Static progressive/dynamic splinting:* Dorsal hand or forearm-based splint extending to the PIP joint level (MP joints extended) with adjustable straps positioning the IP joints in end-range flexion
F. *Patient education*
1. Modify grip to avoid prolonged or repeated intrinsic-plus position as possible.
2. Performance of active and passive stretches frequently during day is recommended if intrinsic plus position is required for daily activities.

Treatment for Weakness of ED

Treatment overloads the muscle progressively as appropriate for the specific strength of the muscle. Exercises should be done every other day, 3 sets of 10 to 15 repetitions each time, once strength is greater than 3+/5.

Exercises can be performed more often at the weaker grades (Figure 5A-20).

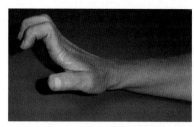

Figure 5A-20. Insufficient finger extension caused by weakness of extensor digitorum. Exercise for MP extension, isolating extensor digitorum.

Treatment for Insufficient Finger and/or Thumb Extension Syndrome Caused by Radial Nerve Injury with Paralysis of Finger and Thumb Extensors[16,29]

A. *Exercises*
  1. AROM and PROM exercises to all affected joints (especially finger, thumb, and wrist flexion and forearm supination).
  2. As motor function returns, begin active and active assistive exercises to affected muscles.
  3. Progress to resistive exercises as appropriate.
B. *Splinting*
  1. Dynamic finger MP and thumb extension splint to be worn at all times, except for PROM exercises to be done 3 times a day and for hygiene. A wrist cock-up should be worn at night.
  2. A simple wrist cock-up during the day is preferred by many patients instead of the dynamic extension splint.
C. *Patient education*
  1. The risks caused by decreased sensation
  2. Potential loss of ROM if exercises are not done regularly

Treatment for Insufficient Finger and/or Thumb Extension Syndrome Caused by Severe Weakness of Intrinsic Muscles

Treatment for severe weakness of intrinsic muscles ("clawing" secondary to ulnar nerve injury)[16,29] is as follows:

A. *Anti-claw splints* (used to increase function when there is motor loss)
B. *PROM* (especially MP flexion and IP extension if loss of AROM)
C. *Patient education*
  1. The risks caused by decreased sensation
  2. Potential loss of ROM if exercises are not done regularly

Conservative Treatment for Injury to Extensor Tendons

For conservative treatment for injuries to extensor tendons that do not require surgery, refer to established protocols.[6,30]
- Boutonnière
- Mallet

NOTES

Insufficient Thumb Palmar Abduction and/or Opposition Syndrome

The principal impairment in insufficient thumb palmar abduction and/or opposition syndrome is limited thumb opposition and/or palmar abduction AROM, but the key to prescribing the appropriate intervention is differentiating between the sources causing the limited opposition/abduction. The sources of the limited thumb opposition/palmar abduction can be broadly classified into two main categories: hypomobility (physiological and accessory motion) or force production deficit (decreased strength). Insufficient thumb palmar abduction and/or opposition with hypomobility is most commonly secondary to a trauma or injury or after a period of immobilization to allow for tissue healing.[16] Initially, these patients may be assigned a movement system diagnosis of hand impairment Stage 1, but another underlying movement system diagnosis of insufficient thumb opposition/palmar abduction may help guide treatment. As the tissues heal, the diagnosis may change from hand impairment to another movement system

Symptoms/History

- Difficulty gripping objects
- Pain in hand and/or forearm
- History of median nerve injury/trauma[16]

DJD of CMC of Thumb
- Slowly developing joint pain, stiffness, and limitation of motion
- Pain limiting performance of functional activities
- May have history of trauma to thumb

Activities/Population

DJD of CMC of Thumb
- May have history of a lot of needlework or as a hairdresser
- More common in women than men[32]
- Onset in fifth to seventh decades of life[32]

Common Referring Diagnoses

- S/p fracture after immobilization
- Median nerve injury
- Crush injury
- SCI
- Brachial plexus injury
- DJD of CMC of thumb
- Thumb pain

Key Tests and Signs for Movement Impairment

Alignment Analysis and Appearance

- Decreased first web space: Thumb resting in more adduction than normal
- Scar
- Muscle atrophy

DJD of CMC of Thumb
- Swelling at the CMC joint of thumb may or may not be present
- Prominent CMC joint
- Adduction deformity of thumb
- Joint subluxation/deformity

Movement Impairment Analysis

- During functional activities requiring opening of the hand in preparation for pinch or grip, the CMC of the thumb does not abduct normally
- Loss of the normal longitudinal arch of the thumb[9,31]
- MP joint abducts excessively

Joint Integrity

Range of Motion

- AROM
  - Limited CMC palmar abduction, opposition, or extension
  - Absent thumb palmar abduction or opposition with paralysis due to median nerve injury
- PROM
  - Palmar abduction ROM: Limited
  - Opposition ROM: Limited
  - DJD of CMC of thumb
    - May have crepitus with PROM[31]

Joint Accessory Motion

Muscle Length Tests

- Based on limited joint ROM
- Adductor pollicis short
- Possibly short FPB

Other Special Tests

DJD of CMC of Thumb
- Swanson's crank and grind test (compression)[33]:
  - Positive as articular degeneration advances
  - Pain and crepitus or instability
- Positive shoulder sign[34]
  - Prominence of the radial base of thumb from dorsal subluxation of the metacarpal on the trapezium; flexion stress (ulnar and volar glide) can be applied to metacarpal of thumb with simultaneous axial loading

Median Nerve Injury
- Sensation: Decreased in median nerve distribution

diagnosis. Insufficient thumb palmar abduction and/or opposition with hypomobility may also be secondary to paralysis after a median nerve injury.[16] However, if there is any active function of the median nerve–innervated muscles, then force production deficit instead of hypomobility would guide treatment. A third reason for the insufficient thumb palmar abduction and/or opposition with hypomobility might be joint subluxation and deformity secondary to osteoarthritis of the CMC joint of the thumb.[9,31] The "Source of Signs and Symptoms" column provides key information regarding the cluster of findings identifying the source of the insufficient thumb palmar abduction or opposition. The identified source or cause of insufficient finger and/or thumb extension comprises the second part of the name of the syndrome.

Source of Signs and Symptoms

Force Production Deficit
Median Nerve Injury
- PROM greater than AROM
- Strength 2/5[13]
- If pain is associated with limited PROM, it will be at the end-ROM

Hypomobility
Contracture of thumb adductor muscles, CMC joint structures, or scar
- AROM equals PROM and limited
- Superficial firm and immobile scar in first web space
- Decreased CMC accessory motion
- If pain is associated with the limited PROM, it will be at the end-ROM

Median Nerve Injury
- PROM greater than AROM
- PROM normal
- MMT: 0/5 to 1/5

CMC Subluxation/Deformity
- AROM equals PROM
- Swelling at the CMC[31]
- Prominent CMC joint[35]
- Adduction deformity (Eaton Stages III or IV)[31]
- Variable direction of impaired accessory motion[36]
- Onset of pain during ROM in multiple directions

Associated Signs or Contributing Factors

Alignment Analysis and Appearance
- Stiff hand posture (finger MP joints extended, IP joints flexed, and thumb adducted)

DJD of CMC of Thumb
- May have MP joint hyperextension (swan neck) or MP joint flexion (boutonnière)[37-39]
- May note Heberden's nodes on DIP joints and Bouchard's nodes on PIP joints of fingers[40]

Scar
Appearance/Palpation
- Visible superficial scar blanches when stretched during thumb palmar abduction
- Scar may be firm and immobile and described as red, raised, supple, mature, immature, keloid, hypertrophic, or adherent[19]
  - Scar should be assessed for hypersensitivity, whether it is raised, and mobility

Edema[16,17]
Alignment Analysis and Appearance
- Skin: Shiny with decreased creases
- Size: Enlarged locally or diffuse
- Tends to accumulate on dorsal hand
- Loss of arches with dorsal hand edema. Tends to position joints in their "loose-packed" position
ROM
- Soft end-feel to PROM
Measurement
- Circumference is increased when compared to uninvolved side
- Volumeter is increased when compared to opposite side[17,18]

Palpation
- Edema can be pitting or brawny

Ligament Integrity
- Ligament integrity of ulnar collateral ligament MP joint of thumb: Laxity

Differential Diagnosis

Movement System Impairment Diagnosis
- Hand impairment
- Thumb CMC accessory hypermobility
- Anterior forearm nerve entrapments

Potential Diagnosis Requiring Referral Suggested by Signs and Symptoms
Neuromusculoskeletal*
- Gamekeeper's thumb
- DJD of CMC of thumb (OA)
- Median nerve injury
- Fracture
- Crush injury
- SCI
- Brachial plexus injury
- Cervical radiculopathy
- Joint dislocation
- Chronic ligament sprain (grade III)

Edema Caused by Neuromusculoskeletal Problems[20]
- Hemiplegia
- Cervical rib
- TOS

Visceral
Edema Caused by Visceral Problems[20]
- Neoplasms
- Cardiovascular disease
- Renal disease
- Hepatic disease
- Aneurysm
- Raynaud's phenomenon

Systemic
- Gout[21]
- RA[21]
- Scleroderma[21]

Symptoms/History

**Key Tests and Signs for
Movement Impairment**

Muscle Strength/Performance Impairments
- MMT of thenar muscles[13]
- 3-Point pinch: Weak

DJD of CMC of Thumb
- Decreased pinch strength with collapse of first metacarpal
- Weakness of OP, APL, and APB

Palpation

DJD of CMC of Thumb
- Tenderness of the CMC joint along the entire joint line[31]

*Refer to Magee[20] or Goodman[21] for a comprehensive list of other potential differential diagnoses that might present with neuromuscular changes or edema of the hand.

Source of Signs and Symptoms	Associated Signs or Contributing Factors	Differential Diagnosis
	Muscle Strength/Performance Impairments • May have weakness of more proximal upper extremity muscles with nerve injury	

Treatment

Insufficient Thumb Opposition/Abduction

See Box 5-2 for treatment of scar and edema.

Force Production Deficit

Insufficient Thumb Opposition/Abduction Caused by Median Nerve Injury with Strength 2/5

1. Opposition splint for night use to prevent contracture of first web space[16,29] (Figure 5A-21, *A)*
2. Thumb web active and passive stretching to prevent contracture[29] (Figure 5A-21, *B)*
3. Exercises to strengthen thumb APB and OP[41] (Figures 5A-21, *B* and *C)*

Hypomobility

Insufficient Thumb Opposition/Abduction Caused by Median Nerve Injury with Strength 0/5 to 1/5

1. Opposition splint for functional use[16,29] (Figure 5A-21, *D)*
2. DC electrical stimulation to motor points for paralyzed muscle 3 times/day, 10 repetitions (only if regeneration is anticipated; a controversial treatment [some say it is contraindicated, others say it may be useful initially])
3. Thumb web stretching to prevent or decrease contracture[29]

Insufficient Thumb Opposition/Abduction Caused by Contracture of Thumb Adductor Muscles, CMC Joint Structures, or Scar

1. Progressive stretching of web space using Otoform K or elastomer with splinting to be worn as much of the day as possible[16] (Figure 5A-21, *E* and *F)*
2. Exercises to actively and passively stretch the first web space (e.g., thumb abduction and opposition and extension)
3. Practice grasping objects as a method to stretch the first web space

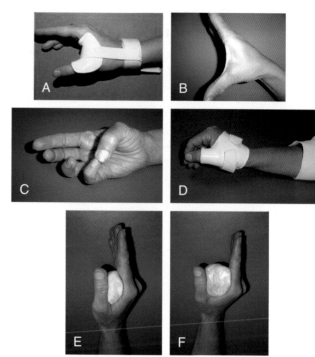

Figure 5A-21. Insufficient thumb opposition/abduction. **A,** Use of custom static splint for stretching of first web space or prevention of contracture. **B,** Palmar abduction exercising the abductor pollicis brevis. **C,** Exercise for the opponens pollicis. **D,** Opposition splint for functional use after median nerve injury. **E** and **F,** Use of Otoform K for progressive stretching of limited first web space.

Insufficient Thumb Opposition/Abduction Caused by CMC Subluxation/Deformity

A. *Patient education/assistive devices*[28,42]

  1. Joint protection/patient education: Instruct patient in good protection principles (e.g., how to use thumb with balanced forces and good alignment).

  2. Adaptive equipment

    a. Provide assistive devices for joint stability as needed.

      1) Build up pencil to facilitate correct movement pattern and decrease range of flexion required during writing.

      2) Avoid strong grip and pinch; key turner, jar opener, and use of Dycem may be helpful.

B. *Splinting*[16,40]: The main purpose of a splint is to decrease pain by providing increased stability to the CMC joint. The CMC joint is most stable in a position of abduction and opposition. However, abduction and opposition will likely not be achievable in the presence of subluxation and deformity. Correcting MP alignment can facilitate correct CMC alignment. Splinting is most effective for patients with Eaton's Stage I or II CMC arthritis but can be tried in the later stages. Although thermoplastic splints provide stability to the CMC, the hard plastic in the palm of the hand inhibits function so compromises often have to be made to insure patient compliance with splint use.

  1. Forearm-based thumb spica for severe pain for total rest of joint and involvement of the scapho-trapezial joint (Eaton Stage IV) (Figure 5A-22, *A*).

  2. Hand-based thumb spica to position thumb in abduction with IP free for functional splint (Figure 5A-22, *B*). Many patients prefer a neoprene thumb spica splint (Comfort Cool, North Coast Medical, Inc.) versus a thermoplastic thumb spica splint because it is easier to use the hand functionally, yet the neoprene splint still provides some support and stabilization to the CMC joint[43] (Figure 5A-22, *C*).

  3. If the MP joint hyperextends, a splint to prevent MP hyperextension may be helpful[44,45] (see Figure 5A-22, *B*).

    Stabilizing the MP joint in 30 degrees of flexion may unload the anterior compartment of the CMC joint, which is often involved.[46]

  4. Some recommend a splint immobilizing the CMC joint only[47] (Figure 5A-22, *D*).

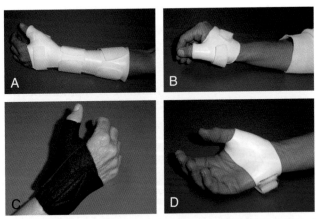

Figure 5A-22. Splinting for insufficient thumb opposition/palmar abduction. **A,** Thermoplastic forearm-based static thumb splint immobilizing the wrist, CMC, and MP. **B,** Thermoplastic hand-based static thumb splint immobilizing the CMC and MP. **C,** Neoprene hand-based Comfort Cool static thumb splint immobilizing the CMC and MP. **D,** Hand-based static thumb splint immobilizing the CMC.

C. Modalities

  1. Paraffin: Can be useful for pain relief and can be done at home after one trial and patient education in clinic.

Thumb Carpometacarpal Accessory Hypermobility Syndrome

In the thumb CMC accessory hypermobility syndrome, pain is located at the CMC joint, but the alignment and movement impairments occur at all joints of the thumb. The CMC joint may be either extended/abducted or adducted/flexed. The impairments at the CMC joint are associated with either (1) MP flexion with IP extension or (2) MP extension with IP flexion and result in loss of the normal longitudinal arch of the thumb. This movement pattern is due to an inability to coordinate the timing and sequencing of the movements between the IP, MP, and

Symptoms and History

- Pain in area of CMC joint of thumb exacerbated by pinching activities
- Weakness secondary to pain noted with use of thumb

If associated with DJD of CMC of thumb, slowly developing joint pain, stiffness, and limitation of motion

Activities/Populations

- May see hairdressers or others that perform activities requiring repetitive pinch or gripping with thumb adducted
- Writing
- Surgeons
- Chronic loading of joint surfaces or alteration in mechanical forces across the joint
- Many patients with this syndrome are young with hypermobile joints
- DJD of CMC of thumb is more common in women than men[9,48]

Common Referring Diagnoses

- Thumb pain
- Wrist pain
- DJD of CMC of thumb
  - Eaton's Stage I or II[31]
- Thumb arthritis
- Basal joint arthritis or pain

Key Tests and Signs for Movement Impairment

Alignment Analysis[37-39,46]

- Thumb CMC resting alignment of:
  - CMC adduction/flexion
  - CMC abduction/extension
- Impairments at CMC joint are associated with either:
  - MP flexion with IP extension
  - MP hyperextension with IP flexion

Movement Impairment Analysis

- Unable to maintain the arc of pinch during functional activities and produces symptoms
  - The CMC joint remains in an extended/abducted position: Associated MP joint flexion and IP joint hyperextension or
  - The CMC joint collapses into adduction/flexion: Associated with MP hyperextension with IP flexion or associated with MP flexion with IP extension
  Correction of arc of pinch decreases or abolishes symptoms at CMC joint.
- During active thumb extension*:
  - CMC extends relatively more (amount and timing) than MP (MP flexion with IP extension looks like boutonnière)[37] or
  - MP extends relatively more than CMC (MP hyperextension with IP flexion looks like swan neck)[1]
- During active thumb flexion:
  - CMC is flexing more readily than MP or
  - CMC remains in abducted and extended position, while the MP joint flexes excessively and the IP joint hyperextends
- During thumb palmar abduction: MP abducts relatively more than CMC
Correction of movement impairments listed in the preceding bullets decreases or abolishes symptoms. Correction of the alignment or movement pattern at the CMC joint may not be optimal without simultaneous correction at adjacent joints such as the MP.

Joint Integrity

Range of Motion/Muscle Length

Generally, in this syndrome, limitation of ROM is not a problem. More commonly, excessive ROM is noted. However, if the ROM is limited, the limitation is slight.
- AROM equals PROM
- During PROM, particular attention is paid to differences in stiffness compared to the opposite side
- Thumb abduction[49] and extension may be slightly limited and painful at CMC
- PROM: Relatively stiff or short adductor pollicis and/or FPB
In some cases:
- Stiff or limited MP extension and excessive IP extension or
- Stiff or limited MP flexion and excessive IP flexion

Joint Accessory Mobility

- Hypermobility of the CMC joint[18]

Ligament Integrity

- Ligament laxity

Other Special Tests

- Swanson's crank and grind test[33,40] (compression):
  - Positive as articular degeneration advances
  - Pain and crepitus or instability
- Distraction and rotation of the MC on the trapezium may reproduce pain in the earlier stages[31]

Muscle Strength/Performance Impairments

Pinch Strength/MMT

- Insufficient muscle performance of OP, APL, and APB relative to adductor pollicis, and FPB may not be detectable on MMT but identified based on functional pattern of use
- Possible insufficient muscle performance of first DI[18]
- Weak EPB

*Refer to Magee, 1997[20] or Goodman, 2007[21] for a comprehensive list of other potential differential diagnoses that might present with neuro-muscular changes or edema of the hand.

CMC joints of the thumb and adaptive changes in the tissues. Correction of the impairments decreases the symptoms. The adductor pollicis and FPB are frequently overused relative to the APL, APB, OP, EPB, and FPL. Patients assigned to this diagnosis must have a modifiable movement pattern. This diagnosis is not intended for patients with neurological injury or those in the later stages of arthritis.

Source of Signs and Symptoms

CMC Joint

- Preferred pattern of movement of thumb CMC adduction/flexion or CMC extension/abduction reproduces pain.
- Correction by restoring the normal arc of the thumb decreases symptoms.
- The thumb CMC joint may be slightly prominent and swollen.
- The thumb CMC joint accessory motion impairments are variable but will likely be decreased in some direction.[36]
- There may be tenderness to palpation of the CMC joint along the entire joint margin but especially over the radiovolar margin of the CMC joint.[31]
- Crepitus may also be palpable with ROM.[31]
- Pinch strength: Decreased and painful.[50]

Associated Signs or Contributing Factors

If associated with DJD of CMC of thumb, may note Heberden's nodes on DIP joints and Bouchard's nodes on PIP joints of fingers.[40]

Differential Diagnosis

Movement System Impairment Diagnosis

- Hand impairment
- Insufficient thumb opposition or abduction

Potential Diagnosis Requiring Referral Suggested by Signs and Symptoms

Neuromusculoskeletal*

- DJD of CMC of Thumb (OA)
- Volar plate injury at MP or IP joints of thumb
- Ligament sprain (grade III)
- Focal dystonia
- de Quervain's tendinopathy
- Fracture
- Dislocation
- CTS

Edema Caused by Neuromusculoskeletal Problems[20]

- Hemiplegia
- Cervical rib
- TOS

Visceral

Edema Caused by Visceral Problems[20]

- Neoplasms
- Cardiovascular disease
- Renal disease
- Hepatic disease
- Aneurysm
- Raynaud's phenomenon

Systemic

- Gout[21]
- RA[21]

Treatment for Thumb CMC Accessory Hypermobility

Patient Education

- Maintain arc of thumb during active, functional, and resisted isometric thumb movements.
- Work with patient during the therapy visits on correcting and practicing the movement pattern during the functional activity that is causing the problem. The symptoms should not be reproduced with correct alignment and movement patterns.
- Joint protection (see below).

Exercises

Exercises are recommended, especially for Stages I and II in which the joint is not already subluxed. The focus of the exercises is increasing the performance (timing) of the underused muscle. In doing so, the extensibility of the antagonistic muscle is simultaneously increased (stretched). The exercises are used to correct the movement patterns, thus balancing the mechanical forces to which the joint is subjected.[40]

Recommendations have been made to begin isometric and then progressive resistive exercises for palmar abduction after the acute symptoms have subsided. The goal is to help to stabilize the thumb CMC joint subluxation.[51]

Strengthening of the APL helps maintain stability of the thumb CMC joint: Work on active contraction in the correct alignment. The APL helps to maintain stability of the joint if the joint is aligned well. The APB places the thumb in the position of maximal stability of the thumb CMC joint.[50-52] The angle of pull of the first dorsal interosseous muscle is such that it would stabilize the base of the first metacarpal from dorsoradial subluxation.[18]

Exercises to correct arc of thumb are as follows (for figures refer to main text of chapter):

During active thumb *extension* if movement impairment is as follows:

- CMC extends relatively more (amount and timing) than MP (boutonnière), then cue to:
  - Avoid excessive CMC extension (decrease use of APL).
  - Increase MP extension (increase use of EPB).
  - Avoid IP extension (increase use of FPL, decrease use of thumb intrinsics).
- MP extends relatively more than CMC (swan neck), then cue to:
  - Increase CMC extension and abduction (increase use of APL).
  - Increase IP extension (increase use of EPL).
  - Avoid excessive MP extension (increase use of FPB).
- CMC adducts; EPL dominates over APL, then cue to:
  - Abduct CMC slightly during extension (increase use of APL).

During active thumb *flexion*, if movement impairment is as follows:

- MP flexes relatively more than IP and CMC (boutonnière), then cue to:
  - Increase flexion at IP (increase use of FPL) and CMC.
  - Avoid excessive MP flexion and IP extension (decrease use of thumb intrinsics).
- CMC is relatively more flexible than MP; CMC flexes and adducts, MP extends, and IP flexes excessively (swan neck), then cue to:
  - Maintain CMC in extension and abduction (increase use of APL).
  - Flex MP (increase use of FPB at longer length). *Correction of proximal joint alignments should correct IP joint alignment.*
- CMC adducts and supinates then cue to:
  - Keep CMC abducted and in neutral rotation by strengthening the OP and APB to help maintain the neutral rotation when the impairment is thumb supination.

During thumb *palmar abduction*, if movement impairment is as follows:

- MP abducts relatively more than CMC then cue to:
  - Block MP abduction with splint and work on CMC palmar abduction (increase extensibility of adductor pollicis with use of APB).

Once patient is able to correct the movement pattern without added resistance, progress by exercising the muscles noted here with resistive putty or rubber bands. Increase extensibility of stiff muscles by instructing the patient to take frequent breaks to stretch throughout the day and especially during the functional activity that is contributing to the impairment.

Purpose of Splinting[16,28,40]

Splint/taping assists maintaining the arc of the thumb. The first priority is usually to correct the movement impairment with patient education and exercises, but splinting may be a helpful adjunct. The main purpose of a splint is to decrease pain by stabilizing the CMC joint in the correct alignment. The CMC joint is most stable in a position of abduction and opposition. Correcting MP alignment can facilitate correct CMC alignment. Splinting is most effective for patients with Eaton's Stage I or II CMC arthritis. Although thermoplastic splints provide stability to the CMC, the hard plastic in the palm of the hand inhibits function so compromises in the type of splint prescribed, often have to be made to ensure patient compliance with splint use. Additional purposes of splinting are as follows:

- Rest the joint to decrease inflammation and pain.
- Support the joint to alter the stresses on the painful structures.
- Allow more pain-free function.

- Position the thumb with the CMC joint abducted because this is the position of maximal congruence of the joint.
- Splinting at night to increase the extensibility of the adductor pollicis.
- Positioning the MP joint in flexion during splinting may offload the anterior aspect of the first CMC joint.[36,46]

Splint/Taping Options

- Static hand-based thumb postsplint immobilizing MP and CMC (see Figure 5A-22, *B*).
- Static hand-based thumb postsplint immobilizing CMC only (see Figure 5A-22, *D*).
- Static forearm-based thumb spica splint immobilizing MP and CMC (see Figure 5A-22, *A*).
- Taping to support thumb CMC.

Joint Protection/Adaptive Equipment

Joint protection/adaptive equipment can facilitate the correct alignment and movement pattern[40] as follows:

- Modify tools used at work when possible (e.g., hairdressers have different options available regarding scissor styles that help in modifying the movement pattern).
- Avoid strong grip and pinch.
- Use jar opener.
- Use Dycem or rubber pad to increase friction when opening jar.
- Use key holder.
- Build up circumference of grip on handles.
- Built-up pencil decreases range of flexion required.

Finger (or Thumb) Flexion Syndrome with or without Finger Rotation

The principal movement impairment of finger (or thumb) flexion syndrome is the inability to maintain the normal alignment of the finger during finger flexion. This includes one or more of the following: the longitudinal arch, neutral rotation, or neutral abduction/adduction of the finger. The movement impairment occurs during the pain-provoking functional or occupational activity involving grip or resisted isometric finger flexion. The movement pattern may be due to an inability to coordinate the timing and sequencing of the movements, an alteration of the relative amount of motion between the IP and MP joints of the finger, or overuse during a repetitive activity. Finger MP or PIP joint pain associated with rotation is due to insufficient performance of one interossei muscle and overuse of the antagonistic interossei muscle at the same joint.[53] The overused muscle is relatively stiffer than its antagonist. This results

Symptoms and History

With Rotation
- History of repetitive activity involving use of the finger intrinsic muscles
- Pain at MP or PIP joints of the finger is most common in index and small fingers

Without Rotation
- Poorly localized hand, wrist, or forearm symptoms

Activities/ Populations

With Rotation
- Typing on a computer
- Carrying a bag by the handle with the finger in ulnar deviation
- Grasping a golf club
- Cutting hair (hairdressers)
- Musicians

Without Rotation
- Musicians: String players and pianists
- Writing
- Any kind of grip or pinch activity

Common Referring Diagnoses

With Rotation
- Finger MP or PIP joint pain

Key Tests and Signs for Movement Impairment

Alignment Analysis

With Rotation
- Finger rests in supinated or pronated position compared to the uninvolved side or another uninvolved finger

Without Rotation
- Normal finger alignment
- Scapular alignment may be impaired: Depressed, abducted, anteriorly tilted, or internally or downwardly rotated

Movement Impairment Analysis

With Rotation
- During pain-provoking functional or occupational activity involving grip or resisted isometric finger flexion, unable to maintain finger in neutral rotation and in normal longitudinal arc
  - Correction of rotation and restoration of normal longitudinal arc of finger decreases or abolishes symptoms
- Pattern of MP flexion with IP extension (loss of normal longitudinal arc of finger) and ulnar deviation of the MP joint during finger flexion (computer keyboard)
  - Interossei on one side of finger overused relative to ED
  - FDP and FDS underused relative to interossei
- Rotation of the finger noted during resisted isometric finger flexion (e.g., string player)
- During index finger flexion with abduction, the MP tends to adduct and supinate versus staying in neutral rotation (string player)
  - First palmar interossei overused relative to first dorsal interossei

Without Rotation
- During pain-provoking functional or occupational activity involving grip or resisted isometric finger flexion, unable to maintain normal longitudinal arc of finger, transverse arch of hand, and normal scapular alignment
  - Correction: Restoration of normal longitudinal arc of finger and ideal scapular alignment
- Scapular depression, abduction, internal rotation, downward rotation, or tilt
  - Correction: Restoration of normal scapular alignment
- MPs flex with IPs in relative extension
  - Interossei overused relative to FDS, FDP, and ED
- MPs flex with PIP in hyperextension and DIP flexed (swan neck)
  - Interossei overused relative to FDS, FDP, and ED
  - Laxity of PIP volar plate
- PIP flexed and DIP in hyperextension (boutonnière)
  - Overuse of FDS relative to FDP
  - Laxity of DIP volar plate
  - Correction: Restoration of normal finger alignment

Joint Integrity

With and without Rotation
- Active finger flexion, extension, abduction, and adduction
  - Identify movement impairments
- Passive ROM
  - Flexion ROM normal
  - Extension ROM normal
  - Abduction and adduction normal

in the principal impairment of rotation at the painful joint and results from a repetitive activity. Finger AROM and strength are usually normal. Correction of the movement impairments does not always modify symptoms immediately but instead over time. Patients assigned this diagnosis must have a modifiable movement pattern. This diagnosis is not intended for patients with neurological injury or later stages of arthritis. This syndrome can be associated with a scapular movement impairment but the symptoms are not referred from shoulder or neck structures. Restoration of normal scapular alignment is believed to provide proximal stability, allowing distal segments to work optimally by decreasing excessive stresses on distal tissues.

Source of Signs and Symptoms

Muscle Length Tests

Without Rotation

- Muscle length may be normal but relatively stiffer than the unaffected side

With Rotation

Interossei length test

- Shortness or relative increased stiffness of interossei on one side of the involved finger
- Long or relatively less stiff interossei on the opposite side of the involved finger

Muscle Strength/Performance Impairments

With Rotation

Resisted tests for soft tissue differential diagnosis

- Painful and weak or strong and painful with resistance to the short interossei muscle on the involved finger

MMT

With Rotation

- Interossei: Relative strength or recruitment differences (timing and amount) on opposite sides of involved finger
- ED, FDS, FDP: Usually strong but recruited relatively less than interossei

Without Rotation

- Interossei, ED, FDS, FDP: Usually strong but depending on the movement impairment, one may be recruited more than the others (timing and amount)

Palpation

With Rotation

- Overused muscle may be tender

Proximal Impairments

With or without Rotation

- Scapular depression, downward rotation, abduction, internal rotation or anterior tilt impairments[57]

Associated Signs or Contributing Factors

Alignment Analysis and Appearance

With Rotation

- May note some edema at the painful joint. Use standard methods to assess the edema[16-18]

With and without Rotation

- May have co-existing MS diagnoses at shoulder and elbow joints
- Generalized characteristics of soft tissue/muscle: Muscles are not well defined and relatively less stiff

Ligament Integrity/Length

Without Rotation

- Oblique retinacular ligament length test
  - May be short with boutonnière-type movement impairment

Differential Diagnosis

Movement System Impairment Diagnosis

With and without Rotation

- Hand impairment
- Insufficient finger flexion
- Insufficient finger extension

Potential Diagnosis Requiring Referral Suggested by Signs and Symptoms

With and without Rotation

*Neuromusculoskeletal**

- OA
- Ligament injury
- Fracture
- Dislocation
- Injury to interossei
- Focal dystonia
- Injury to ED, FDP, FDS

Edema Caused by Neuromusculoskeletal Problems[20]

- Hemiplegia
- Cervical Rib
- TOS

Visceral

Edema Caused by Visceral Problems[20]

- Neoplasms
- Cardiovascular disease
- Renal disease
- Hepatic disease
- Aneurysm
- Raynaud's phenomenon

Systemic

- Gout[21]
- RA[21]

**Symptoms and
History**

Key Tests and Signs for Movement Impairment

Ligament Integrity

With Rotation

• Collateral ligament

Without Rotation

• ORL length test[2,54-56]

• Volar plate

Muscle Length Tests

With and without Rotation

• Interossei muscle length test[2]

• Extrinsic finger flexor length test

• Extrinsic finger extensor length test[2]

Muscle Strength/Performance Impairments

With Rotation

• Resisted tests for soft tissue differential diagnosis[49]

   • Interossei muscle

With and without Rotation

• Strength of pinch: Movement impairments may be evident

• MMT of extrinsic flexors, extensors and intrinsics[13]

   • Relative performance between muscle groups is usually the impairment versus weakness detected
     on a MMT

*Refer to Magee[20] or Goodman[21] for a comprehensive list of other potential differential diagnoses that might present with neuromuscular changes or edema of the hand.

Treatment for Finger (or Thumb) Flexion Syndrome *with Rotation*
Patient Education

- Modifying pattern of grip or finger movement during painful functional activity as follows:
  - Increase the use of the finger flexors versus the interossei if possible.
  - Maintain finger in neutral rotation.
  - Maintain finger in normal longitudinal arc.

Exercises

Stretch or increase the extensibility of the short or stiff interossei—if the first palmar interosseous muscle is short or relatively stiff, abduct the index MP with the MP in extension and the IP joints flexed (Figure 5A-16, *C*).

Work the long or relatively less stiff interossei muscles (e.g., if the first palmar interosseous is short, the first dorsal interosseous muscle may need to be stiffer or strengthened). Working the first DI by abducting the index finger actively while maintaining the MP joint extended and the IP joints flexed would accomplish stretching the first palmar interosseous while strengthening the first DI.

Splinting

Use of a splint to hold the MP joint in extension while the finger is used with the IP joints flexed might be helpful in some instances. (e.g., spring splint used for preventing ulnar deviation at the MP joint).

Treatment for Finger (or Thumb) Flexion Syndrome *without Rotation*
Patient Education

Maintain arc of finger during resisted isometric finger flexion activities while maintaining proper scapular alignment and movement. Work with patient on correcting and practicing the movement pattern during the functional activity that is causing the problem.

Exercises

- Increasing performance (timing) of muscle that is underused (for figures, refer to Chapter 5).
- If movement impairment is the following:
  - MPs flex with IPs in relative extension: Cue to correct arc of finger by increasing MP extension (use of ED) and increasing IP flexion (use of FDP and FDS).
  - MPs flex with PIP in hyperextension and DIP flexed (swan neck): Cue to correct arc of finger by increasing MP extension (use of ED) and increasing PIP flexion (use of FDS).
  - PIP flexed and DIP in hyperextension (boutonnière): Cue to correct arc of finger by increasing DIP flexion (use of FDP).
  - Scapular: Refer to shoulder diagnoses in Sahrmann.[57]
  - Once patient is able to correct the movement pattern without added resistance, progress by exercising the muscles noted above with putty or rubber bands.

Increase extensibility of stiff muscles by taking frequent breaks to stretch throughout the day and especially during the functional activity that is contributing to the impairment.

Splint/taping may be helpful to assist maintaining the arc of the finger. The first priority is usually to correct the movement impairment with patient education and exercises, but splinting may be a helpful adjunct.

- MPs flex with IPs in relative extension: Splint to hold MPs in more extension but allow IP flexion.
- MPs flex with PIP in hyperextension and DIP flexed (swan neck): Splint to prevent PIP hyperextension (oval or buttonhole splint).[28]
- PIP flexed and DIP in hyperextension (boutonnière): Splint to hold PIP in more extension but allow DIP flexion (oval or buttonhole splint).

Source or Regional Impairment of the Hand

The movement system diagnosis "hand impairment" is used when the pathoanatomical source diagnosis is not provided on the referral documentation. The focus of the treatment is protecting the injured tissues. Usually, there is a history of acute trauma or injury to the hand or the patient is in the early in postoperative phase. Medical precautions have been issued, thus the patient's typical movement pattern cannot be assessed at this time. Prognosis is for tissue healing, and normal movement is expected. The determination of the use of component versus compensatory treatment methods depends on the expectations of the final outcome. Initially, while on precautions, compensatory methods may be necessary. The information for the regional impairment of the hand diagnosis in this appendix is intended only as a general guide; therefore the physician's protocol for specific precautions and progression must be consulted. The therapist must be familiar with the tissues that are affected by the surgical procedure and the specific surgical approach.

History

Knowledge of specific surgery, injury, medical diagnosis, and surgical approach

Hand Dominance

Types of Injuries (May Be Treated Initially Conservatively or Surgically)

- Gamekeeper's thumb
- Ligament injuries
- Fractures
- de Quervain's disease
- Boutonnière deformity
- Mallet finger
- OA or DJD of CMC of thumb
- CTS

Types of Surgeries

- *Stabilization:* Indications: Fractures, ligament injuries, pain, instability, deformity, AVN, bony tumors
  - ORIF
  - External fixation
  - Fusion
  - Partial arthrodesis
- *Arthroplasty:* Indications: Joint destruction or deformity secondary to RA, OA, or DJD
  - MP most common
  - LRTI
- *Nerve decompression:* Indications: Median, radial, or ulnar nerve compression resulting in pain, loss of sensation, or motor function
- *Replantation/amputation*
- *Compartment decompression:* Indication: Crush injury with secondary loss of arterial blood flow
- *Repair:* Indications: Tear, avulsion, laceration, rupture
  - Ligament
  - Tendon
  - TFCC
  - Nerve grafts and repair
  - Artery
- *Incision and drainage:* Indication: Infection
- *Tendon transfers:* Indication: Paralysis of a muscle with resultant loss of function
- *Soft tissue release/resection:* Indications: Dupuytren's contracture, adhered tendon resulting in loss of active functional use of hand Synovectomy indicated with prolonged swelling, pain and dysfunction, no evidence of joint destruction
  - Compartment or pulley release (indicated with de Quervain's disease or trigger finger/tenosynovitis)
  - Fasciotomy = compartment release
  - Tenolysis
  - Synovectomy
  - Aspiration or excision (indicated with ganglion)
  - Excision of palmar fascia (indicated with Dupuytren's contracture)
  - Surgical decompression (indicated with intersection syndrome)
  - Skin graft or skin flap with significant loss of soft tissue
- *Medications:* Consider side effects and effects of medications on tissue, examination, and intervention

Key Tests and Assessments

Precautions

- Check physician orders and protocol, including splinting requirements. Respect postoperative positioning.
- Assess patient's ability to adhere to precautions.
- No resisted testing in most cases.

Systemic Signs/Symptoms

- Assess vital signs first visit and then as needed. Avoid taking blood pressure in affected upper extremity. Monitor for hypotension, nausea, and dizziness.

Pain

- Assess pain at rest and with movement:
  - Location
  - Intensity
  - Palpation
- Address regimen of analgesics

Neurological Status

- Establish baseline after surgery

Function

- Assess functional activities that are restricted. With patients who have just had hand surgery, much of this assessment is done initially via the history, but depending on the condition, observation of the specific activity may be appropriate.

Appearance

- *Incision:* May be covered by Steri-Strips, bandages, staples, or may have exposed pins. May have open wound. Note amount and type of drainage.
- *Scar:* Note location, mobility, and sensitivity of scar if incision appears healed (usually after about 10 days).
- *Color:* Note bruising and any other discoloration.
- *Temperature:* Note any deviations from normal.
- *Edema:* Note location and measure extent of edema. Assess whether it is brawny or pitting.

Alignment

- Note resting posture of hand and upper extremity.

Palpation

- Perform once incision is healed.

ROM

- Assess ROM of involved hand and wrist (within precautions) and all other upper extremity joints.

Muscle Recruitment/Strength Impairments

- Impairments in AROM or strength may be significant but are NOT the focus of treatment until precautions are lifted or PROM is increased enough to begin strengthening.

Associated Signs

Variations

- Anthropomorphics

Alignment

- Common for scapula to be abducted, humerus adducted and medially rotated, forearm pronated, and wrist flexed equals guarded posture

Movement Impairments

- Consider the possible underlying movement impairment during the initial phase of recovery; confirmed once the precautions are lifted

Underlying Movement Impairment Syndromes

- Insufficient finger or thumb flexion
- Insufficient finger or thumb extension
- Insufficient thumb opposition/abduction
- Thumb CMC accessory hypermobility
- Finger flexion syndrome with or without rotation

Medical Complications

- Infection
- Nonunion of fracture
- Rupture of surgical repair
- Nerve injuries
- CRPS (RSD)

General Hand Impairment Treatment Guidelines*

Moderators

Age, quality of tissue at repair site and tension on repair, extent of injury (degree of soft tissue involvement), location of injury, duration of immobilization, and surgical approach are moderators that should be considered. The patient may have an increased healing time with osteoporosis, a history of diabetes, or steroid use.

Impairments (Body Functions and Structures)
Pain

Stage 1 (surgical or acute injury): Within the first 2 weeks of the postoperative period, some pain will be associated with the exercises. (In contrast to the nonsurgical patient, in whom pain should not be reproduced with exercise.) Gradually, over the next few weeks, pain associated with the exercise should lessen. Pain should not be severe and should not be increased for more than 1 hour after exercise. Exercise can also help decrease complaints of stiffness. Severe pain can indicate being too aggressive with exercises. After a tenolysis, the patient must be able to work through pain to maintain the tendon glide.[22] Complaints of increasing pain, pain that is not decreasing with treatment, or burning pain are all "red flag" indicators that treatment is too aggressive or there is a disruption in the usual course of healing (e.g., CRPS/RSD, nonunion of fracture, and so on). Coordinating the use of analgesics with exercise sessions is important. Splinting may be used during this period to protect the injured tissue.

Stages 2 to 3: Pain associated with the specific tissue that was involved in the surgery should be significantly decreased by weeks 4 to 6. Precautions may be lifted during or by postoperative weeks 4 to 6. As the exercises and activities of the patient are progressed, pain should be monitored closely. Although the patient may still have some increased pain with activity, the patient should report a decrease in pain overall, despite the increase in activity.

Edema

Stage 1 (surgical or acute injury): *Early management of edema is the key to a successful outcome of therapy for a postoperative hand patient.* The hand must be elevated above the level of the heart as much as possible. AROM, splinting to immobilize and rest the tissue, compressive garments or wraps, milking massage, and/or ice or other modalities may help decrease the edema. Caution must be used in donning a compressive garment when precautions regarding motion are present. An increase in edema or edema that is not decreasing with treatment are indications that exercises are too aggressive. This could also be an indicator of an infection. If infection is suspected, the physician should be contacted immediately.

Stages 2 to 3: Edema should decrease significantly in the first 2 to 4 weeks after surgery. Some edema, however, may persist for several months. As activities and exercises are progressed, the edema should continue to decrease gradually.

Appearance

Stage 1 (surgical or acute injury): Infection should be suspected if the area around the incision or the involved joint appears to be red, hot, and swollen.[58] The physician should be consulted immediately if infection is suspected. The incision will have stitches for the first 7 to 14 days. The patient may also have pins that protrude from the finger. Bruising is not uncommon postoperatively. Changes in hair growth, perspiration, or color may indicate some disturbance to the sympathetic nervous function, especially in combination with the complaint of excessive pain.[59] However, dark hair growth on the arm after casting is very common. *Stages 2 to 3:* The incision should be well healed. Bruising should be diminishing. Signs of increased bruising are a red flag and the patient should be immediately referred to the physician.

Scar

Stage 1 (surgical linear scars): Scarring, although a normal process of healing, must be managed well in the hand or it can severely limit function. Gliding between adjacent structures in the hand must occur to allow good motion and function. Early management of scar contributes to a good outcome. Exercise, massage, compression, silicone gel sheets, and vibration are used in the management of scar. The use of silicone gel is best supported by evidence in the literature. However, clinical experts also commonly use the other methods of scar management. Further research is needed to determine the efficacy of these other methods. The gradual application of stress to the scar or incision helps the scar remodel so that it allows the necessary gliding between structures. A dry incision that has been closed and reopens as a result of the stresses applied with scar massage indicates that the scar massage is too aggressive. Scars may be classified according to type. Linear scars that are immature are confined to the area of the incision. They may be raised and pink or reddish in the remodeling phase. As they mature, they become whitish and flatten. A hypersensitive scar requires desensitization. See Box 5-2 for treatment guidelines on managing scar.

Stages 2 to 3: A scar may continue to remodel for up to 2 years.[19] Scar management techniques may be effective until the scar matures, although they are probably most effective early in the healing process.

---

*These principles of treatment for the hand were developed with input from the following clinical experts: Cheryl Caldwell, PT, DPT, CHT; Renee Ivens, PT DPT; Ann Kammien, PT, CHT; Cindy Glaenzer, PT, CHT; and Marcie Harris Hayes, PT, DPT.

Range of Motion

Stage 1

- *The key to a successful outcome is early motion.* The typical position of a stiff hand is with the MPs extended, IPs flexed, and thumb adducted (loss of first web space). Prevention of the stiff hand is the key.
- Depending on the type of injury, the patient may have ROM precautions per physician order to protect the healing tissues. Splinting is commonly used to adhere to the ROM precautions yet allow initiation of exercise soon after surgery. Generally the exercises are done frequently throughout the day within pain tolerance.
- The typical exercise progression starts with active, progresses to passive to increase the stretch, and then to resistive ROM (tendon injuries are an exception to this rule). Progression through the continuum is based primarily on the healing of the involved tissues. If there has been a tendon repair, the progression may be passive exercise before active. Composite stretches of the repaired tendon must be avoided in the early healing phase. The tissues must be allowed to heal and adapt to gradual application of stress. Active contraction of a repaired tendon is also often avoided, although this depends on several factors such as choice of suture material and method. Communication with the surgeon regarding the repair technique helps direct the choice of exercise.
- When performing ROM exercises on a finger with a fracture attention to finger placement during the exercises can minimize the stresses placed on the healing fracture site. Point tenderness to palpation at the fracture site indicates that the fracture is not well healed.
- When working on ROM at one joint, it is helpful to block the adjacent joints so they cannot move. This is based on the principle that the body takes the path of least resistance. The joint that moves most easily will move first and the most, so to increase the ROM at a stiffer joint, the more flexible joint must be stabilized. This can be done manually, using a splint or a Bunnell block.
- All uninvolved upper extremity joints should be exercised to prevent the development of restricted ROM at those joints.
- Decreasing pain and edema and improving ROM are usually signs that it is okay to progress the exercises. Refer to the specific diagnostic syndrome for guidelines regarding progression of the exercises.
- Joint mobilization may be a useful technique to facilitate increases in ROM. Consult with the physician before initiating joint mobilization after a fracture or joint injury.

Stages 2 to 3: Precautions regarding ROM will usually be lifted sometime in the first 6 weeks after surgery or injury so there are no precautions by this stage. Once precautions have been lifted, if there is a plateau in the improvement of ROM with the use of active exercise, exercises are progressed to passive. If ROM is still not improving by at least 10 degrees per week, then static progressive or dynamic splinting should be initiated. Increasing ROM may still be the primary focus of treatment, although strengthening can begin through increased functional use.

Strength

Stage 1: Generally, strengthening is not done during the first 4 to 6 weeks after an injury or surgery. During Stage 1, focus instead is either on immobilization, decreasing edema, scar management, or on gaining ROM, with the correct movement pattern. Occasionally, light resistance is used to increase the recruitment of a muscle versus overload and strengthening. If this is done, it should not violate any precautions that are still in force.

Stages 2 to 3: It is generally safe to begin strengthening exercises 6 weeks after a surgery or fracture. The specific protocol or the physician should be consulted for the exact time when strengthening can be initiated. Once the physician has lifted any precautions related to strengthening, progression to resistive exercise is based on the patient's ability to perform AROM with a good movement pattern and without a significant increase in pain relative to the pain produced with the same movement without resistance. Refer to specific protocols for guidelines regarding progression to resistance. Vital signs should be monitored when initiating an upper extremity resistive exercise program, particularly at higher levels such as using the BTE.

Coordination

Stage 1: Exercises focusing on coordination are generally not initiated until later in the rehabilitation phase.

Stages 2 to 3: Often, specific exercises for coordination are not necessary. The patient will regain their coordination through increasing the functional use of their hand, as well as through the exercises prescribed for regaining ROM and strength. However, in certain instances, specific exercises for coordination may be useful. One example of this would be a patient who is learning to use his or her nondominant hand as his or her dominant hand. This patient may require specific writing exercises.

Cardiovascular and Muscular Endurance

Stage 1: Patients may become deconditioned after a severe hand injury. Resuming or initiating an exercise program, such as walking, to increase cardiovascular endurance is indicated as soon as pain allows, assuming the exercise does not violate any precautions related to the tissue healing.

Stages 2 to 3: The intensity, duration, and frequency of the exercise can be progressed as tolerated. Cardiovascular endurance exercises may have an added benefit of helping decrease pain and generally increase the patient's feeling of well-being.

Patient Education

Stages 1 to 3: The patient will need to be educated regarding the specific medical precautions, how to maintain precautions during hygiene, and the definition of PROM or assisted AROM. Educate the patient regarding the structures and tissues involved. Use of a hand model, anatomical pictures, handouts, and books are helpful. Also, the patient must be educated regarding the care, use, precautions, schedule for use, and how to don and doff his or her splints.

Changes in Status

Stages 1 to 3: Consider reports of increased pain or edema, decreased strength, or significant change in ROM carefully, especially in combination. The patient should be questioned regarding precipitating events (e.g., time of onset, activity, and so on). If the integrity of the surgery is in doubt, contact the physician promptly. If patient has fever and erythema spreading from the incision, the physician should be contacted because of the possibility of an infection.

Function (Activity Limitations/ Participation Restrictions)

General Guidelines

Stage 1: Early functional use of the hand must be encouraged while protecting the healing tissue. Educate the patient regarding precautions/restrictions and use of the involved extremity during ADLs such as eating, bathing, dressing, work, and so on). Educate patient regarding the use of splint as needed.

Stages 2 to 3: Once any precautions have been lifted, the patient may need to be instructed to specifically return to using the hand functionally since he or she may avoid using the hand because of habit.

Specific Suggestions

Writing

Stage 1: If the dominant hand is involved, the patient will frequently be unable to write in the immediate postoperative period. He or she may need to learn to write with their other hand temporarily.

Stages 2 to 3: Using a pen or pencil with a larger circumference is helpful if ROM is limited or grip is painful. This can be accomplished by purchasing a pen with a larger circumference or building up the pen with foam.

Driving

Stage 1: Patients are usually unable to drive in the immediate postoperative period.

Stages 2 to 3: Most patients will be able to return to driving without special treatment related to driving if they have regained their hand ROM, grip, and pinch strength. The patient should practice in their own driveway before returning to driving on the streets. If needed,

once precautions are lifted, driving can be simulated on the BTE. If weakness is a limiting factor, task-specific strengthening can be done using the BTE.

Work and Sports

Stage 1: Many patients will be off work and unable to participate in sports during the immediate postoperative period. During the postoperative period, their rehabilitation is their "job" because it can be quite time consuming, especially with involved injuries. When the patient is cleared to return to work or sports, he or she should be instructed in gradual resumption of activities.

Stages 2 to 3: If the patient has a job that places high demands on strength or endurance, the BTE is a useful exercise tool. Strengthening can be initiated using the BTE once ROM has plateaued or returned to normal, the patient is able to perform light ADLs without problems and isolated strengthening has been initiated without an increase in pain. Many hand patients will be deconditioned if they have had a severe injury, so vital signs should be monitored when initiating resistive exercises to the upper extremity. Many hand patients also develop shoulder pain. Shoulder alignment and movement should be examined and any movement impairments corrected before initiating overhead resistive exercises. The alignment and movement of the shoulder and trunk should be monitored closely during the exercises on the BTE. Some patients will be able to return to work with "light duty" restrictions before regaining full strength and endurance. Sport-specific exercises can be initiated and progressed gradually once precautions are lifted. The patient may require a protective splint that is acceptable for the sport until full healing and rehabilitation have been completed.

Eating

Stage 1: Patients may require assistance or they may be able to eat independently using the opposite extremity. Foam can be used to build up utensils. During therapy practice sessions, resistive putty can be used to build up the utensil.

Stages 2 to 3: Once precautions have been lifted, the patient should be encouraged to use the affected hand with the normal pattern while eating.

Sleeping

Stage 1: The involved side should be supported with a pillow under the arm, keeping the hand higher than the heart to minimize edema. Sleep is usually significantly disrupted in the immediate postoperative period.

Stages 2 to 3: Once the edema has resolved or is minimal, the patient can return to sleeping in their preferred position without elevating the hand.

Support and Splinting

Stage 1: Splinting is used extensively but judiciously after surgeries or injuries to protect the healing tissue, yet allow as much ROM and functional use of the extremity as possible. It is very important to have a splint that fits well and is appropriate for the diagnosis. The patient must be educated in the use, precautions, and care of the splint. They must be taught how to don and doff the splint. Use of slings with patients with hand injuries is avoided to minimize problems with the shoulder and to minimize edema in the hand.

Stages 2 to 3: Static progressive or dynamic splinting may be used during this stage to help increase ROM. Protective splinting may be required to facilitate an earlier return to sports or work.

Hygiene

Stages 1 to 3: Patients may need assistance with bathing and other hygiene activities or they may be independent using the opposite extremity. Giving suggestions may be appreciated and helpful.

Medications/Modalities
Medications

During the immediate postoperative phase, physical therapy treatment should be timed with analgesics. This is particularly important in the first 2 weeks after tenolysis, so the patient is able to work through pain to maintain the ROM gains achieved during the surgery.

Communication with the physician is vital to provide optimal pain relief for the patient.

Whirlpool Treatment[25]

In general, use of whirlpools for treatment of patients with hand injuries is contraindicated because both the dependent position of the hand in the whirlpool and the warm water temperature encourage increased edema in the hand. If a whirlpool must be used, the water temperature should be no warmer than 98° F.

Paraffin or Hot Pack Treatment[25]

The patient's hand should be elevated while receiving either of these heat modalities to prevent an increase of edema. Paraffin can be used with the hand wrapped in a flexed position with Coban to increase the extensibility of the structures limiting finger flexion.

Electrical Stimulation[25]

Electrical stimulation is used by some clinical hand experts to increase tendon gliding and increase strength.

Tissue Factors

	Muscle/Tendon	Ligament/Capsule	Bone
Stress increased	Resistive ROM End-range stretch AROM PROM Immobilization	End-range stretch, regardless if active, passive, or resistive	Resistive ROM Active or passive depends on the fracture location in relation to the muscle insertion or forces applied during passive motion

Bone

The key to a good outcome is early active motion without compromising the stability of the fracture. Communicate with the physician regarding the adequacy of stabilization of the fracture (e.g., ORIF). Sometimes AROM can be begin as early as 5 to 15 days postoperative. Progression to PROM and static progressive or dynamic splinting is determined by x-ray (once the fracture is fairly well healed). Progression to strengthening is done once ROM is pretty good and fracture is well healed (usually 6 to 8 weeks). Generally, the joints proximal and distal to the fracture are immobilized when using a splint or cast.

Ligament

The key to a good outcome is prevention of shortness or adherence of the ligaments in the joints that are immobilized and maintenance of ROM at the upper extremity joints that are not immobilized. The typical posture of the stiff hand is with the MPs in extension, the IPs flexed, and the thumb adducted. In this position the collateral ligaments at the MPs get short or adhered, and the volar plate and accessory collateral ligaments at the IPs get short or adhered. Whenever possible, immobilize the hand in the functional position (MP flexion, IP extension, and thumb abduction) to maintain the length of the ligaments and to maintain the first web space. Recognize, however, that

this position of immobilization will contribute to the development of intrinsic muscle shortness so exercises to correct this may need to be prescribed once the immobilization is no longer necessary.[16]

Nerve

Postoperatively, the tension on the nerve repair must be avoided, and this is done with immobilization using a splint. Early motion is started while protecting the site of repair. Nerves, whether repaired or normal, are sensitive to stretch so it is better to use an oscillatory motion during exercises rather than a prolonged stretch.[60] Patients may need education regarding skin protection when there is sensory loss, sensory re-education, or desensitization. Return of sensibility and motor function is tested periodically to document progress. Refer to a text on hand rehabilitation for more information about this topic.[61] Another consideration related to nerves is the edematous hand. Edema may cause compression of nerve.

Cartilage

Grinding or crepitus may be a sign of loss of or damage to cartilage in the joint.

Skin

Edema in the hand takes up excess laxity in the dorsal skin, contributing to decreased finger and thumb ROM.[16]

Immobility of the skin caused by edema or scarring must be prevented to maximize ROM.

Wound care: Wound care of the incision or care of pin sites is often an important part of the treatment of the postoperative hand. Pin and suture care may be needed. In some settings, the therapist will remove sutures at the time ordered by the physician. The incision should be monitored for drainage or sutures that have become inflamed. At the time of the first PT visit, bulky dressings may need to be removed and replaced with a lighter dressing. Enough dressing should be used just to absorb any drainage. Generally, the lighter and less restrictive the dressing, the better. A bulky dressing restricts ROM. Check with the physician for his or her preferences regarding wound care and dressing changes. Watch for any maceration of the skin from straps, splints, or wound dressings.

Muscle

Positions of immobilization to protect the healing muscles and/or tendons may result in subsequent muscle shortness or tendon adhesions. After the initial postoperative period of precautions, examination should be done to check for muscle shortness and tendon adhesions. Exercises and splinting should be implemented to correct the impairment as necessary. The first web space is commonly decreased with swelling, resulting in shortness of the thumb adductor. Generally, function after a laceration and repair of a muscle is restored more easily than after laceration and repair of a tendon.

Tendon

The key to a good outcome after tendon repair or tenolysis is preserving tendon gliding by starting early protected ROM.[4,22]

Tendon Repairs

Protocols for treatment s/p tendon repairs depend on the zone of the tendon in which the injury occurred. Healing tendons have their weakest tensile strength between 5 to 15 days after repair. The amount of tension that can be placed on the repaired tendon also depends on the type of suture and repair, the condition of the tendon at the time of repair, and so on. It is important to maintain full finger joint ROM while avoiding placing excessive stresses on the repaired tendon until it has healed sufficiently. Full PIP ROM is important for good differential tendon glide between the FDS and FDP. Splinting is used the first few weeks to prevent excessive stresses on the repaired tendon. If the patient is not getting good tendon gliding and seems to have a lot of scarring, they may need to be progressed faster than the guidelines provide on the protocol. If the patient has good motion and little scarring, the timeframes on the protocol may need to be more conservative.

REFERENCES

1. Knight SL: Assessment and management of swan neck deformity, *Int Congr Ser* 1295:154-157, 2006.

2. Aulicino PL: Clinical examination of the hand. In Mackin EJ, Callahan A, Osterman AL, et al, eds: *Rehabilitation of the hand and upper extremity*, ed 5, St Louis, 2002, Mosby.

3. Culp RW, Taras JS: Primary care of flexor tendon injuries. In Mackin EJ, Callahan A, Osterman AL, et al, eds: *Rehabilitation of the hand and upper extremity*, ed 5, St Louis, 2002, Mosby.

4. Stewart Pettengill KM, van Strien G: Postoperative management of flexor tendon injuries. In Mackin EJ, Callahan A, Osterman AL, et al, eds: *Rehabilitation of the hand and upper extremity*, ed 5, St Louis, 2002, Mosby.

5. Innis PC: Surgical management of the stiff hand. In Mackin EJ, Callahan A, Osterman AL, et al, eds: *Rehabilitation of the hand and upper extremity*, ed 5, St Louis, 2002, Mosby.

6. Rosenthal EA: The extensor tendons: anatomy and management. In Mackin EJ, Callahan A, Osterman AL, et al, eds: *Rehabilitation of the hand and upper extremity*, ed 5, St Louis, 2002, Mosby.

7. Cambridge-Keeling CA: Range-of-motion measurement of the hand. In Mackin EJ, Callahan A, Osterman AL, et al, eds: *Rehabilitation of the hand and upper extremity*, ed 5, St Louis, 2002, Mosby.

8. Tubiana R, Thomine J, Mackin E: *Examination of the hand and wrist*, ed 2, London, 1996, Informa Healthcare.

9. Neumann DA: *Kinesiology of the musculoskeletal system: foundations for physical rehabilitation*, St Louis, 2002, Mosby.

10. Littler JW, Eaton RG: Redistribution of forces in the correction of boutonnière deformity, *J Bone Joint Surg Am* 49(7):1267-1274, 1967.

11. Matev I: The boutonnière deformity, *Hand* 11(2):90-95, 1969.

12. Stanley J: Boutonnière deformity, *J Bone Joint Surg Br* 86(Supp III):216a, 2004.

13. Kendall FP, McCreary EK, Provence PG, et al: *Muscles: testing and function with posture and pain*, ed 5, Baltimore, 2005, Lippincott Williams & Wilkins.

14. Campbell PJ, Wilson RL: Management of joint injuries and intraarticular fractures. In Mackin EJ, Callahan A, Osterman AL, et al, eds: *Rehabilitation of the hand and upper extremity*, ed 5, St Louis, 2002, Mosby.

15. Alter S, Feldon P, Terrono AL: Pathomechanics of deformities in the arthritic hand and wrist. In Mackin EJ, Callahan A, Osterman AL, et al, eds: *Rehabilitation of the hand and upper extremity*, ed 5, St Louis, 2002, Mosby.

16. Colditz JC: Anatomic considerations for splinting the thumb. In Mackin EJ, Callahan A, Osterman AL, et al, eds: *Rehabilitation of the hand and upper extremity*, ed 5, St Louis, 2002, Mosby.

17. Villeco JP, Mackin EJ, Hunter JM: Edema: therapist's management. In Mackin EJ, Callahan A, Osterman AL, et al, eds: *Rehabilitation of the hand and upper extremity*, ed 5, St Louis, 2002, Mosby.

18. Brand PW, Hollister AM: *Clinical mechanics of the hand*, ed 3, St Louis, 1999, Mosby.

19. Mustoe TA, Cooter RD, Gold MH, et al: International clinical recommendations on scar management, *Plast Reconstr Surg* 1102:560-571, 2002.

20. Magee DJ: *Orthopedic physical assessment*, ed 3, Philadelphia, 1997, Saunders.

21. Goodman CC, Snyder TEK: *Differential diagnosis for physical therapists: screening for referral*, ed 4, St Louis, 2007, Saunders.

22. Mackin EJ, Callahan A, Osterman AL, et al, eds: *Rehabilitation of the hand and upper extremity*, ed 5, St Louis, 2002, Mosby.

23. Fess EE: Documentation: essential elements of an upper extremity assessment battery. In Mackin EJ, Callahan A, Osterman AL, et al, eds: *Rehabilitation of the hand and upper extremity*, ed 5, St Louis, 2002, Mosby.

24. Evans RB: Clinical management of extensor tendon injuries. In Mackin EJ, Callahan A, Osterman AL, et al, eds: *Rehabilitation of the hand and upper extremity*, ed 5, St Louis, 2002, Mosby.

25. Michlovitz SL: Ultrasound and selected physical agent modalities in upper extremity rehabilitation. In Mackin EJ, Callahan A, Osterman EL, et al, eds: *Rehabilitation of the hand and upper extremity*, ed 5, St Louis, 2002, Mosby.

26. LaStayo PC: Ulnar wrist pain and impairment: a therapist's algorithmic approach to the triangular fibrocartilage complex. In Mackin EJ, Callahan A, Osterman AL, et al, eds: *Rehabilitation of the hand and upper extremity*, ed 5, St Louis, 2002, Mosby.

27. Sandoval R, Kare JA, Washington IE, et al: Swan neck deformity. Available at http://www.emedicine.com/orthoped/topic562.htm. Accessed June 29, 2010.

28. Biese J: Therapist's evaluation and conservative management of rheumatoid arthritis in the hand and wrist. In Mackin EJ, Callahan A, Osterman AL, et al, eds: *Rehabilitation of the hand and upper extremity*, ed 5, St Louis, 2002, Mosby.

29. Skirven TM, Callahan AD: Therapist's management of peripheral nerve injuries. In Mackin EJ, Callahan A, Osterman AL, et al, eds: *Rehabilitation of the hand and upper extremity*, ed 5, St Louis, 2002, Mosby.

30. Cannon NM, Beal BG, Walters KJ, et al: *Diagnosis and treatment manual for physicians and therapists: upper extremity rehabilitation*, ed 4, Indianapolis, 2001, The Hand Rehabilitation Center of Indiana.

31. Eaton RG, Glickel SZ: Trapeziometacarpal osteoarthritis. Staging as a rationale for treatment, *Hand Clin* 3(4):455-471, 1987.

32. Wajon A, Ada L, Edmunds I: Surgery for thumb (trapeziometacarpal joint) osteoarthritis, *Cochrane Database Syst Rev* (4):CD004631, 2005.

33. Swanson AB: Disabling arthritis at the base of the thumb: treatment by resection of the trapezium and flexible (silicone) implant arthroplasty, *J Bone Joint Surg Am* 54(3):456-471. 1972.

34. Tomaino MM, Pellegrini VD Jr, Burton RI: Arthroplasty of the basal joint of the thumb. Long-term follow-up after ligament reconstruction with tendon interposition, *J Bone Joint Surg Am* 77(3):346-355, 1995.

35. Eaton CJ, Lister GD: Radial nerve compression, *Hand Clin* 8(2):345-357, 1992.

36. Kovler M, Lundon K, McKee N, et al: The human first carpometacarpal joint: osteoarthritic degeneration and 3-dimensional modeling, *J Hand Ther* 17(4):393-400, 2004.

37. Nalebuff EA: Diagnosis, classification and management of rheumatoid thumb deformities, *Bull Hosp Joint Dis* 29(2):119-137, 1968.

38. Terrono AL: The rheumatoid thumb, *J Am Soc Surg Hand* 1(2):81-92, 2001.

39. Tomaino MM: Classification and treatment of the rheumatoid thumb, *Int Congr Ser* 1295:162-168, 2006.

40. Melvin JL. Therapists' management of osteoarthritis in the hand. In Mackin EJ, Callahan A, Osterman AL, et al, eds: *Rehabilitation of the hand and upper extremity*, ed 5, St Louis, 2002, Mosby.

41. Hayes EP, Carney K, Wolf JM, et al: Carpal tunnel syndrome. In Mackin EJ, Callahan A, Osterman AL, et al, eds: *Rehabilitation of the hand and upper extremity*, ed 5, St Louis, 2002, Mosby.

42. Terrono AL, Nalebuff EA, Philips CA: The rheumatoid thumb. In Mackin EJ, Callahan A, Osterman AL, et al, eds: *Rehabilitation of the hand and upper extremity*, ed 5, St Louis, 2002, Mosby.

43. Weiss S, LaStayo P, Mills A, Bramlet D: Splinting the degenerative basal joint: custom-made or prefabricated neoprene? *J Hand Ther* 17(4):401-406, 2004.

44. Wajon A: Clinical splinting successes: the thumb "strap splint" for dynamic instability of the trapeziometacarpal joint, *J Hand Ther* 13(3):236-237, 2000.

45. Galindo A, Lim S: A metacarpophalangeal joint stabilization splint: the Galindo-Lim thumb metacarpophalangeal joint stabilization splint, *J Hand Ther* 15(1):83-84, 2002.

46. Moulton MJ, Parentis MA, Kelly MJ, et al: Influence of metacarpophalangeal joint position on basal joint-loading in the thumb, *J Bone Joint Surg Am* 83(5):709-716, 2001.

47. Colditz JC: The biomechanics of a thumb carpometacarpal immobilization splint: design and fitting, *J Hand Ther* 13(3):228-235, 2000.

48. Pellegrini VD Jr: Pathomechanics of the thumb trapeziometacarpal joint, *Hand Clin* 17(2):175-184, vii-viii, 2001.

49. Cyriax J: *Textbook of orthopaedic medicine*, ed 7, London, 1978, Bailliere Tindall.

50. Poole JU, Pellegrini VD Jr: Arthritis of the thumb basal joint complex, *J Hand Ther* 13(2):91-107, 2000.

51. Pellegrini VD Jr: Osteoarthritis at the base of the thumb, *Orthop Clin North Am* 23(1):83-102, 1992.

52. Neumann DA, Bielefeld T: The carpometacarpal joint of the thumb: stability, deformity, and therapeutic intervention, *J Orthop Sports Phys Ther* 33(7):386-399, 2003.

53. Schreuders TAR, Brandsma JW, Stam HJ: The intrinsic muscles of the hand: function, assessment and principles for therapeutic intervention, *Phys Med Rehab Kuror* 17:20-27, 2007.

54. Landsmeer JM: The anatomy of the dorsal aponeurosis of the human finger and its functional significance, *Anat Rec* 104(1):31-44, 1949.

55. Shrewsbury MM, Johnson RK: A systematic study of the oblique retinacular ligament of the human finger: its structure and function, *J Hand Surg Am* 2(3):194-199, 1977.

56. Dell PC, Sforzo CR: Ulnar intrinsic anatomy and dysfunction, *J Hand Ther* 18(2):198-207, 2005.

57. Sahrmann SA: *Diagnosis and treatment of movement impairment syndromes*, St Louis, 2002, Mosby.

58. Nathan R, Taras JS: Common infections in the hand. In Mackin EJ, Callahan A, Osterman AL, eds: *Rehabilitation of the hand and upper extremity*, ed 5, St Louis, 2002, Mosby.

59. Koman LA, Smith BP, Smith TL: Reflex sympathetic dystrophy (complex regional pain syndromes: types 1 and 2). In Mackin EJ, Callahan A, Osterman AL, et al, eds: *Rehabilitation of the hand and upper extremity*, ed 5, St Louis, 2002, Mosby.

60. Butler DS: *Mobilisation of the nervous system*, Melbourne, 1994, Churchill Livingstone.

61. Mackin EJ, Callahan A, Osterman AL, eds: *Rehabilitation of the hand and upper extremity*, ed 5, St Louis, 2002, Mosby.

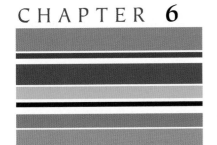

C H A P T E R 6

Movement System Syndromes of the Elbow

Cheryl Caldwell, Lynnette Khoo-Summers

INTRODUCTION

Elbow dysfunctions may be caused by an acute injury or as a result of prolonged or repetitive activities. Effective treatment requires managing the acute tissue injury as well as the underlying movement impairments. Based on years of clinical observations, we have classified the patterns of movement deviations associated with elbow dysfunctions. The classifications are labeled as movement system syndromes. This chapter describes two categories of movement system syndromes: (1) those based on the source or region of the injury and (2) those based on the principal movement system impairment (Box 6-1).

A diagnosis based on the source or pathoanatomy is most commonly used for acute elbow dysfunction and is often provided in the referral. In these cases, a complete movement system examination is not possible. The source diagnosis guides physical therapy treatment is based on established protocols. These protocols are based on stages of tissue healing because they identify the source (pathoanatomical tissue) that is affected and the degree of the injury. The regional diagnosis, elbow impairment is used when the referral does not state the pathoanatomical or source diagnosis for an acute injury (see Box 6-1). After resolution of this early or severe stage of tissue injury, a complete movement system examination should be performed to establish a diagnosis of the principal movement impairment.

A diagnosis based on the principal movement system impairment should also be used for elbow dysfunction caused by prolonged or repetitive activities. These types of slowly developing conditions do not have a protocol for treatment or even an established standardized examination, particularly one that assesses precise movement. The repetitive movements that induce the pain conditions result in slight deviations from precise movement and thus an examination to assess movement characteristics is essential.

The movement system syndromes in this chapter are named for the movement, which produces the symptoms

that when modified decreases the symptoms. This preferred movement pattern is believed to be the cause of the tissue injury. Much of the content within the syndromes is not unique to the experienced therapist, but the content is organized in a unique way by focusing on the movements that are the cause of the symptoms and identifying the cluster of impairments contributing to the imprecise movement pattern. A major objective of the systematic examination of the elbow and forearm is to identify and treat the cause of the dysfunction instead of identifying and treating isolated impairments. For example, if treatment is based on goniometric measurement of active range of motion (AROM) without taking into account precision of the movement, the treatment may not be the most effective and efficient.

In addition to the movement system or source or regional diagnosis, assignment of a stage of rehabilitation helps guide the development of the treatment plan. The staging system is described in Chapter 2.

Knowledge of normal alignment, movement, and muscle function guides the therapist in identifying alignment and movement impairments and prescribing treatment to correct those impairments. Unique to the movement system examination of the elbow and forearm is the emphasis on first evaluating the patient's preferred pattern of movement and correlating this with the onset of symptoms (primary test). The examiner's focus is on identifying the joint that is relatively most flexible and is the cause of the patient's chief complaint. The primary test is immediately followed by a secondary test in which the symptom-provoking preferred pattern of movement is modified to determine the effect on the symptoms. This sequence of testing is performed throughout the examination, as well as during the observation of functional activities. Identifying and modifying the functional activities is critical.

Additional key elements in the examination and treatment of the elbow and forearm for all diagnostic groups presented in this chapter that may be unique are as follows:

BOX 6-1

Movement System Diagnoses for the Elbow

- Wrist extension with forearm pronation (lateral epicondylosis) syndrome
- Elbow hypomobility syndrome
- Elbow flexion syndrome (cubital tunnel syndrome) syndrome
- Elbow valgus syndrome: With or without extension syndrome
- Elbow extension syndrome
- Posterior forearm nerve entrapment syndromes (radial tunnel and posterior interosseous nerve)
- Anterior forearm nerve entrapment syndromes (pronator syndrome and anterior interosseous nerve syndrome)
- Wrist flexion with pronation (medial epicondylosis) syndrome
- Ulnohumeral and radiohumeral multidirectional accessory hypermobility syndrome
- Source or elbow impairment

Conditions that may fall under the regional impairment diagnosis of the elbow when the pathoanatomical or source diagnosis is not provided on the referral documentation are as follows:

INJURIES
- Injuries that may be treated conservatively or surgically initially include ligament or joint injuries, dislocations, fractures, nerve, muscle, and tendon

POSTOPERATIVE
- Stabilization: Indications: Fractures, ligament injuries, pain, instability, deformity, bony tumors
  - ORIF, external fixation, fusion
- Arthroplasty: Indications: Joint destruction or deformity secondary to RA, OA, or DJD
- Nerve decompression: Indications: Median, radial, or ulnar nerve compression resulting in pain, loss of sensation, or motor function
- Replantation/amputation
- Compartment decompression: Indication: Crush injury with secondary loss of arterial blood flow
- Repair: Indications: Tear, avulsion, laceration, rupture
  - Ligament, tendon, nerve (grafts and repair), and artery
- Incision and drainage: Indication: Infection
- Tendon and nerve transfers: Indication: Paralysis of a muscle with resultant loss of function
- Soft tissue release/resection: Indications: Synovectomy with prolonged swelling, pain, and dysfunction, no evidence of joint destruction
  - Compartment release, synovectomy, aspiration or excision, surgical decompression, and skin graft or skin flap with significant loss of soft tissue

DJD, Degenerative joint disease; *OA,* osteoarthritis; *ORIF,* open reduction internal fixation; *RA,* rheumatoid arthritis.

- Identifying the joint that is relatively most flexible[1] and training the patient to move less at the flexible joint and more at the stiffer joint.
  - Example: The concept of relative flexibility is applied in the examination of patients that can be given the

movement system diagnosis elbow hypomobility syndrome. The joint or structure that is stiffest is the least likely to move. Therefore, for treatment to be most effective, the structure or joint that is relatively most flexible (often the shoulder) must be stabilized or made stiffer. The goal is the normal balance of stiffness around the joints and between joints.

- Identifying the repeated or prolonged functional activity that has caused the adaptations in joint flexibility.
- Identifying the specific muscle impairments contributing to the movement dysfunction of the affected joints. Muscle impairments include recruitment, stiffness, changes in length, or weakness.
  - Assessing stiffness[1] throughout the ROM when assessing muscle length instead of solely making a determination of length at the end-range. Stiffness is assessed by comparing muscles on opposite sides of the body, as well as on opposing sides of a joint. A balance of stiffness around the joint is a prerequisite for precise motion at that joint.
  - Increased stiffness or decreased muscle length can cause increased joint compression contributing to the patient's symptoms.
- Identifying the site that is relatively most flexible and alterations in the normal muscle recruitment patterns such as overuse of one synergist compared to another. These are identified both during the individual tests of the examination, functional, work, leisure, and sports activities.
- Identifying alignment and movement impairments in the proximal upper extremity and relating these impairments to the symptomatic elbow and forearm. Proximal impairments may result in increased muscle exertion distally and may place distal nerves at increased risk for injury.[2]
- Restoring the precise pattern of movement in degenerating painful joints to decrease symptoms and the rate of degeneration.[1] This is most effective in the early stages of degeneration. The inevitable process of degeneration progresses through stages, from hypermobility to eventual hypomobility.[3,4] Degeneration occurs because of both intrinsic (genetic) and extrinsic (mechanical) factors. Although it is not possible to stop the process of aging and degeneration, it may be possible to slow or delay the effects of degeneration by changing the extrinsic factors such as movement patterns. Imprecise movement at the elbow and forearm rarely occur in isolation but are also associated with movement impairments at the shoulder.
- Practice during treatment modifying the movement pattern during functional activities and specific exercises.[1]
- Training muscles to stabilize the joint that is relatively too flexible.[1]
  - Increasing or decreasing muscle stiffness to restore the balance of stiffness around a joint.

- Modifying patterns of muscle recruitment (timing, duration, and magnitude).
- If necessary, splints are useful to prevent the site that is relatively most flexible from moving and encouraging movement at the less flexible site.

Symptoms in the elbow and forearm may be referred from the neck, thoracic outlet, or wrist.[2] Therefore the examination of the elbow and forearm should include differentiating whether the source of the symptoms is from the elbow and forearm versus referred from one of these regions.[5]

Edema and scar are impairments that may exist in any of the syndromes and must be addressed for treatment to be effective, but identification of the edema and scar is not critical for assigning the movement system diagnosis.

EXAMINATION AND KEY TESTS

Subjective Examination

During the history, particular attention is paid to questioning the patient regarding the daily activities that are performed repeatedly and those that are associated with increasing and decreasing the symptoms.

Objective Examination

I. Screening[6]
II. Posture and alignment
III. Palpation and appearance: Skin, scar, circulation, edema, atrophy, hypertrophy, and nodules
IV. Functional activities: Work, writing, eating, and dressing
V. Movement analysis*
   A. AROM
      1. Onset of pain
      2. Quality of motion: Movement at one joint more than another
   B. Passive ROM (PROM)
      1. Ligament integrity
      2. Limited ROM caused by shortness of joint structures
      3. Muscle length tests (Box 6-2): When assessing muscle length, particular attention is paid to stiffness throughout the ROM, as well as the end-feel and quantity of motion. Comparison of stiffness and length is made to the same muscle on the uninvolved side and to synergists and antagonists on the involved side.
         a. Biceps
         b. Triceps
         c. Wrist and finger flexors and extensors

      d. Pronators
      e. Supinators
VI. Strength
   A. Manual muscle testing (MMT)[7]
   B. Resisted tests for soft tissue differential diagnosis[8]
   C. Grip test with dynamometer[9]
   D. Motor function:
      1. Ulnar nerve: Froment's sign and crossing fingers[10-12]
      2. Median nerve
      3. Radial nerve
VII. Sensory testing[2,13,14]
   A. Tinel's sign
VIII. Special tests (Box 6-3)

ALIGNMENT OF THE ELBOW

Prolonged postures or repeated movements performed by patients result in adaptations in their tissues (tissue impairments). These tissue impairments (e.g., short, stiff, long, overused, or weak muscles) result in imprecise movement patterns that eventually result in tissue injury. The identification of impairments in alignment provides insight into possible existing impairments in the tissues that will be verified later in the examination.

Normal Standing Alignment

Normal standing alignment gives an indication of the preferred patterns of muscle use and resting muscle lengths. Normal alignment of the elbow and forearm at rest includes (1) slight flexion of the elbow and (2) neutral rotation of the forearm so that the thumb is oriented anteriorly and the palm of the hand is oriented towards the body (Figures 6-1, 6-2, and 6-3 on p. 291).

Although the carrying angle is not evident during resting alignment in standing, the carrying angle should be assessed by having the subject supinate the forearm with the elbow in full extension,[5] while maintaining normal resting alignment of the humerus. The normal carrying angle varies from 2 to 26 degrees[15] and is slightly less in males and greater in females. Normally, the carrying angle should be symmetrical side to side (Figure 6-4, p. 291).

With the elbow flexed to 90 degrees, the medial and lateral epicondyles and the olecranon should form a triangle with sides of equal lengths. With the elbow in full extension, the medial and lateral epicondyles and the olecranon should be aligned in a straight line[5,16] (Figure 6-5, p. 292).

Examining the alignment of the shoulder girdle is an important component of evaluation of elbow and forearm dysfunction. Any impairments in the shoulder girdle alignment must first be corrected to correctly assess the alignment of the elbow and forearm.

Text continues on p. 292

---

*Synthesize the findings from the movement testing (AROM and PROM movement impairments, effect on symptoms, and resistive tests) to determine the reason for the loss of motion and symptoms. Refer to description of syndromes in the Chapter 6 Appendix for specific test findings.

BOX 6-2

Procedures for Testing Muscle Length

Muscle length tests should be performed passively. During testing, identify sites that are relatively most flexible and feel for relative differences in stiffness.

LENGTH TEST FOR WRIST EXTENSORS

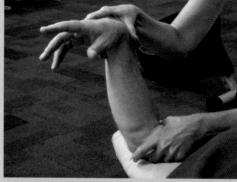

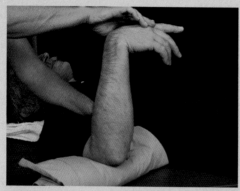

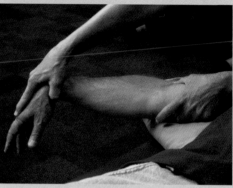

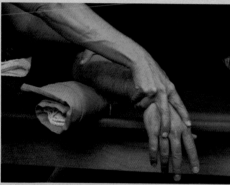

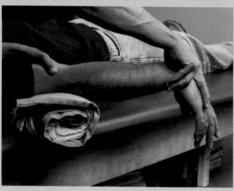

- *Patient starting position:* Supine with humerus in about 30 degrees abduction and towel roll under distal humerus, elbow flexed 90 degrees and forearm neutral.
- *Motion:* Passive wrist flexion followed by forearm pronation followed by elbow extension while maintaining each of the other motions (equals end position). Stabilize the humerus in neutral rotation.
- *Normal:* When comparing the amount of wrist flexion in the starting position to the amount of wrist flexion in the end position, the range of motion (ROM) is the same.
- *Impaired:* Shortness is indicated by a decrease in wrist flexion in the end position compared to the starting position. Comparing relative stiffness on the involved side to the uninvolved side and to other muscle groups should be assessed.
- *Substitutions:* Forearm supination, humeral medial rotation.

BOX 6-2

Procedures for Testing Muscle Length—cont'd

LENGTH TEST FOR WRIST FLEXORS

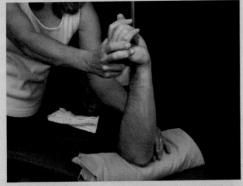

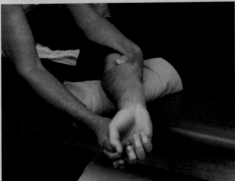

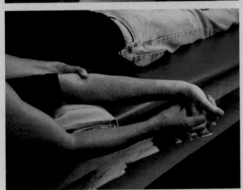

position. Comparison of relative stiffness on the involved side to the uninvolved side and to other muscle groups should be assessed.
- *Substitutions:* Forearm pronation, humeral lateral rotation.

LENGTH TEST FOR PRONATORS

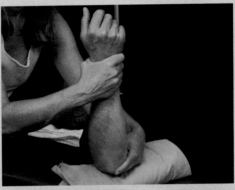

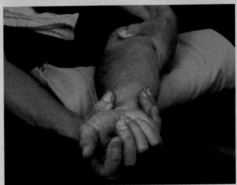

- *Patient starting position:* Supine with humerus in about 30 degrees abduction and towel roll under distal humerus, elbow flexed 90 degrees and forearm neutral.
- *Motion:* Passive wrist extension followed by forearm supination followed by elbow extension while maintaining each of the other motions (equals end position). Stabilize the humerus in neutral rotation.
- *Normal:* When comparing the amount of wrist extension in the starting position to the amount of wrist extension in the end position, the ROM is the same.
- *Impaired:* Shortness is indicated by a decrease in wrist extension in the end position compared to the starting

- *Patient starting position:* Supine with humerus in about 30 degrees abduction and towel roll under distal humerus, elbow flexed 90 degrees and forearm, wrist and fingers in neutral position.
- *Motion:* Passive forearm supination followed by elbow extension while maintaining the supination (equals end position). Stabilize the humerus in neutral rotation.
- *Normal:* When comparing the amount of forearm supination in the starting position to the amount of forearm supination in the end position, the ROM is the same.
- *Impaired:* The muscle is short if forearm supination is more limited with the elbow extended than with the elbow flexed. Elbow extension ROM would be greater with the forearm pronated than supinated if the pronator teres is short. Comparison of relative stiffness on the involved side to the uninvolved side and to other muscle groups should be assessed.
- *Substitutions:* Forearm pronation, humeral lateral rotation.

Continued

BOX 6-2

Procedures for Testing Muscle Length—cont'd

LENGTH TEST FOR SUPINATOR

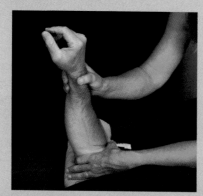

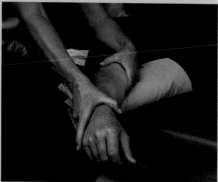

- *Patient starting position:* Supine with humerus in about 30 degrees abduction and towel roll under distal humerus, elbow flexed 90 degrees and forearm, wrist, and fingers in neutral position.
- *Motion: Passive* forearm pronation followed by elbow extension while maintaining the pronation (equals end position). Stabilize the humerus.
- *Normal:* The same amount of forearm pronation in the starting position as in the end position.
- *Impaired:* If the supinator is short, forearm pronation should be decreased with the elbow flexed, as well as extended. If the biceps brachii is short, pronation will decrease as the elbow is extended and/or the elbow will not extend through full ROM. Comparison of relative stiffness on the involved side to the uninvolved side and to other muscle groups should be assessed.
- *Substitutions:* Forearm pronation, humeral lateral rotation.

LENGTH TEST FOR BICEPS BRACHII

Make sure to stabilize the scapula when testing the length of the biceps. Also watch for humeral medial rotation as the forearm is pronated.[1,2]

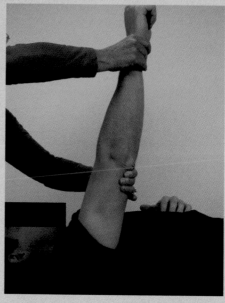

Method 1A.

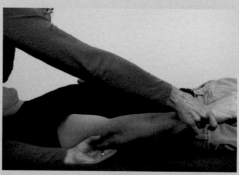

Method 1B.

- *Patient starting position:* Supine with arm at side, elbow flexed, and forearm supinated. Towel roll placed on table for support to distal humerus during test.
- *Motion:*
  - *Method 1:* Flex the shoulder 90 degrees. While maintaining the shoulder flexion, passively extend the elbow while pronating the forearm while maintaining shoulder flexion. Compare the amount of elbow extension with the shoulder flexed and the forearm pronated to the amount of elbow extension with the shoulder extended and the forearm pronated. Avoid wrist being fully flexed.

BOX 6-2

Procedures for Testing Muscle Length—cont'd

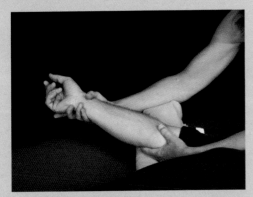

Method 2A.

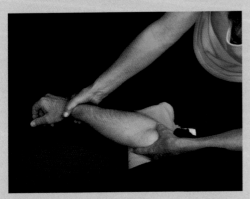

Method 2B.

- *Method 2:* Passively extend the elbow with the forearm supinated. Then pronate the forearm while maintaining full elbow extension.[2]
- *Normal:* Full elbow extension to 0 degrees with forearm pronated and scapula stable.
- *Impaired:*
  - *Method 1:* Less elbow extension with shoulder extended and the forearm pronated than with the shoulder flexed and the forearm supinated.
  - *Method 2:* Decreased range of forearm pronation with the elbow extended or less elbow extension with the forearm pronated than with the forearm supinated.[2]
- Comparing relative stiffness on the involved side to the uninvolved side and to other muscle groups should be assessed.

- *Substitutions:* Scapular anterior tilt, forearm supination, elbow flexion.

LENGTH TEST FOR TRICEPS BRACHII

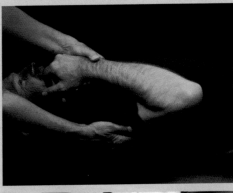

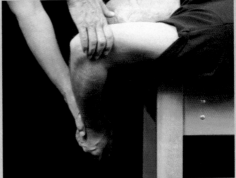

- *Patient position:* Supine close to edge of table or sitting
- *Motion:* Passive shoulder flexion to end ROM followed by elbow flexion while maintaining the shoulder flexion. Avoid trunk extension.
- *Normal:* 170 degrees shoulder flexion and 140 to 150 degrees elbow flexion (simultaneously).
- *Impaired:* The triceps is short if elbow flexion is less with the shoulder at end range flexion than with the shoulder at 0 degrees of flexion. Comparing relative stiffness on the involved side to the uninvolved side and to other muscle groups should be assessed.
- *Substitutions:* Shoulder extension or adduction, trunk extension.

REFERENCES

1. Davila SA, Johnston-Jones K: Managing the stiff elbow: operative, nonoperative, and postoperative techniques, *J Hand Ther* 19(2):268-281, 2006.
2. Bankov S: A test for differentiation between contracture and spasm of the biceps muscle in posttraumatic rigidity of the elbow joint, *Hand* 7(3):262-265, 1975.

BOX 6-3

Procedures for Special Tests

TESTS FOR LIGAMENTOUS INTEGRITY
Valgus (A) and varus (B) stress tests

The position of the forearm may make a difference in laxity. It is recommended to perform the test with the forearm in supination, pronation, and neutral rotation.[1] Posterolateral instability can mimic medial collateral ligament laxity with the forearm supinated. Therefore, if there is laxity when applying a valgus force with the forearm pronated, this would be a positive test for laxity of the medial collateral ligament.[2]

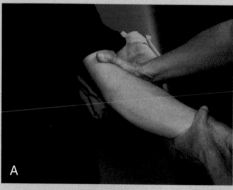

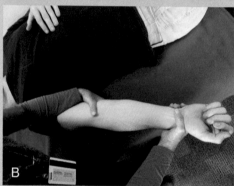

- *Purpose:* To assess the integrity of the medial and lateral collateral ligaments at the elbow.
- *Position:* Sitting, supine, or prone.[2]
- *Procedure*
  - *Valgus stress:* This test should be performed with the elbow flexed 20 to 30 degrees.[2] Apply a *valgus* force to the elbow. Stabilize the distal humerus by gripping it just above the humeral condyles. Use the other hand to apply the valgus force on the distal medial forearm by gripping the forearm just proximal to the wrist.
  - *Varus stress:* This test should be performed with the elbow flexed 20 to 30 degrees.[2] Apply a *varus* force to the elbow. Stabilize the distal humerus by gripping it just above the humeral condyles. Use the other hand to apply the varus force on the distal lateral forearm by gripping the forearm just proximal to the wrist.
  - *Normal:* Firm end-feel and no pain.
- *Positive:* Increased laxity compared to the other side with or without pain, or normal end-feel but with reproduction of symptoms in the area of the ligament being tested.

Moving valgus stress test[3,4]

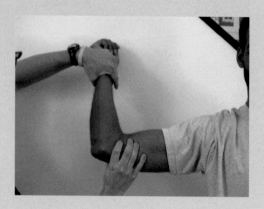

- *Purpose:* Ulnar collateral ligament (UCL) insufficiency, medial elbow pain.
- *Patient position:* Upright, shoulder abducted 90 degrees[3]
- *Procedure:* "Starting with the elbow maximally flexed, a modest valgus torque is applied to the elbow until the shoulder reaches its limit of external rotation. While a constant valgus torque is maintained, the elbow is quickly extended to about 30 degrees."[3]
- *Normal:* No pain and normal end-feel.
- *Positive test:* "The pain generated by the maneuver must reproduce the medial elbow pain at the UCL that the patient has with activities and the pain should be maximal between the position of late cocking (120 degrees) and early acceleration (70 degrees) as the elbow is extended. In the majority of cases the patient will experience the pain very suddenly within the range 70 to 120 degrees."[3]

Milking maneuver test[2,4]

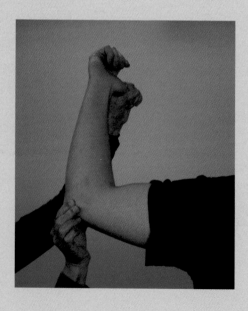

BOX 6-3

Procedures for Special Tests—cont'd
Milking maneuver test—cont'd

- *Purpose:* UCL insufficiency, medial elbow pain.
- *Patient position:* Sitting.[2]
- *Procedure:* "Examiner grasps the thrower's thumb with the arm in the cocked position of 90 degrees of shoulder abduction and 90 degrees elbow flexion and applies valgus stress by pulling down on the thumb."[2] Palpate for tenderness and joint space opening during this maneuver.[5]
- *Normal:* No pain and normal end-feel.
- *Positive test:* Tenderness over the medial collateral ligament and joint space gapping during this maneuver.[5]

Valgus extension overload test

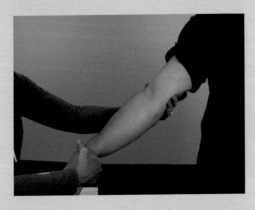

- *Purpose:* "To detect the presence of a posteromedial olecranon osteophyte or olecranon fossa overgrowth."[2]
- *Patient position:* Seated.
- *Procedure:* "The examiner stabilizes the humerus with one hand and with the opposite hand pronates the forearm and applies a valgus force while quickly maximally extending the elbow."[2]
- *Normal:* No pain and normal end-feel.
- *Positive test:* "Pain posteromedially as the olecranon tip osteophyte engages into the olecranon fossa."[2]

Palpation of ulnar collateral ligament of the elbow[2]

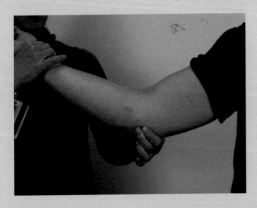

Palpation of ulnar collateral ligament of the elbow—cont'd

- *Purpose:* To implicate the anterior band of the UCL as the source of the patient's symptoms.
- *Position:* Sitting with the examiner supporting the elbow in 70 to 90 degrees of elbow flexion and the forearm supinated.[2]
- *Procedure:* Palpate distal and slightly anterior to the medial epicondyle.[2]
- *Normal:* Painless.
- *Positive:* Tender to palpation.

TEST FOR POSTEROLATERAL ROTARY INSTABILITY OF THE ELBOW
Lateral pivot shift test[6]

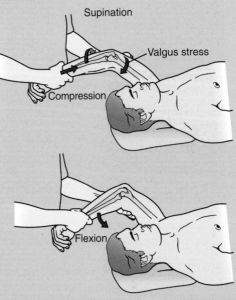

Supination
Valgus stress
Compression
Flexion

(From Magee DI: *Orthopedic physical assessment,* ed 5, Philadelphia, 2008, Saunders.)

- *Purpose:* To determine if there is posterolateral instability of the elbow.
- *Patient position:* Supine with the arm overhead with the forearm supinated.
- *Procedure:* Apply a mild-to-moderate valgus force while flexing the elbow past 40 degrees[6] to attempt to rotate and sublux the humeroulnar joint.
- *Normal:* No pain or instability during the test.
- *Positive test:* As the elbow flexes past about 30 to 60 degrees, it reduces with a palpable clunk. The test is also positive if there is apprehension without subluxation.[6]

TESTS FOR ULNAR NERVE COMPRESSION AT THE ELBOW
Test to reproduce subluxing of ulnar nerve[7]
- *Purpose:* To detect subluxation of the ulnar nerve in patients that have aching of the medial elbow that radiates proximally or distally and paraesthesia in ring and small fingers.
- *Patient position:* Seated.
- *Procedure:* Palpate for subluxation of the ulnar nerve at the cubital tunnel during elbow flexion and extension.[7]
- *Normal:* No subluxation or tenderness.

Continued

BOX 6-3

Procedures for Special Tests—cont'd

Test to reproduce subluxing of ulnar nerve—cont'd

- *Positive test:* Subluxation, tenderness, or positive Tinel's sign.
  - *Note:* Presence of dorsal hand symptoms in the ulnar nerve distribution rules out ulnar nerve entrapment at the wrist.[8]

Elbow flexion test[9]

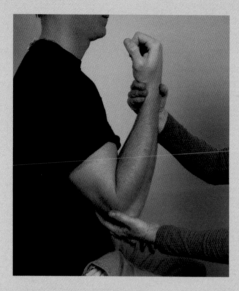

- *Purpose:* To increase the pressure on the ulnar nerve in the cubital tunnel. Used in diagnosis of cubital tunnel syndrome.
- *Patient position:* Patient seated with the shoulder resting in adduction by the side.
- *Procedure:* Passively flex the elbow with the forearm supinated and wrist in neutral position,[9] maintaining the arm by the side. Maintain end-range elbow flexion for 60 seconds[9] or until onset of symptoms, whichever comes first.
- *Normal:* No symptoms in 60 seconds.
- *Positive:* Numbness/tingling are reproduced in the ulnar nerve distribution.[9]
- *Note:* The elbow flexion test combined with the pressure provocative test (see next test) improves the sensitivity, specificity, and positive predictive value of the tests.

Pressure provocative test used for cubital tunnel syndrome[9]

- *Purpose:* To increase pressure on the ulnar nerve just proximal to the cubital tunnel. This test can also be used to aid in the diagnosis of compression of other nerves.
- *Patient position:* As noted for elbow flexion test.
- *Procedure:* Same as for elbow flexion test. While in the position for the elbow flexion test, manual pressure is placed on the ulnar nerve just proximal to the cubital tunnel.
- *Normal:* Same as for elbow flexion test.
- *Positive:* Same as for elbow flexion test.

TESTS FOR RADIAL NERVE COMPRESSION IN THE FOREARM
Middle finger test[8,10,11]

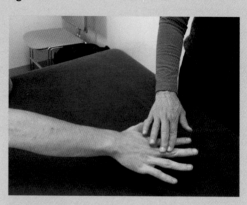

- *Purpose:* To transfer force from the middle finger to the medial border of the extensor carpi radialis brevis (ECRB) and therefore increase the pressure on the deep branch of the radial nerve. Used to diagnose radial tunnel syndrome.
- *Patient position:* Sitting with the shoulder flexed to 90 degrees, the elbow in extension, the wrist neutral, and the fingers extended.
- *Procedure:* Resist middle finger extension.
- *Normal:* No pain.
- *Positive:* Reproduction of the symptoms the patient is complaining about at the radial tunnel.

Supination test with elbow extended[8]

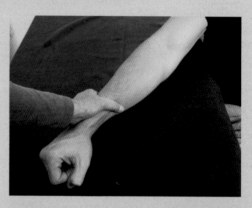

- *Purpose:* To contract the supinator and by doing so apply increased pressure to the deep branch of the radial nerve as it passes under the supinator muscle. Used to diagnose radial tunnel syndrome.
- *Patient position:* Sitting with the shoulder flexed to 90 degrees, the elbow in extension, forearm pronated, the wrist neutral, and the fingers relaxed.
- *Procedure:* Resist forearm supination with forearm pronated and elbow extended.
- *Normal:* No pain and strong.
- *Positive:* Reproduction of the symptoms the patient complaining about at the radial tunnel.

BOX 6-3

Procedures for Special Tests—cont'd

TESTS FOR MEDIAN NERVE COMPRESSION IN THE FOREARM
Pinch: Three jaw chuck (circle sign)[12]

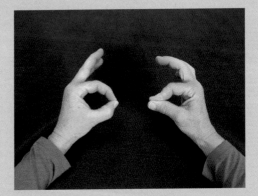

- *Purpose:* To test the strength of the flexor pollicis longus (FPL) and flexor digitorum profundus (FDP) to index. Used to diagnose anterior interosseous nerve syndrome.
- *Patient position:* Sitting.
- *Procedure:* Ask the patient to touch the tip of the index finger with the tip of the thumb, forming a circle with those digits.[8,12,13]
- *Normal:* Thumb interphalangeal (IP) joint should be in slight flexion; index distal interphalangeal (DIP) joint should be flexed (see left hand in figure above).
- *Positive:* An impaired movement pattern is noted during pinch with the thumb IP joint and the DIP joint of the index finger hyperextending or an inability to form a circle with the thumb and index fingers[8,12,13] (see right hand in figure above).

Resisted pronation with elbow extended[14]

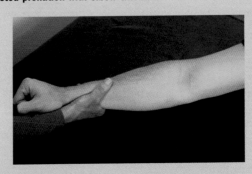

- *Purpose:* To increase the pressure on the median nerve by contracting the pronator teres. Used in diagnosis of pronator syndrome.
- *Patient position:* Patient seated with shoulder in about 45 degrees of flexion and elbow extended. Wrist and fingers in neutral position.
- *Procedure:* Resist forearm pronation with the forearm in neutral rotation.[14]
- *Normal:* No reproduction of symptoms and strong.
- *Positive:* Reproduction of pain, numbness, and tingling in the median nerve distribution.

Resisted elbow flexion between 120 and 130 degrees
- *Purpose:* To increase the pressure on the median nerve at the ligament of Struthers just proximal to elbow joint. Used in diagnosis of pronator syndrome.[14]
- *Patient position:* Patient seated with humerus by the side and the elbow flexed 120 degrees. Wrist and fingers in neutral position.
- *Procedure:* Resist elbow flexion.[14]
- *Normal:* No reproduction of symptoms and strong.
- *Positive:* Reproduction of pain, numbness, and tingling in the median nerve distribution.

Resisted elbow flexion
- *Purpose:* To increase the pressure on the median nerve by contracting the biceps and therefore increasing tension on the lacertus fibrosus. Used in diagnosis of pronator syndrome.[14]
- *Patient position:* Patient seated with humerus by the side and the elbow flexed 90 degrees. Wrist and fingers in neutral position.
- *Procedure:* Resist elbow flexion with the forearm in pronation[14] or with supination.[15]
- *Normal:* No reproduction of symptoms and strong.
- *Positive:* Reproduction of pain, numbness, and tingling in the median nerve distribution.

Resisted flexion of middle finger proximal interphalangeal joint

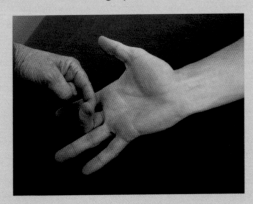

- *Purpose:* To increase the pressure on the median nerve at the superficialis arch by contracting the flexor digitorum superficialis (FDS). Used in diagnosis of pronator syndrome.[13-15]
- *Patient position:* Patient seated with humerus by the side and the elbow flexed 90 degrees. Wrist and fingers in neutral position; forearm supinated.
- *Procedure:* Resist flexion of the middle finger proximal interphalangeal (PIP) joint.[13-15]
- *Normal:* No reproduction of symptoms and strong.
- *Positive:* Reproduction of pain, numbness and tingling in the median nerve distribution.

Continued

BOX 6-3

Procedures for Special Tests—cont'd

TEST FOR WRIST EXTENSION WITH FOREARM PRONATION (LATERAL EPICONDYLOSIS)

Wrist extension (resisted) with elbow flexed and extended (tennis elbow test)[16-18]

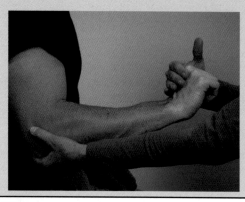

- *Purpose:* To implicate the contractile structures (wrist extensors) as the source of the patient's symptoms.
- *Patient position:* Tennis elbow test (testing ECRL more than ECRB)[19]: Sitting with the shoulder in about 70 degrees of flexion, the elbow extended, the forearm pronated, and the wrist in slight extension. Tennis elbow test (testing ECRB more than ECRL)[19]: Sitting with the humerus next to the side, the elbow flexed greater than 90 degrees, the forearm pronated, and the wrist in slight extension.
- *Procedure:* Resist wrist extension while preventing movement of the joint (isometric).
- *Normal:* Strong and pain free.
- *Positive:* Strong and painful at the lateral epicondylar region.

REFERENCES

1. Pomianowski S, O'Driscoll SW, Neale PG, et al: The effect of forearm rotation on laxity and stability of the elbow, *Clin Biomech* 16(5):401-407, 2001.
2. Cain EL Jr, Dugas JR: History and examination of the thrower's elbow, *Clin Sports Med* 23(4):553-566, 2004.
3. O'Driscoll SW, Lawton RL, Smith AM: The "moving valgus stress test" for medial collateral ligament tears of the elbow, *Am J Sports Med* 33(2):231-239, 2005.
4. ElAttrache NS, Ahmad CS: Diagnosis and treatment of ulnar collateral ligament injuries in athletes. In Morrey BF, Sanchez-Sotelo J, eds: *The elbow and its disorders*, ed 4, Philadelphia, 2009, Saunders.
5. Safran MR: Ulnar collateral ligament injury in the overhead athlete: diagnosis and treatment. *Clin Sports Med* 23(4):643-663, 2004.
6. O'Driscoll SW, Jupiter JB, King GJ, et al: The unstable elbow, *Instr Course Lect* 50:89-102, 2001.
7. Keefe DT, Lintner DM: Nerve injuries in the throwing elbow, *Clin Sports Med* 23(4):723-742, 2004.
8. Mackinnon S, Dellon A: *Surgery of the peripheral nerve*, New York, 1988, Thieme.
9. Novak CB, Lee GW, Mackinnon SE, et al: Provocative testing for cubital tunnel syndrome, *J Hand Surg Am* 19(5):817-820, 1994.
10. Eaton CJ, Lister GD: Radial nerve compression, *Hand Clin* 8(2):345-357, 1992.
11. Roles NC, Maudsley RH: Radial tunnel syndrome: resistant tennis elbow as a nerve entrapment, *J Bone Joint Surg Br* 54(3):499-508, 1992.
12. Andreisek G, Crook DW, Burg D, et al: Peripheral neuropathies of the median, radial, and ulnar nerves: MR imaging features, *Radiographics* 26(5):1267-1287, 2006.
13. Lee MJ, LaStayo PC: Pronator syndrome and other nerve compressions that mimic carpal tunnel syndrome, *J Orthop Sports Phys Ther* 34(10):601-609, 2004.
14. Eversmann WW: Proximal median nerve compression, *Hand Clin* 8(2):307-315, 1992.
15. Spinner RJ. Nerve entrapment syndromes. In Morrey BF, Sanchez-Sotelo J, eds: *The elbow and its disorders*, ed 4, Philadelphia, 2009, Saunders.
16. Hoppenfeld S: Physical examination of the spine and extremities, Norwalk, CT, 1976, Appleton-Century-Crofts.
17. Piligian G, Herbert R, Hearns M, et al: Evaluation and management of chronic work-related musculoskeletal disorders of the distal upper extremity, *Am J Ind Med* 37(1):75-93, 2000.
18. Fedorczyk JM: Tennis elbow: blending basic science with clinical practice, *J Hand Ther* 2006 April;19(2):146-153, 2006.
19. Kendall FP, McCreary EK, Provance PG, et al: *Muscles: testing and function with posture and pain*, ed 5, Baltimore, 2005, Lippincott Williams & Wilkins.

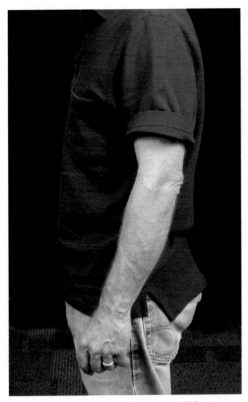

Figure 6-1. Normal alignment: Side view.

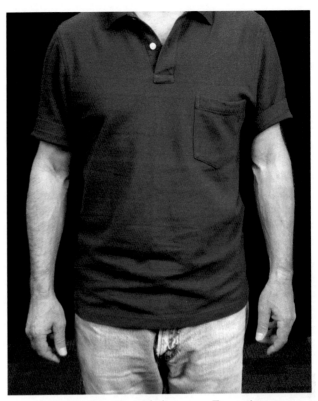

Figure 6-2. Normal alignment: Front view.

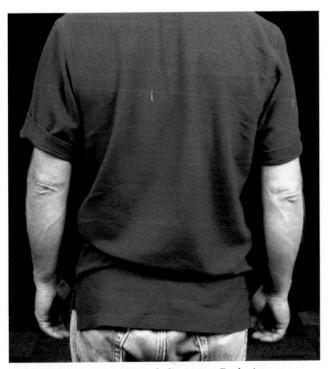

Figure 6-3. Normal alignment: Back view.

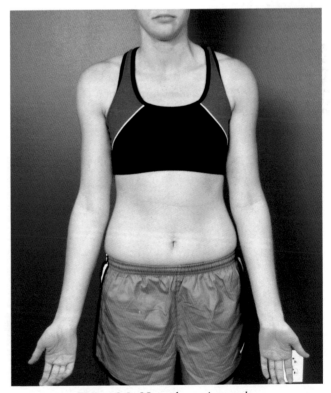

Figure 6-4. Normal carrying angle.

Visual appraisal of muscle and tendon development should also be part of assessing alignment. Muscles should be equally defined between muscles on the same side and symmetrical compared to the same muscle on the opposite side. Muscles may be slightly more hypertrophied on the dominant versus nondominant arm.

Impaired Alignment

Impaired alignment provides important clues regarding the source of the signs or symptoms and gives an indication of the preferred patterns of muscle use and resting muscle stiffness or lengths. However, assessment of alignment is only the first step in the objective examination and any clues obtained need to be confirmed during the rest of the tests in the examination.

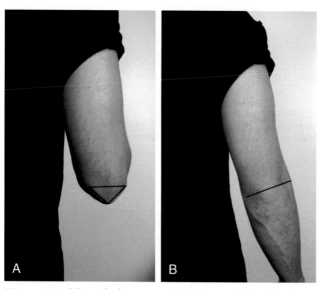

Figure 6-5. Normal alignment of olecranon (**A**) and epicondyles (**B**).

Alignment impairments of the elbow and forearm include increased or decreased elbow extension or flexion,[17,18] increased or decreased carrying angle,[5,19] and forearm pronation (Figures 6-6 to 6-10). Shoulder alignment must be considered in making the determination of elbow and forearm alignment impairments. If distal impairments are noted, then scapular and humeral alignment should first be corrected to determine if the origin of the elbow and forearm malalignment is distal or proximal (see Figure 6-10).

The impaired alignments as described may be a result of acute injury or a chronic disease process. Some impaired alignments may be the result of a prolonged position of immobilization required for tissue healing after an injury or surgery. However, patients who have not had a significant injury nor have a chronic disease may have pain caused by mild alignment impairments. These mild impairments are the result of tissue adaptations from repeated or sustained postures or movements used in daily activities. The tissues affected include capsule, bone, ligaments, nerve, or muscle. Modification of these impaired alignments that are the result of repeated activities may help prevent tissue injury or alleviate pain in the presence of tissue injury. Other factors affecting alignment include age, gender, race, genetics, and structural variations. Although these factors cannot be modified, they must be considered during examination and treatment.

A resting alignment of elbow extension (see Figure 6-7) indicates relative decreased stiffness, underuse, weakness, or paralysis of the elbow flexors or laxity of anterior capsule. Elbow extension may also indicate a normal anatomical variation of a short olecranon.

An alignment impairment of elbow flexion (see Figure 6-6) indicates relative increased stiffness,[20] strength, or

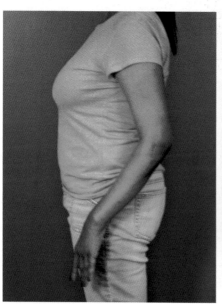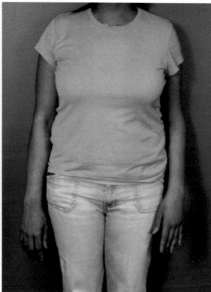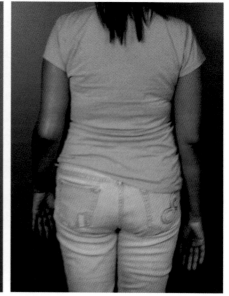

Figure 6-6. Alignment impairments: Increased elbow flexion.

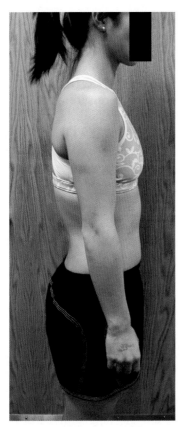

Figure 6-7. Alignment impairments: Decreased elbow flexion.

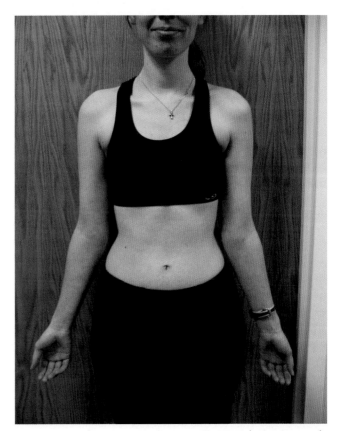

Figure 6-9. Alignment impairments: Increased carrying angle (structural).

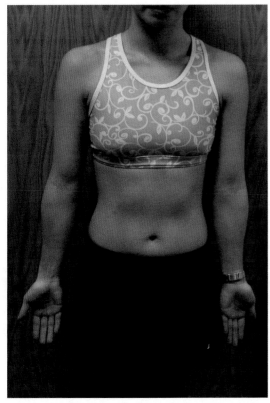

Figure 6-8. Alignment impairments: Decreased carrying angle (structural).

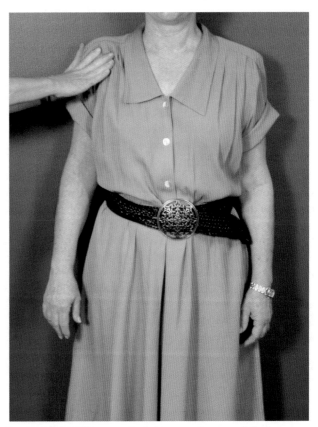

Figure 6-10. Alignment impairments: Increased forearm pronation on right noted with corrected scapular alignment.

overuse of the elbow flexors and short ligaments or anterior capsule.[21] The elbow flexion alignment can also be caused by posterior structures limiting full elbow extension.[22] A resting alignment impairment of increased elbow flexion may result in a compensatory shoulder alignment impairment of glenohumeral joint extension with scapular anterior tilt (see Figure 6-6). Likewise, shoulder alignment impairments can also contribute to the alignment impairment of elbow flexion.

Alteration of the normal bony relationships between the medial and lateral epicondyles and the olecranon with the elbow flexed 90 degrees and in full extension indicates dislocation, fracture, or growth disturbance.[5]

The normal carrying angle is altered by a variety of factors. Some of the muscles that attach to the lateral epicondyle create valgus forces at the elbow joint.[23] Repeated valgus movements may be associated with relatively overused or stiff wrist and finger extensors relative to the flexors contributing to an increase in the carrying angle.[18] Repeated valgus stresses at the elbow may also result in laxity of the medial collateral ligament and bony or articular changes on the lateral side of the elbow.[24,25] A decreased versus an increased carrying angle is a less common impairment in alignment[19] and may also be a normal structural variation (see Figures 6-8 and 6-9). Some of the muscles that attach to the medial epicondyle create varus forces at the elbow joint.[23] In theory, a decreased carrying angle may also indicate relative increased use or stiffness of the wrist and finger flexors compared to extensors.

Obesity may result in impaired standing alignments of increased elbow flexion and forearm pronation.

Shoulder alignment must be considered in making the determination of elbow and forearm alignment impairments. Impairments in shoulder girdle alignment may affect patterns of muscle use in the forearm and elbow or cause proximal or distal nerve compression with symptoms radiating distally into the hand.[2]

Visual appraisal of muscle and tendon development should also be examined when assessing alignment.[24] Asymmetry of muscle bulk between muscles on the same side or compared to the same muscle on the opposite side is another indicator of impaired patterns of muscle use or of nerve injury.

An important component of examination of the elbow and forearm is assessment of appearance, including skin, creases, scar, circulation, temperature, edema, and nodules[5,26-28] (see Box 5-2 for more information on scar and edema).

NORMAL MOTIONS OF THE ELBOW

Elbow Flexion

Elbow flexion occurs in the sagittal plane about a medial-to-lateral axis.[19,29] Normal active elbow flexion ROM is 145 degrees.[21,29] Passive elbow flexion is 160 degrees.[30] The end-feel of passive elbow flexion is that of soft tissue

approximation.[27] Passive elbow flexion may also be limited by the radius impacting on radial fossa, the coronoid process on coronoid fossa, tension from the posterior capsule, and passive tension of the triceps.[29,30] The size of the cubital tunnel decreases about 50% with elbow flexion, increasing the pressure on the ulnar nerve.[31,32] During elbow flexion starting from the fully extended position, the ulna and the head of the radius glide anteriorly and superiorly on the trochlea and capitellum of the humerus, respectively.[19]

Elbow Extension

Elbow extension occurs in the sagittal plane about a medial-to-lateral axis.[19] Normal active and passive extension is +5 degrees of hyperextension.[19,33] Elbow hyperextension beyond +5 degrees may be due to a structurally short olecranon. Active and passive elbow extension is limited by the impact of the olecranon on olecranon fossa, tension on the anterior capsule and ligament, and the elbow flexor muscles.[21,30] During elbow extension beginning from the fully flexed position, the ulna and radius glide posteriorly on the trochlea and capitellum of the humerus.[19,34]

Forearm Pronation and Supination

Forearm pronation and supination occur in the horizontal plane about a longitudinal or superior-to-inferior axis.[19,29,30] Normal supination is 85 degrees, and normal pronation is 75 degrees.[19,33,35] Pronation is limited by the impact of the radius on the ulna, tension on the dorsal radioulnar and quadrate ligaments, short or stiff supinator or extensor carpi radialis longus (only when the wrist is flexed), and decreased accessory motions at the ulnohumeral joint.[19,30,36] Forearm pronation is accompanied by slight internal rotation of the ulna and supination by external rotation of the ulna.[29] Supination is limited by tension on the oblique cord, anterior radioulnar, and quadrate ligaments and short or stiff pronators.[19,30,36] At the distal radioulnar joint, during supination the radius glides in a posterolateral direction on the ulna and during pronation in an anteromedial direction.[34] At the proximal radioulnar joint, the primary accessory motion of the radius on the ulna is spinning,[19] although there may be some posterior glide of the head of the radius on the ulna during pronation and anterior glide during supination.[34]

During forearm pronation and supination the position of the ulna relative to the radius changes. This is referred to as negative or positive ulnar variance. During forearm pronation, the ulna shifts distally relative to the radius, increasing the compressive forces on the ulnar wrist structures.[21,37-39] Forearm pronation results in a change in the position of the ulna relative to the radius so that the ulna protrudes distally relative to the radius more than with the forearm in the neutral and supinated positions (positive ulnar variance).[38] Strong grip also results in positive ulnar variance because of the compressive forces across the wrist.[37] The clinical significance of movements that result in an increase in positive ulnar variance is that with ulnar-sided wrist pain (e.g., triangular fibrocartilage complex injuries), strengthening grip may aggravate the symptoms, especially with the forearm pronated. The least compression on the ulnar side of the wrist is with the wrist radially deviated, forearm supinated, and avoiding strong gripping.

Pronation[33,40] of the forearm and elbow flexion[29,33,41] increase the contact of the radius on the capitellum, whereas supination decreases the contact. The position of forearm rotation also affects varus and valgus stability at the elbow[29]; however, studies vary regarding the position that provides most laxity.[33]

MUSCULAR ACTIONS OF THE ELBOW

The three primary flexors of the elbow include the biceps, brachialis, and brachioradialis. As a whole, the elbow flexors are more powerful than the extensors.[19,35] The elbow flexors have their best mechanical advantage with the elbow flexed at 90 degrees.[19,30,35] With the elbow at 90 degrees of flexion, the angle of the tendon to the bone is almost perpendicular so most of the force contributes to elbow flexion. However, when the elbow is in extension, the force generated by the elbow flexors is almost parallel to the bone, so the mechanical advantage is less for flexing the elbow instead contributing more to compressing or stabilizing the joint.[30]

The biceps brachii is an elbow flexor and forearm supinator. With the insertion fixed, the biceps flexes the elbow, moving the humerus toward the forearm, as in a pull-up or chin-up exercise.[7] The active function of the biceps at the shoulder is unclear. Some investigators have stated that the biceps compresses the head of the humerus into the glenoid, prevents humeral superior glide, and serves a role in glenohumeral joint stability.[42] However, these roles have been disputed by others. Although the active role of the long head of the biceps is unclear, passively it may contribute to preventing humeral superior and anterior translation.[43,44] Distally, the biceps is attached to the bicipital aponeurosis or the lacertus fibrosis.[45] The median nerve can be compressed under the bicipital aponeurosis, so active or resisted elbow flexion may reproduce symptoms.[46,47,48] The biceps has the best moment arm for elbow flexion with the elbow flexed at 90 degrees.[29] The biceps can rupture either from its proximal or distal attachment, causing symptoms in the region of the anterior elbow and shoulder.[49] The biceps is important in decelerating the forearm in throwing[43] and increases valgus stability at the elbow via compressive forces when the elbow is extended.[50] The compressive forces created by the biceps can also increase varus stability in the lateral collateral ligament (LCL)–deficient elbow.[51]

The biceps is less active when the elbow is flexed with the forearm pronated or when the forearm is supinated with the elbow extended.[29,52] Therefore patients that repeatedly use the arm with the elbow flexed and the forearm in pronation may have underused biceps. The extensor carpi radialis longus (ECRL) has a good moment arm to be an elbow flexor with the forearm pronated.[11,23] Thus the ECRL may become overused, stiff, short, or painful if used repeatedly during elbow flexion with the forearm pronated. Treatment of this impairment includes educating the patient to increase the use of the biceps by flexing the elbow with the forearm supinated when possible and increasing the flexibility of the ECRL if needed (see Chapter 6 Appendix).

Contraction of the biceps exerts a force in an anterior direction on the head of the radius.[30] If there is laxity of the annular ligament, biceps muscle contraction may cause anterior instability of the radius on the ulna.

Proper scapular alignment is critical for optimal function of the biceps. During elbow flexion, if scapular muscle performance is insufficient to stabilize the scapula, contraction of the biceps may cause scapular anterior tilt and internal rotation. Resisted elbow flexion is often associated with glenohumeral joint extension and scapular anterior tilt and internal rotation as commonly observed in weight lifters (Figure 6-11). The movement impairment of glenohumeral joint extension and scapular anterior tilt and internal rotation during elbow flexion may also contribute to excessive anterior gliding of the humerus on the glenoid. Performing resisted elbow flexion exercises with impaired scapular alignment decreases the subacromial space, potentially causing increased wear and tear on the long head of the biceps tendon as it travels through this space. In addition, the biceps works at a shorter length with the scapula anteriorly tilted than with proper scapular alignment, potentially resulting in shortness or increased stiffness of the biceps. The biceps may not generate as much tension in a shortened position as in a longer position, so correcting the scapular alignment may increase the tension-generating ability of the biceps. When modifying the alignment and movement pattern of the glenohumeral joint and scapula during resisted elbow flexion, initially the load must be decreased, allowing the scapular muscles to maintain the correct scapular alignment during elbow flexion.

Shortness or stiffness of the biceps results in scapular anterior tilt with passive stretch to the biceps as the elbow is extended and the forearm is pronated or decreased elbow extension with the forearm pronated and the shoulder extended. Caution should be used in stretching the biceps. Stretching performed with the glenohumeral joint in hyperextension can create excessive stretch on the anterior structures of the shoulder contributing to humeral anterior glide and shoulder symptoms. In most cases, the length of the biceps is adequate if full elbow extension can be achieved with the forearm pronated and the glenohumeral joint at zero degrees of flexion (see Box 6-2).

When trying to differentiate between the contractile structures that flex the elbow and that are the source of the symptoms, it is useful to resist elbow flexion with the

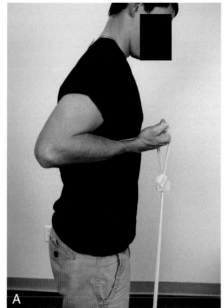

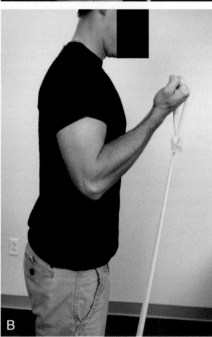

Figure 6-11. Movement impairment. **A,** Scapular anterior tilt and shoulder extension during contraction of the biceps brachii. **B,** Corrected movement pattern.

forearm supinated and pronated. Reproduction of symptoms with resisted elbow flexion with the forearm supinated would implicate the biceps, whereas with pronation, the ECRL may be implicated. Careful observation of the alignment and movement of the scapula during resisted elbow flexion tests is helpful to identify scapular impairments. Correction of the scapular impairments may improve the performance of the biceps or decrease symptoms.

The brachialis flexes the elbow joint regardless of whether the forearm is pronated or supinated.[19,29] Its sole function is elbow flexion. The brachialis has a large volume and cross-sectional area and thus can generate a lot of force compared to the other elbow flexors.[19] Kendall[7] states that with the insertion fixed, the brachialis flexes the elbow by moving the humerus toward the forearm as in a pull-up or chin-up exercise.[7] The brachialis increases valgus stability at the elbow via compressive forces when the elbow is extended.[50] The compressive forces created by the brachialis can also increase varus stability in the LCL–deficient elbow.[51] The brachialis lies immediately anterior to the elbow joint capsule. With trauma to the elbow, myositis ossificans occasionally affects the brachialis.[53]

The brachioradialis flexes the elbow joint. In addition, with resistance to forearm movements, the brachioradialis assists with pronation and supination.[7] The brachioradialis has increased activity with faster movements and with the forearm in semipronation versus in supination.[52]

The triceps brachii extends the elbow. The long head also assists in adducting and extending the shoulder.[7] The triceps may be implicated as the source of symptoms at the posterior elbow.[54] The long head of the triceps has the largest volume and physiological cross-sectional area of the muscles at the elbow besides the brachialis.[19] The triceps has the best moment arm for elbow extension at near full extension.[29] However, the triceps produces maximum torque at 90 degrees of elbow flexion.[19] Of the three heads of the triceps, the medial head is the most active, unless resistance is applied.[55] The triceps can generate more force with the shoulder flexed versus extended. The triceps increases valgus stability at the elbow via compressive forces when the elbow is flexed.[50] The compressive forces created by the triceps can also increase varus stability in the LCL–deficient elbow.[51] Shortness or stiffness results in elbow extension with the shoulder in full abduction or flexion.

The anconeus extends the elbow. The anconeus helps to stabilize the elbow with any elbow motion.[7,29] The anconeus may be implicated as the source of symptoms at the posterior elbow.

Muscles of the Wrist and Hand Affecting the Elbow

The ECRL and extensor carpi radialis brevis (ECRB) cross the elbow joint and can be implicated as the source of symptoms at the lateral elbow.[54] Although these muscles are named as wrist extensors and radial deviators,[7] the ECRL may also help supinate the forearm[19] and has a very good moment arm for flexing the elbow.[7,23,56] In addition, the ECRL may provide some force in the direction of valgus at the elbow joint.[23] The ECRL is a better radial deviator of the wrist than the ECRB. During finger flexion, gripping, or pinching, the ECRL and ECRB are active to ensure the correct length tension capabilities of the finger flexors.[19,57,58] During contraction of the finger flexors as with attempted gripping or pinching, weakness of the wrist extensors results in the wrist flexing.

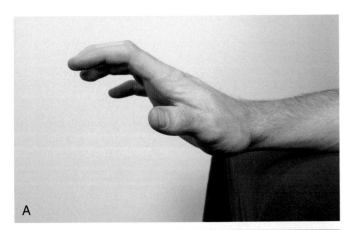

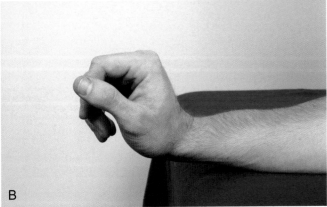

Figure 6-12. **A,** Movement impairment: Finger extensors substituting for wrist extensors. **B,** Corrected: Wrist extension without finger extension.

During active wrist extension, if the wrist extensors are weak, the fingers may extend, indicating substitution by the extensor digitorum (ED). This is common after a wrist fracture. To strengthen the wrist extensors, it is critical to keep the fingers relaxed in flexion to avoid substitution by the ED (Figure 6-12).

The ECRL may often become overused, stiff, short, or painful. The ECRL has a good moment arm for elbow flexion[11] in any forearm position but is the greatest with the forearm pronated.[23] Repeated flexion of the elbow with the forearm pronated contributes to overuse of the ECRL. This is often the case with patients with lateral epicondylosis. During forearm pronation, compensatory humeral medial rotation allows the ECRL to remain stiff or short. Humeral medial rotation should be avoided during exercises designed to increase the extensibility of the ECRL. If the ECRL is overused because the elbow is repeatedly flexed with the forearm in pronation, an important part of treatment is educating the patient to increase the use of the biceps by flexing the elbow with the forearm supinated instead of pronated. In addition, the ECRL tends to be overused because it is active as a synergist during any gripping or pinching functional activities.[19]

When performing resisted tests to differentiate between the ECRL and ECRB as the source of the symptoms, modification of elbow position can be helpful.[7]

Symptomatic resisted wrist extension with the elbow flexed implicates the ECRB, whereas the elbow extended implicates the ECRL.

Shortness or stiffness of the ECRL may be a contributing factor to limited elbow extension ROM if the wrist is flexed. Therefore elbow extension range should be checked with and without a stretch on the ECRL.[17] Combined wrist flexion, forearm pronation, and elbow extension[54] with the humerus stabilized in neutral rotation places maximum stretch on the ECRL and ECRB. Shortness or stiffness of the ECRL and ECRB results in wrist extension and radial deviation[7] when the forearm is pronated with the elbow extended and the humerus stabilized in neutral rotation (see Box 6-2). When the goal is to avoid excessive stresses on the ECRL and ECRB, progression of exercises should take into consideration the position in which the muscle is on maximum stretch.[59] For example, performing wrist extension and flexion exercises with the forearm in neutral rotation and the elbow flexed places less tensile stress on the ECRL than with the forearm pronated and elbow extended.

The extensor carpi ulnaris (ECU) extends and ulnarly deviates the wrist.[7] Although the ECU crosses the elbow, in our experience, it is rarely implicated as the source of elbow pain. The ECU may provide some force in the direction of valgus at the elbow joint.[23] It is a better wrist extensor with the forearm supinated than with the forearm pronated because the tendon slips anteriorly during forearm pronation.[11,60] The ECU is active as an antagonist during wrist flexion[52] and stabilizes the wrist during thumb abduction.[57] The ECU works along with the ECRL and ED during wrist extension. Shortness of the ECU results in a resting alignment of ulnar deviation with slight wrist extension.[7] As the wrist is passively flexed, stiffness of the ECU is identified as increased resistance through the motion.

The flexor carpi radialis (FCR) flexes and radially deviates the wrist. The FCR may also assist in pronation of the forearm and elbow flexion.[7,56] It may contribute to the dynamic stability of the elbow, particularly against valgus forces.[23] The FCR contracts during radial deviation to counterbalance the extensor component of the ECRL.[19] The FCR may be implicated as a source of symptoms at the medial elbow (wrist flexion with pronation or medial epicondylosis). Shortness or stiffness of the FCR may be a contributing factor to limited elbow extension ROM, especially if the wrist is extended. Therefore elbow extension range should be checked with and without a stretch on the FCR.[17] Shortness of the FCR results in a resting alignment of wrist flexion and radial deviation.[7] As the wrist is passively extended, stiffness of the FCR is identified as increased resistance through the motion.

The flexor carpi ulnaris (FCU) flexes and ulnarly deviates the wrist[7] but may be a source of symptoms at the medial elbow.[54] The FCU assists with elbow flexion[7,60] and may provide some force in the direction of varus at the elbow joint,[23] thereby contributing to dynamic stability of the elbow.[29,61,62] The FCU may also assist elbow extension.[23] The FCU is a very strong muscle with a large cross-sectional area.[11,19] It is less active as an ulnar deviator than the ECU.[11] Because the ulnar nerve travels through the FCU, overuse, stiffness, or shortness of the FCU may contribute to ulnar nerve compression at the elbow.[54] Shortness or stiffness of the FCU may be a contributing factor to limited elbow ROM, especially if the wrist is extended. Therefore elbow extension and flexion range should be checked with and without a stretch on the FCU.[17] Shortness of the FCU results in a resting alignment of wrist flexion with ulnar deviation.[7] As the wrist is extended, stiffness of the FCU is identified as resistance through the motion.

The flexor digitorum superficialis (FDS) crosses the elbow and provides some force in the direction of varus at the elbow joint,[23] thereby contributing to dynamic stability of the elbow against valgus forces.[29,61,62] The median nerve may become compressed as it travels under the proximal edge of the FDS, producing symptoms in the anterior forearm and hand. Contraction of the FDS to the middle finger increases the compression, aggravating the symptoms.

Muscles of Forearm Pronation and Supination

In general, the supinators are stronger than the pronators of the forearm.[19] However, pronation can be more easily compensated for than supination, using shoulder abduction or medial rotation. Most patients who have had a traumatic injury affecting the elbow region have more difficulty regaining supination than pronation ROM.

The pronator teres pronates the forearm and assists with elbow flexion.[7,63] It may contribute to the dynamic stability of the elbow, particularly against valgus forces.[61] The pronator teres is often overused, stiff, or short in patients with wrist extension with pronation (lateral epicondylosis) and anterior forearm nerve entrapment syndromes such as pronator syndrome. Focusing on alignments and movements involving forearm supination instead of pronation is beneficial for these patients. Shortness or stiffness of the pronator teres in these patients may also be associated with shortness or stiffness of the finger flexors. In these instances, therefore, exercises for increasing extensibility should incorporate forearm supination with wrist and finger extension. Of all the elbow flexors, the pronator teres is the most medial. If the pronator teres is more dominant, stiffer, or shorter than the other elbow flexors, a rotatory impairment at the elbow may result (e.g., relative humeral lateral rotation and pronation of the forearm). In other words, when the patient attempts forearm supination and elbow extension, if the pronator teres is stiff, and the ulnohumeral joint is relatively most flexible, the humerus may laterally rotate slightly. In these cases, the medial humeral condyle appears more prominent than normal during elbow extension with forearm supination (Figure 6-13).

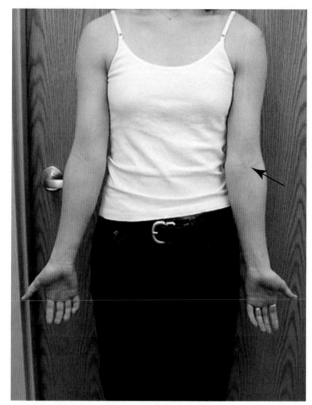

Figure 6-13. Movement impairment during elbow extension. Excessive humeral lateral rotation during forearm supination on left side.

The pronator quadratus pronates the forearm.[7] It is also a stabilizer of the distal radioulnar joint (DRUJ).[19] According to Kendall,[7] the pronator quadratus can be isolated by working on forearm pronation with the elbow at end-range flexion.

The supinator supinates the forearm.[7] The supinator is a weaker supinator than the biceps but is not influenced by elbow position.[63] Patients with wrist extension with pronation (lateral epicondylosis) usually have overused forearm pronators relative to the supinator and the biceps. To isolate the supinator, strengthening exercises should be done with the shoulder flexed at 90 degrees and elbow at end-range flexion.[7] In cases in which there is laxity of the ligaments stabilizing the head of the radius on the ulna, the supinator may counteract the anterior force exerted on the head of the radius by contraction of the biceps brachii. The finger and wrist extensors assist with forearm supination.[64]

MOVEMENT SYSTEM SYNDROMES of the Elbow

The proposed movement system syndromes of the elbow have been developed based on clinical experience and examination of the literature but are still a "work in progress" and need testing and refining through feedback from other clinicians with expertise in treating patients with elbow problems.

To our knowledge, no other classification systems have been described to guide physical therapy management of the patient with elbow dysfunction. Commonly, it is the physician's diagnoses related to the pathoanatomical source of pain, established protocols, and isolated impairments that guide treatment. The premise of this chapter is that clusters of impairments comprise syndromes that when identified more effectively guide physical therapy management of patients with elbow problems than if only a pathoanatomical problem is identified. This is especially true in patients with elbow problems who are referred to physical therapy and have not recently had surgery. In many cases, the physician's diagnosis, while important and helpful, is not sufficient to guide the physical therapy management of the patient with elbow problems.

Some patients with elbow symptoms have problems that are not guided by established protocols. Based on the premise that the physical therapist has primary expertise in analysis of the movement system, a set of diagnoses were developed for the elbow to guide physical therapy treatment of these patients. The proposed diagnoses are named either for the alignments and movements that appear to be related to the patient's symptom behavior or for the primary cause of the patient's impairments. The focus of the diagnoses is on the movement that produces the pain rather than the pathoanatomical source of the pain. In many cases, the pain is associated with movement, thus alterations in the precision of movement are the cause of the tissue irritation and need to be corrected to achieve optimal outcomes.

This section of the text focuses on the overall description of each syndrome and on the information in the first three columns in the Chapter 6 Appendix. Refer to the Chapter 6 Appendix for the complete description of the syndromes. It is possible that a patient might be assigned more than one syndrome, but usually one syndrome is primary.

WRIST EXTENSION WITH FOREARM PRONATION SYNDROME

Wrist extension with forearm pronation syndrome (lateral epicondylosis) is characterized by lateral elbow pain provoked by gripping and lifting activities resulting in overuse of the wrist extensors. It is described in the literature that the extensor carpi radialis brevis (ECRB) tendon is most involved as evidenced by microscopic tears.[65-67] However, clinically, the lateral elbow pain is usually aggravated most when the wrist extensors are used with the forearm pronated and the elbow extended. This may also implicate the ECRL.[7,68] In this syndrome, the biceps and supinator may be underused and wrist extensors and pronators overused during elbow flexion. Overuse comes about not solely as the result of the primary aggravating job or sporting activity but because of other activities that are performed with a similar movement pattern during the day. Supinating the forearm

during elbow flexion decreases the symptoms by increasing performance of the biceps brachii and decreasing the overuse of the ECRL. The overused muscles are often relatively stiffer than the underused synergist. Modification of associated impairments in shoulder girdle alignment and movement is often necessary to decrease the stresses on the injured tissues at the elbow.[69] Modification of symptoms may also be achieved by changing the movement pattern to decrease the stresses on the wrist extensors by avoiding use of the muscle when it is lengthened[59] and/or in the extremely shortened range.

Symptoms and History

The patient with wrist extension with forearm pronation syndrome reports pain in the area of the lateral epicondyle that sometimes radiates distally into the forearm. The pain is aggravated by gripping activities such as lifting or pouring a gallon of milk, lifting a coffee cup, carrying a brief case, intensive manual labor,[70,71] performance-related movements in musicians,[72] computer keyboard use, and sports such as baseball, tennis, swimming, and fencing.[70] Patients with this syndrome have pain with repetitive gripping or prolonged positioning in wrist extension, forearm pronation, and elbow flexion. The onset of symptoms is usually gradual.[65] This syndrome is more common in the dominant extremity,[65] and the incidence or prevalence is 1% to 3%[73] of the population. It occurs equally in men and women.[67] Studies have shown that it is a self-limiting condition resolving in 18 months to 2 years.[74]

Common referring diagnoses for this syndrome include lateral epicondylitis, tennis elbow, and grade I or II LCL sprain.

Key Tests and Signs

Alignment/Appearance Analysis

It is common for patients with this syndrome to have finger and wrist extensors that appear better developed or defined than the biceps brachii (Figure 6-14).

Movement Impairments Analysis

Aggravating functional activities. For patients with this syndrome, the performance of individual functional activities (based on the history) must be examined for the movement impairment that has been identified across the examination. Particular attention is paid to the movement patterns of the shoulder, elbow, forearm, and wrist. Movement impairments are commonly identified with gripping used during reaching and lifting or during elbow flexion and extension. The most common preferred pattern of reaching and lifting is with the forearm pronated. During this motion, the humerus medially rotates and abducts more readily than the forearm pronates. Modification of the preferred movement pattern by reaching and gripping with the forearm supinated decreases the symptoms. Less commonly a movement impairment of excessive wrist extension ROM during elbow extension has been identified while statically gripping an object. This impaired movement pattern was noted on the bowing arm of a musician playing the violin. A contributing factor to the excessive wrist extension ROM that was identified in this musician was excessive

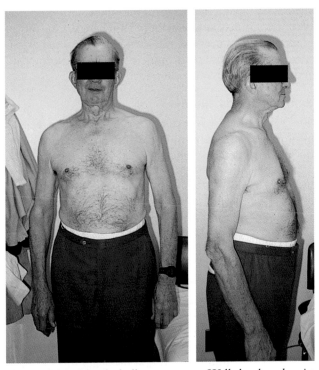

Figure 6-14. Muscle bulk asymmetry: Well-developed wrist extensors; atrophy of biceps brachii.

glenohumeral joint abduction. Modification of the preferred alignment by slightly decreasing the glenohumeral abduction and maintaining the wrist in a more neutral position decreased the patient's symptoms (Figure 6-15). Another less commonly observed movement impairment is excessive wrist extension during elbow flexion with forearm aligned in neutral rotation, the glenohumeral joint in 90 degrees of abduction, and the scapula abducted. This impairment was noted in a musician playing the harp. Modification of her preferred movement pattern by adducting the scapula slightly resulted in less wrist extension ROM and decreased her symptoms.

Joint Integrity

Active and passive finger, wrist, forearm, and elbow ROM should be assessed. Active wrist extension may or may not be painful, depending on level of irritability of the tissues. Passive wrist extension ROM will be normal[67] and painless, whereas combined wrist flexion, elbow extension, and forearm pronation may be slightly limited and painful as the result of increased tension on the injured tissues. Active and passive finger ROM will be normal.

Muscle Length

Tests of muscle length for the wrist and finger extensors should be performed. The tests of muscle length should be performed passively with particular attention paid to the amount of resistance to passive stretch (stiffness) throughout the ROM during the test and to which joint

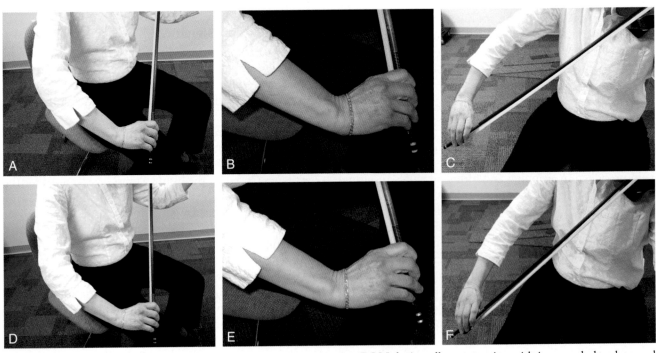

Figure 6-15. Movement impairment. **A** to **C**, Excessive wrist extension ROM during elbow extension with increased glenohumeral abduction. **D** to **F**, Decreasing the amount of glenohumeral abduction decreases the wrist extension ROM. Contributing factor to elbow pain was excessive shoulder abduction.

moves most easily. The purpose of the tests is to identify whether decreased muscle length or increased stiffness is contributing to the movement pattern causing the symptoms. Mill's test is similar to a length test of the wrist extensors. A positive Mill's test stretches the wrist extensors by a combined movement into forearm pronation, wrist flexion, and elbow extension and results in reproduction of the patient's lateral elbow pain.[54,65,75] See Box 6-2 for specific procedures recommended for the length tests. During the wrist extensor length test, the amount of resistance to passive stretch is noted as the elbow is extended with the wrist flexed and the forearm pronated. If the wrist extensors are relatively stiff or short, the humerus usually medially rotates more readily than the forearm pronates. Stiffness or shortness of the finger and wrist extensors is a common finding relative to the uninvolved extremity.

Muscle Strength and Performance Impairments

Resisted tests for soft tissue differential diagnosis should be performed when examining the patient with wrist extension with forearm pronation syndrome to help determine the source and irritability of the patient's symptoms. Muscle groups that should be tested include the wrist flexors and extensors, forearm pronators and supinators, and elbow flexors and extensors. The classic sign for this syndrome is increased pain with resisted wrist extension with the elbow extended[71] and no pain with resisted wrist flexion. The resisted wrist extension test has been named the *Cozen's test.*[76] Classically, this test is done with the elbow flexed about 90 degrees and the forearm pronated. In addition, we recommend performing the test with the elbow flexed greater than 90 degrees and with the elbow extended to differentiate between the ECRB and ECRL as the greater source of the symptoms.[7] Resisted wrist extension is often more painful with the elbow extended than with the elbow flexed.

Resisted forearm pronation and supination are usually strong and do not aggravate the symptoms. When the tissues are very irritable, these motions may be painful, but resisted wrist extension is the most painful.

Resisted elbow flexion and extension may or may not be painful, depending on the level of tissue irritability. We recommend testing the elbow flexors with the forearm pronated and supinated. Resisted elbow flexion with the forearm pronated is usually more painful than with the forearm supinated presumably because of the contribution of the ECRL to elbow flexion with the forearm pronated.[23] Resisted elbow extension is usually strong and painless.

MMT of the wrist extensors provides useful information but usually cannot be accurately assessed initially because of pain. Wrist extensor strength is usually at least 3/5.

Grip strength tested with a grip dynamometer is usually decreased because the patient's symptoms are associated with gripping activities. The source of the symptoms in this syndrome, the wrist extensors, automatically contract during gripping to maintain the length of the finger flexors, thus maximizing the ability of the finger flexors to generate tension. Testing grip strength can be used as an outcome measure to identify changes in symptoms with gripping.[77] Patients with lateral epicondylosis (tennis elbow) have been found to have decreased grip strength with the elbow extended compared to grip strength with the elbow flexed.[78] Therefore comparing grip strength with the elbow flexed versus extended may be useful for confirming the presence of this syndrome.

Palpation

Palpation reveals point tenderness over the lateral epicondyle or just distal to it over wrist extensor muscles.[68,71]

Source of Signs and Symptoms

The source of the signs and symptoms for wrist extension with forearm pronation syndrome is muscle and tendon. The ECRB is the muscle most commonly involved, but less often there is involvement of the ED and ECRL (common extensor origin where it originates at the lateral epicondyle).[67,68] The Chapter 6 Appendix includes the complete listing of associated signs or contributing factors, differential diagnoses, and treatment for this syndrome. The primary focus of the treatment is discussed in the next section.

Treatment

The primary focus of treatment is to decrease the stresses imposed on the wrist extensors by modifying the patient's preferred movement pattern during the functional activities they perform repeatedly. Modifications include not only the alignment and movement patterns of the wrist but also the forearm, elbow, and shoulder.[70,79-81] The patient is educated to perform gripping activities involving lifting and reaching with the elbow flexed and the forearm supinated when possible. When performing repeated gripping activities associated with elbow flexion and extension, the end-ranges of wrist flexion and extension should be avoided. The therapist must work with the patient during the therapy visits on correcting and practicing the movement pattern during the functional activity causing the problem.

Patient education regarding the need and strategies used for decreasing the stresses on the injured tissues is an essential component of the initial treatment.[82] As the pain decreases, indicating healing of tissues, the progression of stressing the tissues must be done very gradually. During performance of home exercises or functional activities, the symptoms should be no greater than 2/10 intensity and should resolve within 30 minutes to 1 hour after exercise.

Specific exercises are prescribed to increase the extensibility of the muscles that are stiff or short, most often the wrist and finger extensors and finger flexors. Particular attention is paid to avoiding subtle substitutions, such as humeral medial rotation, during the wrist and finger extensor stretching exercises (see Box 6-2). If stretching is indicated for the finger flexors, it is often helpful to stretch them passively (wrist extension with the palm flat on the table) to avoid use of the wrist extensors during the stretch. The patient is instructed to take frequent breaks to stretch to help increase the extensibility of stiff muscles. Stretching is performed throughout the day and especially during the functional activity that is contributing to the impairment. The focus on stretching is on the muscles that are used the most and those found to be short or stiff during the examination. Besides increasing extensibility, stretching helps relax the muscle that is being stretched.

As the pain subsides, strengthening exercises for the wrist extensors and forearm pronators and supinators are usually indicated, but the progression must be very gradual.

The use of a forearm strap during the day is often helpful.[70,83] A splint to immobilize the wrist can be helpful when the tissues are particularly irritable.[68,70] However, the patient must be cautioned not to try to use the wrist normally with the splint on or they will unintentionally be performing isometric-resisted wrist exercises within the splint. The splint is intended to be a reminder to rest the wrist. An active assistive wrist extension splint has also been described and reported as beneficial.[84,85] The Chapter 6 Appendix includes more specific information regarding the examination, findings, and management for this syndrome.

ELBOW HYPOMOBILITY SYNDROME

The principal movement impairment in elbow hypomobility syndrome is significant limitation of accessory and physiological motion of the elbow. Flexion loss is usually greater than extension loss[54] and is usually also associated with a loss of forearm pronation and supination. This is most often the result of the effects of prolonged immobilization after surgery or trauma.

Symptoms and History

The patient with elbow hypomobility complains of stiffness, decreased ROM, and pain, especially at the end-ranges of motion. Patients with this diagnosis usually have no complaints of numbness and tingling.

Patients with elbow hypomobility will have difficulty performing self-care activities such as feeding and personal hygiene. They also frequently report difficulty with turning a key in the ignition, reading, and laundry.

Common referring diagnoses include fractures, dislocations, or associated surgical procedures of the elbow or forearm. Additional referring diagnoses are stiff elbow and elbow pain.

Key Tests and Signs

Alignment Analysis

Patients with elbow hypomobility demonstrate alignment impairments of excessive flexion of the elbow, forearm pronation, and associated extension at the glenohumeral joint (Figure 6-16). The elbow is often swollen and if the patient has had surgery or a trauma, there may be scarring in the elbow region (Figure 6-17).

Movement Impairment Analysis

Patients with elbow hypomobility frequently have movement impairments of the shoulder girdle that compensate for the limited accessory and physiological motion of the elbow and forearm. The compensatory movements of the shoulder girdle include scapular anterior

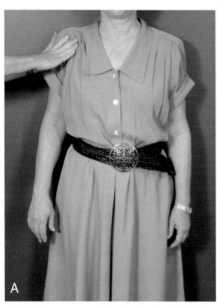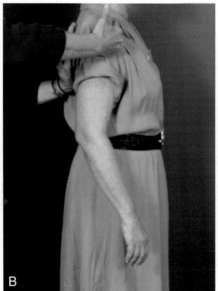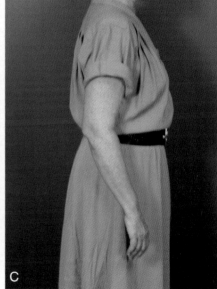

Figure 6-16. Alignment: Elbow hypomobility. **A,** Increased pronation. **B,** Increased elbow flexion. **C,** Glenohumeral extension.

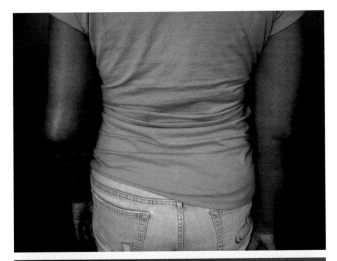

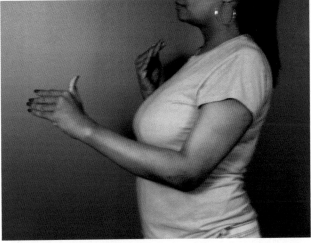

Figure 6-18. Movement Impairment: Scapular posterior tilt and adduction, shoulder flexion, and trunk extension during elbow flexion.

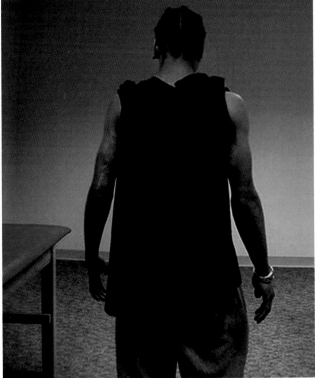

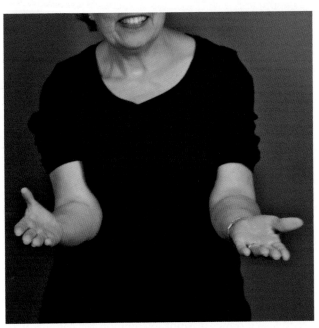

Figure 6-17. Left elbow is edematous compared to right elbow is normal.

Figure 6-19. Movement impairment: Shoulder lateral rotation and adduction during forearm supination.

tilt or shoulder extension during elbow extension (see Figure 6-6); scapular adduction and posterior tilt, shoulder flexion, and trunk extension during elbow flexion (Figure 6-18); shoulder adduction and lateral rotation during forearm supination (Figure 6-19); and shoulder abduction and medial rotation during forearm pronation (Figure 6-20).

Joint Integrity
AROM and PROM of the elbow and forearm should be assessed. AROM and PROM are approximately equal and limited in a capsular pattern (flexion loss is greater than extension loss).[54] There is a capsular end-feel to PROM, and the onset of pain is often not until the end

of the restricted ROM. The timing of the onset of pain varies, depending on the irritability of the tissues. There is almost always an associated loss of forearm pronation and supination. Shoulder wrist and hand ROM should be assessed, but those findings are not essential for assigning the diagnosis.

Tests for ligament integrity are usually negative. A key finding in patients with elbow hypomobility is decreased joint accessory mobility in all directions.

Muscle Strength and Performance Impairments
General assessment of the strength of the elbow and forearm muscles usually indicates strength of at least 3/5 as graded by Kendall.[7] Formal assessment of strength

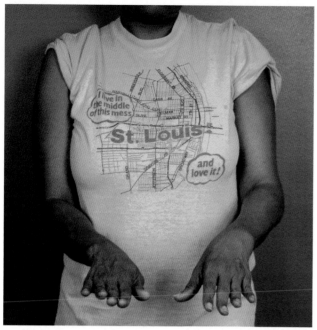

Figure 6-20. Movement impairment: Shoulder medial rotation and slight abduction during forearm pronation on her left.

often cannot be performed at the time of the initial visit because of pain or the stage of healing of the tissues.

Source of Signs and Symptoms

Potential sources of the signs and symptoms for patients with elbow hypomobility include joint structures such as the elbow capsule,[17] ligaments, bone, muscle,[17] tendon, and bursae. Edema and scarring in the elbow or forearm region may also contribute to the hypomobility.[17] Further details regarding the evaluation of edema and scar can be found in Box 5-2. Neurapraxia, compression, or adhesions of the nerves in the elbow and forearm regions may be additional sources of hypomobility.[17]

The Chapter 6 Appendix includes the complete listing of associated signs or contributing factors and treatment for this syndrome. It is not uncommon for patients with elbow hypomobility to develop shoulder pain, presumably as the result of the associated compensatory movement impairments of the shoulder previously described in the movement impairment section. Thus associated shoulder impairments should be addressed in treatment. It is also common for patients with an injury resulting in elbow hypomobility to have associated edema in the forearm, wrist, and hand. Therefore the wrist and hand should be carefully evaluated and treated as indicated. The primary focus of treatment for elbow hypomobility is discussed in the next section.

Treatment

The primary focus of treatment for patients with elbow hypomobility is to increase the AROM and PROM of the elbow and forearm with the goal of at least −30 degrees of extension to 130 degrees of flexion and 50 degrees each

for pronation and supination.[86] Since improved surgical methods allow the initiation of therapy earlier in the healing process, full ROM can often be obtained. However, with complex injuries, these guidelines can be used for the minimally acceptable ROM needed for function. Gains in ROM are made using edema and scar management techniques, active and passive exercises, hold-relax and contract-relax relaxation techniques, joint mobilization techniques, and splinting.[17] Heat modalities may be used as needed.[17] Caution should be used to avoid forced manipulation that may lead to muscle tears in the muscle before complete healing so myositis ossificans does not develop.[53] The patient should be encouraged to use the involved arm functionally and increase activities by incorporating weight bearing as tolerated.[17]

The therapist must educate the patient regarding the compensatory movement patterns used during elbow and forearm motions and how to move without the compensatory strategies. In cases in which the onset of symptoms is not until the end of the restricted range, the patient may need to push through an increase in symptoms to gain ROM. However, the increase in symptoms should not be severe and the symptoms should subside quickly when stopping the exercise.

Splinting can be a helpful adjunct to treatment, facilitating adaptations in the length of tissues because of the prolonged stretch applied to the tissues.[17,87] Static progressive splints used during the day to improve elbow and forearm motion and static extension splinting at night are often helpful as indicated (Figure 6-21). We recommend initiating exercise before splinting, but if improvements in ROM start to plateau, splinting should be initiated without delay while the tissues are still in the early remodeling phase.

The Chapter 6 Appendix includes further details regarding the examination, findings, and management for this syndrome.

ELBOW FLEXION SYNDROME (CUBITAL TUNNEL SYNDROME)

The principal movement impairment in elbow flexion syndrome (cubital tunnel syndrome) is elbow flexion. Prolonged or repetitive elbow flexion places excessive stresses on the ulnar nerve at the medial elbow, causing symptoms.[47] Ulnar nerve injury may be caused by compression, traction, or friction.[88] Elbow flexion may be associated with forearm pronation, wrist flexion or extension, and shoulder abduction.[89-91] Shoulder abduction, forearm pronation, and wrist extension contribute to elongation of the nerve, whereas contraction of the FCU during wrist flexion may aggravate symptoms as the result of compression of the nerve. The ulnar nerve travels through the cubital tunnel, which is formed by the elbow joint and medial collateral ligament (MCL) laterally and the aponeurosis between the two heads of the FCU medially[92] (Figure 6-22).

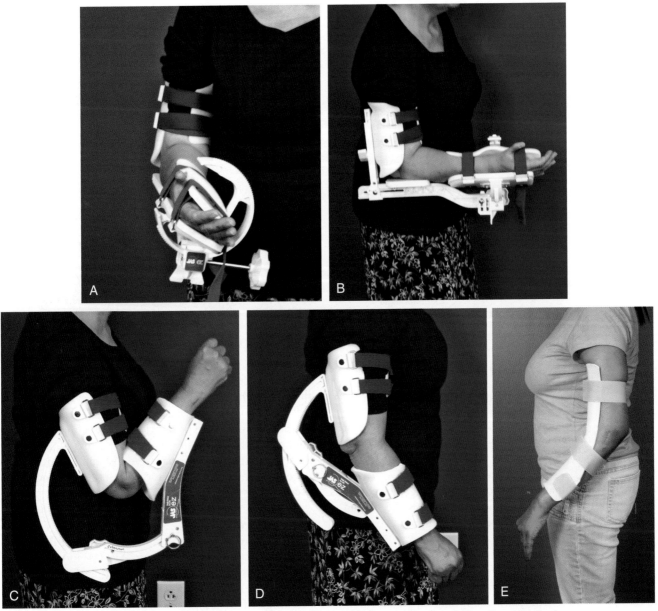

Figure 6-21. Splinting. **A** and **B**, Static progressive forearm supination splint. **C** and **D**, Static progressive elbow flexion and extension splint. **E**, Static progressive extension splint for night use.

Symptoms and History

Patients with elbow flexion syndrome complain of numbness and tingling in the small and ring fingers and on the palmar and dorsoulnar side of the hand. In the early stages of compression, symptoms are typically intermittent.[90] Loss of sensation usually occurs before loss of motor function. Patients may also complain of pain in the medial elbow, a deep ache in the medial aspect of the proximal forearm, and, in the later stages, weakness of grip.[90]

Elbow flexion syndrome is associated with repetitive activities or prolonged postures involving flexion of the elbow. When the elbow is flexed, there is a 55% decrease in the size of the tunnel[90] and significant elongation of the nerve.[91] Additional tensile stresses are applied to the

ulnar nerve if elbow flexion is associated with valgus forces at the elbow,[93,94] shoulder abduction, forearm pronation, and wrist extension.[89] Symptoms may be aggravated by sleeping with the elbow flexed,[90] direct pressure to the medial elbow,[47,90] and resisted exercises involving elbow flexion and wrist flexion. Other populations that are associated with elbow flexion syndrome are carpenters, painters, and musicians.[94] In the later stages of compression, patients may report difficulty with handwriting or using a key or hammer caused by loss of motor function. People with diabetes and alcoholism are at higher risk for developing elbow flexion syndrome.[90]

Common referring diagnoses for patients with elbow flexion syndrome are cubital tunnel syndrome, ulnar

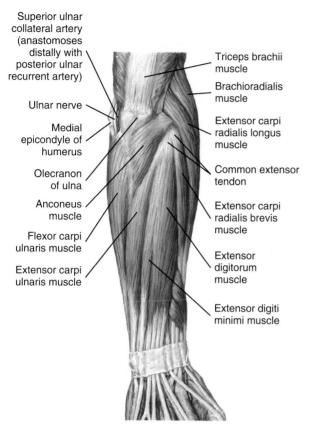

Superior ulnar
collateral artery
(anastomoses
distally with
posterior ulnar
recurrent artery)

Ulnar nerve

Medial
epicondyle of
humerus

Olecranon
of ulna

Anconeus
muscle

Flexor carpi
ulnaris muscle

Extensor carpi
ulnaris muscle

Triceps brachii
muscle

Brachioradialis
muscle

Extensor carpi
radialis longus
muscle

Common extensor
tendon

Extensor carpi
radialis brevis
muscle

Extensor
digitorum
muscle

Extensor digiti
minimi muscle

Figure 6-22. Location of the ulnar nerve at the elbow. (Netter medical illustrations used with permission of Elsevier. All rights reserved.)

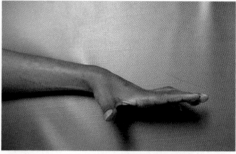

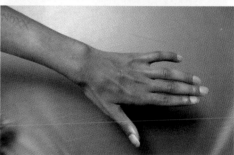

Figure 6-23. Clawing posture, atrophy of interossei, and Wartenberg's sign.

neuritis, and ulnar nerve compression at the elbow. Elbow flexion or cubital tunnel syndrome is the second most frequent nerve entrapment in the upper extremity after carpal tunnel syndrome.[71,90]

Key Tests and Signs

Alignment Analysis

The most common impairment in alignment in elbow flexion syndrome is habitual elbow flexion used in a variety of positions or activities. Avoiding elbow flexion greater than 70 degree decreases or abolishes the symptoms over time. Habitual alignment of wrist flexion with ulnar deviation (contraction of FCU) may also be noted, and correction of this also decreases symptoms. In the later stages of nerve compression, atrophy of the interossei and hypothenar muscles, a "claw-hand posture," and a positive Wartenberg's sign (abduction of small finger secondary to unopposed ED) may be present[90,92] (Figure 6-23).

Movement Impairment Analysis

The principal movement impairment for elbow flexion syndrome is habitual, repetitive, or prolonged elbow flexion. Elbow flexion may be associated with shoulder abduction, forearm pronation, and wrist flexion or extension. Forearm pronation and wrist extension contribute to elongation of the nerve, whereas contraction of the FCU during wrist flexion may aggravate symptoms

caused by compression of the nerve.[90,91] Avoidance of these movements decreases or abolishes symptoms. The "elbow flexion test" is used as a provocative test to confirm the elbow as the site of injurious stresses that are being applied to the ulnar nerve.[90,91,95] The test is positive if sensory symptoms in ulnar nerve distribution are reproduced within 1 minute.[95] Box 6-3 includes the procedures used for this test.

Joint Integrity

Joint integrity is assessed using AROM and PROM and joint accessory mobility testing. AROM and PROM of the elbow, wrist, and hand are normal in the earlier stages, but in the later stages of nerve compression, "clawing" of the ring and fifth fingers may occur with attempted active finger extension (see Figure 6-23). If left untreated in the later stages, PROM and joint accessory mobility may be limited for metacarpal (MP) flexion and interphalangeal (IP) extension of the ring and fifth fingers.

Muscle Length

Examination of the stiffness and length of the wrist flexors is important, since one of the potential sites of compression of the ulnar nerve is between the two heads of the FCU. The FCU may be stiff or short, contributing to compression of the nerve (see Box 6-2).

Muscle Strength and Performance Impairments

Strength testing should include MMT of the muscles innervated by the ulnar nerve distal to the cubital tunnel, grip, lateral, three-point pinch, and Froment's sign. Froment's sign is a test designed to test the strength of the adductor pollicis during key pinch[11] (Figure 6-24, C). Strength will be normal in the earlier stages of

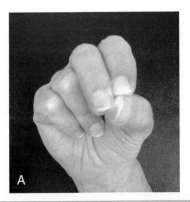

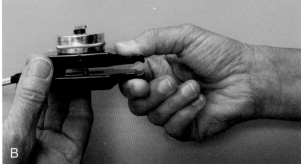

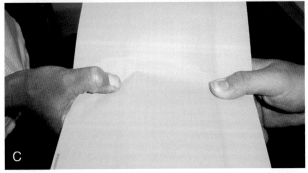

Figure 6-24. **A,** 3-point pinch. **B,** Lateral or key pinch. **C,** Froment's sign; positive on *left*, normal on *right*.

compression but weak or absent in the later stages. Muscles that may be weak include the palmar and dorsal interossei, fourth and fifth lumbricals, adductor pollicis, flexor digitorum profundus (FDP) of the ring and fifth fingers, and the FCU. The weakness of grip strength is secondary to the weakness of the intrinsics.[90]

Other Special Tests

Special tests are used to confirm the region in which excessive stresses are being applied to the nerve or the severity of the nerve compression. Four special tests that may be indicated with patients with this syndrome are (1) pressure provocative testing,[95] (2) Tinel's sign,[89,90,95] (3) sensory testing of light touch using the Semmes-Weinstein monofilaments,[90] and 4) two-point discrimination.[90] Pressure provocative testing of the ulnar nerve at the elbow and Tinel's sign may produce symptoms distal to the ulnar groove at the elbow.[90,95] Light touch may be decreased in the ulnar nerve distribution in the hand. No sensory loss should be present in the forearm. In the later stages of

compression, two-point discrimination may be impaired in the ring and small fingertips.[90] Specific procedures for these tests (except pressure provocative test) are not described in this text but have been well described previously.[13,14,95] Box 6-3 includes the pressure provocative test.

Source of Signs and Symptoms

The source of the signs and symptoms for patients with elbow flexion syndrome is the ulnar nerve. The Chapter 6 Appendix includes the associated signs or contributing factors, differential diagnoses, and treatment for this syndrome. It is common for patients with elbow flexion syndrome to have associated impairments of the shoulder girdle, such as scapular depression, imposing additional injurious tensions on the nerve tissues and thus contributing to the patient's symptoms. Therefore associated shoulder impairments must be addressed in treatment. The primary focus of treatment for elbow flexion syndrome is discussed in the next section.

Treatment

Conservative treatment is indicated for patients with milder involvement,[89,90,94] intermittent symptoms, and no muscle weakness or sensory loss. If symptoms worsen or weakness develops during the course of physical therapy treatment, the patient should be referred to the physician for possible surgery. Fifty percent of patients with mild involvement recover with conservative methods of treatment.[89] It is recommended that conservative treatment should be attempted for 4 weeks[88] to 6 months.[91]

The primary focus of treatment is patient education regarding avoiding repetitive activities or prolonged postures involving elbow flexion greater than 70 degrees, direct pressure to the medial elbow, forearm pronation, and wrist flexion.[88-91] Minimizing valgus forces to the elbow also decreases the stresses on the ulnar nerve.[94] See the Chapter 6 Appendix for further details regarding the examination, findings, and management of the patient with elbow flexion syndrome.

ELBOW VALGUS SYNDROME WITH AND WITHOUT ELBOW EXTENSION

The principal movement impairment in elbow valgus syndrome, with and without elbow extension (valgus extension overload syndrome), is excessive valgus of the elbow resulting in the laxity of or sprain of the medial/ulnar collateral ligament (MCL) at the elbow[96] (Figure 6-25). This syndrome is common in baseball pitchers and athletes who play racquet sports because of the repetitive valgus stresses on the elbow[96] (Figure 6-26). The repetitive valgus forces result in increased tensile forces on the medial structures of the elbow and increased compressive forces on the lateral structures of the elbow.[97] This syndrome is often associated with ulnar nerve injury at the elbow (elbow flexion syndrome) and may also be associated with and progress to pain with elbow extension.[98]

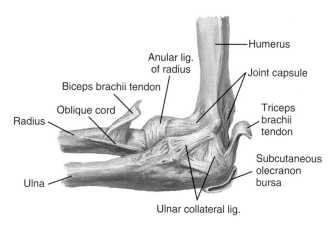

In 90° flexion: medial view

Figure 6-25. Medial or ulnar collateral ligament at the elbow. (Netter medical illustrations used with permission of Elsevier. All rights reserved.)

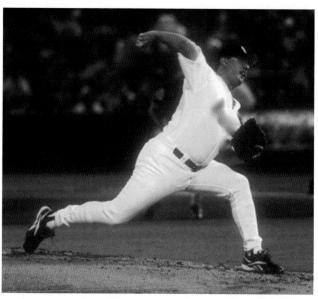

Figure 6-26. Valgus forces on the elbow with throwing. (From Rockwood CA, Matson FA, Wirth MA, et al: *The shoulder*, ed 4, Philadelphia, 2009, Saunders.)

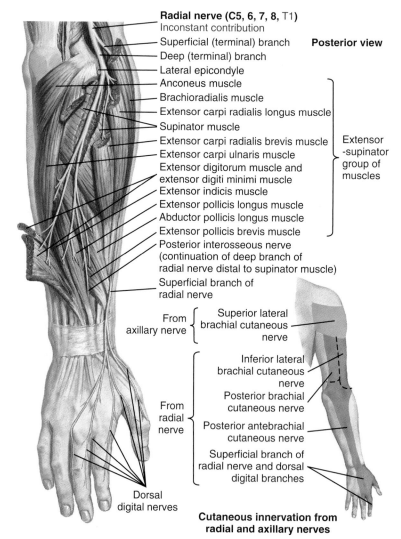

Figure 6-27. Anatomical path of radial nerve in forearm. (Netter medical illustrations used with permission of Elsevier. All rights reserved.)

This syndrome is not discussed further here because our clinical practice has limited experience with patients that fall into this category. Although valgus extension overload syndrome has been described previously, we have chosen to include this syndrome in the chapter altering the name to be consistent with the naming of the other movement system diagnoses presented in this text. We have also added impairments that theoretically may contribute to the syndrome. See the Chapter 6 Appendix for further details regarding the examination, findings, and management of this syndrome.

ELBOW EXTENSION SYNDROME

Elbow extension syndrome is characterized by posterior elbow pain provoked at the end-range of elbow extension. Two subcategories of this syndrome are as follows:
1. Normal or excessive elbow joint extension ROM (source of pain is joint structures).
2. Limited elbow joint extension (source of pain is muscle, tendon, or joint).

This syndrome is not discussed further in the text because it is in the early stages of development and our clinical practice has limited experience with patients with this syndrome. The Chapter 6 Appendix includes further details regarding the examination, findings, and management of this syndrome.

NERVE ENTRAPMENT SYNDROMES

The next two diagnostic categories are related to nerve entrapment syndromes. Nerve entrapment syndromes in the forearm have been described well by other others. We have organized the information to be consistent with the clinical decision-making process used with the other syndromes in this text. These syndromes are not discussed in detail in the text because our clinical practice currently does not see a large number of patients in this category; however, we have included some movement system impairments that in our experience and knowledge of anatomy may be associated with the nerve compressions and may contribute to the syndrome. See the Chapter 6 Appendix for further details regarding the examination, findings, and management of these syndromes.

Posterior Forearm Nerve Entrapment Syndromes

Posterior forearm nerve entrapment syndromes include radial tunnel (RT) syndrome and posterior interosseous nerve syndrome (PINS) and both of these are associated with compression of the deep branch of the radial nerve in the forearm[99] (Figure 6-27). With RT syndrome, the main complaint is pain with minimal loss of strength or the loss of strength is primarily a result of pain. Although the patient with PINS may also have pain in the forearm, with PINS, the compression has progressed so that there is significant muscle weakness but no loss of sensation.[99,100] Repetitive use of the wrist extensors or

supinator may contribute to compression of the radial nerve in these syndromes.

Anterior Forearm Nerve Entrapment Syndromes

Anterior forearm nerve entrapment syndromes include pronator syndrome (PS) and anterior interosseous nerve syndrome (AINS). PS is compression of the main branch of the median nerve in the proximal forearm[46,101] (Figure 6-28). AINS is compression of a motor-only branch of the median nerve. The AINS arises from the median nerve in the area of the pronator teres muscle. With PS, there is usually minimal loss of strength or loss of strength is primarily the result of pain and there may be changes in sensation.[46] In AINS, there is significant muscle weakness and there are no sensory changes. Weakness of the flexor pollicis longus (FPL), the FDP to the index finger, and the pronator quadratus are characteristic signs of AINS.[46] Anterior forearm nerve entrapment syndromes

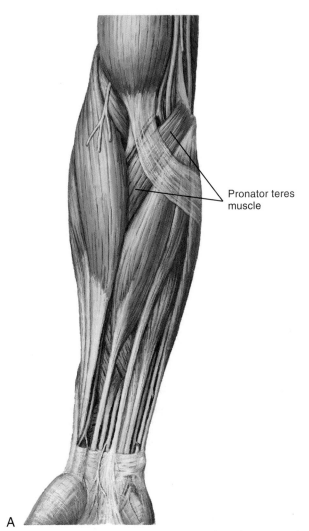

Pronator teres muscle

A

Figure 6-28. A to **C,** Anatomical path of median nerve in forearm (superficial to deep). (Netter medical illustrations used with permission of Elsevier. All rights reserved.) *Continued*

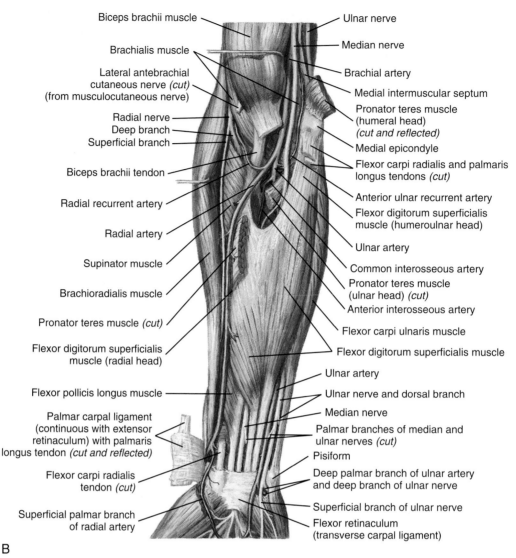

Biceps brachii muscle

Brachialis muscle

Lateral antebrachial
cutaneous nerve *(cut)*
(from musculocutaneous nerve)

Radial nerve
Deep branch
Superficial branch

Biceps brachii tendon

Radial recurrent artery

Radial artery

Supinator muscle

Brachioradialis muscle

Pronator teres muscle *(cut)*

Flexor digitorum superficialis
muscle (radial head)

Flexor pollicis longus muscle

Palmar carpal ligament
(continuous with extensor
retinaculum) with palmaris
longus tendon *(cut and reflected)*

Flexor carpi radialis
tendon *(cut)*

Superficial palmar branch
of radial artery

Ulnar nerve

Median nerve

Brachial artery

Medial intermuscular septum

Pronator teres muscle
(humeral head)
(cut and reflected)

Medial epicondyle

Flexor carpi radialis and palmaris
longus tendons *(cut)*

Anterior ulnar recurrent artery

Flexor digitorum superficialis
muscle (humeroulnar head)

Ulnar artery

Common interosseous artery

Pronator teres muscle
(ulnar head) *(cut)*

Anterior interosseous artery

Flexor carpi ulnaris muscle

Flexor digitorum superficialis muscle

Ulnar artery

Ulnar nerve and dorsal branch

Median nerve

Palmar branches of median and
ulnar nerves *(cut)*

Pisiform

Deep palmar branch of ulnar artery
and deep branch of ulnar nerve

Superficial branch of ulnar nerve

Flexor retinaculum
(transverse carpal ligament)

B

Figure 6-28, cont'd. A to **C,** Anatomical path of median nerve in forearm (superficial to deep).
(Netter medical illustrations used with permission of Elsevier. All rights reserved.)

may result from repetitive use of the forearm pronators
and finger flexors.

WRIST FLEXION WITH FOREARM PRONATION SYNDROME

Wrist flexion with forearm pronation syndrome (medial
epicondylosis or golfer's elbow) is seen much less frequently than wrist extension with forearm pronation.[102]
It is characterized by medial elbow pain[102] provoked by
repetitive or sustained activities resulting in overuse of
the wrist flexors and forearm pronators. Modification of
symptoms may be achieved by changing the movement
pattern in order to decrease the stresses on the wrist
flexors and pronators by avoiding use of the muscles
when they are lengthened and/or in the extremely shortened range. The overused muscles are often relatively
stiffer than the underused synergist.

This syndrome is not discussed in the text because in
our current clinical practice we have few patients that fall

into this category. We have chosen to include this syndrome here, altering the name to be consistent with the
naming of the other movement system diagnoses presented in this text. We have added some content and
impairments that theoretically may contribute to this
syndrome. See the Chapter 6 Appendix for further details
regarding the examination, findings, and management of
this syndrome.

ULNOHUMERAL AND RADIOHUMERAL MULTIDIRECTIONAL ACCESSORY HYPERMOBILITY SYNDROME

The principal impairment in ulnohumeral and radiohumeral multidirectional accessory hypermobility syndrome is elbow joint pain associated with impaired
rotation of the elbow joint (increased rotation of the
ulna and radius relative to the humerus) in a variety of
directions associated with excessive flexibility of the
elbow joint structures. Patients with the diagnosis of

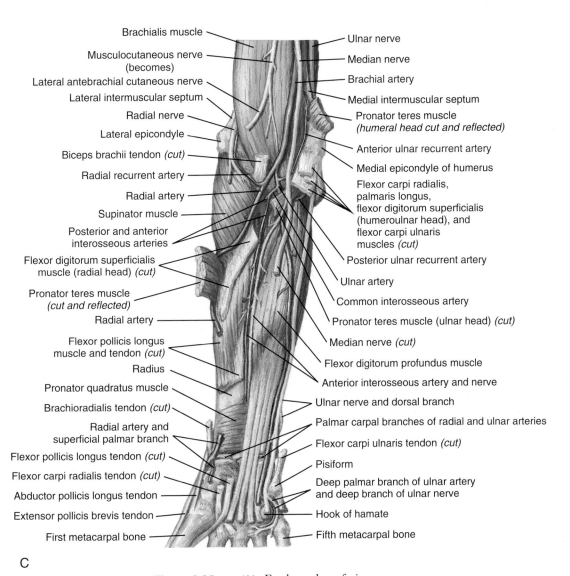

Brachialis muscle

Musculocutaneous nerve (becomes)

Lateral antebrachial cutaneous nerve

Lateral intermuscular septum

Radial nerve

Lateral epicondyle

Biceps brachii tendon *(cut)*

Radial recurrent artery

Radial artery

Supinator muscle

Posterior and anterior interosseous arteries

Flexor digitorum superficialis muscle (radial head) *(cut)*

Pronator teres muscle *(cut and reflected)*

Radial artery

Flexor pollicis longus muscle and tendon *(cut)*

Radius

Pronator quadratus muscle

Brachioradialis tendon *(cut)*

Radial artery and superficial palmar branch

Flexor pollicis longus tendon *(cut)*

Flexor carpi radialis tendon *(cut)*

Abductor pollicis longus tendon

Extensor pollicis brevis tendon

First metacarpal bone

Ulnar nerve

Median nerve

Brachial artery

Medial intermuscular septum

Pronator teres muscle *(humeral head cut and reflected)*

Anterior ulnar recurrent artery

Medial epicondyle of humerus

Flexor carpi radialis, palmaris longus, flexor digitorum superficialis (humeroulnar head), and flexor carpi ulnaris muscles *(cut)*

Posterior ulnar recurrent artery

Ulnar artery

Common interosseous artery

Pronator teres muscle (ulnar head) *(cut)*

Median nerve *(cut)*

Flexor digitorum profundus muscle

Anterior interosseous artery and nerve

Ulnar nerve and dorsal branch

Palmar carpal branches of radial and ulnar arteries

Flexor carpi ulnaris tendon *(cut)*

Pisiform

Deep palmar branch of ulnar artery and deep branch of ulnar nerve

Hook of hamate

Fifth metacarpal bone

C

Figure 6-28, cont'd. For legend see facing page.

posterolateral rotary instability[103-105] may be included in this category. A clinical test for posterolateral rotary instability is the lateral pivot shift test (see Box 6-3).

This syndrome is not discussed in the text because our clinical practice has limited experience with patients that fall into this category. However, we have chosen to include this syndrome in the chapter using a naming system consistent with the naming of the other movement system diagnoses presented in this text.

ELBOW IMPAIRMENT SYNDROME

Patients that fall into this category will usually have a history of acute trauma or injury to the elbow or forearm or the patient is in the early postoperative phase. When known, the diagnosis assigned by the physician or the name of the operative procedure provided on the referral is used as the diagnosis that will guide the physical therapy treatment, for example, cubital tunnel syndrome, status/post anterior submuscular transposition, Stage 1. If the

referral does not state the diagnosis or the procedure that was performed by the physician, the diagnosis "elbow impairment" will be used.

The focus of the treatment is protecting the injured tissues. Medical precautions have often been issued. Because of the acuity of the condition, the patient's typical movement pattern cannot be assessed at this time. The prognosis of tissue healing and normal movement is expected. The determination of the use of component versus compensatory treatment methods depends on the expectations of the final outcome. Initially, while precautions are required, compensatory methods may be necessary. The guidelines provided in the Chapter 6 Appendix are intended to be general, therefore the consulting physician's protocols for specific precautions and progressions are necessary. Appropriate application of the protocols, however, requires that the therapist be familiar with the tissues that are affected by the surgical procedure and the specific surgical approach and that he or she understands the variables that need to be considered while applying stresses to the healing tissues. This knowledge, as well as collegial communication with the physician, allows the therapist to make appropriate adjustments in the protocol as needed.

The Chapter 6 Appendix has more specific information regarding common referring diagnoses, examination, and general treatment guidelines for this diagnosis. Underlying movement system syndromes that should be considered are wrist extension with forearm pronation syndrome, elbow hypomobility syndrome, elbow flexion syndrome, anterior or posterior nerve entrapment syndromes of the forearm, elbow valgus syndrome with or without extension, elbow extension syndrome, wrist flexion with pronation syndrome, or ulnohumeral and radiohumeral multidirectional accessory hypermobility syndrome.

See Chapter 2 and the Chapter 6 Appendix for further details regarding this diagnosis.

REFERENCES

1. Sahrmann SA: *Diagnosis and treatment of movement impairment syndromes*, St Louis, 2002, Mosby.
2. Novak CB, Mackinnon SE: Evaluation of nerve injury and nerve compression in the upper quadrant, *J Hand Ther* 182:230-240, 2005.
3. Fujiwara A, Lim TH, An HS, et al: The effect of disc degeneration and facet joint osteoarthritis on the segmental flexibility of the lumbar spine, *Spine* 2523:3036-3044, 2000.
4. Eaton RG, Littler JW: Ligament reconstruction for the painful thumb carpometacarpal joint, *J Bone Joint Surg Am* 558:1655-1666, 1973.
5. Regan WD, Morrey BF: Physical examination of the elbow. In Morrey BF, Sanchez-Sotelo J, eds: *The elbow and its disorders*, Philadelphia, 2009, Saunders.
6. Magee DJ: *Orthopedic physical assessment*, ed 3, Philadelphia, 1997, Saunders.
7. Kendall FP, McCreary EK, Provance PG, et al: *Muscles: testing and function with posture and pain*, ed 5, Baltimore, 2005, Lippincott Williams & Wilkins.
8. Cyriax J: *Textbook of orthopaedic medicine*, ed 7, London, 1978, Bailliere Tindall.
9. Bechtol C: Grip test: the use of a dynamometer with adjustable handle spacings, *J Bone Joint Surg Am* 36(4):820-824, 1954.
10. Earle AS, Vlastou C: Crossed fingers and other tests of ulnar nerve motor function, *J Hand Surg Am* 56:560-565, 1980.
11. Brand PW, Hollister AM: *Clinical mechanics of the hand*, ed 3, St Louis, 1999, Mosby.
12. Mannerfelt L: Studies on the hand in ulnar nerve paralysis. A clinical-experimental investigation in normal and anomalous innervation, *Acta Orthop Scand*, Suppl 87:19-53, 1966.
13. Callahan A: Sensibility assessment for nerve lesions-in-continuity and nerve lacerations. In Mackin EJ, Callahan A, Skirven TM, et al, eds: *Rehabilitation of the hand and upper extremity*, ed 5, St Louis, 2002, Mosby.
14. Bell-Krotoski J: Sensibility testing with the Semmes-Weinstein monofilaments. In Mackin EJ, Callahan A, Skirven TM, et al, eds: *Rehabilitation of the hand and upper extremity*, ed 5, St Louis, 2002, Mosby.
15. Beals RK: The normal carrying angle of the elbow. A radiographic study of 422 patients, *Clin Orthop Relat Res* 119:194-196, 1976.
16. Hoppenfeld S: *Physical examination of the spine and extremities*, Norwalk, CT, 1976, Appleton-Century-Crofts.
17. Davila SA, Johnston-Jones K: Managing the stiff elbow: operative, nonoperative, and postoperative techniques, *J Hand Ther* 192:268-281, 2006.
18. Cain EL Jr, Dugas JR: History and examination of the thrower's elbow, *Clin Sports Med* 234:553-566, 2004.
19. Neumann DA: *Kinesiology of the musculoskeletal system: foundations for physical rehabilitation*, St Louis, 2002, Mosby.
20. Chleboun GS, Howell JN, Conatser RR, et al: The relationship between elbow flexor volume and angular stiffness at the elbow, *Clin Biomech Bristol Avon* 126:383-392, 1997.
21. Zimmerman NB: Clinical application of advances in elbow and forearm anatomy and biomechanics, *Hand Clin* 181:1-19, 2002.
22. Vardakas DG, Varitimidis SE, Goebel F, et al: Evaluating and treating the stiff elbow, *Hand Clin* 181:77-85, 2002.
23. An KN, Hui FC, Morrey BF, et al: Muscles across the elbow joint: a biomechanical analysis, *J Biomech* 1410:659-669, 1981.
24. Dines JS, ElAttrache NS: Articular injuries in the athlete. In Morrey BF, Sanchez-Sotelo J, eds: *The elbow and its disorders*, ed 4, Philadelphia, 2009, Saunders.
25. Schickendantz MS: Diagnosis and treatment of elbow disorders in the overhead athlete, *Hand Clin* 181:65-75, 2002.
26. Luthra HS: Rheumatoid arthritis. In Morrey BF, Sanchez-Sotelo J, eds: *The elbow and its disorders*, ed 4, Philadelphia, 2009, Saunders.
27. MacDermid JC, Michlovitz SL: Examination of the elbow: linking diagnosis, prognosis, and outcomes as a framework for maximizing therapy interventions, *J Hand Ther* 192:82-97, 2006.
28. McAuliffe JA: Clinical and radiographic evaluation of the elbow. In Mackin EJ, Callahan A, Skirven TM, et al, eds: *Rehabilitation of the hand and upper extremity*, ed 5, St Louis, 2002, Mosby.
29. An K, Zobitz ME, Morrey BF: Biomechanics of the elbow. In Morrey BF, Sanchez-Sotelo J, eds: *The elbow and its disorders*, ed 4, Philadelphia, 2009, Saunders.
30. Kapandji AI: *The physiology of the joints*, ed 6, Edinburgh, 2007, Churchill Livingstone.
31. Gelberman RH, Yamaguchi K, Hollstien SB, et al: Changes in interstitial pressure and cross-sectional area of the cubital tunnel and of the ulnar nerve with flexion of the elbow. An experimental study in human cadaver, *J Bone Joint Surg Am* 804:492-501, 1998.
32. Polatsch DB, Melone CP Jr, Beldner S, et al: Ulnar nerve anatomy, *Hand Clin* 233:283-289, 2007.
33. Lockard M: Clinical biomechanics of the elbow, *J Hand Ther* 192:72-80, 2006.
34. Kisner C, Colby LA: *Therapeutic exercises: foundations and techniques*, ed 5, Philadelphia, 2007, FA Davis.
35. Morrey B, An K: Functional Evaluation of the Elbow. In Morrey BF, Sanchez-Sotelo J, eds: *The elbow and its disorders*, ed 4, Philadelphia, 2009, Saunders.

36. Spinner M, Kaplan EB: The quadrate ligament of the elbow–its relationship to the stability of the proximal radio-ulnar joint, *Acta Orthop Scand* 416:632-647, 1970.

37. LaStayo PC, Lee MJ: The forearm complex: anatomy, biomechanics and clinical considerations, *J Hand Ther* 192:137-144, 2006.

38. Palmer AK, Glisson RR, Werner FW: Ulnar variance determination, *J Hand Surg Am* 74:376-379, 1982.

39. Jaffe R, Chidgey LK, LaStayo PC: The distal radioulnar joint: anatomy and management of disorders, *J Hand Ther* 92:129-138, 1996.

40. McGinley JC, Hopgood BC, Gaughan JP, et al: Forearm and elbow injury: the influence of rotational position, *J Bone Joint Surg Am* 85-A12:2403-2409, 2003.

41. Wolff AL, Hotchkiss RN: Lateral elbow instability: non-operative, operative, and postoperative management, *J Hand Ther* 192:238-243, 2006.

42. Pagnani MJ, Deng XH, Warren RF, et al: Role of the long head of the biceps brachii in glenohumeral stability: a biomechanical study in cadaver, *J Shoulder Elbow Surg* 54:255-262, 1996.

43. Krupp RJ, Kevern MA, Gaines MD, et al: Long head of the biceps tendon pain: differential diagnosis and treatment, *J Orthop Sports Phys Ther* 392:55-70, 2009.

44. Rodosky MW, Harner CD, Fu FH: The role of the long head of the biceps muscle and superior glenoid labrum in anterior stability of the shoulder, *Am J Sports Med* 221:121-130, 1994.

45. Netter FH: *Atlas of human anatomy*, ed 4, Philadelphia, 2006, Saunders.

46. Eversmann WW: Proximal median nerve compression, *Hand Clin* 82:307-315, 1992.

47. Andreisek G, Crook DW, Burg D, et al: Peripheral neuropathies of the median, radial, and ulnar nerves: MR imaging features, *Radiographics* 265:1267-1287, 2006.

48. Laha RK, Lunsford D, Dujovny M: Lacertus fibrousus compression of the median nerve. Case report, *J Neurosurg* 485:838-841, 1978.

49. Hughes JS, Morrey BF: Injury of the flexors of the elbow: biceps tendon injury. In Morrey BF, Sanchez-Sotelo J, eds: *The elbow and its disorders*, ed 4, Philadelphia, 2009, Saunders.

50. Morrey BF, Tanaka S, An KN: Valgus stability of the elbow. A definition of primary and secondary constraints, *Clin Orthop Relat Res* 265:187-195, 1991.

51. Dunning CE, Zarzour ZD, Patterson SD, et al: Muscle forces and pronation stabilize the lateral ligament deficient elbow, *Clin Orthop Relat Res* 388:118-124, 2001.

52. Basmajian JV, DeLuca CJ: *Muscles alive: their functions revealed by electromyography*, ed 5, Baltimore, 1985, Williams & Wilkins.

53. Casavant AM, Hastings H: Heterotopic ossification about the elbow: a therapist's guide to evaluation and management, *J Hand Ther* 192:255-266, 2006.

54. Dutton M: *Orthopaedic examination, evaluation, and intervention*, New York, 2004, McGraw-Hill.

55. Travill AA: Electromyographic study of the extensor apparatus of the forearm, *Anat Rec* 144:373-376, 1962.

56. Steindler A: Arthritic deformities of the wrist and fingers, *J Bone Joint Surg Am* 33-A(4):849-862, 1951.

57. Tubiana R, Thomine J, Mackin E: *Examination of the hand and wrist*, ed 2, London, 1996, Informa Healthcare.

58. Hazelton FT, Smidt GL, Flatt AE, et al: The influence of wrist position on the force produced by the finger flexors, *J Biomech* 85:301-306, 1975.

59. Cannon NM: A therapist's perspective on the conservative management of lateral epicondylitis, *Lecture at Indiana hand care course*, Indianapolis, 2004.

60. Levangie PK, Norkin CC: *Joint structure & function: a comprehensive analysis*, ed 3, Philadelphia, 2001, FA Davis.

61. Park MC, Ahmad CS: Dynamic contributions of the flexor-pronator mass to elbow valgus stability. *J Bone Joint Surg Am* 86-A10:2268-2274, 2004.

62. Davidson PA, Pink M, Perry J, et al: Functional anatomy of the flexor pronator muscle group in relation to the medial collateral ligament of the elbow, *Am J Sports Med* 232:245-250, 1995.

63. Morrey BF: Anatomy of the elbow joint. In Morrey BF, Sanchez-Sotelo J, eds: *The elbow and its disorders*, ed 4, Philadelphia, 2009, Saunders.

64. Alcid JG, Ahmad CS, Lee TQ: Elbow anatomy and structural biomechanics, *Clin Sports Med* 234:503-517, 2004.

65. Whaley AL, Baker CL: Lateral epicondylitis, *Clin Sports Med* 234:677-691, 2004.

66. Faro F, Wolf JM: Lateral epicondylitis: review and current concepts, *J Hand Surg Am* 328:1271-1279, 2007.

67. Nirschl RP, Ashman ES: Elbow tendinopathy: tennis elbow, *Clin Sports Med* 224:813-836, 2003.

68. Plancher KD, Halbrecht J, Lourie GM: Medial and lateral epicondylitis in the athlete, *Clin Sports Med* 152:283-305, 1996.

69. Kibler WB, Sciascia A: Kinetic chain contributions to elbow function and dysfunction in sports, *Clin Sports Med* 234:545-552, 2004.

70. Nirschl RP, Alvarado GJ: Muscle tendon and trauma. In Morrey BF, Sanchez-Sotelo J, eds: *The elbow and its disorders*, ed 4, Philadelphia, 2009, Saunders.

71. Piligian G, Herbert R, Hearns M, et al: Evaluation and management of chronic work-related musculoskeletal disorders of the distal upper extremity, *Am J Ind Med* 371:75-93, 2000.

72. Pascarelli EF, Hsu YP: Understanding work-related upper extremity disorders: clinical findings in 485 computer users, musicians, and others, *J Occup Rehabil* 111:1-21, 2001.

73. Martinez-Silvestrini JA, Newcomer KL, Gay RE, et al: Chronic lateral epicondylitis: comparative effectiveness of a home exercise program including stretching alone versus stretching supplemented with eccentric or concentric strengthening, *J Hand Ther* 184:411-419, 2005.

74. Buchbinder R, Green S, Struijs P: Tennis elbow, *Am Fam Physician* 755:701-702, 2007.

75. Mills GP: The treatment of "tennis elbow," *Br Med J* 7:12-13, 1928.

76. Fedorczyk JM: Therapist's management of elbow tendinitis. In Mackin EJ, Callahan A, Skirven TM, et al, eds: *Rehabilitation of the hand and upper extremity*, ed 5, St Louis, 2002, Mosby.

77. Verhaar JA, Walenkamp GH, van MH, et al: Local corticosteroid injection versus Cyriax-type physiotherapy for tennis elbow, *J Bone Joint Surg Br* 781:128-132, 1996.

78. De Smet L, Fabry G: Grip strength in patients with tennis elbow. Influence of elbow position, *Acta Orthop Belg* 621:26-29, 1996.

79. Kraushaar BS, Nirschl RP: Tendinosis of the elbow tennis elbow. Clinical features and findings of histological, immunohistochemical, and electron microscopy studies, *J Bone Joint Surg Am* 812:259-278, 1999.

80. Kibler WB: Biomechanical analysis of the shoulder during tennis activities, *Clin Sports Med* 141:79-85, 1995.

81. Ellenbecker TS: Rehabilitation of shoulder and elbow injuries in tennis players, *Clin Sports Med* 141:87-110, 1995.

82. Smith J, Morrey BF: Principles of elbow rehabilitation. In Morrey BF, Sanchez-Sotelo J, eds: *The elbow and its disorders*, ed 4, Philadelphia, 2009, Saunders.

83. Froimson AI: Treatment of tennis elbow with forearm support band, *J Bone Joint Surg Am* 531:183-184, 1971.

84. Faes M, van den AB, de Lint JA, et al: Dynamic extensor brace for lateral epicondylitis, *Clin Orthop Relat Res* 442:149-157, 2006.

85. Faes M, van EN, de Lint JA, et al: A dynamic extensor brace reduces electromyographic activity of wrist extensor muscles in patients with lateral epicondylalgia, *J Orthop Sports Phys Ther* 363:170-178, 2006.

86. Morrey BF, Askew LJ, An KN, et al: A biomechanical study of normal functional elbow motion, *J Bone Joint Surg* 636:872-877, 1981.

87. Morrey BF: Splints and bracing at the elbow. In Morrey BF, Sanchez-Sotelo J, eds: *The elbow and its disorders*, ed 4, Philadelphia, 2009, Saunders.

88. Spinner RJ: Nerve entrapment syndromes. In Morrey BF, Sanchez-Sotelo J, eds: *The elbow and its disorders*, ed 4, Philadelphia, 2009, Saunders.

89. Lund AT, Amadio PC: Treatment of cubital tunnel syndrome: perspectives for the therapist, *J Hand Ther* 192:170-178, 2006.

90. Rayan GM: Proximal ulnar nerve compression. Cubital tunnel syndrome, *Hand Clin* 82:325-336, 1992.

91. Idler RS: General principles of patient evaluation and nonoperative management of cubital syndrome, *Hand Clin* 122:397-403, 1996.

92. Omer GE: Diagnosis and management of cubital tunnel syndrome. In Mackin EJ, Callahan A, Skirven TM, et al, eds: *Rehabilitation of the hand and upper extremity*, ed 5, St Louis, 2002, Mosby.

93. Keefe DT, Lintner DM: Nerve injuries in the throwing elbow, *Clin Sports Med* 234:723-742, 2004.

94. Szabo RM, Kwak C: Natural history and conservative management of cubital tunnel syndrome, *Hand Clin* 233:311-313, 2007.

95. Novak CB, Lee GW, Mackinnon SE, et al: Provocative testing for cubital tunnel syndrome, *J Hand Surg Am* 195:817-820, 1994.

96. El Attrache NS, Ahmad CS: Diagnosis and treatment of ulnar collateral ligament injuries in athletes. In Morrey BF, Sanchez-Sotelo J, eds: *The elbow and its disorders*, ed 4, Philadelphia, 2009, Saunders.

97. Safran MR: Ulnar collateral ligament injury in the overhead athlete: diagnosis and treatment, *Clin Sports Med* 234:643-663, 2004.

98. Ahmad CS, El Attrache NS: Valgus extension overload syndrome and stress injury of the olecranon, *Clin Sports Med* 234:665-676, 2004.

99. Huisstede B, Miedema HS, van Opstal T, et al: Interventions for treating the radial tunnel syndrome: a systematic review of observational studies, *J Hand Surg Am* 331:72-78, 2008.

100. Eaton CJ, Lister GD: Radial nerve compression, *Hand Clin* 82:345-357, 1992.

101. Lee MJ, LaStayo PC: Pronator syndrome and other nerve compressions that mimic carpal tunnel syndrome, *J Orthop Sports Phys Ther* 3410:601-609, 2004.

102. Gabel GT, Morrey BF: Medial epicondylitis. In Morrey BF, Sanchez-Sotelo J, eds: *The elbow and its disorders*, ed 4, Philadelphia, 2009, Saunders.

103. Singleton SB, Conway JE: PLRI: Posterolateral rotatory instability of the elbow, *Clin Sports Med* 234:629-662, 2004.

104. O'Driscoll SW, Jupiter JB, King GJ, et al: The unstable elbow, *Instr Course Lect* 50:89-102, 2001.

105. Field LD, Savoie FH 3rd: Management of loose bodies and other limited procedures. In Morrey BF, Sanchez-Sotelo J, eds: *The elbow and its disorders*, ed 4, Philadelphia, 2009, Saunders.

APPENDIX

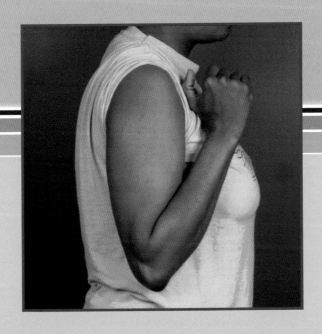

Wrist Extension with Forearm Pronation Syndrome

Wrist extension with forearm pronation (lateral epicondylosis) syndrome is characterized by lateral elbow pain provoked by gripping and lifting activities, resulting in overuse of the wrist extensors. The extensor carpi radialis brevis (ECRB) tendon is most involved as evidenced by microscopic tears.[1-3] However, clinically, the lateral elbow pain is usually aggravated most when the wrist extensors are used with the forearm pronated and the elbow extended, which may also implicate the extensor carpi radialis longus (ECRL).[4,5] In this syndrome, the biceps and supinator may be underused and wrist extensors and pronators overused during elbow flexion. Overuse comes about not solely as the result of the primary aggravating job or sporting activity but because of other activities performed

Symptoms and History

- Pain location: Lateral epicondyle, sometimes radiating down forearm
- Pain with repetitive gripping or prolonged positioning with wrist extended, forearm pronated, and elbow flexed
- Usually gradual onset[1] caused by overuse[8]
- Onset usually in third, fourth, or fifth decades[8]

Incidence and Prevalence
- 1%-3% of the population[9]
- More common in dominant extremity[1]
- Occurs equally in men and women[3]

Prognosis
- Self-limiting in 18 months to 2 years[10]

Activities/Population
- Intensive manual labor[8,11]
- Computer keyboard use[8]
- Writing[8]
- Sports such as:
  - Baseball[8]
  - Tennis[8]
  - Fencing[8]
  - Swimming[8]
  - Racquetball[8]
  - Squash[8]
  - Bowling
  - Golf[8]
  - Weightlifting[8]
- Gardening
- Musicians[12] (violinists and harpists)
- Lifting or pouring gallon of milk or coffee cup
- Carrying brief case
- Removing clothes from washer
- Turning door knobs
- Opening jars
- Sweeping
- Using hedge trimmers

Common Referring Diagnoses
- Lateral epicondylitis
- Tennis elbow
- LCL sprain grade I/II
- Elbow pain

Key Tests and Signs for Movement Impairment

Alignment Analysis
- Finger and wrist extensors are more well-developed than biceps brachii.

Movement Impairment Analysis

Aggravating Functional Activities
- Examine performance of individual functional activities (based on the history) for the movement impairment that has been identified across the examination.
- Pay particular attention to the movement patterns of the shoulder, elbow, forearm, and wrist.
- Gripping during reaching and lifting:
  - Reaching and lifting is performed with forearm pronated; during this motion, the humerus medially rotates and abducts more readily than the forearm pronates.
  - Correction is to reach and grip with forearm supinated to decrease symptoms.
- Gripping during elbow flexion and extension is less commonly observed.
  - Excessive range of wrist extension during elbow extension with excessive glenohumeral abduction (e.g., violinist).
    - Correction: Small decrease in glenohumeral abduction and maintaining wrist in more neutral alignment.
  - Excessive wrist extension during elbow flexion with the forearm aligned in neutral rotation, the glenohumeral joint in 90 degrees of abduction, and the scapula abducted (e.g., harpist).
    - Correction is to avoid extreme range of wrist extension by a small increase in scapular adduction.

Joint Integrity

AROM
- Active wrist extension may or may not be painful, depending on level of irritability.

PROM
- Wrist flexion normal but may be painful.
- Wrist extension ROM normal[3] and painless.
- Elbow extension, forearm pronation, and wrist flexion may be slightly limited and painful secondary to increased tension on injured tissues.
- Finger ROM normal.

Muscle Length Tests

Wrist and Finger Extensor Length Tests
- Positive Mill's test: Stretch to wrist extensors (forearm pronation, wrist flexion, and elbow extension) reproduces pain lateral elbow pain.[1,13,14]
- During length test, resistance to forearm pronation is felt as the elbow is extended with the wrist flexed. The humerus medially rotates more readily than the forearm pronates.
  - May have stiffness or shortness of finger and wrist extensors relative to opposite side.
  - Forearm tends to supinate with stretch to wrist and finger extensors.

with a similar movement pattern during the day. Supinating the forearm during elbow flexion decreases the symptoms by increasing performance of the biceps brachii and decreasing the overuse of the ECRL. The overused muscles are often relatively stiffer than the underused synergist. Modification of associated impairments in shoulder girdle alignment and movement is often necessary to decrease the stresses on the injured tissues at the elbow.[6] Modification of symptoms may also be achieved by changing the movement pattern to decrease the stresses on the wrist extensors by avoiding use of the muscle when it is lengthened[7] and/or in the extremely shortened range.

Source of Signs and Symptoms

Muscle/Tendon

- Microscopic tears of the ECRB with secondary involvement of the ED and ECRL (common extensor origin where it originates at the lateral epicondyle)[3,5]

Associated Signs or Contributing Factors

Alignment Analysis

- May have increased carrying angle.

Movement Impairment Analysis

- Often associated with scapular abduction and limited shoulder medial rotation[19,20] (refer to Chapter 5 in Sahrmann[21]).

Aggravating Functional Activities

- During reaching with palm up, the humerus laterally rotates and adducts more readily than the forearm supinates.

Joint Integrity

AROM

- Active elbow, forearm, wrist, and finger ROM may be normal or decreased.
- Elbow extension may be limited.

PROM

- Elbow extension and forearm pronation may be limited.

Joint Accessory Mobility Test

- May have decreased lateral glide at UH joint.[22]
- May have increased compression/proximal glide at RH/UH joints (gripping and muscle stiffness or shortness increase compression at these joints).
  - Correction: Long axis distraction of forearm and wrist decreases symptoms.

Muscle Length Tests

- Finger flexors may be stiff or short.
- Triceps and/or biceps and pronator teres may be short or stiff.

Muscle Strength/Performance Impairments

Resisted Tests

- Finger extensors often painful.

Isokinetic Testing

- Normal ratio of wrist extension/flexion (1:2) may be altered.[23]

MMT

- Supinator may be weak, but strength at least 3/5.

Differential Diagnoses

Movement System Diagnosis

- Posterior forearm nerve entrapment syndrome
- Elbow impairment

Potential Diagnoses Requiring Referral Suggested by Signs and Symptoms

Neuromusculoskeletal

- Cervical radioculpathy (C5-C6)[8,24]
- Synovitis proximal RU joint[3]
- Radial tunnel syndrome[8,25,26]
- Chronic extensor compartment syndrome[25]
- Annular ligament impingement or inflammation[24]
- LCL sprain grade II/III[24]
- Fracture of radial head, capitellum, or lateral epicondyle[26,27]
- AVN of lateral epicondyle (osteochondritis dissecans)[3,26]
- Tumor in the supinator muscle[26]
- Inflammation at attachment of triceps at olecranon[26]
- CTS[8,26]
- Shingles
- Entrapment of the musculocutaneous nerve, as it exits between the biceps and brachialis[5]
- Rotator cuff tendinosis[8]

Systemic

- RA[26]

APL, Abductor pollicis longus; *AROM*, active range of motion; *AVN*, avascular necrosis; *CRPS*, complex regional pain syndrome; *CTS*, carpal tunnel syndrome; *DIP*, distal interphalangeal; *DJD*, degenerative joint disease; *ECRB*, extensor carpi radialis brevis; *ECRL*, extensor carpi radialis longus; *ECU*, extensor carpi ulnaris; *ED*, extensor digitorum; *EDC*, extensor digitorum communis; *EMG*, electromyography; *EPB*, extensor pollicis brevis; *FDP*, flexor digitorum profundus; *FDS*, flexor digitorum superficialis; *FPB*, flexor pollicis brevis; *FPL*, flexor pollicis longus; *IP*, interphalangeal; *LCL*, lateral collateral ligament; *MCL*, medial collateral ligament; *MMT*, manual muscle testing; *NCV*, nerve conduction velocity; *OA*, osteoarthritis; *ORIF*, open reduction internal fixation; *PROM*, passive range of motion; *RA*, rheumatoid arthritis; *RH*, radiohumeral; *ROM*, range of motion; *RSD*, reflex sympathetic dystrophy; *RU*, radioulnar; *TOS*, thoracic outlet syndrome; *UH*, ulnohumeral.

Symptoms and History	Key Tests and Signs for Movement Impairment
	Muscle Strength/Performance Impairments

Muscle Strength/Performance Impairments

Resisted Tests (Soft Tissue Differential Diagnosis)

- Wrist flexors and extensors
  - Pain increased with resisted wrist extension with elbow extended[11] or flexed (Cozen's test[15]).
    - Testing resisted wrist extension with elbow extended and flexed helps differentiate between involvement of ECRL and ECRB.[4]
    - Resisted wrist extension is often more painful with the elbow extended versus flexed.[8]
  - Resisted wrist flexion is not painful.
- Forearm pronators and supinators
  - Usually not painful and should be strong.
  - If painful, not as painful as wrist extension.
- Elbow flexors and extensors
  - Depends on level of irritability; elbow flexors may or may not be painful and should be strong.
    - Resisted elbow flexion more likely to increase pain with forearm pronated (presumably to the result of contribution of ECRL with forearm pronated[16]); less pain with forearm supinated.
  - Elbow extensors strong and painless.

MMT

- Wrist extensors
  - Unable to accurately assess strength initially as the result of pain.
  - Usually wrist extensor strength at least 3/5.

Grip Strength[17]: Decreased Because of Pain

- Increased pain and decreased strength with elbow extended compared to with elbow flexed.[18]

Palpation

- Tender over lateral epicondyle or 5 mm distal to the lateral epicondyle[8] over wrist extensor muscles.[5,11]

NOTES

Treatment

Therapy: Conservative

According to Buchbinder et al,[28] the effectiveness of exercise, mobilization, and bracing is unknown for the treatment of lateral epicondylosis. Others have stated that conservative treatment is effective for 90% of patients.[29] According to Nirschl,[8] patients most likely to respond to nonoperative treatment are those with minor pain only after heavy activity or those with pain at rest and during activity, but they are able to perform functional activities without too much pain after periods of rest. If pain at night and at rest make performance of functional activities difficult, Nirschl states surgical treatment is most often necessary.[8]

Patient Education

- Patient to avoid painful activities by correcting alignment and movement impairments during daily activities, work, and sports as described:
  - Train elbow flexion with forearm supinated versus pronated as possible to increase use of biceps and decrease use of wrist extensors.
  - Grip objects with forearm supinated versus pronated when possible.
- Modify work and sports activities as appropriate[8,30]:
  - May need to change tools; alter grip throughout the day.
  - Take breaks to stretch frequently throughout the day.
  - Sitting at computer: Support arm using mouse to decrease use of ECRL as an elbow flexor.
- Importance of and methods of resting wrist extensors:
  - Splint (see "Orthotic Devices" section on next page)
  - Alternate gripping methods
  - Total rest
  - Use of opposite upper extremity

Exercises

Gradual progression is the key to maximizing successful treatment. These patients need gradual increased stresses to the wrist extensor tissues to increase threshold for injury or increase tolerance for activity. The exercises should be performed without aggravating symptoms.

- *Increase flexibility/decrease stiffness:* It is important to manually prevent rotation of the humerus during the following stretching exercises. When stretching the extensors, the humerus tends to medially rotate, whereas when stretching the finger flexors, the humerus laterally rotates.
  - Wrist and finger extensors: Initial visit instruct in stretching exercises as appropriate (Figures 6A-1 and 6A-2). Usually, wrist and finger extensors are "short" or stiff.
    - Wrist extensors: Stabilize humerus in neutral rotation during stretch. Progression of stretching is as follows: First, wrist flexion with elbow at 90 degrees flexion and forearm neutral; then wrist

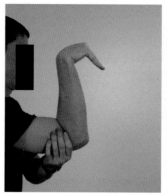
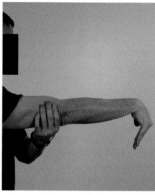

Figure 6A-1. Wrist extensor stretch.

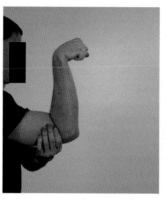
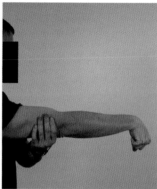

Figure 6A-2. Finger extensor stretch.

flexion with elbow at 90 degrees flexion with forearm pronated; then wrist flexion with forearm neutral and elbow extended; then wrist flexion with forearm pronated and elbow extended; last, wrist flexion with forearm pronated, elbow extended, and wrist ulnarly deviated.[7]
  - Finger extensors: The same progression could be followed as described under wrist extensors with the addition of finger flexion. Usually, the fingers are the first to be flexed during the sequence of movements.
- Finger flexors are also often stiff or short; stretch passively to avoid use of wrist and finger extensors. Stabilize humerus during stretch (Figure 6A-3).
- Joint mobilization: More research is necessary; few studies are available.
  - Mobilization with movement (lateral glide of UH joint).[22,31,32]
- *Improve muscle strength/performance[33]:*
  - Wrist extensors, forearm supinators, and biceps brachii: Ratio of wrist extensor strength to wrist flexor strength normally is 1:2.
  Progression of exercises as follows:
  - If pain is decreasing, progress to isometric exercises for wrist flexion and extension in various parts of the ROM; isometric forearm supination/pronation, elbow flexion with supination for biceps, and elbow extension. Exercises should be pain-free or with

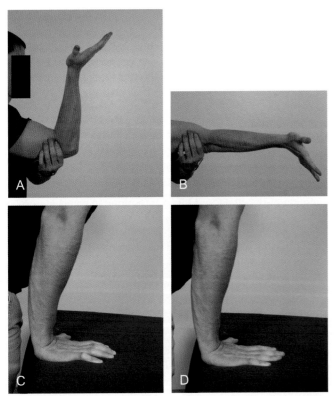

Figure 6A-3. Active Finger flexor stretch. **A** and **B**, Passive finger flexor stretch. **C**, Incorrect with PIP flexion. **D**, Correct with PIP extension.

minimal pain (no greater than 2/10 intensity) that subsides quickly after exercise.

- If pain is no greater than 2/10 and does not worsen with isometric exercises, progress to isotonic resisted exercises for wrist extension/flexion, forearm supination/pronation, elbow flexion with supination for biceps, and elbow extension. Progress resistance as tolerated. Exercises should be done without pain greater than 2/10. The goal for resistive exercises should be 70% maximum voluntary contraction (MVC) and be done 3 to 4 times/week. When working on isotonic wrist extension strengthening, start with the elbow flexed and progress to doing the exercises with elbow extended.[20] If supinator is weak, perform resisted supination exercises with elbow extended.

- Eccentric exercises instead of concentric is the new trend for treating tendinopathy, but the evidence is lacking supporting eccentric exercise over other types of exercises for lateral epicondylosis.[34] Isokinetic exercises: Tennis players may need 2:3 ratio of wrist extension to flexion strength (increased wrist extension strength).[24]

- Shoulder girdle musculature[6,8,30,35]: Refer to Chapter 5 in Sahrmann[21] for correct impaired shoulder alignment and movement.

- Return to work: The more difficult cases may benefit from conditioning using BTE Technologies (Hannover, Md.).

Orthotic Devices

According to Struijs et al,[36] there are no definitive conclusions on their effectiveness.

- Forearm strap[8,33] (also called *counterforce brace*[8]) provided at initial visit.[1-3,33] Straps that are 3 or 3.5 inches wide are better than narrower ones. Their purpose is to absorb and dissipate forces to wrist extensor mass and prevent full muscle contraction.[8] Patient should be careful not to wear the strap too tight as that might cause compression and injury to the nerves in the elbow region[37] (Figure 6A-4).

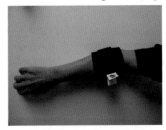

Figure 6A-4. Elbow strap.

- Wrist cock up splint with wrist in 10 to 25 degrees extension will help rest the wrist extensor muscles. Not first-choice treatment unless very acute/inflamed.[8] Immobilize joint just long enough to decrease pain. According to Faro,[2] no definitive conclusions can be drawn regarding the effectiveness of orthotic devices for this condition (Figure 6A-5).

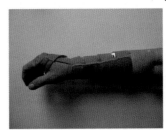

Figure 6A-5. Wrist splint.

- Dynamic extensor assist brace: splint that assists the wrist into extension but allows wrist flexion might be helpful.[38,39]
- Taping the elbow has also been found to be helpful.[40]

Modalities

Modalities may be helpful but "exercise is the mainstay of the treatment."[1,3,33]

- Iontophoresis to lateral epicondyle area[33]
- High-voltage electrical stimulation (4 to 6 sessions over 2 to 3 week period)[8]
- Ice or hot pack may be useful for pain relief at home.

Massage

Massage to the painful extensor muscle mass such as cross-friction massage may be helpful.[1,33] However, in our experience, rest, exercises and correction of movement impairment during specific activities is the key to conservative management.

Elbow Hypomobility Syndrome

The principal movement impairment in elbow hypomobility syndrome is significant limitation of accessory and physiological motion of the elbow. Flexion loss is usually greater than extension loss[13] and is usually also associated with a loss of forearm pronation and supination. This is most often the result of the effects of prolonged immobilization after surgery or trauma.

Symptoms and History

- Complaints of stiffness and decreased ROM
- Complaints of pain, especially at end ROM[41]
- No complaints of numbness and tingling

Activities/Population

- Difficulty with self-care activities such as feeding, turning key in ignition, reading, personal hygiene

Common Referring Diagnoses

- Fracture
- Dislocation
- Any surgical procedure of elbow or forearm
- Stiff elbow
- Elbow pain

Key Tests and Signs for Movement Impairment

Alignment Analysis

- Elbow in excessive flexion, forearm pronated
- Glenohumeral extension

Movement Impairment Analysis

- Limited accessory and physiological motion of the elbow and forearm resulting in compensatory movements:
  - May note scapular anterior tilt with elbow extension
  - Scapular adduction and posterior tilt and trunk extension with elbow flexion
  - Shoulder adduction and lateral rotation with forearm supination
  - Shoulder abduction and medial rotation with forearm pronation
  - Shoulder extension during elbow extension
  - Shoulder flexion during elbow flexion

Joint Integrity

ROM

- Pain increased at end of restricted AROM and PROM with capsular end-feel
- Loss of PROM in capsular pattern, flexion loss greater than extension loss (ulnohumeral)[13]
- Associated decreased ROM of pronation/supination of forearm

Ligament Integrity

- Negative

Joint Accessory Mobility

- Decreased accessory ROM

Muscle Strength/Performance Impairments

- Strength: Generalized weakness of elbow flexion, extension, forearm pronation/supination (strength usually >3/5)

Source of Signs and Symptoms

Joint/Bone
- Elbow capsule,[41] ligaments, bone

Muscle/Tendon/Bursae
- Co-contraction[41]
- Inhibition
- Stiffness develops secondary to weakness
- Muscle or tendon contracture or adhesions

Edema[41]

Alignment/Appearance
- Skin: Shiny with decreased creases; loss of the concavities on either side of the olecranon
- Size: Enlarged locally or diffuse
- Tends to accumulate around elbow but may also be associated with edema of the hand

Measurement
- Circumference: Increased when compared to uninvolved side

Palpation
- Edema: Can be pitting or brawny

Scar[41]

Appearance/Palpation
- Visible superficial scar
- Scar is described as red, raised, supple, mature, immature, keloid, hypertrophic, adherent; should be assessed for hypersensitivity, whether it is raised, and mobility

Nerve[41]
- Stiffness develops secondary to:
  - Neurapraxia
  - Nerve compression
  - Adhesions

Associated Signs or Contributing Factors

Alignment Analysis

Posture
- May be associated with stiff hand and wrist posture (metacarpal joints extended, interphalangeal joints flexed, thumb adducted, and wrist flexed)

Movement Impairment Analysis
- May be associated with scapular anterior tilt
- May have associated loss of ROM at shoulder, wrist, and hand[41]
- May develop secondary shoulder pain and impingement caused by faulty movement imposed by limited elbow ROM

Muscle Length
- May have secondary shortness of elbow, wrist, and finger flexors and extensors, supinator or pronator muscles[41]

Differential Diagnoses

Movement System Diagnosis
- Elbow impairment

Potential Diagnoses Requiring Referral Suggested by Signs and Symptoms

Neuromusculoskeletal
- Synovitis proximal RU joint
- Fracture or dislocation[41]
- Arthrogryposis (persistent contracture of a joint)
- Myositis ossificans[24]
- Heterotopic ossification[41]
- Compartment syndrome[24]
- Osteochondrosis (AVN)[24]
- Osteophytes
- Intraarticular incongruity[41]

Systemic
- RA[24]
- Osteoarthrosis (any disease involving the joints)[24]
- Chondromatosis (tumor)[24]
- Gout[24]
- Chondrocalcinosus[24]

Treatment
Therapy: Conservative
- Nonoperative treatment is indicated with mild contractures present 6 months or less.[42]
- Focus for treatment is to increase AROM and PROM of elbow and forearm with goal of at least −30 to 130 degrees elbow extension/flexion and 50 degrees pronation and 50 degrees supination for acceptable function.

Patient Education
- During elbow and forearm exercises or functional use of upper extremity, avoid substituting movement of the scapula or glenohumeral joint.
- Guidelines regarding pain during exercises: To gain ROM, the patient must work through some discomfort, especially at the end-ranges, but the pain should not be severe and should not last for more than 1 hour after exercise.
- The patient should be encouraged to use the involved arm functionally and increase activities by incorporating weight bearing as tolerated.
- Avoid use of sling.

Treatment of Edema and Scar
Refer to general guidelines for treatment of edema and scar in Box 5-2.

Exercises
- *Increase flexibility/decrease stiffness:*
  - Stretching should be low load, within tissue tolerance, and prolonged duration. Aggressive stretching can increase inflammation, contributing to increased contracture.[43] Caution should be used to avoid forced manipulation that may lead to muscle tears in the muscle before complete healing so myositis ossificans does not develop.[44]
  - AROM and PROM[41] exercises to RU and UH joints with attention to correct stabilization of scapulothoracic joints and glenohumeral joints.
  - Muscle length: May need stretching of wrist and finger extensors and flexors to increase elbow extension, as well as primary elbow flexors. Hold 20 to 30 seconds.
  - Proprioceptive neuromuscular facilitation (PNF): Hold-relax and contract-relax may be helpful to reduce co-contraction.[41]
  - Joint mobilization[41,45]:
    - Distraction of UH joint at 90 degrees.
    - Anterior to posterior and posterior to anterior glides at radioulnar joints.
  - Some advocate continuous passive motion (CPM),[42] whereas others say it helps maintain motion but does not help increase motion.[43]
- *Improve muscle strength/performance* (initiate strengthening when ROM gains begin to plateau, beginning with physiological movements and progressing to functional and sport movements):
  - Wrist[41]
  - Forearm pronation/supination[41]
  - Elbow flexion and extension[41]
  - Initiate active triceps exercises early after injury to prevent adhesions (supine with shoulder flexed 90 degrees, active elbow extension)[41]
  - Shoulder, with attention to correct scapular alignment

Splinting
- Prolonged gentle stretch is most effective to increase ROM[33, 41] (see Figure 6-21).
- At night, use static extension splinting or custom-made static progressive extension splint to increase extension if end-feel is soft.
- During the day, use prefabricated static progressive or dynamic splint if end-feel is firm. Static progressive splint is used 3 to 6 times/day for 30 to 60 minutes each time.

Modalities
Using heat (ultrasound, fluid therapy, or hot packs) on the tissues, as well as stretching, can be helpful.[41]

NOTES

Elbow Flexion Syndrome

The principal movement impairment in elbow flexion syndrome (cubital tunnel) is habitual, repetitive, or prolonged elbow flexion. Prolonged or repetitive elbow flexion places excessive stresses on the ulnar nerve at the medial elbow, causing symptoms.[46] Ulnar nerve injury may be caused by compression, traction, or friction.[47] Elbow flexion may be associated with forearm pronation, wrist flexion or extension, and shoulder abduction.[48-50] Shoulder abduction,

Symptoms and History

- Numbness and tingling in the small and ring fingers and on the palmar and dorsoulnar side of the hand
- Typically, symptoms are intermittent initially, with sensory loss occurring before motor[49]
- Sometimes elbow pain (medially) with deep ache in medial aspect of proximal forearm[49]
- Weak grip in later stages[49]

Activities/Population

- Elbow flexion activities (get 55% decrease in size of tunnel with elbow flexion[49] and significant elongation of nerve[50])
- Activities involving valgus forces to elbow[52,53] (e.g., baseball players, tennis players)
- Carpenters, painters, musicians[53]
- Sleeping (usually with elbow flexed)[49]
- Difficulty using a key, hammer, or handwriting with motor loss
- Chronic repetitive trauma to the flexed elbow via direct pressure to medial elbow (e.g., habitually leaning on the elbow)[46,49]
- Resistive upper extremity exercises (especially elbow flexion)
- Diabetic[49]
- Alcoholic[49]

Common Referring Diagnoses

- Cubital tunnel syndrome
- Ulnar neuritis
- Ulnar nerve compression at the elbow

Second most frequent nerve entrapment in the upper extremity after CTS[11,49]

Key Tests and Signs for Movement Impairment

Alignment Analysis
Posture/Muscle Development
- Habitual prolonged elbow flexion
  - Correction decreases or abolishes symptoms
- Habitual contraction of FCU (wrist flexion with ulnar deviation)
  - Correction decreases or abolishes symptoms
- "Claw" hand in severe cases
- Positive Wartenberg's sign[49,51] (abduction of small finger secondary to unopposed ED in later stages)
- Atrophy of interosseus, especially first dorsal interosseus and hypothenar eminence in later stages[49]

Movement Impairment Analysis
- Habitual repetitive or prolonged elbow flexion, forearm pronation and wrist flexion or extension
  - Correction decreases or abolishes symptoms

Elbow Flexion Test[49,50,54]
- Positive if sensory symptoms in ulnar nerve distribution within 1 minute
- Best sensitivity (0.98) and specificity (0.95),[54] if combined with pressure provocation test

Joint Integrity
AROM
- Initially normal, then "clawing" of the ring and fifth fingers with attempted active finger extension (in later stages)

PROM
- Initially normal, then restricted metacarpalphalangeal flexion and interphalangeal extension of the ring and fifth fingers if untreated (in later stages)

Joint Accessory Mobility
- May be limited in later stages related to decreased PROM

Muscle Length Tests
Wrist Flexor Length
- Shortness or stiffness of FCU[55]

Muscle Strength/Performance Impairments
- Later stages only
- Strength: Weak grip, lateral, and three-point pinch when compared to the uninvolved side; intrinsic weakness usually noted first, then grip weakness noted due to the intrinsic weakness[49]
- Froment's sign[56]: Positive (with motor loss); initially negative

MMT
- Weak[49]
  - Palmar and dorsal interosseous
  - Fourth and fifth lumbricals
  - Adductor pollicis
  - FDP of ring and fifth fingers
  - FCU

Other Special Tests
Pressure Provocative Test[54]
- Can produce symptoms distal to ulnar groove
- Can be used in combination with the elbow flexion test

Tinel's Sign[48,49,54]
- Positive in ulnar groove at the elbow (may be present in 24% of normals).[49]
- 4 to 6 taps proximal to cubital tunnel found to have sensitivity (true positive) of 0.70 and specificity (true negative) of 0.98[54]

Test to Reproduce Subluxing of Ulnar Nerve
- May or may not be positive[52]

Sensation
- Monofilaments[49]: Can see diminished sensation in the ulnar nerve distribution; sensory loss usually occurs before overt weakness; no sensory loss in forearm
- Two-point discrimination[49]: Can be altered in ring and small volar tips (this occurs later)

forearm pronation, and wrist extension contribute to elongation of the nerve, whereas contraction of the flexor carpi ulnaris (FCU) during wrist flexion may aggravate symptoms as the result of compression of the nerve. The ulnar nerve travels through the cubital tunnel, which is formed by the elbow joint and medial collateral ligament (MCL) laterally, and the aponeurosis between the two heads of the FCU medially.[51]

Source of Signs and Symptoms

Ulnar nerve

Associated Signs or Contributing Factors

Alignment Analysis

Posture
- Increased carrying angle or repetitive valgus forces to elbow[53,57]

Structural Variations
- Bony compression from old fracture[53]
- Shallow cubital tunnel
- Cubitus valgus[52,53]
- Ganglion[53]
- Anomalous muscles: Anconeus epitrochlearis[50]

Predisposing Factors
- Acute trauma to the nerve
- Subluxing nerve[51]
  - Palpation for subluxing nerve as elbow is flexed and extended
  - Test to reproduce subluxing of ulnar nerve
- Thin (no padding for nerve)
- Obese
- Hypertrophy of medial head of triceps or FCU compressing ulnar nerve[52]
- Double crush[58]

Associated Movement Diagnosis
- Related to TOS
  - Scapular depression
  - Scapular downward rotation
  - Scapular abduction
  - Faulty scapular alignment and shoulder motion contributing to increased tension on neurovascular bundle with overhead activities

Differential Diagnoses

Movement System Diagnosis
- Elbow impairment
- Elbow valgus syndrome with or without extension
- Wrist flexion with forearm pronation (medial epicondylosis)
- Insufficient finger flexion or extension (at the MPs and IPs) causing a "claw" appearance.

Potential Diagnoses Requiring Referral Suggested by Signs and Symptoms

Neuromusculoskeletal
- Cervical radiculopathy (C8-T1)[48,49,59]
- TOS[48,49,59] (may have co-existent TOS: "double crush")
- Compression of ulnar nerve at Guyon's canal[48,49] (FDP and FCU not affected; no sensory change on dorsum of hand; Tinel's sign positive at wrist, not elbow; Phalen's test might produce ulnar nerve symptoms)
- Intraspinal pathology[51]
- Amyotrophic lateral sclerosis (ALS)[51]
- Hansen's disease[51]
- Chronic alcoholism[51]
- Hemophilia[51]
- Renal disease[51]
- MCL sprain or laxity[60]
- Fracture medial epicondyle[27,60]
- Medial epicondylosis[27]
- Flexor pronator strain[27]

Systemic
- OA (any disease involving the joints)
- Pancoast tumor[48,49]

Treatment

Nonoperative Treatment

Indicated for patients with milder involvement of intermittent symptoms,[48,49,53] without muscle weakness or sensory loss. If symptoms worsen or weakness develops, refer for possible surgery. Fifty percent of patients with mild involvement recover with conservative methods of treatment.[48] It is recommended that conservative treatment be attempted for 4 weeks[47] to 6 months.[50]

Patient Education

- The primary focus of patient education is to teach the patient to avoid repetitive activities or prolonged postures involving elbow flexion greater than 70 degrees, direct pressure to the medial elbow, forearm pronation, and wrist flexion. Minimizing valgus forces to the elbow also decreases the stresses on the ulnar nerve.[47-50,53] Correcting proximal impairments is also important.
- Modifications to work and functional activities:
  - Avoid leaning on elbows (Figure 6A-6).

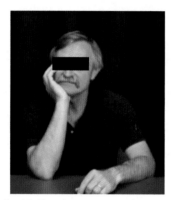

Figure 6A-6. Avoid direct pressure to ulnar nerve (leaning on elbows).

  - Avoid prolonged or repeated elbow flexion and pronation and wrist flexion.
  - Avoid frequent of prolonged contraction of FCU.
  - Avoid positions or activities placing valgus forces at the elbow with the shoulder abducted because this position places the ulnar nerve on maximum tension.[53]
  - Arrange keyboard so that elbows are flexed 70 degrees or less (Figure 6A-7).

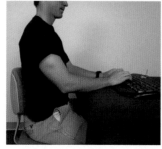

Figure 6A-7. Place keyboard so elbows are flexed 70 degrees or less and arms are supported for correct shoulder alignment.

- Support arms so shoulders are aligned correctly but with care to avoid direct pressure to medial elbow (Figure 6A-8).

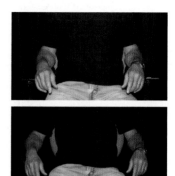

Figure 6A-8. Suggestions for sitting. Support arms so shoulders are aligned correctly but with care to avoid direct pressure to medial elbow.

- Pad edges of table.
- Support arms on pillows at night for sleep to align shoulders correctly but with care to avoid elbow flexion greater than 70 degrees (Figure 6A-9).

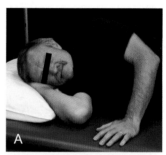

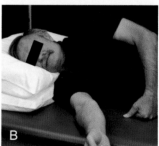

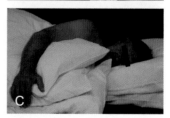

Figure 6A-9. Suggestions for sleeping. **A,** Avoid elbow flexion. **B,** Keep elbow extended or flexed only slightly. **C,** Support arm for sleep to maintain ideal shoulder girdle alignment.

- Avoid crossing arms in front. Correction: Sit with forearm resting in lap and forearm supinated[53] (Figure 6A-10).

- Elbow pad worn volarly to limit elbow flexion at night (see Figure 6A-11, *B*).
- Rigid elbow flexion–block splint; allows 0 to 70 degrees. Only worn at night and as needed daily (Figure 6A-12).

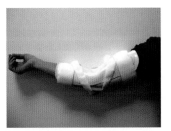

Figure 6A-12. Rigid elbow flexion–block splint.

- For motor loss:
  - Anti-claw splints, if motor loss to increase function (Figure 6A-13).

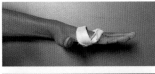
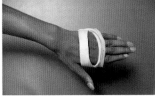

Figure 6A-13. Anti-claw splint.

Postoperative treatment is not be covered in this text; see other sources.[48]

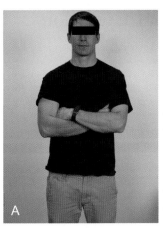
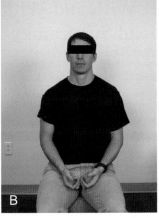

Figure 6A-10. **A,** Avoid crossing arms in front of you. **B,** When sitting rest forearms supinated and arms resting in lap.

- Use phone head set.
- Replace hammering with nail gun.

Exercises
- For transient symptoms with no motor loss:
  - Increase flexibility of FCU.[55]
  - Nerve gliding exercises.
    - Some advocate use of upper limb tension test (ULTT) for gentle gliding and stretching of a peripheral nervous system component or its associated structures.[48]
    - Careful to use oscillating movements versus prolonged stretches and avoid reproducing symptoms.
  - Correct proximal impairments contributing to neural tension.[55]
    - Correct faulty movement and alignment of neck and shoulder girdle.
- For motor loss:
  - PROM (especially metacarpalphalangeal flexion and interphalangeal extension if loss of AROM)

Splint/protective padding[48,53,61]
- For transient symptoms with no motor loss:
  - Elbow pad worn medially to avoid direct pressure to ulnar nerve (Figure 6A-11, *A*).

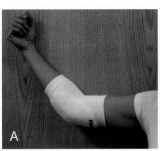
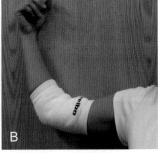

Figure 6A-11. Elbow pad **(A)** worn with pad posteromedially to avoid pressure to ulnar nerve. **B,** Worn with pad anteriorly to prevent excessive elbow flexion at night.

Elbow Valgus Syndrome: With and Without Extension (Valgus Extension Overload Syndrome)

The principal movement impairment in elbow valgus syndrome is excessive valgus of the elbow, resulting in the laxity of or sprain of the medial/ulnar collateral ligament (MCL) at the elbow.[62] This is common in athletes that are baseball pitchers and that play racquet sports due to the repetitive valgus stresses on the elbow.[62] The repetitive valgus forces result in increased tensile forces on the medial structures of the elbow and increased compressive forces on the lateral structures of the elbow.[63] This syndrome is often associated with ulnar nerve injury at the elbow (elbow flexion syndrome) and may also be associated with and progress to pain with elbow extension.[64]

Symptoms and History

Without Extension
- Pain primarily in medial elbow but may also have lateral elbow pain[60,63]

With Extension
- Pain posterior or medial elbow as the elbow extends[64]
- Onset may be gradual or acute
- If acute, may report popping that occurs during valgus stresses to elbow[63]

Activities/Population
- May be worse with pitching, throwing, or overhead serves as in tennis or squash[63]

Common Referring Diagnoses

Without Extension
- Medial epicondylitis (golfer's elbow)
- MCL sprain (pitcher's elbow)
- Cubital tunnel syndrome
- Ulnar neuritis

With Extension
- Olecranon bursitis
- Triceps tendinopathy
- Anconeus tendonipathy
- Valgus extension overload[64]
- Elbow sprain

Key Tests and Signs for Movement Impairment

Alignment Analysis
- If acute, may have ecchymosis medial elbow and forearm[63]

Movement Impairment Analysis
- Pain with repetitive motion causing valgus force at elbow joint[60,63]
  - Correction: Avoiding valgus forces at the elbow and increasing glenohumeral lateral rotation decreases symptoms
- May have decreased humeral lateral rotation ROM (normal lateral rotation for baseball player is 95 to 105 degrees, 115 degrees is too much)
  - Decreased lateral rotation ROM may increase valgus forces at elbow during throwing[65]

Joint Integrity

Active ROM

With and without Extension
- ROM may change along continuum:
  - Acute: Some decreased elbow flexion or extension
  - Early chronic: Elbow and forearm ROM usually full
  - Late chronic: May have elbow flexion contracture[64]

With Extension
- Onset of pain at end ROM elbow extension[64]
  - Correction: Limiting the range of elbow extension abolishes symptoms

PROM

With and without Extension
- Normal elbow extension range

With Extension
- Painful at end-range extension
- May lose elbow extension if associated with osteophytes[57,63,64]

Ligament Integrity Tests

With and without Extension
- Moving valgus stress test[62,66]
  - Increased laxity in MCL compared to opposite side and reproduces pain, especially with valgus stress at 70 to 120 degrees of flexion
  - May not be able to feel this laxity even with large tear without anesthesia
- Milking maneuver test[57,62,64]
  - Tenderness and joint space opening
- Valgus stress test[57,63]
  - Increased laxity and pain on involved side
- Valgus extension overload test[57]
  - Increased pain posteromedial elbow toward the end of the test

Muscle Strength/Performance Impairments

With and without Extension
- Resisted tests (soft tissue differential diagnosis)
  - Elbow extensors strong and painless
  - Wrist flexors strong and painless[63]

Palpation

With and without Extension
- Point tenderness over origin or insertion of ulnar collateral ligament, commonly on ulna where ligament inserts or on humeral condyle[62,63]
- May also have lateral joint line tenderness or crepitus at radiohumeral joint[57]

With Extension
- Tender posterior medial elbow[57,64]

Source of Signs and Symptoms

With and without Extension
- MCL

With Extension
- Joint, bone, or bursae
  - Olecranon or osteophytes

Associated Signs or Contributing Factors

Alignment Analysis
With and without Extension
- Posture: May have increased carrying angle and increased elbow flexion[57]

Structural Variations
With Extension
- Posterior osteophytes on ulna[57,64]

With and without Extension
- Cartilage changes medially
- RH joint problems secondary to compression[57,64]

Movement Impairment Analysis
With and without Extension
- Faulty scapular motion (e.g., decreased scapular adduction, posterior tilt, or external rotation during cocking in throwing may cause increased valgus stresses at elbow)[67]

Muscle Length Tests
With and without Extension
- Pronator teres length test: Often short or stiff
- Wrist and finger flexor length test: Possible increased wrist and finger flexor length or decreased stiffness (increased carrying angle)
- Wrist and finger extensor length test: Possible decreased wrist and finger extensor length or increased stiffness (increased carrying angle)

Muscle Strength/Performance Impairments
- Possible decreased wrist and finger flexor strength (related to increased carrying angle)

Differential Diagnoses

Movement System Diagnosis
- Elbow flexion syndrome
- Elbow extension syndrome
- Elbow impairment

Potential Diagnoses Requiring Referral Suggested by Signs and Symptoms

Neuromusculoskeletal

With and without Extension
- Cubital tunnel[57,60,63,64]
- AVN (osteochondritis dissecans) lateral elbow[57]
- Epiphysitis of medial epicondyle (Little Leaguer's elbow)[57]
- Avulsion of medial epicondyle in adolescents before epiphyseal closure[57]
- Osteophytes or loose bodies or traction spurs[57,63,64]
- Medial epicondyle stress fracture, bone bruise, or edema
- Ligament sprains grades 2 and 3[63]
- Tendinopathy or avulsion of flexor pronator muscles[60,63]

With Extension
- Stress fracture of olecranon[64]
- Cervical radiculopathy[57]

Treatment for Elbow Valgus Syndrome

With and without Extension

- For second and third degree sprains, surgery may be indicated.[60]
- It is unknown how much the dynamic elements contribute to elbow stability. The contribution is probably low, but typically, rehabilitation includes increasing the endurance and strength (both concentric and eccentric) of the wrist flexors and forearm pronators.
- The initial focus of treatment is rest, but exercises can be introduced once the initial discomfort resolves.
- Elbow extension is limited initially with first-degree sprains and postoperatively with more severe sprains to decrease the stress on the anterior bundle of the MCL, which is the primary structure that resists valgus forces at the elbow.[60]

With Extension

- Treatment is the same as for elbow valgus syndrome plus an increased emphasis on eccentric control of the biceps brachii to decrease the forces on the posterior elbow.[65]

Patient Education

With and without Extension

- In the early healing stages, avoid activities or exercises producing valgus forces such as the following:
  - Resisted horizontal adduction
  - Resisted shoulder medial rotation
- Correct movement pattern used during sport or functional activity to decrease valgus forces at the elbow[64]

With Extension

- In the early healing stages, avoid end-ROM elbow extension

Exercises (First-Degree Sprain)

With and without Extension

- *Increase flexibility/ROM*
  - Restore normal elbow, forearm, and wrist ROM.[65] Minimize elbow flexion contractures.[65]
  - Joint mobilization may be helpful.[65]
  - Wrist and finger extensors: If short or stiff, stretch.
- *Improve muscle strength/performance:*
  - The initial exercises are strengthening of the wrist flexors with a gradual progression to forearm pronators. The FCU and FDS are dynamic stabilizers of the medial elbow.[62,63] Exercises causing any valgus loading are avoided for about 6 weeks.[60]

- As pain and tenderness decrease, strengthening exercises for elbow flexion/extension, wrist flexion/extension, forearm pronation/supination are progressed from isometric to concentric to eccentric.[65]
- As pain and tenderness decrease, exercises for neuromuscular control are also recommended (PNF).[65]
- About 6 weeks postinjury, gradual progression to valgus loading exercises (e.g., resistive horizontal adduction and shoulder medial rotation exercises) is done if the patient is going to return to an activity causing valgus loading forces at the elbow. Strengthening exercises may be more aggressive focusing on speed, plyometric activities, and progression into a throwing program.[65]
- The criteria for gradual progression into valgus loading exercises are as follows[60]:
  - Normal strength in shoulder and forearm muscles: Isokinetic testing may be useful to determine full strength.[65]
  - Ligament stress tests are negative.
  - No tenderness with palpation over the ligament.
- Correct shoulder girdle impairments that may contribute to increasing valgus forces across the elbow,[60,65] especially increasing glenohumeral lateral rotation or scapular adduction, posterior tilt, and external rotation.

With Extension

- Biceps brachii: Eccentric control[64,65]

Bracing[60] (Figure 6A-14)

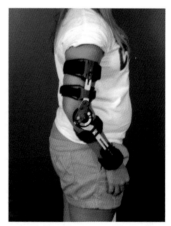

Figure 6A-14. Brace after ulnar collateral ligament injury to prevent valgus forces at elbow.

Without Extension
- For first-degree sprain, bracing may be used to prevent valgus of elbow[60]:
  - A hinged brace is used that limits the elbow from extending fully during the first 2 weeks.[60]
  - After the first 2 weeks, the brace is adjusted to gradually allow full elbow extension.[60]
  - The brace is worn for 6 weeks.[60]

With Extension
- In early healing stage, taping or splinting to block end-range of motion elbow extension (Figure 6A-15).

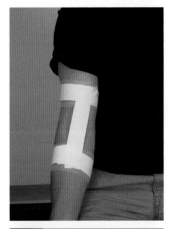
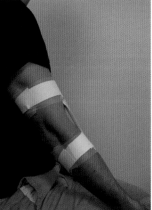

Figure 6A-15. Taping to block end-range elbow extension.

Elbow Extension Syndrome

Elbow extension syndrome is characterized by posterior elbow pain provoked at the end-range of elbow extension. Two subcategories are normal or excessive elbow joint extension ROM (source of pain is joint structures) and limited elbow joint extension (source of pain is muscle, tendon, or joint).

Symptoms and History

Excessive and Limited Extension
- Pain with end-ROM elbow extension

Activities/Population

Excessive Extension
- May be involved in sports (e.g., swimmers)
- More common at younger ages

Limited Extension
- Trauma: Falling off ladder, bicycle, or roof, resulting in fracture or dislocation

Common Referring Diagnoses

Excessive and Limited Extension
- Olecranon bursitis
- Triceps tendinopathy
- Anconeus tendinopathy
- Elbow sprain

Limited Extension
- S/p dislocation, fracture, or stiff elbow (overuse of anconeus with pain over anconeus from overexertion trying to regain elbow extension)

Key Tests and Signs for Movement Impairment

Alignment Analysis

Limited extension
- Standing: Increased elbow flexion

Movement Impairment Analysis

Joint Integrity

Excessive Extension

AROM
- Elbow extension ROM may be increased (hyperextension)
- Onset of pain at end-ROM elbow extension
  - Correction: Limiting the range of elbow extension abolishes symptoms

PROM
- Normal or increased elbow extension range and painful at end-range

Limited Extension

AROM and PROM
- Elbow extension ROM limited 10 to 15 degrees
- Forearm supination ROM slightly limited
- Active extension painful, but PROM not painful at end-ROM
- Onset of pain at end-ROM elbow extension
  - Correction: Avoid forceful end-range elbow extension; passive instead of active

Joint Accessory Mobility

Limited Extension
- Decreased accessory ROM for elbow extension

Ligament Integrity Test
- Valgus extension overload test: Negative

Muscle Strength/Performance Impairments

Excessive Extension
- Elbow extensors strong and painless

Limited Extension
- Elbow extensors strong and painful

Palpation

Excessive Extension
- Tender posterior medial elbow

Limited Extension
- Tender posterior elbow over triceps tendon or anconeus

Source of Signs and Symptoms

Excessive Extension
- Joint, bone, and bursae

Limited Extension
- Muscle, tendon, and joint

Associated Signs or Contributing Factors

Alignment Analysis
Excessive Extension
- May have generalized decreased muscle bulk and stiffness

Structural Variations
Excessive Extension
- May have short olecranon (structural)

Differential Diagnoses

Movement System Diagnosis
- Elbow valgus with and without extension
- Elbow hypomobility

Potential Diagnoses Requiring Referral Suggested by Signs and Symptoms

Neuromusculoskeletal
- Olecranon fracture[27]
- Olecranon apophysitis[27]
- Triceps strain[27]
- Olecranon bursitis[27]
- Loose bodies[27]
- Synovitis[27]
- Posteromedial spurs[27]
- Cervical radiculopathy (C7)
- Ligament sprains grades 2 and 3

Treatment for Elbow Extension Syndrome: Excessive Extension

Treatment emphasizes eccentric control of the biceps brachii to decrease the forces on the posterior elbow.[65]

Patient Education
- Avoid end-ROM active or passive elbow extension.

Exercises
- Improve muscle strength/performance:
  - Biceps brachii: Eccentric control

Splinting/Bracing/Taping
- Taping or splinting to block end-ROM elbow extension (see Figure 6A-15).

Treatment for Elbow Extension Syndrome: Limited Extension

Patient Education
- Avoid forceful active end-ROM elbow extension.

Exercises
- Increase flexibility/ROM:
  - Focus on passive stretching into elbow extension instead of active.

Splinting/Bracing
- Splinting to apply low-load prolonged stretch into elbow extension (see Figure 6-21).

NOTES

Posterior Forearm Nerve Entrapment Syndromes

Contraction or stretch of the supinator or ECRB muscles result in the compression of the deep branch of the radial nerve. With radial tunnel (RT) syndrome, the main complaint is pain, and there is usually minimal loss of strength or loss of strength is primarily due to pain. With posterior interosseous nerve (PINS) syndrome, the compression has progressed so that there is significant muscle weakness but no loss of sensation. Repetitive use of the wrist extensors may contribute to compression of the radial nerve in these syndromes.

Symptoms and History

- RT: Main complaint is pain[25,68]
- PINS: Main complaint is weakness of finger, thumb, and wrist extension[25,68]
  - Onset of weakness may be rapid

In both RT and PINS:
- Aching pain in extensor muscles just below elbow, sometimes radiating to the dorsum of wrist[25]
- May also complain of pain over lateral epicondyle
- Pain worse with use of arm[68]

Activities/Population
- Occupation may play a role if repetitive movements required (baseball pitching, pianist)
- Repeated activities involving forearm pronation/supination[25,68]
- Often work in a position of elbow flexion with forearm pronation, fingers flexed and poor alignment of the shoulders
- May be caused by trauma or inflammation
- Incidence is 1% to 2% of all nerve entrapments[69]
- 2:1 ratio of men to women[25]
- 2:1 ratio of dominant to nondominant arm[25]

Common Referring Diagnoses
- Tennis elbow (lateral epicondylitis)
- Lateral elbow pain
- PINS or RT syndrome
- Ligament sprain

Key Tests and Signs for Movement Impairment

Movement Impairment Analysis
Palpation[25,58]
- RT: Tenderness of radial nerve over anterior radial head
- RT: Lateral epicondyle may also be tender but less so than radial nerve over radial head

Joint Integrity
- ROM: No significant loss except possibly forearm pronation

Muscle Length Tests
Pain
- For both RT and PINS, pain may be increased over radial tunnel with wrist flexion and forearm pronation, which stretches the supinator and wrist extensors compressing the nerve

Wrist Extensor Length Test
- During length test, observe humeral medial rotation versus forearm pronation
- Wrist extensors stiff or short
- May reproduce symptoms over radial nerve at elbow

Supinator Length Test
- Based on ROM tests: Short or stiff supinator

Muscle Strength/Performance Impairments
MMT
- No significant motor loss in RT[25,58]
- PINS has motor loss in the following muscles: EDC, ECU, EPL, EPB, and APL[58]
- PINS: BR, ECRL, ECRB, and supinator should have intact strength

Resisted Tests (Soft Tissue Differential Diagnosis)
- Middle finger test[25,58,68,70]:
  - RT: Resisted extension of middle finger with elbow extended is painful over radial tunnel, since ECRB inserts base of middle finger metacarpal
  - This test is traditionally described for RT, but it may also be positive in lateral epicondylitis
- Supination test[25,58,68]:
  - RT: Pain over radial tunnel increased with resisted wrist extension or forearm supination with elbow extended

Other Special Tests
Pressure Provocative Testing
- Positive

Sensation
- No sensory loss in RT or PINS[25,58]

Tinel's Sign
- Negative (motor nerve)

Source of Signs and Symptoms

Radial Nerve

In both RT and PINS:

- The nerve may be compressed under[25,58]:
  - Fibrous bands
  - ECRB at its sharp fibrous medial border as it rises from common extensor origin
  - A "fan" of vessels from the radial recurrent artery
  - The arcade of Frohse, which is the free-fibrous proximal margin of the supinator

Associated Signs or Contributing Factors

Alignment Analysis

Posture

- Forward shoulders
- May have increased carrying angle
- May have elbow flexion contracture

PINS

- Consider "double crush" [58,71] from faulty shoulder (especially scapular depression) and cervical alignment

Movement Impairment Analysis

Both RT and PINS

- ECRB, ECRL, and supinator tend to be overused for elbow flexion rather than the biceps
- During reaching with palm down, the humerus medially rotates more readily than the forearm pronates
- During reaching with palm up, the humerus laterally rotates more readily than the forearm supinates

Muscle Length Tests

Finger extensor and flexor length tests

- Short or stiff finger extensors
- Short or stiff finger flexors potentially increase work required of wrist and finger extensors

Differential Diagnoses

Movement System Diagnosis

- Wrist extension with forearm pronation syndrome (lateral epicondylosis)

Potential Diagnoses Requiring Referral Suggested by Signs and Symptoms

Neuromusculoskeletal

- Lateral collateral ligament sprain
- PINS or RT syndrome[69]
- Fracture or dislocation of radial head[25]
- Lateral epicondyle avulsion
- Cervical radiculopathy (C6-C7, C8)[58,69]
- Proximal radial nerve palsy at midshaft of humerus[58]
- Loose bodies
- AVN of lateral epicondyle
- OA or synovitis of radiocapitellar joint[69]
- Impingement of articular branch of radial nerve[69]
- Muscle tear of ECRB[69]
- Posterior plica impingement[69]
- deQuervain's disease[69]
- Brachial plexus neuritis[69]
- Finger extensor tendon ruptures[58]
- Lateral epicondylosis[58]
- Anconeus tendonitis[69]
- Posterolateral rotatory instability of the elbow[72]

Systemi c

- RA[58]
- Tumor[25]
- Lead poisoning with toxic neuropathy[58]

Treatment for Posterior Forearm Nerve Entrapment Syndromes: Radial Tunnel Syndrome

Nonsurgical treatment may be tried for 2 to 6 months.[25,72] The effectiveness of nonsurgical treatment is unknown.[68]

- Avoid aggravating symptoms because of nerve compression.[25,71]
- If stretches reproduce symptoms, avoid prolonged stretch and instead use oscillatory movement.
- Use of forearm strap is contraindicated and may make patient worse because it adds to the compression of the nerve.

Patient Education

- Patient to avoid painful activities by correcting movement impairments as described as follows:
  - Patient to increase use of biceps and decrease use of wrist extensors.
    - Train elbow flexion with forearm supinated versus pronated as possible.
    - Grip objects with forearm supinated versus pronated.
    - Caution with supination to avoid aggravating symptoms because of nerve compression.
  - Avoid prolonged positioning or repeated movements of the following:
    - Wrist extension[71,73]
    - Forearm pronation or supination[71,73]
    - Elbow extension[71]
- Modify work and sports activities as appropriate.
  - May need to change tools; alter grip throughout the day.
  - Take breaks to stretch frequently throughout the day.
  - Sitting at computer: Support arm using mouse to decrease use of ECRL as an elbow flexor.
  - Decrease force required by elbow and wrist muscles by maximizing use of proximal joints.
    - Vacuuming: Use body and legs to help exert force versus using just arms (basic rules of body mechanics will help decrease stress on elbow).
    - Correct alignment and movement of shoulder girdle.
  - Avoid static pinching or gripping.[71]
- Methods of resting wrist extensors
  - Splint (see "Splint" section)
  - Alternate gripping methods
  - Total rest
  - Use of opposite upper extremities

Exercises:

- Key is gradual progression.
- Increasing the flexibility of the wrist extensors and the supinator may help decrease compression of the nerve. The exercises should be performed without aggravating symptoms.

- *Increase flexibility/decrease stiffness:* It is important to manually prevent rotation of the humerus during the following stretching exercises. When stretching the finger and wrist extensors, the humerus will tend to medially rotate, whereas when stretching the finger flexors, the humerus will laterally rotate.
  - Wrist and finger extensors and supinator[73]: On initial visit, instruct in stretching exercises as appropriate. Usually wrist and finger extensors are "short" or stiff.
    - Wrist extensors and supinator: Stabilize humerus during stretch. Progression of stretching is as follows: First, wrist flexion with elbow at 90 degrees flexion and forearm neutral, then wrist flexion with elbow at 90 degrees flexion with forearm pronated; then wrist flexion with forearm neutral and elbow extended; then wrist flexion with forearm pronated and elbow extended; last, wrist flexion with forearm pronated, elbow extended, and wrist ulnarly deviated.[7]
    - Finger extensors: The same progression could be followed as described under wrist extensors with the addition of finger flexion.
  - Finger flexors are also often stiff or short: Stretch passively to avoid use of wrist and finger extensors. Stabilize humerus during stretch.
  - Correct impairments of cervical and scapular regions.[55]
  - Nerve gliding exercises are theorized to be helpful by some experts.[71]
- *Improve muscle strength/performance*
  - Shoulder girdle musculature: Refer to Chapter 5 in Sahrmann[21] to correct impaired shoulder alignment and movement.

Splint

- To rest from repetitive movements and used for several weeks.[73]
- Positioning the arm in elbow flexion, forearm supination, and wrist extension (long arm posterior splint with elbow flexed 90 degrees, wrist extended, and forearm supinated) places the least stress on the structures of the radial tunnel, but patients may be more compliant with a smaller wrist splint holding the wrist in extension.[71]

Modalities

- Ultrasound 1 mHz (duty cycle 25%) at 1.0 watt/cm^2 for 15 minutes over proximal forearm.[71]
- Other modalities recommended are transcutaneous electrical nerve stimulation (TENS), high-voltage pulsed current electrical stimulation, iontophoresis, and cryotherapy.[73]

Posterior Interosseous Nerve Syndrome

- The effectiveness of conservative treatment for PINS is unknown.[68]

Patient Education

- Modify activities as needed to decrease stress and/or overuse to area (see "Patient Education" section on previous page).

Exercises

- PROM to fingers for flexion and extension and to thumb for all its motions
- AROM and strengthening to involved muscles as innervation returns

Splint

- Dynamic thumb and finger extension splint to facilitate functional use of hand and prevent overstretch of weak extensors[25]

Surgical

- Decompression of nerve should be considered if no improvement after 3 months of conservative treatment.[25]

Anterior Forearm Nerve Entrapment Syndromes

Pronator syndrome (PS) is compression of the main branch of the median nerve in the proximal forearm, which may result from repetitive use of the forearm pronators and finger flexors. Compression of the anterior interosseous nerve, which is a motor-only branch of the median nerve, is anterior interosseous nerve syndrome (AINS). With PS, there is usually minimal loss of strength or loss of strength is primarily a result of pain, and there may be changes in sensation. In AINS, there is significant muscle weakness, with no sensory changes.

Symptoms and History

- PS: If main trunk of median nerve is compressed in areas described:
  - Aching pain in the proximal anterior forearm[74,75]
  - Numbness or paresthesias in the distribution of the median nerve,[46,74,75] including the palm of the hand
  - Onset usually insidious[75]
- AINS
  - Pain in proximal forearm increased with exercise and decreased with rest[74]
  - No sensory complaints[46,74,75]
  - Acute onset muscle weakness[46,74]
  - May have difficulty writing or picking up small objects[75]

Activities/Population

- Repetitive movements of the elbow and forearm that involve forearm pronation and supination[46,58,74,75]
- Repetitive grasping[75]
- Unusual upper extrenity exertion
- More common in women than men[75]
- Usually presents in fifth decade[75]

Common Referring Diagnoses

- CTS
- PS
- AINS
- TOS
- Hand weakness
- Tendinopathy of flexor muscles

Etiology

- Acute injury to forearm[46]
- Prolonged external compression[46]

Key Tests and Signs for Movement Impairment

Movement Impairment Analysis
- PS: Repetitive forearm pronation resulting in overuse of the pronator teres

Muscle Length Tests

Pronator Teres Length Test

PS:
- Stretch to pronator teres reproduces tingling (e.g., forearm supination with elbow extension)
- Decreased length or increased stiffness of pronator teres[55]

Finger Flexor Length Test
- Stiffness or shortness of finger flexors
- Symptoms may be reproduced

Biceps Length Test
- Short or stiff biceps increasing tension on lacertus fibrosus
- Symptoms may be reproduced

Muscle Strength/Performance Impairments

Resisted Tests (Soft Tissue Differential Diagnosis)

PS
- Resisted elbow flexion at 120 to 130 degrees of elbow flexion implicates compression of the nerve at the ligament of Struthers.[74]
- Resisted forearm pronation with the forearm neutral stresses the pronator teres muscle.[47,74,75]
- Resisted elbow flexion with the forearm in pronation[74] or supinated[47,75] stresses the lacertus fibrosus.
- Resisted flexion of the long finger PIP joint stresses the FDS arch[47,74,75].
- If any of the resisted tests above reproduce symptoms, they are positive.

MMT

PS:
- Usually no muscle weakness.[46] If compression is severe, possible weakness of forearm and thenar muscles

AINS:
- Weakness or paralysis of FPL, FDP to index, long and pronator quadratus[46,74]
- In later stages: Unique pinch pattern, hyperextension of thumb IP and DIP of index and middle[46,74,75]

Palpation

Both PS and AINS:
- Tenderness, firmness, or enlargement of the pronator teres muscle[46]
- Tenderness over proximal forearm

PS:
- Positive pronator compression test[75]

Special Tests

PS:
- Tinel's sign: Positive over distal margin of pronator teres[46,58,75]
- Pressure: Provocative test positive over proximal forearm[58]

AINS:
- Positive "circle sign": Unable to make circle with thumb and index finger[46]

Sensation
- Normal in AINS, but may be decreased in median distribution with compression of main median nerve in PS[46,74,75]

Source of Signs and Symptoms

Median Nerve

- Sites of compression for main branch for PS
  - Ligament of Struthers
  - Lacertus fibrosus
  - Pronator teres
  - Arch of FDS
  - Anterior interosseous nerve

Associated Signs or Contributing Factors

Structural Variations

- Anomalous musculotendinous structures[45]

Joint Integrity and Muscle Length Tests

- Impairments of the shoulder girdle may contribute to increased use of forearm pronators

Special Tests

- Phalen's test negative[75]

Consider "double crush"[58,75]

Differential Diagnoses

Movement System Diagnosis

- Elbow impairment
- Elbow valgus syndrome
- Elbow flexion syndrome (cubital tunnel)

Potential Diagnoses Requiring Referral Suggested by Signs and Symptoms

Neuromusculoskeletal

- Cervical radiculopathy[46,75]
- Brachial plexopathy[46,75]
- TOS[46,75]
- Median nerve compression at wrist (CTS)[46,75]
- Compartment syndrome[74]
- Mononeuritis (neuralgic amyotrophy)[46]
- Isolated lesion of FPL tendon[46]
- Radial, ulnar, or humeral fractures[46]
- Anomalous musculotendinous structures[46]
- Vascular abnormality[46]
- Hematoma[46]

Systemic

- Tumor, lipoma, or gangion[46]
- RA[46]

Treatment for PS and AINS

Little research is available regarding the most effective intervention.[75]

Treatment for Pronator Syndrome

- If no change in symptoms after nonsurgical treatment for 8 to 12 weeks, refer back to physician for further evaluation.[75]
- Avoid aggravating symptoms because of nerve compression.
- If stretches reproduce symptoms, avoid prolonged stretch and instead use oscillatory movement.

Patient Education

- Modify activities of daily living, leisure, and work that increase the symptoms.
- Avoid repeated grasping and forearm pronation and supination.[75]
- Stretch frequently throughout the day.

Exercises

- *Increase flexibility and nerve gliding, and decrease stiffness:*
  - Pronator teres[55]
  - Finger flexor
  - Biceps brachii
  - Median nerve gliding[75]
- *Improve muscle strength/performance:*
  - Supinator
  - Shoulder girdle musculature: Refer to Chapter 5 in Sahrmann[21] for correct impaired shoulder alignment and movement.

Splinting

- Static splint with elbow flexed at 90 degrees, forearm in neutral,[75] and wrist in 25 degrees extension.
  - Purpose of splint is to avoid stretch to pronator teres and therefore compression of the nerve.
  - The splint is worn initially most of the time, and use is gradually decreased as symptoms decrease.[75]

Modalities[75]

Usually not the mainstay of treatment by this author
- Ultrasound
- Electrical stimulation
- Iontophoresis

Treatment for Anterior Interosseous Nerve Syndrome

If motor weakness is present, conservative treatment seems to be controversial and not well described. Seki et al[76] described conservative treatment for patients with spontaneous onset of AINS. Conservative treatment was described as electrical stimulation therapy and vitamin B$_{12}$. This same author recommends nonoperative treatment for patients under 40 years of age. The time to signs of recovery was reported as usually 12 months or under in this age range but longer for older patients. No further description of the conservative treatment was provided. Refer the patient with AINS to physician for further evaluation if motor weakness is present. Lee et al[75] recommend the same treatment for AINS as for PS.

NOTES

Wrist Flexion with Forearm Pronation Syndrome

Wrist flexion with forearm pronation syndrome (medial epicondylosis or golfer's elbow) is characterized by medial elbow pain provoked by repetitive or sustained activities resulting in overuse of the wrist flexors and forearm pronators. Modification of symptoms may be achieved by changing the movement pattern to decrease the stresses on the wrist flexors and forearm pronators by avoiding use of the muscles when they are lengthened and/or in the extremely shortened range. The overused muscles are often relatively stiffer than the underused synergist.

Symptoms and History

- Pain located at the medial epicondyle sometimes radiating distally into anterior forearm[60,77]
- Onset of symptoms usually gradual and insidious[59,60]
- Only 10% to 20% of all epicondylitis diagnoses are medial[59,77]

Activities/Population

- Activites involving repetitive use of wrist flexor and forearm pronator muscles[77]
- Weightlifters
- Overhead athletes such as baseball players, especially the acceleration phase of pitching[60,77]
- Golf, tennis, bowling, racquet ball, football, archery, javelin throwing, carpentry, plumbing, meat cutting[77]
- Therapist performing treatment techniques using fingers in flexion with wrist flexed
- Less often can be due to trauma[77]
- Occurs most in fourth and fifth decades[77]
- 2:1 male:female[59]
- Usually in dominant arm[59,77]

Common Referring Diagnoses

- Medial epicondylitis[59]
- Golfer's elbow[59]
- Flexor pronator strain[60]
- Ulnar nerve symptoms associated with medial epicondylosis[59]

Key Tests and Signs for Movement Impairment

Alignment Analysis

- Hypertrophy of anterior forearm muscles in throwing athletes[77]
- Swelling medial elbow may be present[77]

Movement Impairment Analysis

Aggravating Functional Activities

- Examine performance of individual functional activities (based on the history) for the movement impairment that has been identified across the examination.
- Pay particular attention to the movement patterns of the shoulder, elbow, forearm, and wrist.
  - Gripping with reaching:
    - Golfer's flex wrist excessively during swing to compensate for decreased shoulder motion.
    - Correction: Minimizing the range of wrist flexion by increasing shoulder motion during gripping decreases symptoms.

Joint Integrity Tests

ROM

- Active wrist flexion: May or may not be painful, depending on level of irritability
- Active forearm pronation: May or may not be painful, depending on level of irritability
- Passive elbow, forearm, wrist, and finger ROM:
  - ROM usually normal initially[59,77]
  - Passive wrist and/or wrist and finger extension painful
  - Wrist extension may be painful
  - Wrist flexion painless

Muscle Length Tests

- Wrist and finger flexors:
  - May have shortness or stiffness of finger and wrist flexors relative to opposite side[60,77]
- Stretch to wrist flexors (forearm supination, wrist extension, and elbow extension) reproduces pain, medial elbow pain, forearm tends to pronate and humerus laterally rotates

Muscle Strength/Performance Impairments

Resisted Tests (Soft Tissue Differential Diagnosis)

- Forearm pronation: Pain increased with resisted forearm pronation[59,77]
- Wrist flexors and extensors: Pain increased with resisted wrist flexion[59,77]

MMT

- Wrist flexors and forearm pronators: Unable to assess strength initially because of pain. Usually wrist flexor and forearm pronator strength at least 3/5
- Grip strength: Decreased as a result of pain

Palpation

- Tender over medial epicondyle or just distal to it over wrist flexor muscles[59,77]

Source of Signs and Symptoms

Muscle/Tendon

- Degenerative changes of the common flexor tendon at the elbow where it originates at the medial epicondyle. The following muscles may be involved[77]:
  - Pronator teres
  - FCR
  - PL
  - FDS
  - FCU

Associated Signs or Contributing Factors

Alignment Analysis

- Increased carrying angle.[77]

Joint Integrity

- Check for shoulder girdle impairments.
- ROM: May develop elbow flexion contractures.[77]

Muscle Length Tests

- Check for shoulder girdle impairments.

Muscle Strength/Performance Impairments

- Check for shoulder girdle impairments.
- Resisted FDS may reproduce symptoms greater than wrist flexors or FDP.

Differential Diagnoses

Movement System Diagnosis

- Elbow flexion
- Elbow valgus syndrome with or without extension

Potential Diagnoses Requiring Referral Suggested by Signs and Symptoms

Neuromusculoskeletal

- Cervical radioculpathy[59] (C8,T1)
- TOS[59]
- Ulnar neuropathy (cubital tunnel syndrome)[59,77]
- MCL sprain grade II/III[59,77]
- Avulsion fracture of medial epicondyle[60]
- Triceps tendonopathy[59]
- Flexor pronator rupture[60]
- Olecranon spur[59]

Systemic

- RA

Treatment

There is a lack of evidence regarding the most effective treatment but nonsurgical treatment is usually recommended.[77] Nonsurgical treatment is tried for up to 6 to 9 months before considering surgery.[59] The treatment principles are the same as for wrist extension with forearm pronation (lateral epicondylosis) but applied instead to the wrist flexors and forearm pronators.

Patient Education

- Patient to avoid painful activities[59,77] by correcting alignment and movement impairments during daily activities, work, and sports as described later.
- Modify work and sports activities as appropriate.[65,77]
  - May need to change tools; alter grip throughout the day.
  - Take breaks to stretch frequently throughout the day.
- Importance of and methods of resting wrist flexors and forearm pronators:
  - Splint (see "Orthotic Devices" section on this page)
  - Alternate gripping methods
  - Total rest
  - Use of opposite UE

Exercises

- Stretching and strengthening of the involved muscles may be helpful to regain full muscle length and wrist and elbow joint range of motion.[59,60,65,77]
- Strengthening can progress from isometric to isotonic concentric and eccentric exercises followed by a gradual return to sport activities. Initially, the elbow should be flexed while working on wrist ROM, but as pain decreases, the wrist exercises should be done with the elbow in more extension.[77]
- Conditioning of the entire body is strongly recommended.[77]

Orthotic Devices

- Forearm strap or counterforce bracing may be helpful.[59,60,77]
- Wrist splinting (see Figure 6A-5).[59,77]

Modalities

- Modalities may be helpful,[60] including ultrasound, high voltage galvanic stimulation,[65,77] iontophoresis,[65] phonophoresis,[65] and ice.[65,77]

NOTES

Elbow Impairment

Acutely, the movement system diagnosis of elbow impairment is used when the pathoanatomical or source diagnosis is not provided on the referral documentation. The focus of the treatment is protecting the injured tissues. Usually, there is a history of acute trauma or injury to elbow or forearm or early in postoperative phase. Medical precautions have been issued. A patient's typical movement pattern cannot be assessed at this time. The determination of the

History

- Knowledge of specific surgery, injury, medical diagnosis and surgical approach.

Hand Dominance

Types of Injuries

- May be treated initially conservatively or surgically:
  - Medial or lateral collateral ligament sprain
  - Other ligament injuries
  - Elbow dislocation
  - Radial head dislocation
  - Fractures
  - Cubital tunnel syndrome
  - RT syndrome
  - PS
  - Muscle or tendon tears
  - Tendinopathies
  - Myositis ossificans
  - RA
  - Compartment syndrome

Types of Surgeries

- Stabilization: Indications: fractures, ligament injuries, pain, instability, deformity, AVN, bony tumors)
  - ORIF
  - External fixation
  - Fusion
  - Partial arthrodesis
- Arthroplasty: Indications: Joint destruction or deformity secondary to RA, OA, DJD
- Nerve decompression/transposition: Indications: Median, radial or ulnar nerve compression resulting in pain, loss of sensation or motor function)
- Amputation
- Compartment decompression: Indication: Crush injury with secondary loss of arterial blood flow
- Repair: Indications: Tear, avulsion, laceration, rupture)
  - Ligament repair/reconstruction
  - Tendon
  - Nerve (grafts and repair)
  - Artery
- Incision and drainage: Indication: Infection
- Tendon transfers: Indication: paralysis of a muscle with resultant loss of function
- Soft tissue release/resection: Indications: Synovectomy indicated with prolonged swelling, pain and dysfunction, no evidence of joint destruction
  - Fasciotomy equals compartment release
  - Capsular release
  - Synovectomy
  - Aspiration or excision
  - Surgical decompression
  - Debridement
  - Release of tendon
  - Skin graft or skin flap with significant loss of soft tissue
- Medications: Consider side effects and effects of medications on tissue, examination, and intervention

Key Tests and Assessments

Precautions

- Check physician orders and protocol, including splinting requirements. Respect postoperative positioning.
- Assess patient's ability to adhere to precautions.
- No resisted testing in most cases.

Systemic Signs and Symptoms

- Assess vital signs first visit and then as needed. Avoid taking blood pressure in affected upper extremity. Monitor for hypotension, nausea and dizziness.

Pain

- Assess pain at rest and with movement:
  - Location
  - Intensity
  - Palpation
- Address regimen of analgesics

Neurologic Status

- Establish baseline after surgery.

Function (Usually After About 10 Days)

- Assess functional activities that are restricted. With patients that have just had surgery, much of this assessment is done initially via the history, but depending on the condition, observation of the specific activity may be appropriate.

Appearance

Incision: May be covered by steristrips, bandages, staples or exposed pins. May have open wound. Note amount and type of drainage.

Scar: Note location, mobility and sensitivity of scar if incision appears healed.

Color: Note bruising and any other discoloration.

Temperature: Note any abnormalities.

Edema: Note location and measure extent of edema. Assess whether it is brawny or pitting.

Alignment

- Note resting posture of UE.

Palpation

- Performed once incision is healed.

ROM

- Assess ROM of involved hand, wrist, forearm and elbow (within precautions).
- Also assess shoulder ROM.

Impairments in Muscle Recruitment/Strength

- Impairments in active ROM or strength may also be significant but are NOT the focus of treatment until precautions are lifted or PROM is increased enough to begin strengthening.

use of component versus compensatory treatment methods depends on the expectations of the final outcome. Initially, while on precautions, compensatory methods may be necessary. This grid is intended as a general guide, consult the physician's protocol for specific precautions and progression. The therapist must be familiar with the tissues that are affected by the surgical procedure and the specific surgical approach.

Associated Signs

Variations
- Anthropomorphics

Alignment
- Common for scapula to be abducted, humerus adducted and medially rotated, elbow flexed, forearm pronated, wrist flexed. This is the typical guarded posture.

Movement Impairments
- Consider the possible underlying movement impairment during the initial phase of recovery. This is confirmed once the precautions are lifted.

Underlying Movement Impairment Syndromes
- Elbow hypomobility (most likely)
- Wrist extension with forearm pronation
- Elbow flexion
- Posterior forearm nerve compression syndromes
- Anterior forearm nerve compression syndromes
- Wrist flexion with forearm pronation
- Ulnohumeral and radiohumeral multidirectional accessory hypermobility

Medical Complications

- Infection
- Nonunion of fracture
- Rupture of surgical repair
- Nerve injuries
- CRPS (RSD)
- Myositis ossificans
- Instability/redislocation

REFERENCES

1. Whaley AL, Baker CL: Lateral epicondylitis, *Clin Sports Med* 234:677-691, 2004.
2. Faro F, Wolf JM: Lateral epicondylitis: review and current concepts, *J Hand Surg Am* 328:1271-1279, 2007.
3. Nirschl RP, Ashman ES: Elbow tendinopathy: tennis elbow, *Clin Sports Med* 224:813-836, 2003.
4. Kendall FP, McCreary EK, Provance PG, et al: *Muscles: testing and function with posture and pain*, ed 5, Baltimore, 2005, Lippincott Williams & Wilkins.
5. Plancher KD, Halbrecht J, Lourie GM: Medial and lateral epicondylitis in the athlete, *Clin Sports Med* 152:283-305, 1996.
6. Kibler WB, Sciascia A: Kinetic chain contributions to elbow function and dysfunction in sports, *Clin Sports Med* 234:545-552, 2004.
7. Cannon NM: A therapist's perspective on the conservative management of lateral epicondylitis, *Lecture at Indiana hand care course*, Indianapolis, 2004.
8. Nirschl RP, Alvarado GJ: Muscle tendon and trauma. In Morrey BF, Sanchez-Sotelo J, eds: *The elbow and its disorders*, ed 4, Philadelphia, 2009, Saunders.
9. Martinez-Silvestrini JA, Newcomer KL, Gay RE, et al: Chronic lateral epicondylitis: comparative effectiveness of a home exercise program including stretching alone versus stretching supplemented with eccentric or concentric strengthening, *J Hand Ther* 184:411-419, 2005.
10. Buchbinder R, Green S, Struijs P: Tennis elbow, *Am Fam Physician* 75(5):701-702, 2007.
11. Piligian G, Herbert R, Hearns M, et al: Evaluation and management of chronic work-related musculoskeletal disorders of the distal upper extremity, *Am J Ind Med* 37(1):75-93, 2000.
12. Pascarelli EF, Hsu YP: Understanding work-related upper extremity disorders: clinical findings in 485 computer users, musicians, and others, *J Occup Rehabil* 11(1):1-21, 2001.
13. Dutton M: *Orthopaedic examination, evaluation, & intervention*, New York, 2004, McGraw-Hill.
14. Mills GP: The treatment of "tennis elbow", *BMJ* 7:12-13, 1928.
15. Fedorczyk JM: Therapist's management of elbow tendinitis. In Mackin EJ, Callahan A, Skirven TM, et al, eds: *Rehabilitation of the hand and upper extremity*, ed 5, St Louis, 2002, Mosby.
16. An KN, Hui FC, Morrey BF, et al: Muscles across the elbow joint: a biomechanical analysis, *J Biomech* 14(10):659-669, 1981.
17. Verhaar JA, Walenkamp GH, van MH, et al: Local corticosteroid injection versus Cyriax-type physiotherapy for tennis elbow, *J Bone Joint Surg Br* 78(1):128-132, 1996.
18. De Smet L, Fabry G: Grip strength in patients with tennis elbow. Influence of elbow position, *Acta Orthop Belg* 62(1):26-29, 1996.
19. Laban MM, Iyer R, Tamler MS: Occult periarthrosis of the shoulder: a possible progenitor of tennis elbow, *Am J Phys Med Rehabil* 84(11):895-898, 2005.
20. Ellenbecker TS: Rehabilitation of shoulder and elbow injuries in tennis players, *Clin Sports Med* 14(1):87-110, 1995.
21. Sahrmann SA: *Diagnosis and treatment of movement impairment syndromes*, St Louis, 2002, Mosby.
22. Mulligan BR: *Manual therapy: "NAGS", "snags", "mwms" etc*, ed 4, New Zealand, 1999, Plane View Services.
23. Vanswearingen J: Measuring wrist muscle strength, *J Orthop Sports Phys Ther* 4(4):217-228, 1983.
24. Reid DC, Kushner S: The elbow region. In Donatelli RA, Wooden MJ, eds: *Orthopaedic physical therapy*, ed 3, New York, 2001, Churchill Livingstone.
25. Eaton CJ, Lister GD: Radial nerve compression, *Hand Clin* 82:345-357, 1992.
26. Noteboom T, Cruver R, Keller J, et al: Tennis elbow: a review, *J Orthop Sports Phys Ther* 19(6):357-366, 1994.
27. Dines JS, ElAttrache NS: Articular injuries in the athlete. In Morrey BF, Sanchez-Sotelo J, eds: *The elbow and its disorders*, ed 4, Philadelphia, 2009, Saunders.
28. Buchbinder R, Green SE, Struijs P: Tennis elbow, *Clin Evid* (online): http://clinicalevidence.bmj.com/ceweb/conditions/msd/1117/1117-get.pdf. Accessed July 22, 2010.
29. Morrey BF: Surgical failure of tennis elbow. In Morrey BF, Sanchez-Sotelo J, eds: *The elbow and its disorders*, ed 4, Philadelphia, 2009, Saunders.
30. Smith J, Morrey BF: Principles of elbow rehabilitation. In Morrey BF, Sanchez-Sotelo J, eds: *The elbow and its disorders*, ed 4, Philadelphia, 2009, Saunders.
31. Herd CR, Meserve BB: A systematic review of the effectiveness of manipulative therapy in treating lateral epicondylalgia, *J Man Manip Ther* 16(4):225-237, 2008.
32. Paungmali A, O'Leary S, Souvlis T, et al: Hypoalgesic and sympathoexcitatory effects of mobilization with movement for lateral epicondylalgia, *Phys Ther* 83(4):374-383, 2003.
33. Badia A, Stennett C: Sports-related injuries of the elbow, *J Hand Ther* 19(2):206-226, 2006.
34. Woodley BL, Newsham-West RJ, Baxter GD: Chronic tendinopathy: effectiveness of eccentric exercise, *Br J Sports Med* 41(4):188-198, 2007.
35. Kraushaar BS, Nirschl RP: Tendinosis of the elbow (tennis elbow). Clinical features and findings of histological, immunohistochemical, and electron microscopy studies, *J Bone Joint Surg Am* 81(2):259-278, 1999.
36. Struijs PA, Smidt N, Arola H, et al: Orthotic devices for the treatment of tennis elbow, *Cochrane Database Syst Rev* (1):CD001821, 2002.
37. Enzenauer RJ, Nordstrom DM: Anterior interosseous nerve syndrome associated with forearm band treatment of lateral epicondylitis, *Orthopedics* 14(7):788-790, 1991.
38. Faes M, van den AB, de Lint JA, et al: Dynamic extensor brace for lateral epicondylitis, *Clin Orthop Relat Res* 442:149-157, 2006.
39. Faes M, van EN, de Lint JA, et al: A dynamic extensor brace reduces electromyographic activity of wrist extensor muscles in patients with lateral epicondylalgia, *J Orthop Sports Phys Ther* 36(3):170-178, 2006.
40. Vicenzino B, Brooksbank J, Minto J, et al: Initial effects of elbow taping on pain-free grip strength and pressure pain threshold, *J Orthop Sports Phys Ther* 33(7):400-407, 2003.
41. Davila SA, Johnston-Jones K: Managing the stiff elbow: operative, nonoperative, and postoperative techniques, *J Hand Ther* 19(2):268-281, 2006.
42. Vardakas DG, Varitimidis SE, Goebel F, et al: Evaluating and treating the stiff elbow, *Hand Clin* 18(1):77-85, 2002.
43. Morrey BF: Splints and bracing at the elbow. In Morrey BF, Sanchez-Sotelo J, eds: *The elbow and its disorders*, ed 4, Philadelphia, 2009, Saunders.

44. Casavant AM, Hastings H: Heterotopic ossification about the elbow: a therapist's guide to evaluation and management, *J Hand Ther* 19(2):255-266, 2006.

45. Kisner C, Colby LA: *Therapeutic exercises: foundations and techniques*, ed 5, Philadelphia, 2007, FA Davis.

46. Andreisek G, Crook DW, Burg D, et al: Peripheral neuropathies of the median, radial, and ulnar nerves: MR imaging features, *Radiographics* 26(5):1267-1287, 2006.

47. Spinner RJ: Nerve entrapment syndromes. In Morrey BF, Sanchez-Sotelo J, eds: *The elbow and its disorders*, ed 4, Philadelphia, 2009, Saunders.

48. Lund AT, Amadio PC: Treatment of cubital tunnel syndrome: perspectives for the therapist, *J Hand Ther* 19(2):170-178, 2006.

49. Rayan GM: Proximal ulnar nerve compression. Cubital tunnel syndrome, *Hand Clin* 8(2):325-336, 1992.

50. Idler RS: General principles of patient evaluation and nonoperative management of cubital syndrome, *Hand Clin* 12(2):397-403, 1996.

51. Omer GE: Diagnosis and management of cubital tunnel syndrome. In Mackin EJ, Callahan A, Skirven TM, et al, eds: *Rehabilitation of the hand and upper extremity*, ed 5, St Louis, 2002, Mosby.

52. Keefe DT, Lintner DM: Nerve injuries in the throwing elbow, *Clin Sports Med* 23(4):723-742, 2004.

53. Szabo RM, Kwak C: Natural history and conservative management of cubital tunnel syndrome, *Hand Clin* 23(3):311-313, 2007.

54. Novak CB, Lee GW, Mackinnon SE, et al: Provocative testing for cubital tunnel syndrome, *J Hand Surg Am* 19(5):817-820, 1994.

55. Novak CB: Upper extremity work-related musculoskeletal disorders: a treatment perspective, *J Orthop Sports Phys Ther* 34(10):628-637, 2004.

56. Brand PW, Hollister AM: *Clinical mechanics of the hand*, ed 3, St Louis, 1999, Mosby.

57. Cain EL Jr, Dugas JR: History and examination of the thrower's elbow, *Clin Sports Med* 23(4):553-566, 2004.

58. Mackinnon S, Dellon A: *Surgery of the peripheral nerve*, New York, 1988, Thieme.

59. Gabel GT, Morrey BF: Medial epicondylitis. In Morrey BF, Sanchez-Sotelo J, eds: *The elbow and its disorders*, ed 4, Philadelphia, 2009, Saunders.

60. Schickendantz MS: Diagnosis and treatment of elbow disorders in the overhead athlete, *Hand Clin* 18(1):65-75, 2002.

61. Apfel E, Sigafoos GT: Comparison of range-of-motion constraints provided by splints used in the treatment of cubital tunnel syndrome—a pilot study, *J Hand Ther* 19(4):384-391, 2006.

62. ElAttrache NS, Ahmad CS: Diagnosis and treatment of ulnar collateral ligament injuries in athletes. In: Morrey BF, Sanchez-Sotelo J, eds: *The elbow and its disorders*, ed 4, Philadelphia, 2009, Saunders.

63. Safran MR: Ulnar collateral ligament injury in the overhead athlete: diagnosis and treatment, *Clin Sports Med* 234:643-663, 2004.

64. Ahmad CS, El Attrache NS: Valgus extension overload syndrome and stress injury of the olecranon, *Clin Sports Med* 234:665-676, 2004.

65. Wilk KE, Reinold MM, Andrews JR: Rehabilitation of the thrower's elbow, *Tech Hand Up Extrem Surg* 7(4):197-216, 2003.

66. O'Driscoll SW, Lawton RL, Smith AM: The "moving valgus stress test" for medial collateral ligament tears of the elbow, *Am J Sports Med* 33(2):231-239, 2005.

67. Kibler WB: Biomechanical analysis of the shoulder during tennis activities, *Clin Sports Med* 14(1):79-85, 1995.

68. Huisstede B, Miedema HS, van OT, et al: Interventions for treating the radial tunnel syndrome: a systematic review of observational studies, *J Hand Surg Am* 33(1):72-78, 2008.

69. Stanley J: Radial tunnel syndrome: a surgeon's perspective, *J Hand Ther* 19(2):180-184, 2006.

70. Roles NC, Maudsley RH: Radial tunnel syndrome: resistant tennis elbow as a nerve entrapment, *J Bone Joint Surg Br* 54(3):499-508, 1972.

71. Cleary CK: Management of radial tunnel syndrome: a therapist's clinical perspective, *J Hand Ther* 19(2):186-191, 2006.

72. Henry M, Stutz C: A unified approach to radial tunnel syndrome and lateral tendinosis, *Tech Hand Up Extrem Surg* 10(4):200-205, 2006.

73. Alba CD: Therapist's management of radial tunnel syndrome. In Mackin EJ, Callahan A, Skirven TM, et al, eds: *Rehabilitation of the hand and upper extremity*, ed 5, St Louis, 2002, Mosby.

74. Eversmann WW: Proximal median nerve compression, *Hand Clin* 8(2):307-315, 1992.

75. Lee MJ, LaStayo PC: Pronator syndrome and other nerve compressions that mimic carpal tunnel syndrome, *J Orthop Sports Phys Ther* 34(10):601-609, 2004.

76. Seki M, Nakamura H, Kono H: Neurolysis is not required for young patients with a spontaneous palsy of the anterior interosseous nerve: retrospective analysis of cases managed non-operatively, *J Bone Joint Surg Br* 88(12):1606-1609, 2006.

77. Ciccotti MC, Schwartz MA, Ciccotti MG: Diagnosis and treatment of medial epicondylitis of the elbow, *Clin Sports Med* 23(4):693-705, 2004.

78. O'Driscoll SW, Jupiter JB, King GJ, et al: The unstable elbow, *Instr Course Lect* 50:89-102, 2001.

79. Field L, Savoie F: Management of loose bodies and other limited procedures. In Morrey BF, Sanchez-Sotelo J, eds: *The elbow and its disorders*, ed 4, Philadelphia, 2009, Saunders.

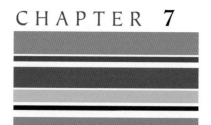

CHAPTER 7

Movement System Syndromes of the Knee

Marcie Harris-Hayes, Suzy L. Cornbleet,
Gregory W. Holtzman

INTRODUCTION

Common knee pain problems seen by physical therapists include overuse injuries, such as patellofemoral pain syndrome (PFPS); traumatic injuries, such as anterior cruciate ligament (ACL) tears; and degenerative conditions, such as osteoarthritis (OA). Treatment directed at the identified source, such as soft tissue injury, may be useful after injury to reduce pain and return to function, however may not address the cause or contributing factors of the condition. One of the proposed contributing factors to injury is abnormal movement patterns or movement impairments. There is growing support that movement impairments may contribute to knee problems such as PFPS,[1-3] iliotibial band (ITB) friction syndrome,[4-5] ACL tears,[6] and OA.[7,8] In addition, studies have shown that addressing movement impairments can improve symptoms, enhance patient function after injury,[9-12] and prevent future injury.[13,14]

In this chapter, we will focus on the syndromes and treatment of movement impairments proposed to contribute to mechanical knee pain and injury. The diagnosis of acute, traumatic injuries, such as ligamentous and meniscal tears is described in Chapter 2. The treatment of acute, traumatic injuries is not discussed in detail here because many excellent sources are available to describe the rehabilitation of these conditions.* The syndromes described in this chapter will, however, assist the therapist in identifying possible underlying movement impairments present during the early stages of rehabilitation.

Movement system syndromes (MSS) are influenced by a variety of factors that are important to consider during examination and treatment. Factors to consider are intrinsic characteristics, such as age, gender, and structural variations, and extrinsic characteristics, such as work or sport activity and work environment. For each patient, the examiner must consider the contribution of individual factors, as well as the possible interaction of these factors. OA provides an example of how multiple factors may contribute to the progression of a musculoskeletal problem. Increased age,[15] high body mass,[15-17] structural alignment,[8,18] knee laxity,[19,20] and participation in activities that involve deep knee flexion[21] have all been shown to increase the risk of knee OA or the progression of knee OA. The interaction of these factors may further compound the risk. For example, Sharma et al[16] found a positive relationship between body mass index (BMI) and the severity of radiographic OA in the varus-aligned knee. How quickly a joint degenerates or an injury occurs is likely determined by the interaction of multiple factors specific to the individual. These factors must be taken into account during the treatment of knee pain problems.

The relationship of the knee to the entire lower quarter should be considered when evaluating individuals with knee pain problems. The knee is the interface between the ankle/foot complex and the hip and is often affected by these neighboring joints. Many muscles crossing the knee joint also cross either the hip or the ankle/foot. Thus alignment faults, structural variations, or movement impairments at the hip or ankle/foot may result in altered stresses at the knee. For example, excessive femoral adduction while performing sit-to-stand may result in increased knee valgus, which is an alignment that has been associated with knee pain and knee injury.[3-5]

Based on the theory of relative stiffness/flexibility, as described in Chapter 1, the body takes the path of least resistance when completing a task. An illustration of relative stiffness/flexibility between the knee and the hip may be seen in a ballet dancer who has a limitation in hip lateral rotation as the result of structural femoral anteversion. To achieve sufficient turn out for first position, the dancer demonstrates lateral rotation of the tibia to

---

*Suggested Readings:

Maxey L, Magnusson J: *Rehabilitation for the postsurgical orthopedic patient*, ed 2, St Louis, Mosby, 2007.

Cioppa-Mosca J, Cahill JB, Cavanaugh JT, et al: *Postsurgical rehabilitation guidelines for the orthopedic clinician*, St Louis, Mosby, 2006.

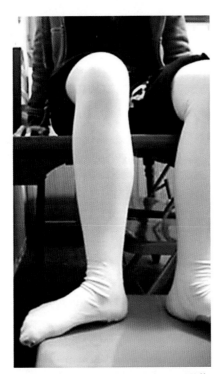

Figure 7-1. Excessive tibial lateral rotation. Ballet dancer in sitting position demonstrating excessive tibial lateral rotation. Excessive tibial lateral rotation may be the consequence of limited hip lateral rotation.

compensate for the lack of hip lateral rotation. The tibiofemoral joint is less stiff than the hip and therefore moves into lateral rotation more easily (Figure 7-1). With continued practice of first position using compensatory rotation of the tibia, the knee undergoes repeated mechanical stresses that accumulate over time, resulting in microtrauma and potentially macrotrauma or injury.

Relative stiffness/flexibility may also occur between a muscle and a joint. The tibiofemoral joint may be relatively less stiff than the tensor fasciae latae-iliotibial band (TFL-ITB). The relative stiffness/flexibility of the TFL-ITB can be observed during the two-joint hip flexor length. If the structures surrounding the tibiofemoral joint do not provide sufficient passive stiffness to stabilize the joint and the TFL-ITB does not easily stretch because of stiffness or shortness, lateral rotation of the tibia may be observed. In a sprinter, this relative stiffness/flexibility could result in repetitive tibial lateral rotation each time the limb initiates swing phase, the position in which the TFL-ITB should be in its most lengthened position. The stresses of repetitive rotation at the tibiofemoral joint may eventually lead to a knee pain problem.

Using the MSS concepts, a standardized examination[22] is performed to determine the movement system syndrome and identify the factors contributing to the syndrome. The movement system syndrome is named for the direction of motion that is associated with an increase in the patient's pain. For example, if the patient reports an increase in symptoms during the primary test of a single-leg squat and demonstrates femoral adduction with knee valgus, then tibiofemoral rotation with valgus (TFRVal) is suspected as the movement impairment. To confirm that TFRVal is associated with the pain complaint, the patient is asked to perform a secondary test by repeating the task while controlling the femoral adduction and knee valgus and keeping the knee aligned properly. If the patient reports a decrease in pain during the secondary test compared to the primary test, the movement system diagnosis of TFRVal is supported. Further substantiation of the diagnosis occurs if the examiner finds that the patient demonstrates the same direction of motion during multiple test items.

Specific to the knee, the movement system syndrome may not be obvious from the standard examination and basic functional activities. This is particularly true in high-level athletes because their impairments and/or symptoms may not be revealed until the knee is physically taxed with higher level activities. Therefore sport-specific or work-specific tasks may need to be assessed. Examples include running, jumping, and landing from a jump. In addition, the specific activity that the patient reports as most problematic should be assessed. Using the concepts of the MSS examination, primary and secondary tests of the higher level activities can be performed to confirm the suspected movement system diagnosis.

Once the movement system syndrome is identified and the stage for rehabilitation is determined, treatment can be provided. Treatment emphasis is on educating the patient in how to restore precise movement during all functional and athletic activities. Therapeutic exercise is also prescribed to address physical impairments, such as poor muscle performance or reduced muscle extensibility, thought to contribute to the movement system syndrome. Traditionally, the focus of rehabilitation of the knee has been placed on strengthening of the thigh musculature in the sagittal plane (quadriceps and hamstrings) with little regard to the influence of transverse or coronal plane motion at the tibiofemoral joint. We have found, however, that many knee pain problems, including PFPS and OA are treated effectively by addressing movement impairments related to excessive rotation or varus/valgus at the tibiofemoral joint. In addition, fitness activities are encouraged; however, modifications may need to be provided during the early stages of rehabilitation.

This chapter describes the normal alignment and movement of the knee and the actions of the surrounding musculature, as well as the structural and acquired faults that affect the knee and must be considered as part of the overall assessment. Finally, the proposed movement system syndrome of the knee and specific treatment recommendations associated with each syndrome are described (Table 7-1). Case examples are used to illustrate the major points.

TABLE 7-1
Movement System Syndromes of the Knee

Symptom	Source of Pain	Treatment
TIBIOFEMORAL ROTATION (TFR) WITH VALGUS (TFRVAL) OR TFR WITH VARUS (TFRVAR) SYNDROME		
Impaired motion at the tibiofemoral joint, transverse or frontal plane		

• Pain location:
  • Joint line
  • Peripatellar region
• Pain associated with tibiofemoral rotation (WB or NWB)
	• Patellofemoral joint
	• Hamstrings
	• Iliotibial band
	• Popliteus
	• Pes anserinus
	• Meniscus
	• Saphenous nerve
	• Subchondral bone
	• Synovium
	• Retinaculum
	• Joint capsule and ligaments
		Both:
		• Education and modification of functional activities that contribute to impaired motion between the femur and tibia
		• Improve muscle performance of hip lateral rotators and abductors
		• Improve extensibility of TFL-ITB
		• Posterior X taping
		• Encourage fitness without increasing symptoms
		TFRVal:
		• Address pronation at foot
		TFRVar:
		• Improve shock absorption—heel to toe pattern

TIBIOFEMORAL HYPOMOBILITY (TFHYPO) SYNDROME		
Physiologic loss of ROM		
• Pain location: • Deep in joint • Pain with WB that decreases with rest • Stiffness	• Collateral ligaments • Subchondral bone • Patellofemoral joint • Meniscus • Joint capsule and ligaments	• Instruct in rolling heel-to-toe gait pattern • Reduce rotation and compressive forces on joint • Improve knee ROM • Mobilization for ROM and pain relief • Strengthen gluteus maximus and gastrocnemius muscles • Improve extensibility of hip flexors • Encourage fitness without increasing symptoms Bracing is an option *In patients with OA:* Caution should be taken to avoid excessive strengthening of quadriceps and hamstrings in patients with malalignment or laxity in the knee[20]
KNEE EXTENSION (KEXT) SYNDROME AND KEXT SYNDROME WITH PATELLAR SUPERIOR GLIDE (KEXTSG) SYNDROME		
Associated with dominance or shortness/stiffness of quadriceps muscle		

Kext
• Pain location:
  • Suprapatellar region
KextSG
• Pain location:
  • Infrapatellar or peripatellar region
	Kext
	• Quadriceps tendon
	• Bursa
	KextSG
	• Patellofemoral joint
	• Fat pad
	• Patellar tendon
	• Plica
		Both
		• Education and modification of functional activities to reduce recruitment of quadriceps (i.e., stairs and fitness activities)
		• Shift weight anteriorly during gait
		• Improve muscle performance of hip extensors
		• Improve extensibility of quadriceps
		• Encourage fitness without increasing symptoms
		KextSG
		• Mobilization: Patellar inferior glide
		• Horseshoe taping of patella may be indicated
		• Patellar strap to reduce stresses on the source of the symptoms (patellar tendon)

KNEE HYPEREXTENSION (KHEXT) SYNDROME		
Associated with dominance of hamstrings		

• Pain location:
  • Anterior or posterior joint line
  • Peripatellar region
	• Patellofemoral joint
	• Fat pad
	• Bursa
	• Plica
	• Meniscus
	• Joint capsule and ligaments
	• Hamstrings
	• Popliteus
		• Education and modification of functional activities to decrease knee hyperextension (i.e., walking and standing): Keep knees unlocked
		• Improve muscle performance of quadriceps and gluteals
		• Improve extensibility of hamstrings and gastrocnemius
		• Posterior X taping
		• Unloader V taping (source: fat pad)
		• Encourage fitness without increasing symptoms

TABLE **7-1**
Movement System Syndromes of the Knee—cont'd

Symptom	Source of Pain	Treatment
PATELLAR LATERAL GLIDE (PLG) SYNDROME		
Impaired alignment or tracking of the patella in the trochlear groove		
• Pain location: • Peripatellar region	• Patellofemoral joint • Patellar tendon • Fat pad • Plica • Subchondral bone • Synovium • Retinaculum • Joint capsule and ligaments	• Limit prolonged knee flexion • Improve muscle performance of quadriceps • Improve extensibility of TFL-ITB • Mobilization—patellar medial glide • Taping of patella may be indicated • Encourage fitness without increasing symptoms
TIBIOFEMORAL ACCESSORY HYPERMOBILITY (TFAH) SYNDROME		
Excessive motion at the tibiofemoral joint		
• May or may not have pain. Instability or giving way	May have deficient ligamentous integrity from previous injury • ACL • PCL • Lateral corner/complex	• Rule out other diagnoses • Neuromuscular retraining • Improve muscle performance of lower extremity musculature • Posterior X taping • Consider bracing • Encourage fitness without increasing symptoms
KNEE IMPAIRMENT		
No movement system syndrome identified or unable to perform a movement examination as occurs in cases of acute trauma or post-surgery		
• Pain is associated with trauma or surgery	Any structure of the knee associated with trauma or surgery	Improve ROM, strength, and neuromuscular control according to the healing of the involved structure. • Stage 1: Tissue protection to reduce stress to injured structure • Stage 2: Gradual progression of activities to gradually increase stress to structure without imposing new injury • Stage 3: Tissue stress progression to prepare tissue for return to normal activities

ACL, Anterior cruciate ligament; *ITB,* iliotibial band; *LR,* lateral rotation; *MR,* medial rotation; *NWB,* non–weight-bearing; *OA,* osteoarthritis; *PCL,* posterior cruciate ligament; *ROM,* range of motion; *TFL,* tensor fascia latae; *WB,* weight-bearing.
Modified from Harris-Hayes M, Sahrmann SA, Norton BJ, et al: Diagnosis and management of a patient with knee pain using the movement system impairment classification system, *J Orthop Sports Phys Ther* 38(4):203-213, 2008.

ALIGNMENT OF THE KNEE

The alignment of the entire lower extremity, including the hip, knee, ankle, and foot must be considered when assessing an individual with knee pain. Alignment of the knee is discussed in detail, and alignment of the hip and the ankle and foot is referred to briefly. Additional information on the ankle and foot can be found in Chapter 8, and additional information on the hip can be found in Sahrmann.[22]

When assessing alignment, one must consider the possibility of structural impairments and distinguish structural from acquired impairments. Structural impairments are related to bony structure and cannot be corrected with training or exercise. Acquired impairments are often the result of postural habits and can be changed with

training. Examples of structural impairments that affect the knee include femoral or acetabular anteversion or retroversion, genu valgus or varus, tibial varum, tibial torsion, and a rigid supinated foot. Although structural impairments cannot be changed or corrected, exercises and activities may need to be modified to accommodate the structural impairment. For example, if an individual's hip lateral rotation is limited by femoral anteversion, the patient should be encouraged not to force hip lateral rotation during posterior gluteus medius strengthening.[22] The patient should also be educated about the problems that can occur if he or she participates in activities that require excessive hip lateral rotation, such as ballet, because compensations often occur at other joints such as the knee. In addition, the patient should be instructed to avoid excessive lateral rotation of the hip during all

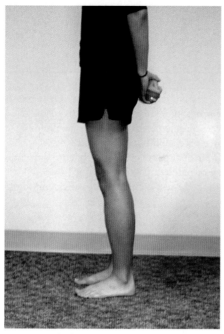

Figure 7-2. Normal alignment of the knee. Tibia and femur should be aligned vertically with the knee angle at approximately 0 degrees of flexion/extension.

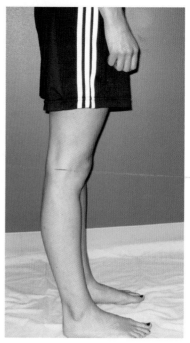

Figure 7-3. Genu recurvatum. Knee extension greater than 5 degrees. Note ankle plantarflexion.

functional activities such as sitting on the floor in the tailor position or stretching during dance warm-ups.

Normal Alignment

Sagittal Plane

Alignment of the lower extremity in the sagittal plane is viewed from the lateral aspect of the individual. The tibia and femur should be aligned vertically with the knee angle at approximately 0 degrees of flexion/extension (Figure 7-2). The angle of the hip joint, measured by a line bisecting the pelvis and a line bisecting the femur, should be 0 degrees in normal alignment. The ankle should be in a neutral position, with 0 degrees of dorsiflexion in relaxed standing.

Impairments

Genu recurvatum or knee hyperextension, defined as knee extension greater than 5 degrees, is commonly observed in children or young adults (Figure 7-3). Genu recurvatum may lead to many other impairments, including tibial bowing in the frontal or sagittal plane, altered compressive forces at the tibiofemoral joint, functional weakness of the quadriceps and gluteus maximus along with possible overrecruitment of the hamstrings, and posterior capsule stretching with ligamentous laxity.[22-24] The knee may appear hyperextended when there is significant posterior bowing of the tibia in the sagittal plane.[22] Standing with the knees in flexion is most typically seen in older individuals with end-stage OA or individuals with an acute injury (Figure 7-4).

Alignment of the knee may be related to alignment deviations of the hip and ankle. For example, knee

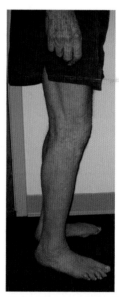

Figure 7-4. Excessive knee flexion.

hyperextension is often associated with posterior pelvic tilt, hip extension, and ankle plantarflexion.[22,23] Knee flexion is often present with anterior pelvic tilt, hip flexion, and ankle dorsiflexion.

Frontal Plane

Normal Alignment

Frontal plane alignment is viewed from the anterior and posterior aspect. The femoral shaft angles medially as a result of the angle of inclination of the proximal femur. The long axis of the femur diverges about 10 degrees from the long axis of the tibia, therefore knee alignment in the frontal plane is a physiologic valgus angle of 170 to 175 degrees in the adult (Figure 7-5).[25,26]

The amount of physiologic valgus changes with normal aging in children. Newborns demonstrate genu varum until about 20 months. Then the angle progresses toward valgus and peaks at approximately 168 degrees when the child reaches about 3 years.[27] The valgus then gradually decreases and reaches the adult value of approximately 170 to 175 degrees by age 6.[25,27,28]

Impairments

If the described angle is less than 170 degrees, it is considered genu valgum (Figure 7-6), and if the angle is greater than 180 degrees, it is considered genu varum (Figure 7-7).[25] Genu valgum may place excessive tensile stresses or strain on the structures on the medial side of the knee and compressive forces on the lateral compartment of the knee. Genu varum may place excessive tensile stresses or strain on the structures on the lateral side of the knee and compressive forces on the medial compartment of the knee. In the young adult, genu varum appears to be more common in men than women.

Malalignment of the tibiofemoral joint in the frontal plane has been associated with osteoarthritis and functional limitations. People with knee OA and a varus or valgus alignment impairment have an increased risk of progression of tibiofemoral OA[8,18,20] and patellofemoral OA.[29-31] In addition, an alignment change of 5 degrees in the frontal plane is associated with decreased ability to perform sit-to-stand and increased pain in people with knee OA.[18] Alignment impairments may also be associated with compartment-specific OA, such as genu varum with medial compartment OA, and genu valgum with lateral compartment OA, which is discussed in detail in the "Tibiofemoral Rotation Syndrome" section.[32]

The structure of the tibia and femur should be considered when assessing frontal plane alignment. Tibial varum is present if the distal one third of the tibia deviates medially from a vertical reference line. Tibial varum has more commonly been measured from the posterior view in resting calcaneal stance with average amounts ranging from 4.6 degrees to 8.3 degrees.[33,34] Our preference is to observe and measure tibial varum from the anterior view because the tibial shaft is more visible and palpable. Keeping in mind the norms stated above, a reasonable criterion for excessive tibial varum would be a deviation greater than 10 degrees (Figure 7-8). Tibial varum is often associated with subtalar joint pronation,[33,34] although we have seen it occur with a supinated foot. Tibial varum is more commonly observed with genu varum than genu valgum.

The structure of the femur may also be associated with genu valgum and varum; however, studies to confirm this have not been reported. Coxa varum, an angle of inclination at the hip that is notably less than 125 degrees,[26] may contribute to a genu valgum. Coxa valgum, an angle of inclination at the hip that is notably greater than 125

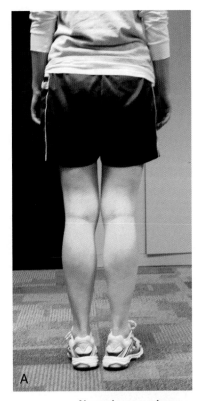

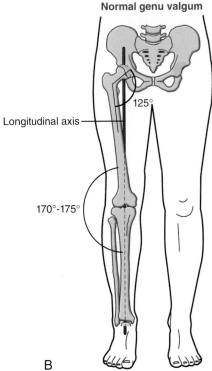

Figure 7-5. A and **B,** Normal physiologic valgus. The normal 125-degree angle of inclination of the proximal femur and the longitudinal axis of rotation throughout the entire lower extremity are also shown. (**B,** From Neuman DA: *Kinesiology of the musculoskeletal system: foundations for rehabilitation,* ed 2, St Louis, 2010, Mosby.)

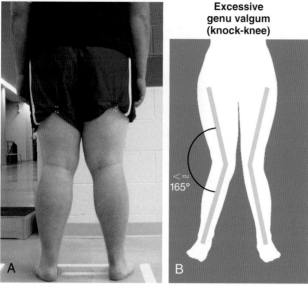

Figure 7-6. **A** and **B**, Genu valgum. Excessive frontal plane deviations. (**B**, From Neuman DA: *Kinesiology of the musculoskeletal system: foundations for rehabilitation*, ed 2, St Louis, 2010, Mosby.)

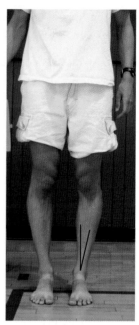

Figure 7-8. Tibial varum. A *line* representing the tibial shaft deviates from a *vertical reference line* greater than 10 degrees.

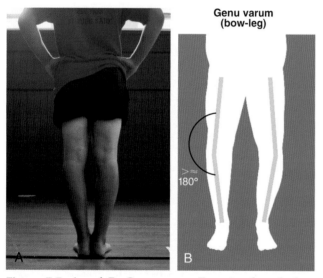

Figure 7-7. **A** and **B**, Genu varum. Excessive frontal plane deviations. (**B**, From Neuman DA: *Kinesiology of the musculoskeletal system: foundations for rehabilitation*, ed 2, St Louis, 2010, Mosby.)

degrees,[26] may contribute to a genu varum through excessive loading on the medial knee compartment that leads to a loss of medial knee joint space.

Transverse Plane

Normal Alignment

Transverse plane alignment is observed from the anterior and posterior aspects. General assessment of the entire lower extremity should be performed, followed by a more specific assessment of each region, such as the hip or knee. Rotation of the femur is assessed from the posterior

view, using the vertical creases that represent the border of the hamstrings and comparing the medial crease to the lateral crease. The distance of the vertical creases should be equal from the medial and lateral aspects of the knee, respectively. Another method would be to palpate the medial and lateral epicondyles and assess the direction of the plane that they are facing (e.g., more medially or more laterally compared to the sagittal plane). The anterior view can also be used to assess for consistency; however, an impaired alignment of the patella can be misleading. See Chapter 8 for a discussion of normal alignment of the foot and ankle in the transverse plane.

Impairments

Femoral medial rotation is a common alignment impairment observed in patients with knee pain (Figure 7-9). When femoral medial rotation is noted in standing alignment, the possibility of a structural femoral anteversion should also be considered and determined with further examination.[22] The appearance of femoral medial rotation may also suggest poor performance of the hip lateral rotators or reduced extensibility of the TFL-ITB. These muscle properties can be assessed with further testing.

When the foot is directed laterally during stance, it may be the result of an acquired postural impairment, such as femoral lateral rotation, or a structural impairment, such as femoral retroversion, tibial external torsion, or foot deformity. The location of the impairment should be assessed (e.g., femur or tibia) and to determine if the impairment is acquired or structural so that treatment may be adjusted accordingly.

Tibial torsion is described as a rotation of the tibial shaft. Although we have observed individuals with

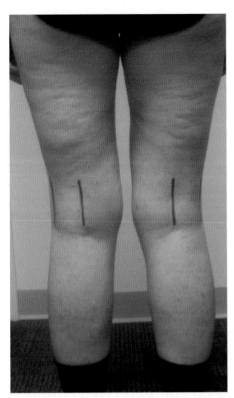

Figure 7-9. Femoral medial rotation. Note the medial and lateral hamstring creases are not an equal distance from the medial and lateral aspects of the knee, respectively. In fact, on the right lower extremity, the lateral hamstring is barely visible.

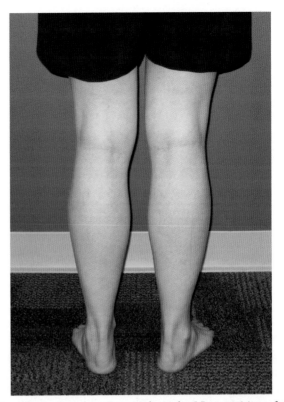

Figure 7-10. Tibial torsion on the right. Note position of the foot relative to the knee. The femur appears to be in medial rotation. However, the foot is laterally deviated, which leads the clinician to suspect torsion or tibial lateral rotation. The specific test for tibial torsion should then be performed.

internal tibial torsion, external tibial torsion is much more common. External tibial torsion is demonstrated when the distal tibia is rotated in the lateral direction greater than 20 to 40 degrees[35-37] compared to the proximal tibia (Figure 7-10). External tibial torsion may be a compensation that develops when femoral anteversion is present and the individual attempts to correct a toe-in alignment. When external tibial torsion is determined to be present, the position of the foot should not be corrected. Trying to align the foot straight ahead will compromise the normal alignment of the ankle/foot and affect the ability of the individual to dorsiflex the ankle.[22] Attempting this correction could also affect the knee by imposing medial rotation of the tibia on the femur.

Alignment of the Patellofemoral Joint

Normal Alignment

Patellar alignment may be viewed anteriorly. In the frontal plane, the patella should be centered in the trochlear groove, although imaging has suggested a slight lateral deviation.[27] In the sagittal plane, patellar alignment is represented by a Insall-Salvati ratio.[38] The Insall-Salvati ratio is the ratio of the patellar tendon length compared to the patellar height with the knee in 60 degrees of flexion. A normal Insall-Salvati ratio is 1±0.2. Although an estimate may be made clinically, measurements are best determined by lateral radiographs.

Impairments

Impaired patellar alignment may lead to abnormal stresses on the patellofemoral joint and surrounding soft tissues that with time may lead to peripatellar pain. The most common alignment impairments of the patella are excessive lateral or excessive superior displacement. Poor performance of the vastus medialis oblique (VMO) muscle and a short, stiff TFL-ITB are thought to contribute to lateral patellar displacement;[39] however, there is limited research to demonstrate this correlation.

By definition, lateral patellar tilt is present when the lateral patellar border is posterior to the medial patellar border and the lateral border cannot be elevated in the anterior direction.[40] The observation of lateral patellar tilt has been shown to be associated with a lateral patellar tilt angle greater than 10 degrees when measured by magnetic resonance imaging (MRI). Further study is needed, however, to assess the association of lateral patellar tilt and the presence of pain.

Excessive superior patellar displacement, also known as *patella alta*, is represented by an Insall-Salvati ratio greater than or equal to 1.2. The superior patellar displacement may indicate that the quadriceps are relatively more stiff than the patellar tendon. This relationship is detailed in the "Knee Extension Syndrome" section. Patella baja, or excessive inferior patellar displacement, has an Insall-Salvati ratio less than or equal to 0.8. Patella baja may be observed as a complication after surgical procedures such as ACL reconstruction, which may be related to the scarring down of the patellar tendon after a surgical procedure.

Although patellar malalignment is believed to be a contributing factor to various knee pain problems, the clinical assessment of patellar alignment is unreliable.[41] Therefore the entire clinical picture must be considered.

MOTIONS OF THE KNEE JOINT

Sagittal Plane

Knee Flexion and Extension

In the sagittal plane, the tibiofemoral joint flexes and extends about a medial-lateral axis passing transversely through the femoral condyles. The axis of rotation does not remain in one location but instead shifts and forms an evolute during the movement. The range of motion (ROM) available varies with age (Table 7-2). Passive ROM (PROM) at the tibiofemoral joint does not change significantly during the adult years[42,43]; however, reduced extensibility of the rectus femoris and hamstring muscles has been shown to significantly contribute to joint limitations in the older individual.[43]

Frontal Plane

In the frontal plane, the tibiofemoral joint abducts and adducts around an anterior to posterior axis. Normal values for tibial adduction and abduction relative to femur are highly variable, with reported mean total values ranging from 2 to 14 degrees.[53-57] There is less motion available when the knee is extended, with only 2 to 6 degrees of total abduction and adduction,[53,54] compared to when the knee is flexed, and motion can increase to 14 degrees.[53-57] Abduction and adduction is typically a passive motion that occurs during activities such as gait.

Transverse Plane

In the transverse plane, the tibiofemoral joint rotates around a vertical axis located approximately at the intercondylar eminence.[58] An individual is expected to have approximately twice the amount of lateral rotation as medial rotation.[59] Reported values for tibiofemoral rotation ROM are highly variable because of the various methods used to assess tibiofemoral rotation. With the knee flexed to 90 degrees, total rotation ROM is between 25 to 57 degrees.[53,59-63] With the knee fully extended, there is essentially no rotation available due to the passive tension of the surrounding ligaments.

During either tibial-on-femoral knee extension or femoral-on-tibial knee extension, conjunct rotation occurs; this is termed the *screw-home mechanism*. This passive rotary-locking mechanism results in approximately 10 degrees of tibial lateral rotation relative to the femur. The major contributing factor to the screw-home mechanism is the shape of the medial femoral condyle that curves approximately 30 degrees laterally, helping to direct the tibia toward its locked position in lateral rotation.[26]

MOTION OF THE PATELLOFEMORAL JOINT

In knee extension, the patella is slightly laterally displaced. With flexion from 0 to 30 degrees, it glides inferiorly and medially. As the knee flexes greater than 30 degrees, the patella continues to glide inferiorly, but changes to a lateral glide.[64,65] During extension from a flexed position, the patellar motion is the reverse of flexion. These motions are so small that they are hardly noticeable to the observer when motion is normal. Tilting and rotation are also reported to occur in the patella. However, there is no consensus in the amount of patellar motion and the reliability in evaluation of position and movement is limited.

KNEE MOTION DURING GAIT

Sagittal Plane

At initial contact (heel strike), the knee flexes 5 degrees, then continues to flex to 10 to 15 degrees during the initial 15% of the gait cycle. During this time, the quadriceps are working eccentrically to provide shock absorption as the body weight is transferred to the limb. The knee reaches almost full knee extension just before heel off, and at heel off, it begins to flex again. Approximately 35 degrees of knee flexion should be noted at toe off and about 60 degrees (maximum flexion) is seen at midswing.[66] The knee then extends again to almost full knee extension just before initial contact. Children demonstrate a similar pattern; however, they tend to walk with more knee flexion. They do not get as much extension as adults during midstance or before initial contact.[67,68]

TABLE 7-2
Knee Flexion and Extension ROM by Age

Age	Passive ROM (Degrees)		Active ROM (Degrees)	
	Extension*	**Flexion**	**Extension**	**Flexion**
Neonate (0-10 days)	20[44-47]	150[46,47]		
3 months	10	145[46]		
6 months	3	140[46]		
Adults up to age 74	5	155[48,49]	0	140[23,49-52]

*Hyperextension is defined as greater than 5 digrees of extension.
ROM, Range of motion.

Frontal Plane

Minimal tibial abduction/adduction may be noted during the gait cycle with a maximum of 5 degrees.[25,69]

Transverse Plane

Generally, during gait, the tibia medially rotates from heel strike until 20 percent of gait cycle (just before midstance). The tibia then laterally rotates until toe off and medially rotates through swing.[25,69] Normal rotation between the tibia and femur during the gait cycle should be approximately 8 to 9 degrees.[25,69] At initial contact, the tibia is laterally rotated about 2 to 3 degrees relative to the femur. From initial contact through midstance, the tibia is medially rotated more than the femur, approaching 5 degrees of tibial medial rotation compared with the femur. During swing, the tibia is laterally rotated relative to the femur.

KNEE MOTION DURING RUNNING

Knee motion during running is similar to walking; however, the knee is relatively more flexed throughout the cycle.[66] On heel strike, the stance knee flexes up to 45 degrees as the quadriceps work eccentrically to aid shock absorption. The knee then extends during stance; however, it never reaches full extension. At midstance, the knee remains flexed approximately 25 degrees. Maximum knee flexion of 90 degrees occurs during swing phase. A similar pattern of knee motion occurs with all speeds of running; however, as speed increases, the amount of knee flexion during swing increases as high as 130 degrees.

MUSCLE ACTIONS OF THE KNEE

Extensors

The quadriceps muscle is the primary extensor of the knee joint and consists of four muscles: vastus intermedius, vastus lateralis, vastus medialis, and rectus femoris (Figure 7-11). The rectus femoris is the only one of these muscles that crosses both the hip and knee, allowing it to also act as a hip flexor.

The quadriceps angle, or Q-angle, represents the line of the resultant force of the quadriceps that tends to pull the patella superiorly and laterally relative to the patellar ligament. The Q-angle is represented by the angle between a line connecting the anterior superior iliac spine (ASIS) to the midpoint of the patella and a line connecting the tibial tubercle to the midpoint of the patella (Figure 7-12). The normal values for Q-angle are less than 10 degrees in men[25,51,70] and less than 15 degrees in women.[25,51,70] A Q-angle larger than normal is proposed to create excessive lateral forces on the patella through a bowstring effect that may predispose the patella to pathological changes. Q-angle can be influenced by excessive femoral anteversion, genu recurvatum, ankle/foot pronation, lateral tibial rotation, genu valgus, patellar alignment, and tibial tubercle anomalies.[2,70,71] The Q-angle should not be confused with the physiologic valgus of the knee.

Quadriceps muscle impairments related to knee pain may include poor performance or overrecruitment. As mentioned previously, the oblique portion of the vastus medialis (VMO) may provide an important restraint to lateral patellar displacement given the angulation of the fibers that attach to the patella. Poor performance of the VMO may contribute to excessive lateral patellar displacement.[39]

With intensive physical training or loading through weight training or sports, the quadriceps may become relatively too stiff or short and contribute to excessive stress on the patella, patellar ligament, or tibial tubercle. This excessive pull superiorly may be associated with patella alta. In contrast, the quadriceps can become functionally weak when habitual alignment of knee hyperextension is present.

The articularis genus is a small muscle located on the anterior distal femur that inserts into the synovial membrane of the knee joint. As the knee is extended, it assists in drawing the synovial membrane upward and preventing folds of the membrane from becoming compressed within the knee joint.

Flexors

The hamstring muscles are comprised of the semimembranosus and semitendinosus muscles medially and the biceps femoris muscle laterally (see Figure 7-16). Their primary actions include knee flexion and hip extension; however, they also assist with hip medial and lateral rotation and may contribute to tibial medial and lateral rotation. The hamstrings are at risk of overuse when synergists, such as the gluteus maximus, are underused.[22] For example, when the foot is fixed on the ground, the hamstrings can extend the knee by pulling the knee back to the body through its action as a hip extensor. Usually, when hamstring dominance such as this occurs, the quadriceps and gluteus maximus are not performing optimally. This movement impairment is commonly seen in individuals with a swayback alignment[22] and genu recurvatum.

Movement impairments in the transverse plane may be the result of impaired hamstrings. The medial hamstrings assist in medial rotation of the hip and can become dominant and shorter in length compared to the biceps femoris. This imbalance in synergists is seen when an individual maintains excessive hip medial rotation or participates in sports or activities that tend to position or encourage hip medial rotation such as cycling. The biceps femoris assists in lateral rotation of the femur and lateral rotation of the tibia. When the primary hip lateral rotators are not performing optimally, the biceps femoris may compensate by increasing its action in an attempt to control hip lateral rotation.[22] The overuse of the biceps in this way may lead to a muscle strain. The biceps femoris may also contribute to lateral rotation or

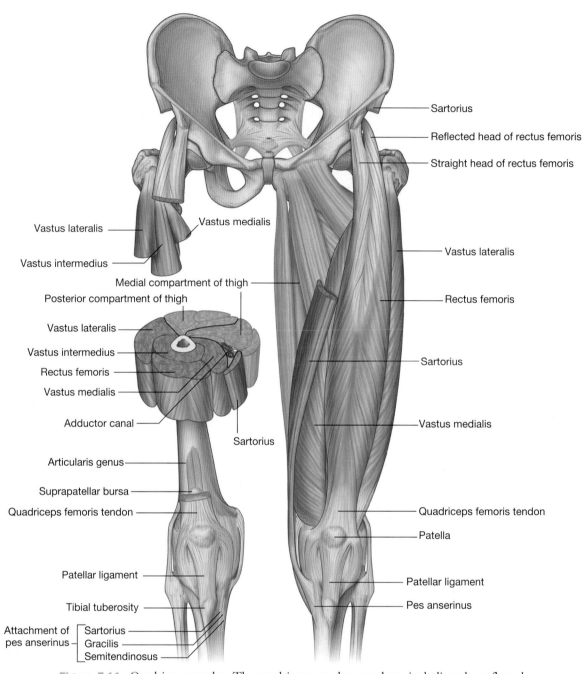

Figure 7-11. Quadricep muscles. The quadriceps can be seen here including the reflected rectus femoris (the only two joint muscle of the quadriceps), along with the vastus lateralis, vastus intermedius and vastus medialis. (From Drake RL, Vogl AW, Mitchell AWM: *Gray's anatomy for students*, ed 2, Baltimore, 2009, Churchill Livingstone.)

posterolateral displacement of the lower leg relative to the femur, given its distal attachment to the fibular head. A patient case demonstrating this phenomena is provided by Sahrmann.[22]

The sartorius muscle flexes, abducts, and laterally rotates the hip and also flexes the knee and rotates it medially. The gracilis acts primarily to adduct the hip and also flexes and medially rotates the knee. Both muscles insert below the medial tibial condyle into the pes anserinus along with the semitendinosus tendon. The pes anserinus insertion may become injured with excessive tibial lateral rotation contributing to medial knee pain.

The gastrocnemius and soleus muscles are powerful ankle plantarflexors; however, the gastrocnemius is also a knee flexor (Figure 7-13). The plantaris also assists with ankle plantarflexion and knee flexion. The gastrocnemius and soleus are described in more detail in Chapter 8. Impairments in length and strength of the gastrocnemius are fairly common. Related to the knee, individuals who stand in knee hyperextension tend to develop shortness

Anterior view

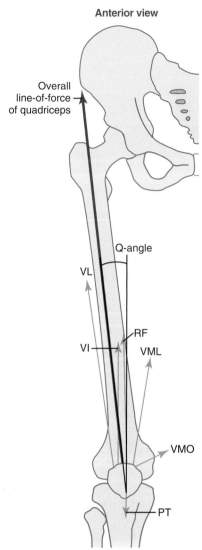

Figure 7-12. Q-angle. The overall line-of-force of the quadriceps is shown as well as the separate line-of-force of the muscles within the quadriceps. The vastus medialis is divided into its two predominant fiber groups: the obliquus and the longus. The net lateral pull exerted on the patella by the quadriceps is indicated by the Q-angle. *PT,* Patellar tendon; *RF,* rectus femoris; *VI,* vastus intermedius; *VL,* vastus lateralis; *VML,* vastus medialis ("longus"); *VMO,* vastus medialis ("obliquus"). (From Neuman DA: *Kinesiology of the musculoskeletal system: foundations for rehabilitation,* ed 2, St Louis, 2010, Mosby.)

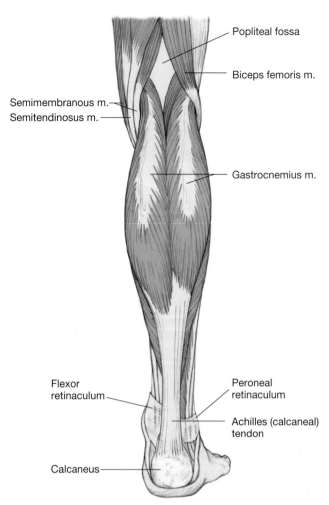

Figure 7-13. Posterior muscles of the lower leg. The gastrocnemius is cut to allow visualization of the soleus muscle. (From Mathers, et al: *Clinical anatomy principles,* St Louis, 1996, Mosby.)

of the gastrocnemius as a result of the alignment of relative plantarflexion. In movement impairments of the knee, poor performance of the ankle plantarflexors may be observed as a lack of push-off during gait, a delayed heel rise, or excessive dorsiflexion during foot flat.

The popliteus muscle is a knee flexor and tibial medial rotator (see Figure 7-13). The popliteus is also known as the key to the knee, because it "unlocks" the knee as it moves from the fully extended (locked) position into flexion. The popliteus unlocks the knee either by medially rotating the tibia in a non–weight-bearing activity or laterally rotating the femur in a weight-bearing activity.

The popliteus is mostly active during crouching and may help the posterior cruciate ligament (PCL) prevent anterior dislocation of the femur.[23,26]

Other Important Hip Muscles That Can Affect the Knee

Lateral Rotators of the Hip

The primary hip lateral rotators include the deep (sometimes referred to as short or intrinsic) lateral rotators and the gluteus maximus. The intrinsic or deep lateral rotators of the hip include the piriformis, gemellus superior and inferior, obturator internus and externus, and quadratus femoris muscles (Figure 7-14). The obturator externus, however, is generally considered a secondary lateral rotator of the hip because its line of force is so close to the longitudinal axis of rotation when the hip is in the anatomical position. As primary lateral rotators of the hip, the deep lateral rotators serve to provide precise control of rotation of the femoral head in the acetabulum, thus maintaining the integrity and stability of the hip

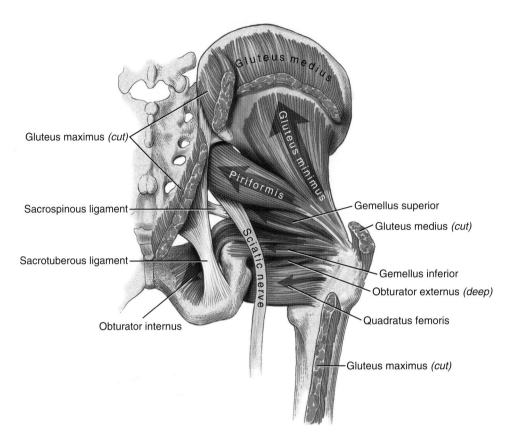

Figure 7-14. Hip lateral rotators. Some of the deep lateral rotators of the hip are depicted here—obturator internus, obturator externus and piriformis. They help to maintain control and stability of the hip joint. When lengthened or weak, they can contribute to femoral medial rotation and knee pain. (From Neuman DA: *Kinesiology of the musculoskeletal system: foundations for rehabilitation,* ed 2, St Louis, 2010, Mosby.)

similar to the way that the rotator cuff muscles provide control of the humeral head in the glenoid. In patients with knee pain syndromes, these muscles often become lengthened and weak, thus losing the precise control of the hip and allowing hip medial rotation to occur.

In addition to being a primary lateral rotator, the gluteus maximus muscle is also a primary hip extensor (Figures 7-15 and 7-16). Individuals who stand in a sway-back alignment commonly have atrophy of the gluteus maximus because their weight line is posterior to their center of mass.[22,23] In these cases, when the gluteus maximus becomes functionally weak, the hamstrings may become the dominant hip extensors instead of the gluteus maximus.

A large portion of the gluteus maximus muscle attaches into the ITB. Therefore shortness or stiffness of the gluteus maximus can contribute to relative stiffness/flexibility issues involving the ITB. Relative stiffness/flexibility as a result of shortness or stiffness of the gluteus maximus through the ITB seems to be more common in males than females and should be suspected if the patient sits in excessive hip abduction.

The secondary lateral rotators of the hip include the sartorius, the biceps femoris, and the posterior fibers of the gluteus minimus and medius (Figure 7-16).

The posterior gluteus medius acts to abduct, extend, and laterally rotate the hip. The length and strength of the posterior gluteus medius is often affected by postural changes at the pelvis and hip. If an individual stands with the right iliac crest higher than the left or with the right hip in medial rotation, the posterior gluteus medius on the right may be lengthened and possibly weak, particularly if tested in the shortened position. Poor performance of this muscle is often a key factor in knee pain problems.

Because control of the knee is needed throughout the range of hip flexion to hip extension in activities such as sit to stand and cutting, the muscle performance of the hip lateral rotators should be tested with the hip flexed and with the hip extended. A number of the hip lateral rotators change their action when the hip is flexed. Although they are hip lateral rotators when the hip is in 0 degrees of flexion, the piriformis and portions of the gluteal muscles change to medial rotators of the femur as the hip is flexed to 90 degrees. This switch in action is due to a change in the location of the muscles' moment arms relative to the axis of rotation.[72,73] Once identified, muscle performance deficits can then be targeted with specific exercises, with the hip flexed or hip extended. Given their likely role in providing stability of the hip,

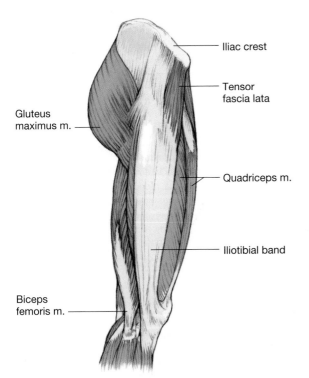

Figure 7-15. Gluteus maximus and tensor fasciae latae–iliotibial band. The TFL-ITB is a major contributor to impairments of the lower extremity. When it is too short or too dominant, it often contributes to femoral medial rotation. Also, the attachment of the TFL-ITB to the patella and the lateral tibial tuberosity may result in impairments of the patella and lateral rotation of the tibia. From this figure, also note the large contribution of the gluteus maximus into the ITB. (From Mathers LH, Chase RA, Dolph J, et al: *Clinical anatomy principles*, St Louis, 1996, Mosby.)

specific attention to the deep lateral rotators (hip flexed position) is warranted.

Medial Rotators of the Hip

The TFL-ITB is a two-joint muscle complex that flexes, abducts, and medially rotates the hip and laterally rotates the tibia through its insertion onto the lateral tibial tubercle (see Figure 7-15). The TFL-ITB also assists in stabilizing the knee when the knee is extended, although it does not actively extend the knee.[23,26] When the TFL-ITB becomes short or too stiff, it can cause a compensatory motion such as lateral tibial rotation or valgus at the knee. The TFL-ITB can also contribute to patellar lateral glide as a result of its insertion onto the lateral patella.[22]

The anterior fibers of the gluteus medius abduct, flex, and medially rotate the hip. Because the anterior fibers of the gluteus medius tend to be stronger than the posterior fibers, the imbalance often results in excessive medial rotation. The anterior gluteus minimus also abducts, flexes, and medially rotates the hip, contributing further to the potential for excessive medial rotation of the hip.[22] When testing performance of the medial rotators of the hip, it is important to remember that muscle function may be increased when the hip is flexed, compared to when the

hip is extended.[72,73] When the hip is extended, there are no primary medial rotators of the hip.[26]

MOVEMENT SYSTEM SYNDROMES
of the Knee

TIBIOFEMORAL ROTATION SYNDROME

Tibiofemoral rotation (TFR) syndrome is characterized by knee pain associated with impaired rotation of the tibiofemoral joint. Excessive rotation between the tibia and femur can be seen during tests of alignment, tests of movement, and performance of functional activities. There are two subcategories of TFR syndrome: TFR with valgus (TFRVal) syndrome and TFR with varus (TFRVar) syndrome. This text focuses on the most common TFR syndrome, TFRVal, and only briefly discusses TFRVar.

Symptoms and History

Individuals that have the diagnosis of TFR syndrome (with valgus or varus) report pain along the tibiofemoral joint line, the peripatellar regions, or at the insertion of the ITB. Pain is often associated with activities that contribute to rotation between the tibia and femur, including weight-bearing activities, such as walking and stair climbing, or non–weight-bearing activities, such as sitting with the lower leg placed in a rotated position relative to the femur. Individuals that demonstrate this movement fault may include ballet dancers, runners, equestrians, and sedentary workers. Those with OA who report instability[74] are also likely to fall into the TFR category.

TIBIOFEMORAL ROTATION WITH VALGUS SYNDROME

Individuals with TFRVal syndrome demonstrate excessive medial rotation or adduction of the femur relative to the tibia, or excessive lateral rotation or abduction of the tibia relative to the femur resulting in knee valgus. This motion has also been described as medial collapse[2,75] or poor dynamic knee stability.[6,76] Clinically, it appears that females are more likely to demonstrate TFRVal than men, and this observation appears to be supported in the literature as well.[76-78] Although it is more common in women, TFRVal syndrome may be present in males, thus the need to take an individualized approach to examination.

Symptoms and History

Structures that may be injured in an individual with TFRVal syndrome include structures of the tibiofemoral joint, the patellofemoral joint, the ITB, and surrounding musculature. A number of studies have demonstrated an association between the movement impairment associated with TFRVal syndrome and knee injury,[1,4,6,79-84] highlighting the importance of assessing the entire lower extremity. In a prospective study, Hewett et al[6] reported that during the landing phase of a jump,

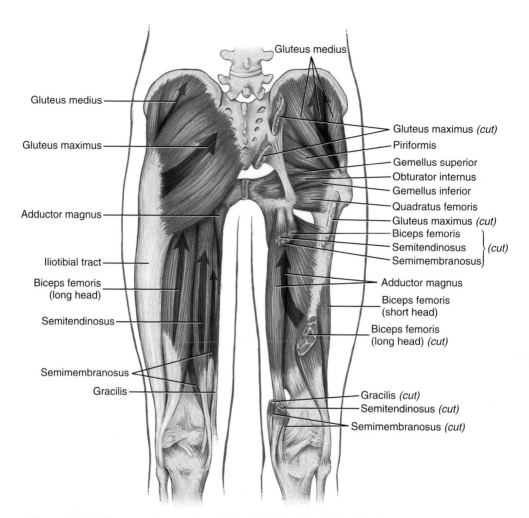

Figure 7-16. The posterior muscles of the hip. The left side highlights the gluteus maximus and hamstring muscles (long head of the biceps femoris, semitendinosus, and semimembranosus). The right side highlights the gluteus medius and five of the six short external rotators, i.e., piriformis, gemellus superior and inferior, obturator internus, and quadratus femoris. (From Neuman DA: *Kinesiology of the musculoskeletal system: foundations for rehabilitation*, ed 2, St Louis, 2010, Mosby.)

young women with a knee valgus angle greater than 8 degrees were more likely to suffer a noncontact ACL injury than those with an angle of less than 8 degrees (Figure 7-17). In addition, Hewett's group demonstrated that the risk of ACL injury is reduced with training to correct the movement impairment.[13,85]

Overuse syndromes, such as PFPS and ITB friction syndrome, have also been associated with TFRVal. Traditional treatment of PFPS has focused on the movement and alignment of the patella[11,86,87]; however, numerous studies have demonstrated that the alignment or movement of the tibia and femur may be associated with PFPS.[1,3,81-84] Although repetitive knee extension-flexion has been implicated in ITB friction syndrome, a recent study demonstrated that increased hip adduction may contribute to the onset of ITB friction syndrome.[4]

An examination that includes the assessment of movement quality and tests of muscle length and

muscle performance, in addition to tests to identify injured structures, is recommended. Key tests and signs of the movement examination are described in the following sections. Tests to assess specific knee structures, such as the ligaments or meniscus, are not the focus of this text; therefore the reader is encouraged to consult other available sources.*

Key Tests and Signs
Alignment Analysis
While the patient is standing, the examiner assesses the overall posture and specific alignment of the lower extremities. Alignment is often not predictive of the movement impairment; however, alignment may contribute to the movement impairment. From the posterior

---

*Suggested reading: Magee DJ: *Orthopedic physical assessment*, ed 4, St Louis, 2002, Saunders.

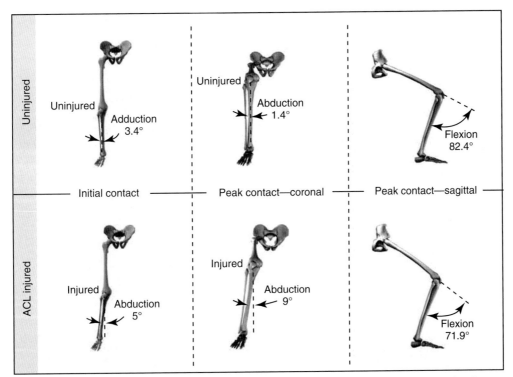

Figure 7-17. Biomechanical model depicting mean knee joint kinematics during the drop vertical jump at initial contact and maximal displacement in the ACL-injured and uninjured groups ($n = 9$ knees and $n = 390$ knees, respectively). *Left,* Coronal plane view of knee abduction angle at initial contact in the ACL-injured and uninjured groups. *Center,* Coronal plane view of maximum knee abduction angle in the ACL-injured and uninjured groups. *Right,* Sagittal plane view of maximum knee flexion angle in the ACL-injured and uninjured groups. (From Hewett TE, Myer GD, Ford KR, et al: Biomechanical measures of neuromuscular control and valgus loading of the knee predict anterior cruciate ligament injury risk in female athletes: a prospective study, *Am J Sports Med* 33:492, 2005.)

view, the patient may demonstrate medial rotation of the femur or lateral rotation of the tibia (Figure 7-18). The patient may also demonstrate knee valgus. From the lateral view, posterior pelvic tilt with hip extension and knee hyperextension might indicate poor performance of the gluteals. A lordotic posture might suggest short or stiff hip flexors and poor abdominal control. Excessive pronation or supination of the foot should also be noted.

Movement Impairments

Standing tests. Single-leg stance should be assessed by comparing both lower extremities. During single-leg stance on the involved limb, the patient will demonstrate excessive medial rotation of the involved femur. The patient may also demonstrate excessive ankle pronation. During single-leg stance on the uninvolved limb, tibial lateral rotation may be noted in the involved limb when the knee is flexed to 90 degrees (Figure 7-19). In addition to movement quality, the examiner may observe the patient's ability to maintain balance when standing on one limb. Poor stability may indicate poor proprioception, which may be a contributor to the patient's pain problem.

During hip and knee flexion in stance (partial squat), the patient will demonstrate femoral (hip) adduction/

medial rotation and knee valgus (Figure 7-20, *A*). This motion may increase or produce the patient's symptoms. When the motion is corrected (Figure 7-20, *B*), the pain typically improves, supporting the diagnosis of TFRVal syndrome.

Supine tests. When performing the two-joint hip flexor length test,[88] lateral rotation or abduction of the tibia may be observed when the involved limb is lowered into hip extension (Figure 7-21). If the patient reports pain during the test, the test is repeated with stabilization of the tibia to prevent the observed motion. If the patient's symptoms are improved, then the movement impairment of TFR is supported. Further tests would be needed to determine if the diagnosis is TFRVal syndrome or TFRVar syndrome.

Prone tests. Lateral rotation of the tibia during knee flexion in prone may be observed. If this motion is painful, then the secondary test should be performed by repeating the motion while preventing the tibial rotation. If the patient's symptoms are improved, then the movement impairment of TFR is supported. Further tests would be needed to determine if the diagnosis was TFRVal syndrome or TFRVar syndrome. During the performance of hip medial or lateral rotation, the examiner may

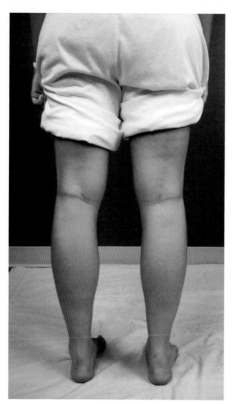

Figure 7-18. Femoral medial rotation. Note the insertion of the medial and lateral hamstrings. The medial hamstrings are more prominent, indicating femoral medial rotation. The lateral hamstring insertion is barely visible on the right lower extremity.

observe excessive rotation or gliding of the tibia relative to the femur. If hip rotation ROM is measured in this position, care should be taken to prevent motion of the tibia relative to the femur, which may inflate the value of hip rotation ROM.[89]

Joint Integrity

In our experience, individuals with TFRVal syndrome often demonstrate an overall laxity in the tibiofemoral joint in the involved and uninvolved joint; however, this laxity has not been quantified. The therapist may suspect ligamentous laxity if there is excessive motion at the tibiofemoral joint while testing hip rotation. In the absence of trauma, tests for ligamentous integrity are often negative with the patient demonstrating equal motion on both limbs.

Muscle Length Impairments

A common muscle impairment includes reduced extensibility of the TFL-ITB,[90] which may contribute to a relative lateral rotation of the tibia through its attachment on the lateral tibial tubercle.

Muscle Strength/Performance Impairments

Impairments of muscle strength and performance include poor performance of the hip lateral rotators and hip

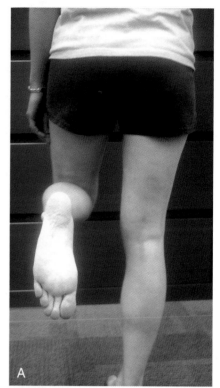

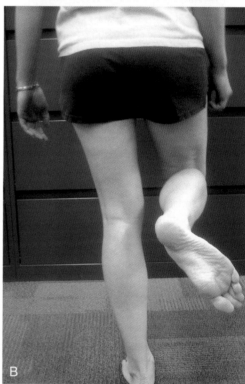

Figure 7-19. Single-leg stance observing the limb being flexed. Note the alignment of the foot. **A,** The left uninvolved foot is vertical relative to the floor. **B,** The right foot is angled away from the vertical indicating tibial lateral rotation.

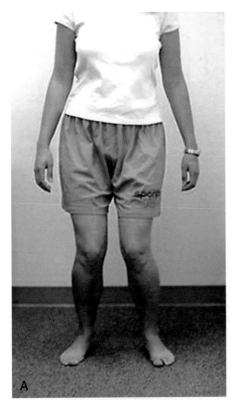

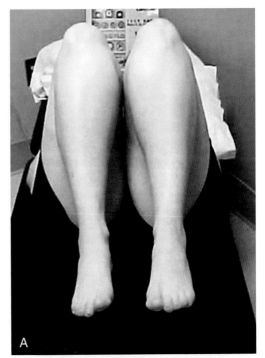

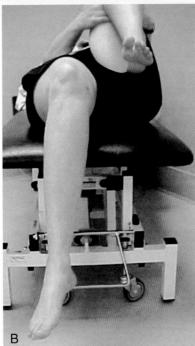

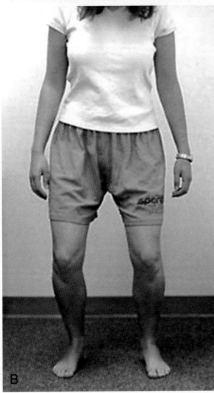

Figure 7-20. Hip and knee flexion in standing. **A,** Note the femoral adduction and medial rotation. There is minimal pronation at the foot, which may contribute to excessive stresses at the knee. **B,** Secondary test of hip and knee flexion in standing. The movement impairment of femoral adduction and medial rotation was corrected.

Figure 7-21. Tibial lateral rotation during two-joint hip flexor length test. **A,** Starting position of the two-joint hip flexor length test. Note position of the right tibia and foot in the sagittal plane. **B,** End position of the two-joint hip flexor length test. Note position of the right tibia and foot. Tibia is now more laterally rotated relative to the femur, secondary to the tension of the TFL-ITB as it is being stretched.

abductors.[91,92] Tibial medial rotators may also be impaired, restricting their ability to control tibial lateral rotation, however these muscles are challenging to assess.

Functional Activities

Gait. During gait, excessive medial rotation or adduction of the femur during stance or tibial lateral rotation during swing may be observed. Excessive pronation of the foot may also be observed.

Step-up and step-down. Most patients with knee pain problems will report an increase in their symptoms with stair ambulation. A step-up and step-down test may be performed to assess the patient's preferred pattern. Patients with TFRVal syndrome will demonstrate femoral adduction and knee valgus with performance of this activity (Figure 7-22). If the movement is painful, a secondary test is performed by repeating the movement and correcting the movement impairment. Because this activity introduces significant stresses on the structures of the knee, reducing the patient's pain significantly may be difficult. If symptoms are not reduced with movement impairment modifications of either the tibiofemoral joint or the patellofemoral joint (see patellofemoral lateral glide syndrome), the patient's pain severity may be too high for the activity being performed.

Tibial lateral rotation may be observed as the patient attempts to clear the toes as they raise the involved foot to the next step (Figure 7-23). This movement impairment may indicate that the medial rotators of the tibia are not sufficiently stabilizing the tibia as the lateral hamstrings contract to flex the knee.

Other Functional Tests

Activities that aggravate the patient's symptoms should be assessed for movement impairments. Patients with TFRVal syndrome exhibit femoral adduction or knee valgus during the symptomatic activities. Common activities include prolonged sitting, squatting, and sit-to-stand. If the patient is an athlete or has low symptom irritability, higher level activities may need to be assessed to determine the movement impairment. These may include running,[1] single-leg squat,[1,93] and various forms of jumping or hopping.[1,76,94]

Summary of Examination Findings

TFRval syndrome presents with the movement impairment of femoral adduction and medial rotation relative to the tibia or tibial abduction/lateral rotation relative to the femur that contributes to a knee valgus. Positions or movements associated with TFRVal syndrome are often painful, and when the movement impairments are corrected, pain is reduced.

Treatment

Primary Objectives

The primary objectives of a treatment program include the following:

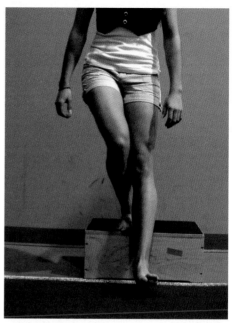

Figure 7-22. Step-down test. Note femoral adduction and knee valgus of the left stance limb.

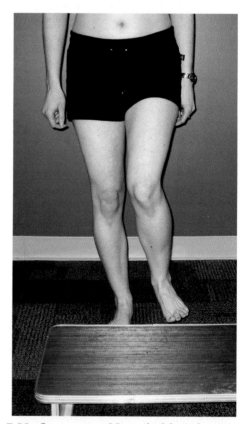

Figure 7-23. Step-up test. Note tibial lateral rotation of the swing leg, indicating movement impairment of tibiofemoral rotation.

1. Correct TFRVal during functional activities.
2. Improve performance of the hip lateral rotators, abductors and tibial medial rotators.
3. Increase extensibility of the TFL-ITB.
4. Address contributions of the foot if necessary.

Corrective Exercise Program

Treatment for this classification includes educating the individual on correcting the postural habits and movements that contribute to the movement impairment and thus the pain problem. The patient is provided with a general description of the impairment: excessive rotation between the tibia and femur. Specific instruction for alignment and functional activities is provided and practiced by the patient. The patient is also instructed in exercises to address the associated muscle impairments.

Alignment. First, the patient is educated in correction of posture and functional activities. To improve alignment between the femur and tibia, the therapist must address impairments in both the sagittal and transverse planes in an effort to achieve a more neutral or ideal alignment. If hyperextension is present, the patient is instructed to unlock the knees. To align the tibia and femur in the transverse plane, the patient is asked to align knees over feet with neutral rotation of hips and tibias by decreasing medial rotation of femur and lateral rotation of tibia. To correct femoral medial rotation, the patient is instructed to contract his or her gluteals and hip lateral rotators to laterally rotate the femur. However, if structural tibial torsion or femoral anteversion is present, normal alignment will not be possible and attempts to "correct" the patient's alignment may result in abnormal stresses to the adjacent joints. Instruction to the patient should emphasize proper alignment that accommodates for these structural impairments. For example, if the patient has tibial torsion, the appearance of a lateral foot progression angle or "turn out" should be allowed. If the patient demonstrates femoral anteversion, the appearance of medial rotation of the femur should be allowed.

Functional activities. Functional activities that contribute to the movement impairment must also be addressed. The functional activity that is most bothersome to the patient should be addressed first, followed by the activities in which the patient spends the most time such as work or school activities. This chapter covers the activities that are useful for most patients; however, the therapist is encouraged to use the principles of the MSI system to address other functional activities that may not be described here.

Gait. To control femoral adduction and medial rotation during gait, the patient is instructed to contract the "buttock muscles" of the stance limb during weight acceptance; the goal is to recruit the hip abductors and lateral rotators. This is sometimes difficult for the patient to achieve on the first visit, therefore an exercise like weight-shifting with unilateral muscle contraction may be useful to assist the patient who is learning to contract the muscles at the appropriate time. The patient should also be instructed to avoid rotating on a fixed foot when making turns.

If the patient is having significant pain in the knee, an assistive device may be suggested to decrease the forces through the affected knee. The cane should be placed in the hand opposite the involved limb. Using the cane in the opposite hand has been shown to significantly reduce external moments[95] across the knee.

Another strategy during gait is to have the patient walk with the feet apart. This change in alignment shifts the adduction moment toward the medial knee and can decrease the pain. As with all recommended alterations in alignment or movement patterns, the change in the symptoms is the guide to the effectiveness and/or appropriateness of the recommendations.

Sit-to-stand; stand-to-sit. The patient should also be instructed to avoid femoral adduction, femoral medial rotation, and knee valgus when transitioning from a sitting position to a standing position. For proper performance of sit-to-stand, the patient is instructed to slide forward in the chair and place the feet hip width apart and aligned behind the knees. On rising, the patient should lean forward to advance the tibias anteriorly over the feet, then use the quadriceps and gluteus maximus muscles to lift the body up and forward out of chair. While performing this, the patient should keep the knee and toes aligned in the transverse plane. Common cues that are useful include "squeeze your seat and keep your knee over your second toe" and "do not let the knees come together." If the patient has difficulty with the correction, a resistive band may be placed around the distal femurs and the patient instructed to gently push into the band to keep it taut as they rise from the chair. If the band becomes loose during the performance of the activity, the patient is provided feedback for the suboptimal performance.

Stairs. The instructions used in the previous paragraph are also useful for stairs. The patient should avoid femoral adduction, femoral medial rotation, and knee valgus while ascending and descending stairs. During stair ascent, the patient may need to shift the weight anteriorly (lean forward over the stairs) to more functionally engage the gluteals.[96]

If the patient has significant pain with stairs, there are a number of methods to reduce symptoms during stair ambulation. These suggestions are useful for all patients with knee pain, despite their movement system syndrome. While ascending stairs, the patient is instructed to use a step-to pattern, leading with the uninvolved extremity and then advancing the involved extremity. As the patient improves and begins to use a step-over-step method, he or she may still be challenged in completing the step-up leading with the involved leg. The patient can use the plantarflexors of the uninvolved leg to help push-up from the lower step. The patient should also be encouraged to use the handrail to reduce the weight bearing on the involved limb.

Descending stairs is often painful for someone with knee impairments. While descending stairs, the patient may use a step-to pattern first leading with the involved extremity and then advancing the uninvolved extremity. Patients who are significantly limited may need to descend the stairs backward; however, this should be assessed

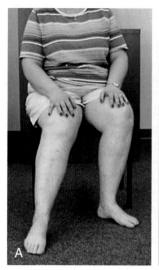
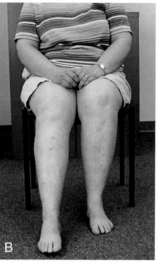

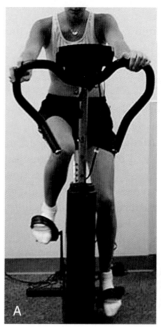
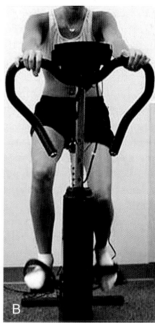

Figure 7-24. Sitting position. **A,** Patient with TFRVal syndrome and knee pain bilaterally demonstrates her working position. She is a transcriptionist and uses a foot pedal regularly. Note position of the feet relative to the knees. **B,** Working position corrected. Patient is instructed in a modified position. (From Harris-Hayes M, Sahrmann SA, Norton BJ, et al: Diagnosis and management of a patient with knee pain using the movement system impaiment classification system, *J Orthop Sports Phys Ther* 38(4):203-213, 2008.)

Figure 7-25. Fitness activity: Cycling. **A,** Note the valgus alignment of the right knee. **B,** Position is modified to correct for TFRVal syndrome.

closely to be sure the patient can perform safely. As the patient improves and begins to use a step-over-step method, a useful method to reduce stress to the involved limb while descending stairs is to use the plantarflexors eccentrically to absorb some of the body weight as the body is lowered onto the lower step.

Other functional activities. Personal activities related to work, school, fitness, and leisure should also be addressed. The patient should be instructed to avoid the TFRVal movement impairment during functional activities. For example, in sitting, the patient may sit with the foot in a relatively lateral position to the knee. The patient should be instructed to modify the position so that the knee and foot are aligned in the transverse plane (Figure 7-24). An impairment may also be demonstrated in the patient's driving. Some patients change from the gas to brake pedal by keeping their heel in contact with the floorboard and rotating the tibia to move the foot, resulting in repetitive rotation between the tibia and the femur. These patients should be instructed to lift the foot from the floor as they change pedals to avoid the repetitive rotation, or they can rotate at the hip rather than the knee. After specific instruction in the performance of key activities, the patient should understand concepts that can be generalized to other activities.

Fitness activities. If the patient does not have a fitness program, then a discussion is warranted to encourage a fitness program as a goal. If the patient participates regularly in fitness, we encourage continued participation in some form of fitness, although the current program

may need to be modified. For example, the patient's aerobic activities may need to be modified by addressing the movement impairment (Figure 7-25) and possibly reducing the intensity. The modified intensity level should be related to the patient's stage of rehabilitation. For example, if the patient's injury is in Stage 1 for rehabilitation, then the patient may use one-leg cycling for aerobic conditioning and progress to activities in the water with the body submerged to reduce stresses to the knee. For Stage 2, the person may be instructed to use a bike or to start with a walking program while concentrating on maintaining proper tibiofemoral alignment. The intensity is then gradually increased as the patient's symptoms improve. Box 7-1 shows an example program to progress an individual back to running after injury.[97] The type of fitness equipment also needs to be considered. For example, if the patient has tibial torsion then Nordic Track or even bicycle pedals that require a fixed forward position of the feet can cause injury to the knee.

Home Exercise Program

In addition to modifying the patient's functional activities, the patient should be instructed in an exercise program to improve muscle performance and extensibility. Exercise prescription should be based on the results of the physical examination and include only exercises that address limitations specific to the patient. In addition, patients should be instructed in the appropriate response to the exercises. Appropriately, patients may feel some muscle soreness or fatigue with activities that overload the muscle. The pain will be in the muscle

BOX 7-1

How to Encourage and Promote Fitness without Injury

STAGE 1 FOR REHABILITATION

- Use of one-leg cycling for aerobic conditioning after surgery.[97]
- Water activities with the body submerged to reduce stresses on the knee.

STAGE 2 FOR REHABILITATION
Example: running

I. Early in the rehabilitation stages, the emphasis is placed on achieving an ideal gait pattern; speed or distance should not be emphasized. Assess gait pattern and instruct as appropriate.

II. Interval training is recommended.

   A. Begin with walking program and gradually mix in short bouts of running. Gradually increase the time running and decrease the time walking.

      1. Example of progression: Patient should be able to walk 30 minutes without an increase in pain or swelling to begin.

         a. Run 1: Walk 4 minutes, run 1 minute, repeat 4 times for a total of 20 minutes

         b. Rest day

         c. Run 2: Walk 3 minutes, run 2 minutes, repeat 4 times for a total of 20 minutes

         d. Rest day

         e. Run 3: Walk 2 minutes, run 3 minutes, repeat 4 times for a total of 20 minutes

         f. Continue to progress running appropriately. (This example will not be appropriate for all patients and must be adjusted as needed.)

         g. Once the patient can run 1 mile without increasing pain or swelling, begin to progress to previous training levels.

   B. It is expected that the patient may experience some generalized discomfort or swelling, particularly after surgery, with the initiation of running. If this generalized pain and swelling persists longer than 48 hours, then the running distance or intensity must be decreased. If the patient describes a stabbing pain or a pain that is consistent with tissue injury, running should be stopped and the patient reevaluated.

III. Modify surface of training if indicated.

   A. Instruct patient to initiate running with surfaces that reduce the ground reaction force on the lower extremities. If available, a track or chip trail would be a good surface to start. Concrete should be avoided if possible.

   B. Running on a street with a camber may contribute to common knee problems such as ITB friction syndrome. Runners should be encouraged to either avoid the camber or alternate the direction of their run.

ITB, Iliotibial band.

regions and not in the joint. However, they should not feel an increase in their symptoms during the performance of their exercises or experience a "pressure sensation" in the knee. This should be made explicit to patients. If either pain or pressure occurs, they should review the instructions to the exercise to be sure that they are performing it correctly and try again. If they still experience pain or pressure, they should discontinue this exercise until they return for their next visit.

Exercises to improve strength and performance of the hip abductors and hip lateral rotators may be prescribed. Many of these exercises are described in detail by Sahrmann.[22] Exercises to improve hip abductor and hip lateral rotator strength, listed from easiest to most difficult, include hip lateral rotator isometrics in prone, hip abduction in prone, progressive hip abduction with lateral rotation in side lying, hip lateral rotation against resistance bands in sitting, and lunges in standing while maintaining proper alignment of the knee. During the performance of these exercises, therapists should check to be sure that the patient is recruiting the correct muscles by palpating the lateral rotators and posterior gluteus medius. In addition, it is important that the patient is able to feel the contraction in the buttock region so that he or she can recreate the exercise at home. To specifically target the gluteus maximus, the patient can perform hip extension in prone with the knee flexed and progress to exercises in standing such as hip extension using resistance bands.

An exercise used to improve the motor recruitment or timing of the hip lateral rotators and abductors is weight shifting with gluteal contraction on the stance lower extremity. Once the patient has demonstrated good performance of the weight-shifting exercise, the exercise may be progressed to standing on one leg with correct alignment. Resisted activities of the opposite leg while standing on the affected leg may also be used to challenge the hip lateral rotators and abductors.

Exercises to improve the extensibility of the TFL-ITB should be prescribed. We recommend the following exercises: (1) prone knee flexion (bilateral [Figure 7-26] or unilateral), (2) prone hip lateral rotation without tibiofemoral motion, (3) two-joint hip flexor length test position, and (4) Ober test position. During the performance of these exercises, the tibiofemoral joint must be stabilized to prevent rotation. The patient is instructed to control tibial rotation by stiffening the necessary musculature at the knee. For example, while performing prone knee flexion, the patient points the foot toward the opposite limb, therefore contracting the tibial medial rotators to help stabilize the joint. If the patient is unable to control the tibial rotation, the exercises will need to be modified. Modifications might include either abducting the hip or placing a pillow under the pelvis to put the TFL-ITB on some slack. During all of these stretching exercises, the patient should have good abdominal support to avoid pelvic anterior tilt or transverse rotation.

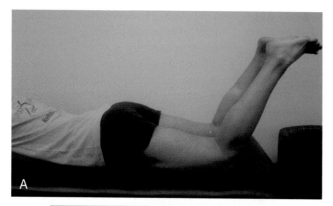

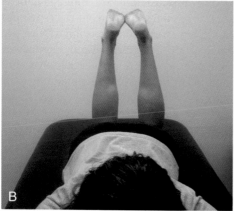

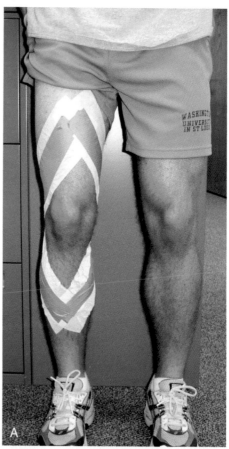

Figure 7-26. Prone knee flexion. **A,** Prone bilateral knee flexion to improve the extensibility of the TFL-ITB. **B,** To prevent tibial lateral rotation during performance of the stretch, the patient is instructed to keep the toes together and the heels in line with the tibias.

Improvement of abdominal performance may be needed. The abdominals assist in keeping the pelvis stable during activities involving the limbs. Some individuals may demonstrate poor performance of the abdominals as evidenced by increased rotation of the pelvis during functional activities such as gait or during performance of exercise (for example, pelvic rotation or tilting while lifting the leg during hip abductor strengthening). If so, he or she should be instructed in exercises to improve strength (lower abdominal progression as described by Sahrmann[22]) and recruitment (encourage patient to pull in abdominals with functional activities).

Taping

If the patient has difficulty correcting the movement impairment, taping may be helpful. The posterior X taping method, developed by our colleague, Debbie Fleming-McDonnell,* has been used as a method to prevent or reduce rotation at the tibiofemoral joint (Figure 7-27). The strips of tape that move from proximal-lateral thigh around the posterior knee to the distal-medial tibia are proposed to assist in reducing femoral medial rotation and

*PT, DPT, Program in Physical Therapy, Washington University School of Medicine, St Louis, Missouri.

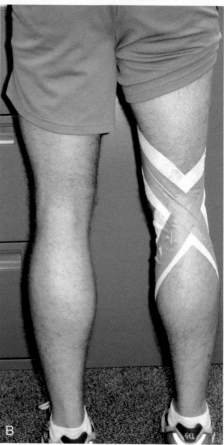

Figure 7-27. Posterior X taping method for TFRVal. **A,** Anterior view. **B,** Posterior view.

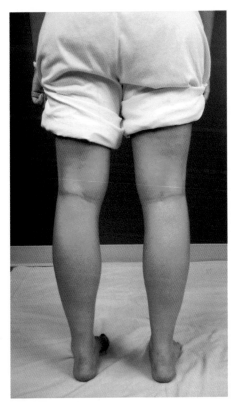

Figure 7-28. Decision-making for orthotics. Patient may not benefit from orthotic. Note excessive femoral medial rotation and foot supination. Recommend correcting hip impairment first.

tibial lateral rotation. We often add other strips of tape for symmetry or to assist in preventing knee hyperextension in patients who tend to hyperextend.

Orthotics

Most patients improve by addressing deficits of the hip only; however, some patients may benefit from orthotics to correct pronation at the foot. A number of articles related to the use of orthotics for knee pain problems have been published; however, the findings are equivocal.[98-102] We believe the inconclusive findings are related to the lack of foot type classification in studies related to knee pain. We believe that some individuals may benefit from correcting impairments of the foot and others may not (Figures 7-28 and 7-29). For example, if a patient demonstrates pronation that is excessive or occurs at an inappropriate time during gait, abnormal rotation at the tibiofemoral joint may result. If pronation is suspected to contribute to the rotation at the tibiofemoral joint, an orthotic may be appropriate.[103] If, however, orthotics do not reduce excessive tibiofemoral rotation or they increase tibiofemoral rotation, they may not be indicated.

A careful assessment of the foot should be done to determine whether the rotation of the femur results in rotation at the tibiofemoral joint or motion at the foot. If excessive medial rotation of the hip occurs and the foot is stiffer than the tibiofemoral joint, whether by foot structure or by using an orthotic, tibiofemoral rotation

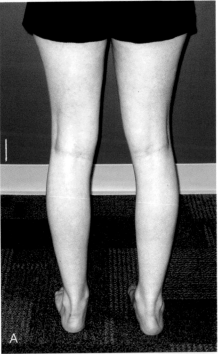

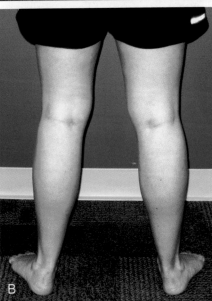

Figure 7-29. Decision-making for orthotics. **A,** Patient may benefit from orthotic. Note excessive femoral medial rotation and foot pronation. Hip may still be a contributor. Recommend correcting contribution of the hip with the addition of orthotics if needed. **B,** Patient may benefit from orthotic; however, correcting standing alignment by reducing hip abduction may improve alignment of the knee and foot.

will be exaggerated. Therefore the therapist must assess if the rotation at the tibiofemoral joint is increased or decreased if a pronation support is provided. When orthotics are indicated, temporary orthotics may be fabricated to assess the usefulness of the orthotic and allow the patient to test the correction before deciding to purchase a customized pair of orthotics.

Neuromuscular Training

Impairments of the neuromuscular system, such as poor balance or proprioception, may be present with any of the movement impairment syndromes. Treatment should include neuromuscular training to address impairments of proprioception and balance and the ability to accommodate to perturbations. When instructing the patient in neuromuscular training exercises, the patient should avoid motions and positions such as excessive knee valgus or femoral medial rotation. Examples of neuromuscular retraining activities are provided in Box 7-2. At time of the writing of this text, there are a number of laboratories studying this topic in patients with knee disorder.[13,14,104,105] The reader is encouraged to review current studies.

TIBIOFEMORAL ROTATION WITH VARUS SYNDROME

Symptoms and History

Individuals with TFRVar syndrome also demonstrate excessive rotation at the tibiofemoral joint; however, it is associated with a knee varus. The patient may demonstrate a varus thrust during gait. A varus thrust has been described in individuals with injury to the posterolateral corner of the knee and recently studied in the osteoarthritic knee.[7] Traditionally, varus thrust has been described as motion that is primarily in the frontal plane and thought to be the consequence of structural changes of the medial compartment in the osteoarthritic knee. We have observed, however, an apparent varus thrust in young individuals without radiological evidence of OA or ligamentous injury. This apparent varus thrust seems to be a result of a combination of hip medial rotation and knee hyperextension.

Structures that may be injured in an individual with TFRVar syndrome include the structures of the tibiofemoral joint, the ITB, and the surrounding musculature. The medial compartment of the tibiofemoral joint may be particularly at risk, given that it is responsible for 60% to 80% of the total load across the knee. Recent interest has been placed on the external knee adduction moment and its contributions to the load on the medial knee compartment.[110] The external knee adduction moment is defined as the product of the ground reaction force and the perpendicular distance to the knee joint (Figure 7-30). Clinically, the alignment associated with the knee adduction moment is genu varus. The knee adduction moment has been associated with the progression of knee OA.[111] An increase in varus alignment of the knee may result in a larger moment arm of the ground reaction force and thus increase the force through the medial compartment.

Several authors have reported that using a "toe-out" gait pattern reduces the knee adduction moment and thus reduces symptoms.[112-114] Two mechanisms have been proposed to explain the reduction of symptoms when a toe-out pattern is used. In their study of individuals with

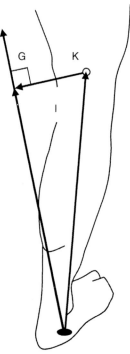

Figure 7-30. The external knee adduction moment is defined as the product of the ground reaction force and the perpendicular distance to the knee joint. *G,* Ground reaction force vector; *I,* momentum of ground reaction force; *K,* knee joint center. (Modified from Jenkyn TR, Hunt MA, Jones IC, et al: Toe-out gait in patients with knee osteoarthritis partially transforms external knee adduction moment into flexion moment during early stance phase of gait: a tri-planar kinetic mechanism, *J Biomech* 41(2):276-83, 2008.)

knee OA, Jenkyn et al[113] demonstrated that a portion of the external knee adduction moment was transformed into a flexion moment during the early phase of stance. Chang et al[115] provided another theory based on their interpretation of a study by Wang et al[116]: A toe-out gait pattern shifts the ground reaction force vector closer to the knee joint center. This shift results in a reduction in the moment arm of the ground reaction force and thus the external knee adduction moment.

Key Tests and Signs

Alignment Analysis

A patient with TFRVar syndrome often presents with femoral medial rotation and knee varus and may demonstrate a supinated or a fixed flat foot. The genu varus may be due to structural problems, such as OA in the medial compartment of the knee, or it may be a postural fault cause by femoral medial rotation along with knee hyperextension (Figure 7-31, *A-D*). The examiner should be careful not to classify by standing alignment alone. An individual may demonstrate a varus alignment in standing but demonstrate knee valgus with activities (Figure 7-31, *E-F*). The examiner must consider the entire movement examination and the symptom behavior to determine the appropriate diagnosis.

BOX 7-2

Neuromuscular Training

When instructing the patient in neuromuscular training exercises, it is important to remind the patient to avoid motions or alignments consistent with his or her specific movement system syndrome.

PROPRIOCEPTION/BALANCE[106]

Activities to improve proprioception of the knee should be incorporated as soon as possible. Begin early in treatment using activities such as weight shifting, progressive increases in weight bearing on the involved LE, and then eventually unilateral stance. As the patient can take full weight on the involved knee, activities are progressed to the use of a balance board.

Progression: Activities should be progressed to prepare patient to return to daily activities, fitness routines, and work or sporting activities. As the patient progresses, proprioception can be challenged by asking the patient to stand on unstable surfaces (pillows, trampoline, or BOSU ball); perturbations can be applied by having the patient catch a ball being thrown to him while standing on one leg or by perturbing the surface on which the patient is standing.[105] Sliding board activities have also been shown to be beneficial to patients after surgery.[107]

SPORT-SPECIFIC TRAINING (IF APPROPRIATE)

In preparation to return to sports, sport-specific activities should be added. The initial phases of these activities will include straight plane activities at a slow pace and then a gradual increase in the level of difficulty by increasing the intensity and patterns to include changes of direction, starts, and stops.

AGILITY EXERCISES

Emphasis is placed on proper movement.

Hopping timed

Within each level, begin with short bouts of hopping and longer rests between (15 seconds on, 30 seconds off), then increase on time and decrease off time (30 seconds on, 15 seconds off).

1. Hopping bilateral LEs with support of the UEs to decrease the amount of stress through the knee
2. Bilateral hopping without support
3. Bilateral hopping in different designs: Side-to-side, back and forth, box, V, zigzag hopping
4. Progress to same activities with unilateral LEs

Jumping from short surface, 2 inches

Emphasis should be placed on landing on both feet evenly with neutral knees over toes (avoid excessive knee valgus or femoral adduction or medial rotation). The patient should also think about landing softly, using the ankle plantarflexors and allowing the knees to flex to help absorb the landing.[13,106]

1. Jump forward, backward, and to each side.
2. Progress by increasing the height of the surface.

Jumping up on to surface

Begin with shorter surface and increase height when appropriate.

Other plyometrics: ladder drills

NOTE: If plyometrics and resistance training are to be performed during the same visit, plyometrics should be performed before the resistance training activities.[106]

RUNNING

See Box 7-1 for initial running program. Once the individual is able to run 1 mile without an increase in symptoms or swelling, cutting activities may begin.

1. Figure 8 running, beginning with a large "8," then gradually decreasing the size of the 8
2. Zigzag running with soft cuts, hard cuts, and cut and spin

NOTE: Care should be taken to evaluate how the patient chooses to cut. Often, particularly in patients who have suffered noncontact injuries, the patient may have adopted an inefficient cutting pattern such as planting the left foot when trying to cut to the left.

JUMPING PROGRAM

Please refer to article by Hewett et al.[13] for description of jumping program. The following are some of the key concepts used in their program.

1. Soft landing: Use plantarflexors to assist in accepting weight
2. Knee flexion: Do not land with knee stiff (remains in extension)
3. Proper knee alignment in the frontal plane: No knee valgus

DRILLS

Once the patient can complete cutting drills without pain or swelling and demonstrates good control of the LE, variations, such as the following, can be added:

1. Drills with sport specific equipment (basketball, hockey stick, soccer ball)
2. Partner drills

BASKETBALL SPECIFIC TRAINING

Please refer to article by Louw et al[108] for description of specific training for basketball.

FUNCTIONAL TESTING

Consider functional tests before the patient's return to sport. There are many functional tests available. The validity of these tests are controversial; however, each test can offer some insight in how the patient may perform in his or her specific sport. It is recommended that a battery of tests be used to assess the aspects of balance, coordination, agility, and strength. Refer to Fitzgerald et al[109] for a proposed system to test patients returning to sports after nonoperative treatment of ACL tear. Common test items for the knee include the following:

1. Single-leg hop for distance
2. Triple-leg hop for distance
3. Six-meter hop for time
4. Crossover hop for distance
5. Six-meter shuttle run
6. Vertical jump
7. Lateral step

LE, Lower extremity; *UE,* upper extremity.

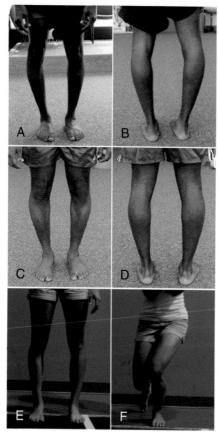

Figure 7-31. TFRVar Alignment. Patient's alignment during examination. Anterior view **(A)** and posterior view **(B).** Patient demonstrates structural faults of genu varum and tibial varum. Genu varum is increased with postural fault of femoral medial rotation and knee hyperextensions. Patient's modified alignment (same patient as **A** and **B**), anterior view **(C),** and posterior view **(D).** Patient has been instructed to correct postural faults by "unlocking his knees" and contracting the hip lateral rotators to reduce femoral medial rotation. Varus alignment in standing **(E)** might suggest TFRVar; however, patient demonstrates valgus positioning of the knee **(F)** during a single leg squat indicating that TFRVal is the likely diagnosis.

Movement Impairments

Standing tests. During single-leg stance on the involved limb, the patient will demonstrate excessive medial rotation of the involved femur with minimal to no movement at the foot. Balance may also be a factor in this syndrome, although clinically it is not as common in TFRVar syndrome as it is in TFRVal syndrome.

Supine tests. Similar to TFRVal syndrome, the patient with TFRVar syndrome may demonstrate rotation or abduction of the tibia during the performance of the two-joint hip flexor length test (see Figure 7-21).

Joint Integrity

The patient may demonstrate mild-to-moderate laxity in the fibular collateral ligament (lateral collateral ligament); however, overall laxity in the tibiofemoral joint is not typically observed in the young individual with

TFRVar syndrome. Older patients with arthritic changes may demonstrate some general joint laxity.

Muscle Length Impairments

Common muscle impairments include reduced extensibility of the TFL-ITB.[90]

Muscle Strength/Performance Impairments

Impairments of muscle strength and performance include poor performance of the hip lateral rotators and possibly hip abductors.[91,92]

Functional Activities

Gait. During gait, excessive femoral medial rotation and knee hyperextension may contribute to the apparent varus thrust during stance. Ankle dorsiflexion and foot pronation are often limited, which may increase stresses to the tibiofemoral joint.

Step-up. During a step-up, the patient does not shift the body weight forward over the foot and demonstrates a faulty movement of pulling the knee back to the body, instead of bringing the body forward over the limb. Because the foot is anchored on the floor during the step-up, hip extension performed by the hamstrings may assist with knee extension, therefore reducing the need to recruit the quadriceps to extend the knee. Gluteal muscles also have a reduced ability to extend the hip when the patient's body weight is kept in a relative posterior position.

Other Functional Tests

Activities that aggravate the patient's symptoms should be assessed for a movement impairment. Common activities include prolonged sitting, squatting, and sit-to-stand. If the patient is an athlete or has low irritability of their symptoms, higher level activities, such as single-leg squat and jumping, may need to be assessed to determine the movement impairment.

Summary of Examination Findings

TFRVar syndrome presents with the movement impairment of excessive rotation between the tibia and femur that is associated with a genu varum. Varum of the tibiofemoral joint may be secondary to structural changes in the medial joint surfaces as in OA; however, an apparent varum may be secondary to acquired impairments of femoral medial rotation and knee hyperextension. Positions or movement associated with TFRVar syndrome are often painful, and when corrected, pain is reduced.

Treatment

Primary Objectives

The primary objectives of a treatment program include the following:
1. Correct TFRVar during functional activities.
2. Improve performance of the hip lateral rotators.
3. Improve shock absorption during gait.

Corrective Exercise Program

Treatment for TFRVar syndrome is similar to the treatment for TFRVal syndrome with a few subtle differences; only the differences are discussed here.

Alignment. Instructions to correct alignment are similar to those for TFRVal syndrome. To improve alignment between the femur and tibia, the therapist must address impairments in both the sagittal and transverse planes in an effort to achieve a more neutral or ideal alignment. If hyperextension is present, the patient is instructed to unlock the knees. To align the tibia and femur in the transverse plane, the patient is asked to align knees over feet with neutral rotation of hips by decreasing medial rotation of femur. To correct femoral medial rotation, the patient is instructed to contract their gluteals and hip lateral rotators to laterally rotate the femur. As described previously, structural impairments, such as tibial varum must be noted and considered when attempting to correct alignment (see Figure 7-31).

Functional activities. Instructions to maintain proper alignment and movement strategies during functional activities are recommended. Cues to correct femoral medial rotation are the same as those provided for patients with TFRVal syndrome. Genu varum is often challenging to correct; however, cues to reduce impact on the knee joint may be useful in reducing stresses on the knee joint. For example, during gait, patients are encouraged to use a heel-to-toe gait pattern and use the rolling of the foot to provide shock absorption. In severe cases, symptoms may be reduced by instructing the patient to walk with a "toe out" pattern.[112-114] If the patient is experiencing medial condyle degenerative changes, the instruction is to walk with the feet closer together and in slight lateral rotation to decrease the stress on the medial condyle.

If the patient could benefit from a cane, typically, the cane is placed in the hand opposite the involved limb. Anecdotally, however, some patients have reported decreased symptoms when the cane is placed in the ipsilateral hand. Using the cane in the ipsilateral hand may decrease the forces on the medial knee. To apply weight onto the cane, the patient shifts the body weight closer to the affected knee, thus reducing the external moment arm of the body weight and possibly the amount of force through the medial compartment of the knee.

Home Exercise Program

Exercises to improve strength and performance of the hip lateral rotators may be prescribed if the patient demonstrates excessive medial rotation. See the "Home Exercise Program" section for "Tibiofemoral Rotation with Valgus Syndrome" for a description of these exercises.

Taping/Bracing

The taping method demonstrated in Figure 7-27 is useful to prevent or reduce rotation and hyperextension at the tibiofemoral joint. In patients with advanced disease, particularly OA, an unloader brace may be useful.[117,118]

Orthotics

Cushioned shoes and an additional cushioned insert may improve shock absorption of the lower extremity, particularly in patients with a rigid, supinated, or structurally (fixed) pronated foot.

CASE PRESENTATION
Tibiofemoral Rotation with Valgus Syndrome

Symptoms and History

A 16-year-old female soccer player is referred to physical therapy for evaluation and treatment of right knee pain. She reports right anteromedial knee pain for 2 months. Her pain began during preseason training and limited her ability to participate in practice. During practice, her pain would increase to 5/10. The pain could be sharp, particularly with cutting and kicking the soccer ball with the involved limb. Her pain improved with rest and ice. Her Knee Outcome Score–Activities of Daily Living (KOS-ADLs)[119] is 74%, and her KOS-Sports score is 57%. Radiographs show no abnormalities of the tibiofemoral or patellofemoral joint.

Alignment Analysis

The patient is 5 feet 10 inches and weighs 150 pounds. In stance, the patient demonstrates medial rotation of the femur and greater foot progression angle (toe out) on the right. In sitting, the tibia is rotated laterally relative to the femur. There are no obvious impairments of patellar alignment.

Movement Analysis

During single-leg stance on the right, the patient demonstrates excessive medial rotation of the femur and pronation of the foot. During a partial squat, the patient demonstrates femoral adduction, knee valgus, and foot pronation. The patient reports an increase in her pain during the performance of the squat. The patient is then instructed to keep her knee in line with her toes and avoid allowing the knees to come together. She is able to correct her performance and reports that her symptoms are decreased compared to the uncorrected movement.

During knee flexion in prone, the patient demonstrates lateral rotation of the tibia and reports an increase in her symptoms at the end of the motion. With manual correction to control tibial lateral rotation, the patient reports a decrease in her symptoms compared to the uncorrected movement.

Joint Integrity

Accessory motions of the patellofemoral joint are excessive in the medial and lateral directions but equal to the uninvolved side. Accessory motions of the tibiofemoral joint are also equal bilaterally. The patient reports no change in her symptoms with the accessory motion testing.

Muscle Length Impairments

During the two-joint hip flexor length test, the patient demonstrates a short, stiff TFL on the right. As the hip is extended, the tibia rotates laterally and the patient reports an increase in her symptoms. With manual correction to control the rotation of the tibia, the patient reports a decrease in her symptoms compared to the first performance.

Muscle Strength/Performance Impairments

On the right, the hip lateral rotators are 4–/5 tested in sitting, the gluteus maximus is 4/5, the TFL is 4/5, and the posterior gluteus medius is 3+/5. While testing the posterior gluteus medius, the patient's hip flexes and medial rotates, indicating that the hip flexors are compensating for performance of the posterior gluteus medius. With cueing, she is able to correct the position but could only maintain the position against minimal pressure to the distal lower extremity.

Stiffness/Extensibility/Flexibility

The TFL-ITB is relatively more stiff than the knee joint causing compensatory lateral tibial rotation during the two-joint hip flexor length test.

Tests for Source

The patient reports tenderness with palpation along the medial and lateral joint lines, as well as the medial patellar facet. McConnell test[120] and the patellofemoral grind test[52,120] for patellofemoral pain are negative. All ligamentous and meniscal tests are negative.

Functional Activities

During sit-to-stand and stair ambulation, the patient demonstrates femoral adduction and knee valgus. She does not report pain with sit-to-stand; however, she is instructed in correcting her movement to reduce femoral adduction and knee valgus. She is able to correct easily. With cutting activities on the right lower extremity, the patient demonstrates femoral adduction and tibial lateral rotation. The cutting maneuvers increase her symptoms. The patient attempts to correct her movement quality during the cutting maneuver; however, she is unable to correct the fault completely.

Diagnosis and Staging

The diagnosis is TFRval syndrome and the stage for rehabilitation is Stage 2. Her prognosis is good to excellent. Positive moderators include her young age, overall good health, high motivation to return to her activities, and her ability to change the simple movement impairments, such as partial squat and sit-to-stand, with instruction only. Negative moderators include her high activity level.

Treatment

The patient was seen once per week for 4 weeks, then once every other week for 2 weeks for a total of 6 visits over 8 weeks. Treatment included instruction in correct performance of functional activities, including her sporting activities. She was also instructed in a home exercise program to improve performance of the hip abductors and hip lateral rotators and exercises to increase the extensibility of the TFL-ITB. Although she reported pain in the right knee only, she was encouraged to perform the exercises bilaterally.

During the first visit, the patient was instructed in correct performance of sit-to-stand, stair ambulation, and squatting. She was instructed to contract her gluteals to control the femoral adduction and knee valgus during the activities. She was able to make these corrections quite easily.

To improve the recruitment of the hip musculature during functional activity, the patient was instructed in the exercises, weight shifting, and single-leg stance. She was encouraged to contract her hip lateral rotators when weight was shifted onto the ipsilateral lower extremity. She was instructed to perform these exercises frequently throughout the day if possible. Daily activities, such as brushing one's teeth or speaking on the phone, provide excellent opportunities to work on weight shifting throughout the day.

To improve performance of the hip lateral rotators and hip abductors, side lying hip abduction/lateral rotation was prescribed with the hip and knee extended (level 2 Sahrmann[22]). The patient was instructed to perform the exercise with her back and leg against the wall. She was instructed to keep the shoulders, hips, and heels on the wall while performing the exercise. The wall provides feedback to remind her to keep her hip in the extended position and avoiding hip flexion.

To more specifically target the hip lateral rotators in hip flexion, she was instructed in lateral rotation in sitting with the feet together.[22] An elastic exercise band was placed around the distal end of the femurs to provide resistance to the hip lateral rotators. These exercises were to be performed once a day, in 3 sets, each set to fatigue. The repetitions depend on her ability to perform the exercise correctly.

Knee flexion in prone was prescribed to improve the extensibility of the TFL-ITB. To prevent tibial lateral rotation, the patient was instructed to flex both knees while keeping her feet together during the exercise.

Although the patient could easily correct her movement impairments during functional activities, it was unlikely that she could correct her movement strategies entirely during her soccer practice, so the patient's knee was taped with the method shown in Figure 7-27. She was instructed to keep the tape in place up to 3 days, as long as she did not develop skin irritation.

At her second visit, 1 week later, the patient reported 50% compliance with the exercises and 70% compliance with the functional activity corrections. She stated that with the tape, she was able to participate in the entire soccer practice. She still had an increase in symptoms, that only increased to a 2/10 maximum. In a subsequent practice after she had removed the tape, she was unable to participate in the entire practice. She demonstrated correct performance of the exercises, therefore the exercises were progressed. Sidelying hip abduction/lateral rotation was progressed to level 3.[22] She was also given prone hip extension with the knee flexed. She was instructed to place pillows under her abdomen while performing prone hip extension, to allow for adequate motion, which was restricted by her short TFL-ITB.

Also, at her second visit, some of her soccer drills were addressed. Recommendations were provided in correcting the movement impairments of hip adduction and tibial lateral rotation during her activities. The patient was taped again.

At 1 month, the patient was able to participate in her practices without a significant increase in her pain and the patient was progressed to Stage 3. Taping was discontinued, and exercises were progressed. The strength and recruitment of her hip musculature improved, thus her program was progressed to exercises in weight bearing. She was given resisted shuffles using an elastic band around the distal femurs. Resisted hip extension and hip abduction in standing were given, using an elastic band for resistance.

Sports-specific drills were practiced while encouraging proper alignment of the knees. Neuromuscular training was also incorporated. The patient was encouraged to incorporate these activities into her regular soccer warm-ups.

Outcome

The patient was seen for a total of 6 visits over 8 weeks. At the time of her last visit, 2 months after her initial visit, the patient reported that she was playing soccer pain-free and continued to use the training drills during her soccer practice. Function was also improved as demonstrated by improved scores: KOS-ADLs is 100% and KOS-Sports is 100%.

TIBIOFEMORAL HYPOMOBILITY SYNDROME

The movement impairment of tibiofemoral hypomobility (TFHypo) syndrome is associated with a limitation in the physiologic motion of the knee. The limitation may result from degenerative changes in the joint or from the effects of prolonged immobilization. OA of the knee may contribute to TFHypo syndrome, although not all individuals with OA have TFHypo syndrome. The diagnosis of tibiofemoral rotation should be considered if a patient has radiographic evidence of OA but no limitation in knee ROM.

Symptoms and History

Individuals with the diagnosis of TFHypo syndrome report knee pain located deep in the joint and often describe their pain as vague. Symptoms are typically increased with weight-bearing activities, such as walking, standing, and stair ambulation, and are relieved with rest. Reports of stiffness after prolonged periods of rest are common. The most common diagnoses used by a referring physician include OA and knee contracture.

Key Tests and Signs
Alignment Analysis
During assessment of standing alignment, the patient often demonstrates knee flexion; however, individuals with OA may demonstrate genu varum or genu valgus. The knee joint may also appear to be enlarged or show signs of inflammation/swelling. In addition to assessing knee alignment, alignment of the hip and foot should also be assessed.

Movement Impairments
Standing tests. During single-leg stance on the involved limb, the patient may demonstrate poor hip and trunk control, which is evidenced by pelvic tilt or trunk lateral bending. This is often described as a positive Trendelenburg sign[121] or a gluteus medius limp when severe (notable lateral trunk flexion over involved side). The patient may also demonstrate poor balance requiring upper extremity support for performance.

Sitting. During sitting knee extension, the patient may demonstrate decreased knee extension ROM. Careful observation of this movement is recommended. Some patients demonstrate co-contraction of the lower extremity muscles, particularly quadriceps and hamstrings, while attempting to extend the knee. If co-contraction is occurring, the limb moves slowly and the patient appears to be using a great deal of effort. If co-contraction is suspected, a cue to reduce effort of the activity often results in ease of the motion and a reduction in symptoms. Passively extending the patient's knee while the patient is sitting in a chair with a backrest will provide information about hamstring length and stiffness.

Joint Integrity
Patients with TFHypo syndrome demonstrate a reduction of ROM in flexion and extension. Limitations in knee ROM may be due to impaired arthrokinematics and/or reduced muscle extensibility, therefore assessment of joint flexibility, accessory motions, and muscle extensibility is recommended. Often, end-range of motion is painful. Patients with TFHypo syndrome associated with OA may report a decrease in their end-range pain with repeated passive motion. Patients with osteoarthritic changes of the joint may demonstrate a capsular pattern, defined as a loss in flexion ROM that is greater than the loss of extension.[122] Recently, however, the validity of using this pattern to detect individuals with OA has been called into question.[123,124]

Muscle Length Impairments
Decreased extensibility of the hip flexors, hamstrings, and ankle plantarflexors may also be associated with the TFHypo syndrome.

Muscle Strength/Performance Impairments

Common muscle impairments include poor performance of the gluteal musculature, hip lateral rotators, gastrocnemius, and quadriceps. As described previously, co-contraction of the quadriceps and hamstrings may be visible during exercise or performance of functional activities. Co-contraction has been shown to increase joint contact pressures that may result in increased injury to the joint surfaces.[125,126]

Functional Activities

Gait. Patients with TFHypo syndrome demonstrate reduced knee ROM throughout their functional activities. During ambulation, there is a reduction of knee excursion in both flexion and extension. Often the knee is maintained in flexion throughout the entire gait cycle. The patient may also demonstrate a decreased stride length and decreased push-off.

Stairs. While descending stairs, the patient may demonstrate reduced knee flexion excursion on the stance limb. This reduced excursion is not solely the result of reduced joint flexibility but may be an impaired movement strategy caused by muscle co-contraction. The patient demonstrates co-contraction of the lower extremity muscles[127] that often results in an increase in symptoms and effort. Follow-up instruction to "let go" of the musculature often results in an improvement in symptoms.

Sit-to-stand. Reduced knee flexion is also seen as the patient moves from a sitting position to standing. Sufficient knee flexion is required to move the tibia anteriorly to bring the patient's center of mass (COM) over their feet. When the anterior movement of the tibia is reduced, the patient compensates with increased hip and trunk flexion to advance their COM anteriorly.

Summary of Examination Findings

Patients with TFHypo syndrome present with a physiologic limitation of knee motion, typically in knee flexion and knee extension. They also demonstrate a limitation of knee joint excursion during functional activities such as gait and stair ambulation. The observed limitation in ROM may be due to limitations in joint flexibility and muscle extensibility or an impaired motor recruitment pattern.

Treatment

Treatment for this syndrome includes first educating the individual on correcting the postural habits and movements that may be contributing to the movement impairment.

Primary Objectives

The primary objectives of a treatment program include the following:

1. Improve knee flexion and extension ROM.
2. Improve muscle performance of gluteals, hip lateral rotators, quadriceps, and gastrocnemius, similar to TFRVal or TFRVar category.
3. Improve aerobic conditioning without an increase in pain or swelling.
4. Educate in performance of functional activities.
5. Caution against repetitive rotation of the knee with the foot fixed.
6. Consider forces created by compression, particularly in knees that are malaligned.
7. Use of an assistive device if necessary during gait to decreases the compressive stresses to the involved knee.

Corrective Exercise Program

The patient is instructed in functional activities and an exercise program to address the associated movement impairments. All patients should be encouraged to participate in regular fitness activities to maintain current weight or reduce weight if the patient is overweight or obese.

Alignment. It is often difficult for patients with TFHypo syndrome to change alignment immediately; however, correct alignment should be encouraged.

Functional activities. In the early stages of rehabilitation, compensatory modifications may be needed to accommodate the lack of ROM or to prevent increased pain. As the patient's ROM and pain improves, the performance of functional activities should focus on teaching the components of ideal motion. If it is determined that the limitation in ROM is structurally fixed, then compensatory techniques should be provided.

Gait. During gait, the patient is instructed to use a "rolling" heel-to-toe gait pattern. This modification's intent is to improve the shock absorption contribution of the foot and encourage improved push-off. If the patient is experiencing severe pain or demonstrates a significant malalignment, such as genu varum, an assistive device should be recommended to redistribute the forces on the affected knee. See the information on the use of a cane in the "Functional Activities" section for "Tibiofemoral Rotation with Varus Syndrome."

Sit-to-stand; stand-to-sit. To rise from a sitting position to standing, the patient should be instructed to slide forward to the edge of the chair. Once at the front of the chair, the patient should position the feet about hip-width apart and slightly posterior to the knees. If knee flexion is significantly limited, the patient may keep the affected knee comfortably extended while placing the unaffected foot appropriately. The patient is instructed to lean forward at the hips to be sure his or her center of mass is moved forward over his or her base of support. The patient is also encouraged to contract the quadriceps and gluteals and avoid femoral adduction when rising from the chair.

When transitioning from standing to a sitting position, the patient is instructed again to contract the gluteals and quadriceps and slowly lower themselves into the chair. Individuals with significant limitations or pain may need to begin practicing these movements with a higher seat surface and use their upper extremities on the armrests to assist with pushing up from the seat and lowering into the seat. Performance of sit-to-stand may be progressed by reducing the use of the upper extremities and lowering the height of the seat.

Stairs

Patients with TFHypo syndrome often have a high severity of symptoms with stair ambulation. Please see the "Treatment" section in the "Tibiofemoral Rotation with Valgus Syndrome" section for methods to reduce symptoms with stair ambulation. If the patient demonstrates co-contraction during the stair descent, cues to "let go" or relax their musculature often results in a reduction of symptoms.

Other functional activities. Activities the patient performs throughout the day that may contribute to the patient's symptoms should be addressed. For example, patients often report increased stiffness and pain after prolonged sitting. They should be instructed to decrease the amount of time that the knee is maintained in one position. They can accomplish this by rising from the chair every 20 to 30 minutes and walking or flexing and extending the knee if the situation will not allow rising from their chair, such as during a business meeting or class.

Fitness activities. Fitness activities should be addressed as soon as possible. The appropriate level of activity demand should be assessed. In the early rehabilitation stages, the patient should begin with non–weight-bearing or reduced weight-bearing activities such as swimming, water exercises, and stationary biking without resistance. As the patient improves, weight bearing should be gradually increased. Using a StairMaster or elliptical cross-trainer can serve as a good transition to walking. While initiating strengthening exercises, it is safer for the patient to begin with high repetitions of relatively low resistance; high levels of resistance are not encouraged because of the high levels of compressive forces through the joint.

Home Exercise Program

The patient should be provided with a home exercise program and instruction on the appropriate response to exercise. Specific exercises should be provided to increase ROM and improve lower extremity muscle strength and muscle extensibility.

Exercises to improve muscle performance, including strengthening and motor recruitment of the hip musculature, are described in detail in the treatment description of TFRVal syndrome. Patients with TFHypo syndrome may also benefit from strengthening of the gastrocnemius muscle, beginning with elastic band resistance and progressing to weight-bearing heel raises. Other muscles that should be considered are the abdominals and the quadriceps, if appropriate.

Historically, quadriceps strengthening has been recommended for patients with knee OA, based on the theory that the quadriceps provide shock absorption at the knee. A recent trial involving patients with knee OA demonstrated that pain can be decreased with the implementation of a strengthening program.[128] However, epidemiological studies specific to knee OA have shown that increased quadriceps strength can actually accelerate the progression of OA in knees with malalignment[16,18,20] or laxity.[20] One must consider the compressive forces that the quadriceps can add to a joint before administering aggressive quadriceps strengthening activities. We recommend that therapeutic exercises to hypertrophy the quadriceps be avoided in patients with malalignment or laxity of the knees. However, the functional performance of the quadriceps may be enhanced through proper performance of functional activities such as sit-to-stand, stand-to-sit, step-up and step-down, and partial wall squats.

Exercises to improve the extensibility of the hip flexors, gastrocnemius, and hamstrings are also prescribed.[22] To improve the extensibility of the hip flexors, the following exercises may be provided: hip and knee extension in supine (heel slide) with the opposite hip held passively flexed to the chest, knee flexion in prone, and hip lateral rotation in prone to specifically stretch the TFL-ITB. To improve the extensibility of the gastrocnemius, the patient may be instructed to perform ankle dorsiflexion in sitting with the knee extended or ankle dorsiflexion in standing. Hamstring extensibility may be increased with knee extension in sitting (see Figure 7-40).

Other Interventions

Accessory and physiologic mobilizations may be used to reduce pain and increase ROM. If the patient is having pain at rest, a distraction mobilization can be taught to the patient for independent use at home. A trial of gentle distraction should be performed to determine if this technique will be appropriate. For the home technique, the patient sits with the knees at 90 degrees, with the lower leg dangling. A small pillow or rolled-up towel is used to elevate the thigh so that the foot is off the floor. A small weight or shoe, approximately 1 to 2 pounds, is applied to the distal limb (Figure 7-32). Patient allows the leg to dangle up to 10 minutes to help relieve discomfort. This may be performed as often as needed to relieve pain.

Bracing may be considered for patients who continue to have symptoms that are limiting their function. Braces range from the simple neoprene sleeve thought to provide warmth and possible improvement in proprioception to customized unloader braces to redistribute forces in the knee. If prescribing a brace, the therapist must consider the patient's goals and motivation, as well as the anthropomorphic characteristics for adequate fit. We recommend a trial of a relatively inexpensive, easy-to-apply brace first. If symptoms are not affected, then a custom brace might be considered.

Finally, neuromuscular training may also improve function of the lower extremity. Activities in Box 7-2 may need to be modified for the patient's skill level. A program

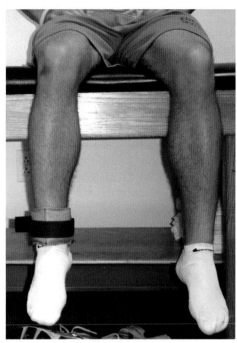

Figure 7-32. Home program for distraction mobilization to reduce pain. Patient is instructed to place light weight or heavy shoe, approximately 1 to 2 pounds, to the distal limb. Patient allows the leg to dangle up to 10 minutes to help relieve discomfort. This may be performed as often as needed to relieve pain.

developed for nonoperative ACL has been modified for use in the older individual and has preliminary evidence indicating success.[104]

KNEE EXTENSION SYNDROME

Knee extension (Kext) syndrome is described as knee pain associated with quadriceps dominance or stiffness that results in an excessive pull on the patella, patellar tendon, or tibial tubercle. This movement system syndrome may be associated with poor performance of the hip extensors. The Kext syndrome has a subcategory of patellar superior glide (KextSG). Although both conditions are a result of quadriceps stiffness, the structures that are involved are related to the location of relative stiffness/flexibility. In KextSG syndrome, the patellar tendon and surrounding retinacula are relatively more flexible than the quadriceps, therefore when the quadriceps contracts, the patellar is displaced superiorly in the trochlear groove. Excessive stresses may be placed on the patellofemoral joint or patella tendon as the patella is pulled superiorly. In Kext syndrome, the patella is thought to be relatively stable and therefore the strain may be placed on the structures superior to the patella. Because the movement impairments of the two conditions are similar, they are described concurrently; movement impairment of Kext syndrome is described and information specific to KextSG syndrome is highlighted.

Symptoms and History

Patients with Kext syndrome report symptoms superior to the patella in structures such as the quadriceps or quadriceps tendon. In contrast, patients with KextSG syndrome report symptoms in the peripatellar region or the infrapatellar region and may involve the patellofemoral joint structures or the patellar tendon and the patellar tendon attachment sites, including the patellar inferior pole and tibial tuberosity. In patients with either syndrome, symptoms are aggravated with activities that require repetitive or forceful knee extension such as jumping. Patients are often athletes such as runners, football linemen, and volleyball players. Common diagnoses used by referring physicians include patellar tendinopathy (often called *jumper's knee*), quadriceps strain, and Osgood-Schlatter disease.

One impairment that might be associated with KextSG syndrome is patella alta. Researchers have identified a clear association between patella alta and increased lateral displacement and lateral tilt of the patella, particularly with a quadriceps contraction.[129-131] Such patellar instability can occur with patella alta because the patella rests superior to the femoral lateral condyle, which typically prevents excessive lateral patellar glide.

In addition, patella alta may also be associated with anterior knee pain or chondromalacia in the absence of patellar instability.[132-136] One potential mechanism underlying the anterior knee pain associated with patella alta is a decrease in contact area between the patella and the femur, which has been demonstrated by Ward and his colleagues.[137,138] Because physical stress to biological tissue is defined as the force per unit area, any decrease in the size of the contact area at a particular joint would increase the stress on that joint, potentially leading to degenerative changes and pain.

Current evidence for the treatment of patella alta is limited to surgical intervention.[131,134,136] In this chapter, we provide a conservative treatment approach for patella alta as related to the diagnosis of knee extension.

Key Tests and Signs
Alignment Analysis
The patient with Kext syndrome or KextSG syndrome may demonstrate a swayback posture with a posterior pelvic tilt. Overdevelopment of the quadriceps musculature may be apparent. In addition, patients with KextSG syndrome often demonstrate patella alta as described by Insall[38] (Figure 7-33).

Movement Impairments
Standing tests. During hip and knee flexion in stance (partial squat), the patient with Kext syndrome often shifts the body weight posteriorly, keeping the tibia perpendicular to the floor (Figure 7-34). The secondary test for this movement is to instruct the patient to shift the body weight anteriorly and allow the tibia to advance

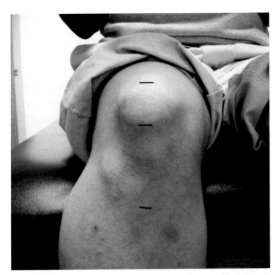

Figure 7-33. Patella alta demonstrated. Insall-Salvati ratio measured clinically: 1.67.

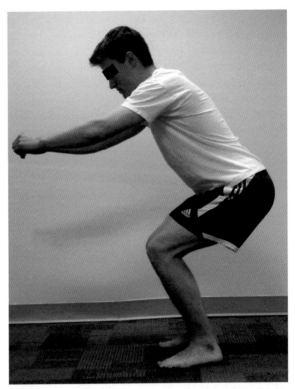

Figure 7-35. Secondary test: Instruct the patient to shift his or her body weight anteriorly and allow the tibia to advance forward over the foot.

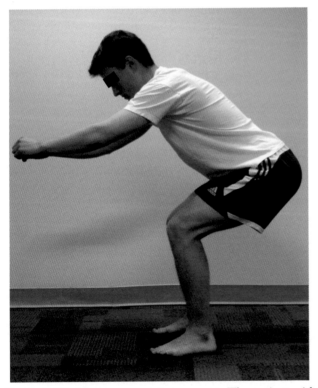

Figure 7-34. Movement test item—squat. The patient with knee extension often shifts the body weight posteriorly, keeping their tibia perpendicular to the floor. If patient reports pain with this movement, perform the secondary test.

forward over the foot (Figure 7-35). If symptoms are reduced, Kext syndrome should be suspected. If KextSG syndrome is suspected (pain located peripatellar or inferior to the patella), the partial squat test may be repeated as the examiner places an inferior glide on the patella. If symptoms are decreased compared to the primary test, KextSG syndrome is supported.

Supine tests. While performing the two-joint hip flexor length test,[88] knee extension may be observed when the involved limb is lowered into hip extension. If the knee extension persists when the hip is brought into abduction, rectus femoris stiffness is implicated. If the patient reports pain during the test, the test may be repeated while the examiner places an inferior glide on the patella. If symptoms decrease, then KextSG syndrome is supported. The patient with Kext (without superior glide) will likely report an increase in symptoms if an inferior glide is placed on the patella, which would place additional stress on the structures superior to the patella.

Prone tests. During knee flexion in prone, patients with KextSG or Kext syndrome will demonstrate a short or stiff rectus femoris and may report pain at the end of their motion. For symptoms in the peripatellar or inferior patellar region, an inferior glide is placed on the patella during the test. A decrease in symptoms with this secondary test supports KextSG syndrome as the diagnosis. Similar to the two-joint hip flexor length test, an increase in symptoms with the inferior glide would implicate Kext syndrome (without superior glide) as the diagnosis.

Sitting tests. The McConnell test[120] for patellofemoral pain may be modified to confirm KextSG syndrome. In sitting, the patient performs an isometric quadriceps contraction against resistance at 120, 90, 60, 30, and 0 degrees of knee flexion. If the patient's pain is produced or increased during any of the contractions, the test is performed again with a manual correction by the examiner. To assess for KextSG syndrome, the examiner places an inferior glide on the patella and asks the patient to again perform the isometric contraction. If the pain is decreased, the patellofemoral joint is implicated as the source of symptoms and KextSG syndrome is implicated as the movement system diagnosis.

Joint Integrity
Patients with KextSG syndrome may demonstrate reduced accessory motion for inferior glide of the patella.

Muscle Length Impairments
Patients with KextSG syndrome or Kext syndrome demonstrate a short or stiff quadriceps during prone knee flexion or the two-joint hip flexor length tests.

Muscle Strength/Performance Impairments
Patients with KextSG syndrome or Kext syndrome often demonstrate poor performance of the gluteus maximus and hamstrings. Quadriceps musculature may compensate for the reduced performance of the hip extensors. The imbalance between the quadriceps and the hip extensors may result in an increased demand on the quadriceps to perform activities that involve extension of the lower extremity.

Stiffness, extensibility, or flexibility. The quadriceps may be short or have increased stiffness due to hypertrophy. In patients with KextSG syndrome, the quadriceps are relatively more stiff than the patellar tendon and the surrounding patellar retinacula and therefore the patella is pulled superiorly excessively. This relative stiffness/flexibility may be observed in a number of tests such as the two-joint hip flexor length test and prone knee flexion.

Functional Activities
During assessment of movements, such as walking and running, patients with Kext syndrome and KextSG syndrome demonstrate decreased knee flexion excursion, particularly between heel strike and foot flat. Reduced knee flexion excursion may also be seen while landing from a jump. While landing from a jump, the knees should flex to assist in absorbing the forces associated with the landing. Patients with Kext or KextSG syndrome often lack this knee flexion and land with a stiff knee, which may be the result of the inability of the quadriceps to elongate appropriately during the landing.

Similar to the partial squat test described earlier, the patient keeps the body weight shifted posteriorly during a step-up or squatting activity. This position may reduce the contribution of the hip extensors and increase the need for quadriceps participation. The increased quadriceps participation may result in an increased load on the patellofemoral joint or peripatellar structures.

Summary of Examination Findings
Kext and KextSG syndromes presents with stiffness of the quadriceps musculature often associated with quadriceps hypertrophy and activities that require repetitive knee extension. The two syndromes differ primarily in location of the structures in which the relative stiffness/flexibility is occurring, thus setting up those structures for injury. KextSG syndrome, the more common of the two, occurs because the quadriceps muscles pull the patella superiorly, resulting in injury in the peripatellar or infrapatellar region. Pain can be reduced by stabilizing the patella in an inferior direction during the aggravating activities. Kext syndrome is less common and often presents as a strain to the quadriceps musculature or the quadriceps tendon.

Treatment
Primary Objectives
The primary objectives of a treatment program for Kext syndrome and KextSG syndrome include the following:
1. Decrease stiffness of quadriceps.
2. Improve gluteal and hamstring contribution to hip extension.
3. Specific to KextSG: Increase inferior glide mobility and decrease superior glide mobility of the patella.

Corrective Exercise Program
Treatment for this classification includes educating the patient in correcting the postural habits and movements that may be contributing to the movement impairment and thus the pain problem. The patient is provided with a general description of the impairment, including dominance/stiffness of the quadriceps and reduced performance of the hip extensors. Then, specific instruction for alignment and functional activities is provided and practiced by the patient. The patient is also instructed in exercises that will address the associated muscle impairments. Treatment described is appropriate for both Kext syndrome and KextSG syndrome, unless otherwise noted.

Functional activities. Functional activities that contribute to the movement impairment must be addressed. The functional activity that is most bothersome to the patient should be addressed first, followed by the activities in which the patient spends the most time such as work or school activities. In this chapter, we cover those activities that are useful for most patients; however, the therapist is encouraged to use the principles of the movement system to address functional activities that may not be described in this chapter.

Sitting. If the patient reports increased symptoms during sitting, he or she should be instructed to reduce the amount of knee flexion while sitting. As symptoms improve, the patient may gradually increase the amount of flexion. If superior patellar glide is contributing, the patient may be instructed to perform a manual inferior glide to the patella to decrease symptoms and to decrease quadriceps stiffness.

Gait. During gait, the patient is encouraged to improve push-off. The patient may also benefit from cues to shift their body weight slightly forward.

Sit-to-stand. To rise from a sitting position to standing, the patient should be instructed to slide forward to the edge of the chair. Once at the front of the chair, the patient should position the feet about hip-width apart and slightly posterior to the knees. The patient is instructed to flex forward at the hips to shift the COM over their feet. The patient should then contract his or her gluteals when rising from the chair while making sure the tibia advances forward over the foot.

Stairs. Similar to rising from a chair, the patient should be instructed in flexing at the hip and shifting the tibia anteriorly to bring the center of mass over the foot. As the patient rises up the step, he or she should use the gluteals to lift the body weight up and forward to ascend stairs. If the patient is unable to ascend or descend stairs without an increase in symptoms, compensatory methods may need to be provided. Please see the "Functional Activities" section in the "Tibiofemoral Rotation with Valgus Syndrome" section for methods to reduce symptoms with stair ambulation.

Fitness activities. Patients with Kext syndrome and KextSG syndrome often participate in fitness, weight training, or sporting activities. These activities may need to be modified to reduce symptoms and reduce quadriceps hypertrophy. If the person participates in weight training, quadriceps strengthening activities should be reduced, and activities to target the gluteals and hamstrings should be substituted. It is important to remember that when a muscle hypertrophies through strengthening, the stiffness of the muscles also increases.

The patient's aerobic activities may be modified by reducing the intensity to a level appropriate for the patient's stage for rehabilitation. The intensity is then increased gradually as the patient's symptoms improve.

If the patient participates in jumping activities on a regular basis, jumping activities should be addressed. The patient should be instructed in achieving sufficient knee flexion during landing and to perform a soft landing. The patient should begin to practice the new strategy at low intensity levels, including small jumps and low impact landing. As the patient improves, the technique may be progressed to higher intensity jumps and landings if symptoms are not aggravated.

Home Exercise Program

Exercises to improve the performance of the gluteus maximus include prone hip extension with the knee flexed, weight shifting, standing on one leg, hip extension in standing with resistance, lunges, and squats. Care should be taken not to increase the patient's knee symptoms with any of these exercises, particularly lunges and squats, which will incorporate quadriceps participation. The appropriate level of exercise depends on

the stage for rehabilitation and the gluteus maximus strength.

Exercises to improve the extensibility of the quadriceps should also be prescribed. We recommend prone knee flexion or the two-joint hip flexor length test position. During all stretching exercises, the patient should have good abdominal support to avoid pelvic anterior tilt or transverse rotation. Patients with KextSG syndrome need to stabilize the patella during these stretches to prevent superior glide and isolate the stretch to the quadriceps. Stabilization of the patella may be accomplished by manual assistance of another person or through taping (Figure 7-36).

If prone knee flexion is prescribed, the patient should flex the knee only as far as he or she can without increased pain. In addition, the therapist needs to be sure the movement of the patella is not restricted by pressure against the supporting surface. In some cases, a folded towel needs to be placed under the thigh so the patella is able to move inferiorly during knee flexion.

Other Interventions

Taping and patellar mobilization may be useful in patients with KextSG syndrome. We have developed a method to reduce the pull of the quadriceps on the patellar tendon and tibial tubercle (see Figure 7-36). Patients who participate in activities that involve repetitive jumping should be taught to reinforce the taping technique, because the

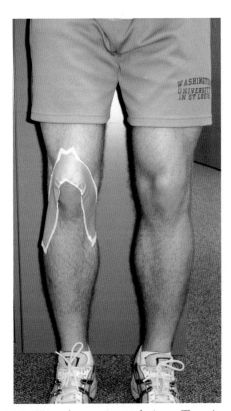

Figure 7-36. Horseshoe taping technique: To assist stabilization of the patella in patients with knee extension with patellar superior glide (KextSG) syndrome.

taping may loosen with the repetitive jumping stresses. Patellar inferior glides and mobilization with movement may be used to help improve the patellar positioning. Based on the concept proposed by Mulligan,[139] a mobilization for KextSG syndrome was developed. While in the sitting position, the patient performs knee extension and flexion. During the eccentric flexion phase, the patient performs a manual inferior glide of the patella.

CASE PRESENTATION
Knee Extension with Patellar Superior Glide Syndrome

Symptoms and History

A 28-year-old male triathlete is referred to physical therapy for evaluation and treatment of left knee pain. He reports left knee pain for 5 months that was located immediately posterior to the patella. His pain began after a recent marathon. He stated that he had no pain during or after the race. He took the recommended rest after the marathon, then approximately 3 weeks after the marathon, he began to increase his running mileage in preparation for his next triathlon. After running a set of intervals, he noticed a sharp pain behind the left kneecap. He had used ibuprofen and ice with minimal relief. At the time of the examination, the patient rated his pain as a 2/10 at rest that increased to 6/10 with running. His symptoms do not appear to increase with cycling or swimming. His KOS-ADL[119] score is 76%, and KOS-Sports score is 71%. No imaging was performed.

Alignment/Appearance

The patient is 6 feet 3 inches and weighs 210 pounds with a fit appearance. In stance, the patient's alignment was unremarkable.

Movement Analysis

Standing

During a partial squat, the patient reports an increase in knee pain. No movement faults are noted. For the secondary test, the partial squat is repeated while the examiner placed a manual patellar glide in the medial direction. The patient reports an increase in knee pain similar to the previous test. The examiner asks the patient to repeat the test while the examiner placed a manual glide in the inferior direction. The patient reports no pain with the test.

Prone

During knee flexion in prone, the patient reports an increase in pain that was resolved with the addition of a patellar inferior glide.

Joint Integrity

Accessory motions of the patellofemoral joint were limited in the inferior direction. The patient reports no change in symptoms with the accessory motions.

Muscle Length Impairments

During the two-joint hip flexor length test, the patient demonstrated a short rectus femoris on the left. As the hip was extended, the knee extended and the patient reports an increase in his symptoms. With a manual glide of the patella in the inferior direction, the patient reports a decrease in his pain compared to the first performance. Hamstrings are short and stiff.

Muscle Strength/Performance Impairments

Using manual muscle testing, the left hip lateral rotators are 4+/5, the gluteus maximus is 4−/5, the iliopsoas is 4/5, and the posterior gluteus medius is 4+/5. Hamstring and quadriceps are strong (5/5); however, the patient reports an increase in his pain when resistance is applied to the quadriceps.

Stiffness/Extensibility/Flexibility

The rectus femoris was relatively more stiff than the patellofemoral joint causing superior glide of the patella during rectus femoris length tests.

Tests for Source

The patient reported tenderness with palpation along the medial and lateral patellar facets. There was no tenderness along the tibiofemoral joint line. The McConnell test[120] and the patellofemoral grind test[52,120] for patellofemoral pain were positive. During the McConnell test, the patient reported pain when resistance is applied with the knee in 60 degrees of flexion. This pain is alleviated with a manual inferior glide. All ligamentous and meniscal tests were negative.

Functional Activities

The patient reports an increase in his symptoms during a stair ascent. As he pushed off of the step with the involved limb, he kept his trunk vertical and did not flex forward at the hip. Cues to lean forward and use his gluteals to push up to the next step resulted in decreased symptoms with the step. Gait was unremarkable. During landing from a jump, he demonstrates reduced knee flexion excursion, giving a stiff knee appearance.

Diagnosis and Staging

The diagnosis is KextSG syndrome, and the stage for rehabilitation is Stage 2. His prognosis is good to excellent. Positive moderators include his young age, overall good health, high motivation to return to his activities, and his ability to change the movement impairments with instruction only. Negative moderators include his high activity level.

Treatment

The patient was seen once per week for 2 weeks, then once every other week for 2 weeks for a total of 4 visits over 7 weeks. Treatment included instruction in correct performance of functional activities, including his sporting activities. He was also instructed in a home exercise program to improve performance of the hip extensors and hip lateral rotators as well as exercises to increase the extensibility of the rectus femoris and hamstrings.

During the first visit, the patient was instructed in shifting his COM forward over the feet during functional activities such as sit-to-stand and ascending stairs. This was accomplished by leaning forward and dorsiflexing the ankle to advance his tibia anteriorly over the foot. He was then instructed to use his gluteals while extending the lower extremity to raise his body weight up to the next step.

To improve performance of the hip lateral rotators and posterior gluteus medius, sidelying hip abduction/lateral rotation with the hip and knee extended was prescribed. To improve gluteus maximus performance, prone hip extension with the knee flexed was prescribed. To accomodate rectus femoris stiffness, he performed this exercise with pillows under his hips to allow greater hip motion. He was instructed to perform the exercises one time per day. He was instructed to perform 3 sets, each set to fatigue. The repetitions depended on his ability to perform the exercise correctly. He was also instructed to stop all of the exercises that he was using to increase quadriceps strength such as resisted knee extension, lunges and squats. He was encouraged instead to substitute gluteal strengthening activities such as hip extension.

To improve extensibility of the rectus femoris, the two-joint hip flexor test position was used as a stretching technique. He was instructed to extend the hip toward the surface of the mat. Once the hip was in the final position, the patient was instructed to flex the knee. The patient was unable to perform the stretch without an increase in symptoms, so the examiner applied the taping method in Figure 7-36 to assist. With the tape applied, the patient could perform the stretch without discomfort behind the patella. He also reported feeling a good stretch in the quadriceps muscles. An alternative stretch, knee flexion in prone, was provided for the times that he could not be taped. He was instructed to flex the knee through the ROM that did not increase his pain.

Regarding his fitness program, the patient was encouraged to continue with cycling and swimming according to his training schedule. For the running component, he was encouraged to avoid interval training that involved sprints for 2 weeks. During these 2 weeks, the distance he runs should be limited to a distance that does not increase his symptoms by more than 2 points. For example, if he rated his pain at rest as 2/10 and increased to 5/10 after the run, he should reduce his distance during the next run. He was encouraged to continue using ice as needed.

The patient was also instructed in how to apply the tape appropriately. He was instructed to at minimum wear the tape during stretching and during his runs. He was encouraged to wear the tape throughout the day if possible.

At his second visit, 1 week later, the patient reported 80% compliance with the exercises and 70% compliance with the functional activity corrections. He reported that his worst pain in the last week was 2/10 after sitting for a prolonged time at a conference. He stated that the tape was helpful and discovered that he could run longer distances if the tape was in place. He demonstrated correct performance of the exercises, therefore the exercises were progressed. Sidelying hip abduction/lateral rotation and prone hip extension were progressed to standing hip abduction/lateral rotation and standing hip extension using resistance. The patient's gym had a pulley resistance system, so he was instructed in the proper performance of the exercises using the pulley system.

He demonstrated proper performance of the two-joint hip flexor length stretch; however, he reported that he had some difficulty finding an appropriate place to perform the stretch. He would like to be able to perform the stretch before and after runs outside. He was instructed in a method to perform the stretch in a half-kneeling position (Figure 7-37). He was encouraged to maintain proper trunk alignment during performance of the stretch.

On review of functional activities, such as sit-to-stand and stair ambulation, the patient was able to demonstrate the activities independently. He reported that he no

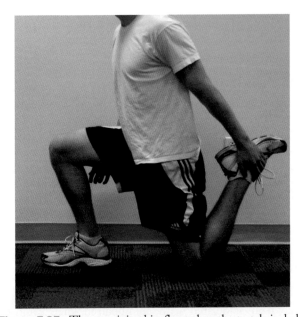

Figure 7-37. The two-joint hip flexor length stretch in half-kneeling position. May be performed in Stage 3 of rehabilitation. The patient is instructed to use the ground to prevent superior glide of the patella while performing the stretch. For patient comfort, this stretch should not be performed on a hard surface. The patient is instructed to maintain proper trunk alignment by using abdominal contraction to prevent lumbar extension and to avoid leaning forward.

longer had pain with stairs, although he was surprised when he had an increase in pain after prolonged sitting. With follow-up questioning, the patient revealed that he did not wear the tape on the day of the conference because he felt it was not needed. To address this relative stiffness/flexibility, the patient was instructed in a self-mobilization using inferior glide of the patella during knee flexion. He was instructed to perform this as often as he could throughout the day, particularly during the days he was sitting for a prolonged period of time.

At 5 weeks, the patient reported that he had no pain at rest or with his training runs. He stated that he had not used tape in the last 2 weeks and felt ready to begin interval training again. He demonstrated independence is his home program and functional activities. He was instructed in how to progress his resistance training for the hip musculature and encouraged to continue performing the stretches on a consistent basis. The strengthening and stretching routine that he typically performed before his injury was reviewed and suggestions were provided. For example, during his hamstring stretch, he demonstrated increased lumbar flexion. He was instructed to avoid lumbar flexion to isolate the stretch to the hamstrings and to avoid unnecessary stress to the lumbar spine.

The examiner agreed that he could initiate his interval training. The patient was encouraged to apply tape during the first few sessions. If he had no increase in symptoms, then he could try a session without tape.

Outcome

At the time of his last visit, 7 weeks later, the patient reported that he had returned to his preinjury training status without tape. Function was also improved as demonstrated by 100% on both KOS-ADL[119] and KOS-Sports scores. He continued to perform his stretching and resistance activities. He also reported beginning a yoga class, which he felt was helpful; however, he wanted to be sure if that was appropriate. Given the patient's inherent stiffness and high activity level, a regular stretching program would be appropriate. The examiner reviewed the poses that the patient was performing and educated him on how to modify particular poses to avoid increased stress to the joints.

KNEE HYPEREXTENSION SYNDROME

Knee hyperextension (Khext) syndrome is described as knee pain associated with an impaired knee extensor mechanism. Dominance of the hamstrings and poor performance of gluteus maximus and quadriceps muscles result in hyperextension of the knee placing excessive stresses on the knee. Differentiating Khext syndrome from TFR syndrome can be a challenge; therefore tests to rule out TFR syndrome should be performed before providing the Khext syndrome diagnosis.

Symptoms and History

Patients report pain located in the peripatellar region or tibiofemoral joint that is aggravated during prolonged standing or with activities that involve rapid knee extension such as swimming or kicking during martial arts. Race walkers also demonstrate Khext syndrome as they repetitively hyperextend their knee to maintain prolonged foot contact during their sport. Common diagnoses used by referring physicians include patellofemoral pain syndrome and fat pad syndrome, also called *Hoffa's disease*.[140]

The articles that are available related to Khext syndrome are limited to describing the effect of knee alignment on structures of the knee. Loudon et al[24] provided a thorough review of the relationship of knee hyperextension alignment and tissue injury. Extension of the knee is not limited by bony anatomy, thus the soft tissues of the posterior knee are primarily responsible for the resistance needed to prevent the knee from further extension. Based on the anatomy and principles of biomechanics, a reasonable assumption is that prolonged knee hyperextension during standing or repetitive hyperextension during gait could result in increased tensile stresses on the ACL and the soft tissues of the posterior knee, as well as compressive stresses on the anterior structures such at the fat pad.[141]

There are a few studies that demonstrate a direct association between knee hyperextension and injury. In a prospective study of female soccer players, Myer et al[142] reported that knee hyperextension alignment increases the odds of sustaining an ACL injury by fivefold. In a case-control study, Loudon et al[143] used conditional stepwise logistic regression to find a significant correlation between knee hyperextension alignment and ACL injury. There is also evidence that women with hyperextension of the knee may have reduced knee joint position sense that may reduce the individual's ability to control end-range knee extension movements.[144]

Although knee hyperextension alignment is implicated in knee injury and pain, an individual with Khext syndrome can demonstrate signs of hyperextension during other tests such as gait and stair ambulation. The diagnosis of Khext syndrome should not be given based on alignment alone.

Key Tests and Signs
Alignment Analysis
Individuals with Khext syndrome often demonstrate knee extension greater than 5 degrees in standing (Figure 7-38). They may also demonstrate a swayback posture with a posterior pelvic tilt and ankle plantarflexion. Correction of the standing alignment may result in a decrease in the patient's symptoms.

Movement Impairments
Standing tests. During single-leg stance on the involved limb, the patient may demonstrate an increase

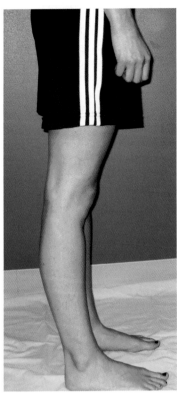

Figure 7-38. Knee hyperextension alignment. Note knee extension greater than 5 degrees and ankle plantarflexion.

in knee hyperextension. If medial rotation of the hip is noted during this test, then a tibiofemoral rotation diagnosis should be considered.

Joint Integrity

Patients in this category may demonstrate a general joint hypermobility as assessed by the Beighton index[145]; however, this is not a requirement. Some patients appear to have general laxity of the ligaments, yet their Beighton index is relatively low. The patient may demonstrate knee extension PROM that is greater than 10 degrees; however, in acute flare-ups of the condition, the patient may actually demonstrate a reduction in knee extension compared to the uninvolved side. This is thought to be a protective mechanism to reduce stresses to the injured structures.

Muscle Length Impairments

The patient may have a short or stiff gastrocnemius; however, these limitations are not seen in all patients with Khext syndrome. Hamstring shortness is often associated with this syndrome.

Muscle Strength/Performance Impairments

Impairments of muscle strength and performance include poor performance of gluteus maximus and quadriceps. The gluteus maximus often tests weak during manual muscle testing (MMT) and demonstrates delayed recruitment during activities such as prone hip extension with the knee extended. The gluteus maximus should contract early in the motion of limb movement during prone hip extension. A notable delay in gluteus maximus contraction may indicate that the hamstrings are acting as the primary hip extensors for the hip movement. The quadriceps often tests strong during a MMT; however, the patient may display poor functional use of the quadriceps during activities such as a step-up or sit-to-stand as evidenced by the patient pulling his or her knees back to the body.

Functional Activities

Gait. During gait, the patient may demonstrate hyperextension from heel strike through late stance. The patient may also demonstrate a prolonged foot flat, keeping their heel in contact with the floor longer than expected. Noyes et al[146] described this gait pattern in patients with posterolateral ligament complex injuries; however, this pattern has been observed in symptomatic patients without documented ligamentous injury.

Step-up. During a step-up, the patient demonstrates a faulty movement of pulling the knee back to the body, instead of shifting the body forward over the limb. This motion is achieved by using the hamstrings more than the quadriceps and gluteus maximus to extend the hip and the knee. Because the foot is anchored on the floor, hip extension performed by the hamstrings results in knee extension and therefore reduces the need to recruit the quadriceps to extend the knee.

Other Functional Tests

Activities that tend to exacerbate the patient's symptoms should be assessed such as sit-to-stand, work requirements, or sporting activities. Typically, the individual demonstrates a knee hyperextension alignment or movement impairment during these aggravating activities.

Summary of Examination Findings

Khext syndrome presents with the movement impairment of knee hyperextension during alignment, movement tests, and functional activities. A special note related to secondary tests for Khext syndrome is that patients with this syndrome often have a chronic condition that does not always modify immediately with secondary tests. The patient may need to try modifications for a period of time to see the effect. For example, the patient may report no change in symptoms with correction of standing alignment; however, if standing alignment is modified while at work, symptoms may improve dramatically.

Differentiating between Khext syndrome and tibiofemoral rotation syndrome can be challenging. If signs for both Khext syndrome and tibiofemoral rotation syndrome are observed, the therapist should follow treatment guidelines for tibiofemoral rotation syndrome, which provides treatment related to the rotation component and also addresses the hyperextension component. Khext syndrome should be reserved for those displaying the movement impairment in the sagittal plane only.

Treatment

Primary Objectives

The primary objectives of a treatment program include the following:

1. Decrease hyperextension of the knee during functional activities.
2. Improve muscle performance of the gluteus maximus and quadriceps.
3. Decrease overrecruitment or dominance of the hamstrings.

Corrective Exercise Program

Treatment for this syndrome includes educating the individual in correcting the postural habits and movements contributing to the movement impairment and thus the pain problem. The patient is provided with a general description of the impairment and specific instruction for alignment and functional activities. Then the functional activities are practiced by the patient. The patient is also instructed in exercises that will address the associated muscle impairments.

Alignment. First, the patient is educated in correction of posture and functional activities. To improve alignment between the femur and tibia, the patient is instructed to relax or unlock the knees to reduce hyperextension of the knee. If the patient stands in a posterior pelvic tilt, this should also be corrected. A mirror is useful during correction of the alignment. Patients often report that their position of hyperextension feels "normal," and the correction feels as if their knees are too flexed as in a partial squat. The mirror reinforces the proper alignment of the knee.

Functional activities

Gait. During ambulation, the patient is encouraged to use a proper heel-to-toe gait pattern and to land softly on the heel at heel strike. The patient is also instructed to avoid knee hyperextension and hip hyperextension during the stance phase of gait cycle. Most patients with knee hyperextension have a delayed heel rise at push-off; therefore a helpful cue is to ask the patient to lift the heel a little earlier than usual. Another useful cue, as described by Noyes et al,[146] is to walk with the knee slightly flexed.

Sit-to-stand/stairs. During sit-to-stand and stairs, the patient is instructed to use the quadriceps and gluteus maximus to lift the body up and forward and to avoid pulling the knee(s) back to meet the body. The final position of the knee should be a neutral position not hyperextended. If the patient is unable to ascend or descend stairs without an increase in symptoms, compensatory methods may need to be provided. Please see the "Functional Activities" section the "Tibiofemoral Rotation with Valgus Syndrome" section for methods to reduce symptoms with stair ambulation.

Standing. Patients with Khext syndrome often report increased symptoms with prolonged standing. They should be instructed in correcting their alignment during stance and to reduce the amount of time that they stand in one position. They should be encouraged to change their activities as often as possible, including sitting, walking and leaning into a support surface. If they are in a situation that does not allow them to change their activity, weight shifting provides some temporary reduction in stresses on the knee.

Fitness activities. If the patient does not have a fitness program, then a discussion is warranted to encourage a fitness program as a goal. If the person participates regularly in a fitness program, modification may be necessary. The patient's aerobic activities may need to be modified by addressing the movement impairment and by reducing the intensity. The intensity level of the aerobic activity should be related to the patient's stage for rehabilitation. For example, if the patient is a speed walker and the injury is Stage 1 for rehabilitation, the patient may be instructed to use a bike, walk in a pool, or start with a slower walking pace or shorter walking distance. The intensity is then gradually increased. As the patient's symptoms improve, the patient should begin to increase the walking distance and then increase the speed.

Home Exercise Program

Exercises to improve strength and performance of the gluteus maximus and quadriceps may be prescribed. To improve gluteus maximus performance, exercises, such as prone hip extension with the knee flexed, weight shifting, single-leg stance, and resisted hip extension, are prescribed. When performing prone hip extension with the knee flexed, the patient should have at least one pillow under the abdomen so that the exercise is performed from some hip flexion to neutral and not into hip hyperextension. Functional activities that can be used as exercise to improve gluteus maximus and quadriceps performance include sit-to-stand, wall sits, step-up/stepdowns, lunges, and squats. Abdominal muscle exercises may also be appropriate if the patient demonstrates poor trunk and/or pelvic control.

Sitting knee extension with ankle dorsiflexion is an exercise that can be performed easily throughout the day to improve the extensibility of the hamstrings and gastrocnemius. The gastrocnemius can be stretched with prolonged passive ankle dorsiflexion in standing, and the hamstrings can be stretched with prolonged knee extension in the sitting position (see Figure 7-40). To properly stretch the hamstrings, be sure that the spine does not flex.

Taping

Taping may be useful in patients with knee hyperextension. The posterior X taping demonstrated in Figure 7-27 to treat TFRVal syndrome will also assist with preventing Khext syndrome. If the fat pad is very irritable, it may be helpful to try the unloading taping technique proposed by McConnell (Figure 7-39).

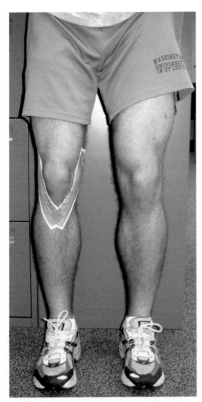

Figure 7-39. Taping technique. Unloading taping technique proposed by Jenny McConnell. This taping method is proposed to reduce stress on the source of symptoms, the fat pad.

Neuromuscular Training

Neuromuscular training to improve proprioception, balance, and the ability to accommodate to perturbations is important (see Box 7-2). During neuromuscular training, the patient is instructed to limit the amount of knee hyperextension.

CASE PRESENTATION
Knee Hyperextension Syndrome

Symptoms and History

A 35-year-old female is referred to physical therapy for evaluation and treatment of left knee pain. She reports two previous bouts of similar pain that resolved fairly quickly without intervention. However, this episode began approximately 3 weeks ago and has not improved. The pain is located in the posterior aspect of her knee and just inferior to the patella deep in the joint. She has participated in competitive race walking for the past 3 years. Initially, her pain would only occur during races or when training, but the pain progressed to occurring with daily walking and stair ambulation. Her pain forced her to stop race walking approximately 2½ weeks ago, and she is very anxious to return to this activity. Her pain rating at the time of the initial visit was 3/10 with daily activities and increases to 6/10 if attempting to race walk. She describes her pain as a deep aching in the posterior

knee that becomes sharper when race walking. Nothing seems to give her relief except taking Ibuprofen. Her KOS-ADL[119] score is 51%, and KOS-Sports score is 40%. Radiographs show no abnormalities of the tibiofemoral or patellofemoral joint. She also states that she has a 2-year-old daughter who she tends to carry on her left hip. She was working part-time as a business consultant.

Alignment Analysis

The patient is 5 feet 6 inches and weighs 135 pounds. In stance, the patient demonstrated tibial varum and genu recurvatum bilaterally; however, both faults were greater on the left compared to the right. She had a flat lumbar spine, posterior pelvic tilt, and hip joint hyperextension with a mild swayback alignment.

Movement Analysis

During single-leg stance on the left, the patient demonstrates increased knee hyperextension. The patient did not report an increase in pain, although she does express a feeling of instability compared to standing on the uninvolved limb. The patient also demonstrates a pelvic lateral tilt (Trendelenburg sign) during single-leg stance bilaterally; however, she demonstrated more tilt during single-leg stance on the left than on the right.

During a step-up onto a 12-inch stool, the patient kept her COM posterior to her base of support and snapped her knee back to her body using her hamstrings. She reported a mild increase in symptoms during this test. She was cued to lean forward to bring her COM over her foot, and to think about using her quadriceps and gluteals as she stepped up. She performed the step-up correctly by following the cues provided. She reported that her symptoms did not increase with the corrected method.

Joint Integrity

Knee extension PROM tested in supine is 15 degrees on the left and 10 degrees on the right. The patient's tibiofemoral joints are mildly lax compared to normal, which was noted particularly during prone hip rotation testing, during which the leg motion was particularly evident.

Muscle Length Impairments

Hamstring length is tested and found to be short bilaterally with 70 degrees passive straight leg raise. Gastrocnemius length was also short bilaterally, measuring 10 degrees ankle dorsiflexion with the knees flexed and 0 degrees with the knees extended.

Muscle Strength/Performance Impairments

On the left side, the gluteus maximus MMT reveals a grade of 4/5 and shows a delayed onset compared to the hamstrings during hip extension with the knee extended. The left quadriceps MMT grade is 5/5, although poor functional performance is suspected. For example, during a wall squat the left quadriceps fatigued more readily than the right, with notable muscle quivering after only 10 seconds. The posterior gluteus medius MMT grade is 4–/5 bilaterally.

Tests for Source

The patient reports tenderness with palpation distal to the inferior pole of the patella in the region of the fat pad on the left. Mild tenderness is also noted on the posterolateral aspect of the knee. All ligamentous and meniscal tests are negative.

Functional Activities

During sit-to-stand and stair ambulation, the patient demonstrates the tendency to pull her knees back to the body using her hamstrings, rather than keep her COM over her feet and use her quadriceps to extend her knees. Increased symptoms are elicited on the left after completing one flight of stairs. The patient is cued to lean forward and to get her shoulders over her feet while concentrating on not hyperextending her knees. Although she has some difficulty performing the stair ambulation correctly with these cues, the patient reports no aggravation of her symptoms. Gait deficits noted are knee hyperextension from heel strike through terminal stance with a delayed heel rise bilaterally. When cued to decrease the knee hyperextension and attempt an earlier heel rise, the patient has trouble trying to change her gait pattern and becomes a little frustrated. A bilateral hip drop is also noted during gait.

Diagnosis and Staging

The diagnosis is Khext syndrome. The stage for rehabilitation is Stage 2. Her prognosis is good to excellent. Positive moderators include her fairly young age, overall good health, and high motivation to return to her activities. Negative moderators include her difficulty making corrections during alignment and functional activities and her anxiety about wanting to return to race walking, a sport that encourages knee hyperextension by demanding that one foot be in contact with the ground at all times.

Treatment

The patient was seen twice per week for 2 weeks secondary to taping needs, then decreased to once per week for 4 weeks for a total of 8 visits over 6 weeks. Treatment included instruction in correct performance of functional activities, including speed walking. She was also instructed in a home exercise program to improve performance of the hip abductors, gluteus maximus, and quadriceps, along with exercises to increase the extensibility of the hamstrings, gastrocnemius, and soleus muscles. Although she reported pain only in the left knee, she was encouraged to perform the exercises bilaterally.

During the first visit, the patient was instructed to correct her standing alignment of knee hyperextension by relaxing her knees. A mirror was needed for visual feedback of her alignment. Her tendency at first was to excessively flex her knees, and she found it very difficult and tiresome to maintain normal alignment. Therefore it was decided to perform the posterior X taping technique to provide an external source of feedback to her when she would start to hyperextend her knees (see Figure 7-27). The patient was instructed to keep the tape on for 1 to 3 days if tolerated and to check her skin carefully when the tape was removed. Assuming there would be no skin reactions, the plan was for her to return at the end of the week to be re-taped.

She was instructed to try alternating the hip she used for carrying her child, instead of always holding her on the left. Holding her child on the left hip resulted in prolonged positioning of hip adduction and pelvic lateral tilt. This prolonged positioning may have contributed to her hip weakness and increased knee hyperextension on the left. The patient was instructed in performance of sit-to-stand, attempting to get her shoulders over her feet and prevent hyperextending her knees when completing the standing maneuver. This task was easier for her to correct than gait or stair climbing during the first session.

To improve the functional performance of the quadriceps, the patient was instructed in a wall squat exercise. She assumed a position of about 45 degrees hip and knee flexion and was instructed to start by maintaining the position for 15 seconds and to perform 5 repetitions. Each day she was to try to add 5 seconds onto her hold time during the first week. She was also cued to avoid hyperextending her knees when returning from the squat position to the hip and knee extended position.

To begin to improve the performance of her gluteus maximus, the patient was instructed to forward bend by hip flexion only with knees flexed and practice returning by contracting her gluteals to lift her upper body. She was also given the exercise of prone hip extension over 3 or 4 pillows to help place her in enough hip flexion so that her knee could stay relaxed in flexion as she extended her hip using her gluteus maximus. She was instructed to perform the exercise one time per day. She was instructed to perform 3 sets, each set to fatigue. The repetitions depended on her ability to perform the exercise correctly.

To improve the recruitment of the posterior gluteus medius, the patient was instructed in weight shifting. She was instructed to avoid pelvic tilting and knee hyperextension as she shifted. The patient had difficulty maintaining the appropriate pelvic position, so she was encouraged to place her hands on her ASIS to monitor the pelvic alignment. She was then able to perform the activity correctly. She was also encouraged to maintain the trunk in a neutral position and avoid sidebending. She was instructed to perform this exercise frequently throughout the day, if possible.

To address her limitations in hamstring extensibility, she was instructed to sit on the edge of a chair with one leg extended and to lean forward from her hips keeping her spine straight until she felt an appropriate stretch to her hamstrings. Because her knee would easily assume a hyperextended position, the patient had to make a conscious effort to keep the knee relaxed in slight flexion during the stretch (Figure 7-40). While stretching her hamstrings, she was also instructed to try to dorsiflex her ankle without toe extension to provide an additional stretch to her gastrocnemius. The patient was instructed in the typical standing wall stretch for the gastrocnemius as well.

At her second visit, she reported 75% compliance with the exercises and about 50% compliance with the functional activity corrections, which were still hard for her. She stated that the tape behind her knees was definitely helpful in relearning how to stand properly. She was able to wear the tape for 2 days and had no skin reaction, so she requested to have the tape applied again at that visit. Her symptoms had decreased to 2/10, and she reported less pain with stair ambulation.

She demonstrated correct performance of the exercises, therefore the exercises were progressed. With the wall squat, she was now able to sustain the position for 30 seconds before fatiguing. This exercise was progressed by having her place her right foot slightly in front of her left, forcing her to increase the load to her left quadriceps. Her weight shifting was progressed to single-leg stance with light upper extremity support and using all the previous cues. An additional exercise was given to her for the posterior gluteus medius. She was instructed in the side lying hip abduction/lateral rotation exercise. Two to three pillows were placed between her legs and her top leg was aligned in 10 to 20 degrees of hip and knee flexion. When the patient attempted to abduct her hip off the pillows, she reported feeling muscles working in her posterior thigh so it was determined that she was substituting with her hamstrings. With much verbal and manual cueing and specific palpation of her posterior gluteus medius, she was able to perform this exercise correctly. The patient was encouraged to start with five repetitions and progress toward ten, only if she could feel the muscle recruitment in the correct location. Because she was performing her prone hip extension exercise correctly, she was encouraged to add more repetitions.

The patient was re-taped and her gait deviations were addressed with the tape applied. The main cues given to her were to lean forward slightly while walking, take smaller strides and lift her heel earlier at terminal stance. Her attempts at these corrections were better than at her first visit, although she felt very awkward. The patient was instructed to continue with the other exercises, trying to be diligent about her hamstring stretching throughout the day.

At the fifth visit during the third week, taping was discontinued because the patient felt she was now able to

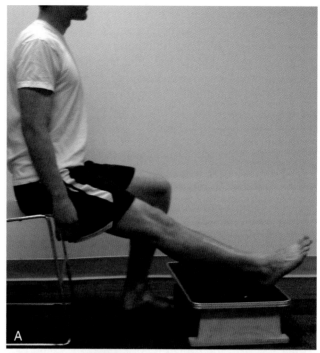

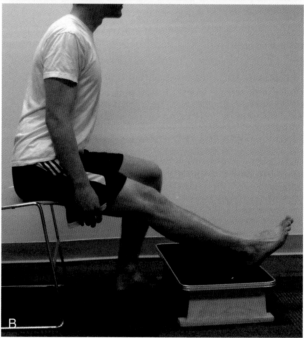

Figure 7-40. Hamstring stretching. Proper performance of hamstring stretch provided to the patient. **A,** The patient sits on the edge of a chair with one leg extended. **B,** The patient then leans forward from the hips, keeping the spine straight until an appropriate stretch is felt.

control the knee hyperextension on her own. The patient reported 0/10 symptoms at that time with walking and with stair ambulation. She admitted to trying to race walk for a short distance but developed low level symptoms so she decided she was not quite ready. At this visit, she was progressed to level 3 of the posterior gluteus medius progression. She was now able to perform single-leg stance without any upper extremity support, so the activity was progressed by performing single-leg stance on an unstable surface starting with pillows and progressing to foam pads and a BOSU ball. She also began standing lunges and step-ups to strengthen her gluteals and quadriceps more functionally, monitoring her movement pattern to be sure she was not using her hamstrings to pull her knee back to her body.

During her sixth visit in the fourth week, she began to practice walking with increased speed while trying to still work on the specific gait cues she had now been practicing for a few weeks. As long as she did not go too fast, she was able to achieve some corrections and did not experience an increase in symptoms. She was progressed to playing catch with a weighted medicine ball while balancing on one leg on the BOSU ball. Also, she now added 5 pound weights in each hand while performing her lunges and step-ups.

Outcome

The patient was seen for a total of 8 visits over 6 weeks. At her last visit, the patient reported that she could race walk for 1 mile without aggravating her symptoms, although she stated that she was not yet up to her previous speed. She reported that it was impossible to prevent the hyperextension as her speed increased. Since she was determined to continue participation in this sport, she was instructed to work on her gait corrections as much as possible throughout the rest of the day, when not race walking. Function was also improved as demonstrated by a KOS-ADL score of 93% and a KOS-Sports score of 84%. She was instructed to continue her home exercise program daily, if possible, even when she was totally pain-free with all activities and to think of it like "brushing her teeth." It was explained to her that if she would stop the exercises, her pain would likely return after a period of time. The patient had no problem with this commitment, and she was discharged from physical therapy.

PATELLAR LATERAL GLIDE SYNDROME

Patellar lateral glide (PLG) syndrome is described as knee pain as a result of an impaired patellar relationship within the trochlear groove. Patients with PLG syndrome have an imbalance between the vastus medialis oblique (VMO) and the vastus lateralis (VL) muscles that may place excessive compressive forces in the lateral patellofemoral joint and tensile forces on the medial joint structures. Shortness or stiffness of the TFL-ITB complex may also contribute to a lateral pull on the patella. A similar syndrome has been described by McConnell.[87]

Symptoms and History

Patients with PLG report peripatellar or retropatellar pain with activities such as stairs, running and squatting.

They may also report an increase in symptoms with prolonged knee flexion when sitting, often called *movie goers syndrome*. PLG rarely occurs in isolation and is often a secondary diagnosis associated with a primary diagnosis of tibiofemoral rotation or knee hyperextension. Common diagnoses used by referring physicians include patellofemoral pain syndrome and patellar chondromalacia.

There is a large body of literature related to the relationship of the VMO and patellofemoral pain; however, the relationship has not been clearly established. A number of authors have reported that patients with patellofemoral pain demonstrate poor performance of the VMO when compared to those without symptoms.[147-151] There are, however, others that report there is no difference in VMO performance between those with and without patellofemoral pain.[152-155] The inconsistent findings demonstrate a need for classification by movement impairment. Subjects with patellofemoral pain are often included in these studies based on pain location; the movement impairment associated with the pain complaint is not considered. Patients with TFRVal syndrome and patients with PLG syndrome may report a similar pain in the peripatellar region, although they may display dissimilar movement impairments. A relationship between VMO performance and patellofemoral pain may exist in individuals with PLG syndrome but may not exist in individuals with TFRVal syndrome. Classification by movement impairments may assist in clarifying the research findings.

Clinical trials of treatment that incorporate VMO strengthening have demonstrated positive results[102]; however, the isolated treatment effects of VMO strengthening are not known. Often these clinical trials include additional treatments, such as stretching and taping, therefore it is difficult to determine the effectiveness of VMO strengthening alone. Recently, authors have demonstrated that increasing the VMO force can decrease the pressure on the lateral patellofemoral joint articular cartilage.[156]

Key Tests and Signs

Alignment Analysis

The patient with PLG syndrome may demonstrate a lateral patellar tilt or lateral patellar glide.

Movement Impairments

Standing tests. During hip and knee flexion in stance (partial squat), the patient may report an increase in their symptoms; however, a movement impairment may not be apparent. A secondary test is performed by asking the patient to repeat the movement while the examiner places a medial glide on the patella. If symptoms are decreased compared to the primary test, PLG is supported.

Supine tests. Patients with PLG syndrome may report an increase in symptoms during the performance of the two-joint hip flexor length test.[88] The test is then repeated while the examiner places a medial glide on the patella. If symptoms decrease, then PLG syndrome is supported. Symptoms may also be decreased by abducting the hip, therefore reducing the stretch on the TFL-ITB.

Prone tests. During knee flexion in prone, patients with PLG syndrome may report pain at the end of their motion. Decreased symptoms when a medial glide is placed on the patella supports the diagnosis of PLG syndrome. Similar to the two-joint hip flexor test, placing the hip into abduction reduces the stretch on the TFL-ITB, which may result in a decrease in the patient's symptoms.

Sitting tests. During knee extension in sitting, the examiner may observe sudden lateral movement of the patella near the end of the knee motion, a motion often referred to as a positive J-sign. This excessive lateral patellar motion may also be seen during an isometric quadriceps contraction.

A McConnell test[120] for patellofemoral pain may be performed to assess for PLG syndrome. In sitting, the patient performs an isometric quadriceps contraction against the therapist's resistance at 120, 90, 60, 30, and 0 degrees of knee flexion. If the patient's pain is produced or increased during any of the contractions, the test is performed again with a manual correction by the examiner. To prevent patellar lateral glide, the examiner places a medial glide on the patella and the resisted test is repeated. If the pain is decreased, the patellofemoral joint is implicated as the source of symptoms and PLG syndrome is implicated as the movement impairment.

Joint Integrity
Patients with PLG syndrome may demonstrate reduced accessory motion for medial glide of the patella.

Muscle Length Impairments
Patients may demonstrate short and/or stiff TFL-ITB and lateral patellar retinaculum. Though not common, sometimes a short and/or stiff gluteus maximus with attachment to the ITB may contribute to the lateral pull of the patella.

Muscle Strength and Performance Impairments
Although weakness of the VMO may contribute to PLG, clinical testing specific to the VMO is not possible. Other characteristics of muscle performance such as muscle timing or endurance have also been suspected to contribute to PLG. Muscle timing and endurance are also difficult to observe clinically. Laboratory measurements, such as electromyography (EMG), may assist in identifying an imbalance in the timing of contraction between the VMO and VL; however, EMG is often not practical in the clinic.

Functional Activities
During performance of functional activities, observation of the movement impairment of PLG syndrome is often difficult; however, secondary tests can be used to support the diagnosis. For example, during activities such as sit-to-stand or step-up, a medial glide may be placed on the patella. If the patient's symptoms are reduced compared to the primary test, then PLG syndrome is supported as the diagnosis.

Treatment

Primary Objectives
The primary objectives of a treatment program include the following:
1. Decrease stiffness of TFL-ITB.
2. Improve quadriceps function.

Corrective Exercise Program
Treatment for PLG syndrome includes educating the individual in correcting the postural habits and movements that may be contributing to the movement impairment and thus the pain problems. The patient is provided with a general description of the impairment and specific instruction for alignment and functional activities. The activities are then practiced by the patient. The patient is also instructed in exercises that will address the associated muscle impairments.

Functional Activities
Sitting. If a patient reports increased symptoms during sitting, the instruction is to reduce the amount of knee flexion while sitting. If the patient has a stiff or short gluteus maximus contributing to the stiffness of the ITB, resulting in PLG, the thighs should be slightly abducted initially. As symptoms improve, the thighs should be gradually adducted until the sitting position is normal and does not cause symptoms. Patients should be encouraged to get out of their chair and flex/extend their knee every 30 minutes to reduce the amount of time the knee is maintained in a flexed position. Patients should also limit the amount of time spent with their legs crossed.

Sit-to-stand. To rise from a sitting position to standing, the patient should be instructed to slide forward to the edge of the chair. Once at the front of the chair, the patient should position the feet about hip-width apart and slightly posterior to the knees. The patient is instructed to contract the quadriceps when rising from the chair. If this motion is painful, the patient may use the hands to assist by pushing up from the armrests of the chair.

Stair ambulation. Similar to rising from a chair, the patient should be instructed to use the quadriceps and gluteals to ascend the stairs. If the patient is unable to ascend or descend stairs without an increase in symptoms, compensatory methods may need to be provided. Please see the "Functional Activities" section in the "Tibiofemoral Rotation with Valgus Syndrome" section for methods to reduce symptoms with stair ambulation.

Fitness activities. Recommendations related to fitness are provided in the "Functional Activities" section in the "Tibiofemoral Rotation with Valgus Syndrome" section.

Home Exercise Program

The patient should be provided with a home exercise program and instruction on the appropriate response to exercise. Exercises specific to PLG syndrome to improve the performance of the quadriceps may be prescribed. We recommend the use of functional activities to improve quadriceps performance. Those exercises, in the order of difficulty beginning with least aggressive, are sit-to-stand transfers, step-ups, lateral step-ups, squats, lunges, and step-downs. Ekstrom et al[157] demonstrated that lunges and lateral step-ups produced greater EMG activity in the VMO compared to other rehabilitation exercises. Biofeedback to improve timing or recruitment of the VMO may be a useful intervention[102,158,159]; however, more clinical studies are needed. In addition, we recommend avoiding open-chain resisted activities in the range of 0 to 45 degrees of flexion and closed-chain activities in the range of 60 to 90 degrees, since these ranges are thought to result in increased stresses to the patellofemoral joint.[160]

Exercises to improve the extensibility of the TFL-ITB should also be prescribed. We recommend prone knee flexion (either unilateral or bilateral) or stretching in the two joint-hip flexor length test position. During prone knee flexion, the patient should initially perform with the involved hip in abduction to reduce the pull of the ITB. As symptoms improve, the amount of hip abduction is reduced.

The two-joint hip flexor stretch position may be used as the patient's symptoms improve. As the involved limb is lowered into extension, the hip should be allowed to abduct. Once the hip is in extension, the hip can then be adducted to add the stretch to the TFL-ITB. Assuming normal anatomy of the femoral lateral condyle, the patella will be secured within the trochlear groove prior to adding the stretch of the TFL-ITB.

Patients must not feel pressure or pain in the location of their symptoms during the stretches. If the symptoms occur, the patella is most likely being mobilized and the stretch will not be effective. Patients with PLG syndrome may need to stabilize the patella during these stretches. Stabilization of the patella may be accomplished by manual assistance of another person or through taping (Figure 7-41). During all stretching exercises, be sure that the patient has good abdominal support to avoid pelvic anterior tilt or rotation. Strengthening the muscles that are antagonists of the TFL-ITB, such as the posterior gluteus medius and gluteus maximus, may also help to improve TFL-ITB extensibility.

Other Interventions

Taping and patellar mobilization may be useful in patients with PLG syndrome. Taping to reduce patellar lateral glide as proposed by McConnell[87] has had clinical success (see Figure 7-41). The evidence consistently supports that taping helps to reduce symptoms,[87,161-165] although the mechanism behind the symptom reduction has not

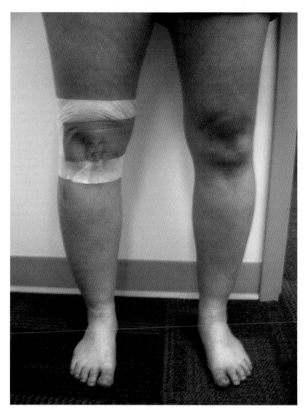

Figure 7-41. Taping technique. Taping to reduce patellar lateral glide as proposed by McConnell.[87] The patella is pushed medially by the tester and strips of tape are placed along the patella, anchored around the medial hamstring muscle bulk.

been determined. Many believe that tape is applied to either change the alignment of the patella or improve the performance of the VMO; however, the literature is mixed.[161,166-172] Although the mechanism is not clear, taping is a safe and relatively convenient intervention that has had clinical success.

Patellar mobilizations in the medial direction may be used to help improve the extensibility of the lateral structures such as the patellar retinaculum and ITB. If the patient is in Stage 1 of rehabilitation, gentle mobilizations may be performed to reduce pain and to initiate mobility in the medial direction. As the patient's symptoms subside, aggressive grades of mobilization should be used to increase extensibility. Patients may be instructed in self-mobilizations to perform along with their home exercise program.

KNEE IMPAIRMENT

Thus far, the focus of this chapter is on the identification and treatment of specific movement system syndromes for the knee. However, patients are commonly referred to physical therapy for rehabilitation of the knee after a surgical procedure or after an acute, traumatic knee injury. When a patient presents to therapy after either a surgical procedure or an acute knee injury, identification of a specific movement system syndrome using a thorough examination may not be possible because of pain, physician-imposed restrictions, or both. In such cases, the physical therapist must recognize the potential pathoanatomical structure(s) involved, perform a limited problem-centered examination to identify specific impairments, and provide treatment that is congruent with the stage for rehabilitation determined according to the guidelines outlined in Chapter 2.

In general, patients for which a movement system syndrome cannot be determined are classified as having a knee impairment, which is a broad term that encompasses a wide array of structural impairments or injuries. An exhaustive discussion of the potential knee injuries a physical therapist might treat and the surgical procedures after which a patient may be referred to physical therapy is beyond the scope of this text. However, to provide optimal care for the patient, the physical therapist must have a thorough understanding of the possible structures of the knee implicated for a particular injury and be familiar with common surgical procedures used by referring physicians. See the Chapter 7 Appendix for additional information regarding specific tissue properties of the structures of the knee, as well as treatment guidelines for each stage of rehabilitation.

Because the knee impairment classification is relatively nonspecific, the physical therapist should provide a source diagnosis, if possible, to guide treatment. Recall from Chapter 2 that if a movement system diagnosis cannot be determined, the diagnosis made by the physical therapist is based on the pathoanatomical structure involved, as identified by the physician; the procedure performed, if any; and the stage for rehabilitation. For example, if a patient presents to physical therapy 3 days after an ACL reconstruction, the diagnosis made by the physical therapist would likely be as follows: ACL tear, status/post ACL reconstruction, Stage 1. If the specific pathoanatomical structure cannot be determined or has not been specified by the physician, the classification of knee impairment should be used to identify the region of the body that is impaired, with an appropriate stage for rehabilitation.

As the patient progresses with physical therapy after an acute injury or surgical procedure, the physical therapist should attend to any underlying movement impairments that either develop or are identified with a more thorough examination. If a movement system syndrome can be determined, the physical therapist should use this diagnosis, with the appropriate stage for rehabilitation, to guide treatment relative to specific movement impairments. If no underlying movement impairment can be determined, the physical therapist should continue to progress treatment as tolerated according to the stage for rehabilitation associated with the source diagnosis provided.[173,174]

CONCLUSION

This chapter offers the reader the diagnostic framework to effectively evaluate and treat chronic, acute, and postsurgical knee pain. By specifically identifying movement impairments and considering the tissue characteristics of pathoanatomical structures in the knee, the physical therapist can be more readily prepared to provide optimal treatment and education to patients who present with knee pain than attempting to develop a program without identifying an underlying syndrome.

REFERENCES

1. Willson JD, Davis IS: Lower extremity mechanics of females with and without patellofemoral pain across activities with progressively greater task demands, *Clin Biomech* 23(2):203-211, 2008.
2. Powers CM: The influence of altered lower-extremity kinematics on patellofemoral joint dysfunction: a theoretical perspective, *J Orthop Sports Phys Ther* 33(11):639-646, 2003.
3. Dierks TA, Manal KT, Hamill J, et al: Proximal and distal influences on hip and knee kinematics in runners with patellofemoral pain during a prolonged run, *J Orthop Sports Phys Ther* 38(8):448-456, 2008.
4. Noehren B, Davis I, Hamill J: ASB Clinical Biomechanics award winner 2006: prospective study of the biomechanical factors associated with iliotibial band syndrome, *Clin Biomech* 22(9):951-956, 2007.
5. Miller RH, Lowry JL, Meardon SA, et al: Lower extremity mechanics of iliotibial band syndrome during an exhaustive run, *Gait Posture* 26(3):407-413, 2007.
6. Hewett TE, Myer GD, Ford KR, et al: Biomechanical Measures of neuromuscular control and valgus loading of the knee predict anterior cruciate ligament injury risk in female athletes: a prospective study, *Am J Sports Med* 33(4):492-501, 2005.
7. Chang A, Hayes K, Dunlop D, et al: Thrust during ambulation and the progression of knee osteoarthritis, *Arthritis Rheum* 50(12):3897-3903, 2004.
8. Cerejo R, Dunlop DD, Cahue S, et al: The influence of alignment on risk of knee osteoarthritis progression according to baseline stage of disease, *Arthritis Rheum* 46(10):2632-2636, 2000.
9. Harris-Hayes M, Sahrmann SA, Norton BJ, et al: Diagnosis and management of a patient with knee pain using the movement system impairment classification system, *J Orthop Sports Phys Ther* 38(4):203-213, 2008.
10. Mascal CL, Landel R, Powers C: Management of patellofemoral pain targeting hip, pelvis, and trunk muscle function: 2 case reports, *J Orthop Sports Phys Ther* 33(11):647-660, 2003.
11. Crossley K, Bennell K, Green S, et al: Physical therapy for patellofemoral pain: a randomized, double-blinded, placebo-controlled trial, *Am J Sports Med* 30(6):857-865, 2002.
12. Selfe J, Richards J, Thewlis D, et al: The biomechanics of step descent under different treatment modalities used in patellofemoral pain, *Gait Posture* 27(2):258-263, 2008.

13. Hewett TE, Lindenfeld TN, Riccobene JV, et al: The effect of neuromuscular training on the incidence of knee injury in female athletes: a prospective study, *Am J Sports Med* 27(6):699-706, 1999.

14. Gilchrist J, Mandelbaum BR, Melancon H, et al: A randomized controlled trial to prevent noncontact anterior cruciate ligament injury in female collegiate soccer players, *Am J Sports Med* 36(8):1476-1483, 2008.

15. Szoeke CEI, Cicuttini FM, Guthrie JR, et al: Factors affecting the prevalence of osteoarthritis in healthy middle-aged women: data from the longitudinal Melbourne Women's Midlife Health Project, *Bone* 39(5):1149-1155, 2006.

16. Sharma L, Lou C, Cahue S, et al: The mechanism of the effect of obesity in knee osteoarthritis: the mediating role of malalignment, *Arthritis Rheum* 43(3):568-575, 2000.

17. Kujala UM, Kettunen J, Paananen H, et al: Knee osteoarthritis in former runners, soccer players, weight lifters, and shooters, *Arthritis Rheum* 38(4):539-546, 1995.

18. Sharma L, Song J, Felson DT, et al: The role of knee alignment in disease progression and functional decline in knee osteoarthritis [erratum appears in JAMA 286(7):792, 2001], *JAMA* 286(2):188-195, 2001.

19. Sharma L, Lou C, Felson DT, et al: Laxity in healthy and osteoarthritic knees, *Arthritis Rheum* 42(5):861-870, 1999.

20. Sharma L, Dunlop DD, Cahue S, et al: Quadriceps strength and osteoarthritis progression in malaligned and lax knees, *Ann Intern Med* 138(8):613-619, 2003.

21. Cooper C, McAlindon T, Coggon D, et al: Occupational activity and osteoarthritis of the knee, *Ann Rheum Dis* 53(2):90-93, 1994.

22. Sahrmann SA: *Diagnosis and treatment of movement impairment syndromes*, St Louis, 2002, Mosby.

23. Kendall FP, McCreary EK, Provance PG, et al: *Muscles: testing and function with posture and pain*, ed 5, Baltimore, 2005, Lippincott Williams & Wilkins.

24. Loudon JK, Goist HL, Loudon KL: Genu recurvatum syndrome, *J Orthop Sports Phys Ther* 27(5):361-367, 1998.

25. Neumann DA: *Kinesiology of the musculoskeletal system: foundations for physical rehabilitation*, St Louis, 2002, Mosby.

26. *Gray's anatomy*, ed 38, Edinburgh, 1999, Churchill Livingstone.

27. Oatis CA: *Kinesiology: the mechanics and pathomechanics of human movement*, Philadelphia, 2004, Lippincott Williams & Wilkins.

28. Gajdosik CG, Gajdosik RL. Musculoskeletal development and adaptation. In Campbell SK, Palisano RJ, Vander Linden DW, eds: *Physical therapy for children*, Philadelphia, 1994, Saunders.

29. Teichtahl AJ, Wluka AE, Cicuttini FM: Frontal plane knee alignment is associated with a longitudinal reduction in patella cartilage volume in people with knee osteoarthritis, *Osteoarthritis Cartilage* 16(7):851-854, 2008.

30. Elahi S, Cahue S, Felson DT, et al: The association between varus-valgus alignment and patellofemoral osteoarthritis, *Arthritis Rheum* 43(8):1874-1880, 2000.

31. Cahue S, Dunlop D, Hayes K, et al: Varus-valgus alignment in the progression of patellofemoral osteoarthritis, *Arthritis Rheum* 50(7):2184-2190, 2004.

32. Teichtahl AJ, Cicuttini FM, Janakiramanan N, et al: Static knee alignment and its association with radiographic knee osteoarthritis, *Osteoarthritis Cartilage* 14(9):958-962, 2006.

33. Tomaro J: Measurement of tibiofibular varum in subjects with unilateral overuse symptoms, *J Orthop Sports Phys Ther* 21(2):86-89, 1995.

34. Mahar SM, Livingston LA: Bilateral measurement of resting calcaneal stance position and tibial varum using digital photography and standardized positioning protocols, *J Am Podiatr Med Assoc* 99(3):198-205, 2009.

35. Seber S, Hazer B, Kose N, et al: Rotational profile of the lower extremity and foot progression angle: computerized tomographic examination of 50 male adults, *Arch Orthop Trauma Surg* 120(5-6):255-258, 2000.

36. Schneider B, Laubenberger J, Jemlich S, et al: Measurement of femoral antetorsion and tibial torsion by magnetic resonance imaging, *Br J Radiol* 70(834):575-579, 1997.

37. Yoshioka Y, Siu DW, Scudamore RA, et al: Tibial anatomy and functional axes, *J Orthop Res* 7(1):132-137, 1989.

38. Insall J, Salvati E: Patella position in the normal knee joint, *Radiology* 101(1):101-104, 1971.

39. Lin YF, Lin JJ, Cheng CK, et al: Association between sonographic morphology of vastus medialis obliquus and patellar alignment in patients with patellofemoral pain syndrome, *J Orthop Sports Phys Ther* 38(4):196-202, 2008.

40. Grelsamer RP, Weinstein CH, Gould J, et al: Patellar tilt: the physical examination correlates with MR imaging, *Knee* 15(1):3-8, 2008.

41. Watson CJ, Propps M, Galt W, et al: Reliability of McConnell's classification of patellar orientation in symptomatic and asymptomatic subjects, *J Orthop Sports Phys Ther* 29(7):378-385, 1999.

42. Roach KE, Miles TP: Normal hip and knee active range of motion: the relationship to age, *Phys Ther* 71(9):656-665, 1991.

43. Nonaka H, Mita K, Watakabe M, et al: Age-related changes in the interactive mobility of the hip and knee joints: a geometrical analysis, *Gait Posture* 15(3):236-243, 2002.

44. Drews JE, Vraciu JK, Pellino G. Range of motion of the joints of the lower extremity of newborns, *Phys Occup Ther Pediatr* 4(2):49-63, 1984.

45. Waugh KG, Minkel JL, Parker R, et al: Measurement of selected hip, knee, and ankle joint motions in newborns, *Phys Ther* 63(10):1616-1621, 1983.

46. Broughton NS, Wright J, Menelaus MB: Range of knee motion in normal neonates, *J Pediatr Orthop* 13(2):263-264, 1993.

47. Schwarze DJ, Denton JR: Normal values of neonatal lower limbs: an evaluation of 1,000 neonates, *J Pediatr Orthop* 13(6):758-760, 1993.

48. Ekstrand J, Wiktorsson M, Oberg B, et al: Lower extremity goniometric measurements: a study to determine their reliability, *Arch Phys Med Rehabil* 63(4):171-175, 1982.

49. Rothstein JM, Miller PJ, Roettger RF: Goniometric reliability in a clinical setting: elbow and knee measurements, *Phys Ther* 63(10):1611-1615, 1983.

50. Roach KE, Miles TP: Normal hip and knee active range of motion: the relationship to age, *Phys Ther* 71(9):656-665, 1991.

51. Johnson LL, van Dyk GE, Green JR III, et al: Clinical assessment of asymptomatic knees: comparison of men and women, *Arthroscopy* 14(4):347-359, 1998.

52. Hoppenfeld S: *Physical examination of the spine and extremities*, Norwalk, CT, 1976, Appleton & Lange.

53. Markolf KL, Mensch JS, Amstutz HC: Stiffness and laxity of the knee—the contributions of the supporting structures. A quantitative in vitro study, *J Bone Joint Surg Am* 58(5):583-594, 1976.

54. Markolf KL, Graff-Radford A, Amstutz HC: In vivo knee stability. A quantitative assessment using an instrumented clinical testing apparatus, *J Bone Joint Surg Am* 60(5):664-674, 1978.

55. Lundberg M, Messner K: Decrease in valgus stiffness after medial knee ligament injury. A 4-year clinical and mechanical follow-up study in 38 patients, *Acta Orthop Scand* 65(6):615-619, 1994.

56. Mills OS, Hull ML: Rotational flexibility of the human knee due to varus/valgus and axial moments in vivo, *J Biomech* 24(8):673-690, 1991.

57. Zhang LQ, Wang G: Dynamic and static control of the human knee joint in abduction-adduction, *J Biomech* 34(9):1107-1115, 2001.

58. Matsumoto H, Seedham BB, Suda Y, et al: Axis location of tibial rotation and its change with flexion angle, *Clin Orthop* 371:178-182, 2000.

59. Mossberg KA, Smith LK: Axial rotation of the knee in women, *J Orthop Sports Phys Ther* 4(4):236-240, 1983.

60. Osternig LR, Bates BT, James SL: Patterns of tibial rotary torque in knees of healthy subjects, *Med Sci Sports Exerc* 12:195-199, 1980.

61. Shoemaker SC, Markolf KL: In vivo rotatory knee stability, *J Bone Joint Surg Am* 164(2):208-216, 1982.

62. Buford WL Jr, Ivey FM Jr, Nakamura T, et al: Internal/external rotation moment arms of muscles at the knee: moment arms for the normal knee and the ACL-deficient knee, *Knee* 8:293-303, 2001.

63. Gollehon DL, Torzilli PA, Warren RF: The role of the posterolateral and cruciate ligaments in the stability of the human knee, *J Bone Joint Surg Am* 69(2):233-242, 1987.

64. Powers CM, Shellock FG, Pfaff M: Quantification of patellar tracking using kinematic MRI, *J Magn Reson Imaging* 8(3):724-732, 1998.

65. Sikorski JM, Peters J, Watt I: The importance of femoral rotation in chondromalacia patellae as shown by serial radiography, *J Bone Joint Surg Br* 61(4):435-442, 1979.

66. Novacheck TF: The biomechanics of running, *Gait Posture* 7(1):77-95, 1998.

67. Stansfield BW, Hillman SJ, Hazlewood ME, et al: Regression analysis of gait parameters with speed in normal children walking at self-selected speeds, *Gait Posture* 23(3):288-294, 2006.

68. Cupp T, Oeffinger D, Tylkowski C, et al: Age-related kinetic changes in normal pediatrics, *J Pediatr Orthop* 19(4):475-478, 1999.

69. Lafortune MA, Cavanagh PR, Sommer HJ III, et al: Three-dimensional kinematics of the human knee during walking, *J Biomech* 25(4):347-357, 1992.

70. Greenfield BH: *Rehabilitation of the knee: a problem-solving approach*, Philadelphia, 1993, FA Davis.

71. Grelsamer RP, McConnell J: *The patella: a team approach*, Gaithersburg, MD, 1998, Aspen Publishers.

72. Delp SL, Hess WE, Hungerford DS, et al: Variation of rotation moment arms with hip flexion, *J Biomech* 32(5):493-501, 1999.

73. Lindsay DM, Maitland M, Lowe RC, et al: Comparison of isokinetic internal and external hip rotation torques using different testing positions, *J Orthop Sports Phys Ther* 16(1):43-50, 1992.

74. Schmitt LC, Fitzgerald GK, Reisman AS, et al: Instability, laxity, and physical function in patients with medial knee osteoarthritis, *Phys Ther* 88(12):1506-1516, 2008.

75. Levinger P, Gilleard W: Tibia and rearfoot motion and ground reaction forces in subjects with patellofemoral pain syndrome during walking, *Gait Posture* 25(1):2-8, 2007.

76. Ford KR, Myer GD, Hewett TE: Valgus knee motion during landing in high school female and male basketball players, *Med Sci Sports Exerc* 35(10):1745-1750, 2003.

77. Pollard CD, Sigward SM, Powers CM: Gender differences in hip joint kinematics and kinetics during side-step cutting maneuver, *Clin J Sport Med* 17(1):38-42, 2007.

78. Sigward SM, Powers CM: The influence of gender on knee kinematics, kinetics and muscle activation patterns during side-step cutting, *Clin Biomech* 21(1):41-48, 2006.

79. Krosshaug T, Nakamae A, Boden B, et al: Estimating 3D joint kinematics from video sequences of running and cutting maneuvers—assessing the accuracy of simple visual inspection, *Gait Posture* 26(3):378-385, 2007.

80. Olsen OE, Myklebust G, Engebretsen L, et al: Injury mechanisms for anterior cruciate ligament injuries in team handball a systematic video analysis, *Am J Sports Med* 32(4):1002-1012, 2004.

81. Lee TQ, Yang BY, Sandusky MD, et al: The effects of tibial rotation on the patellofemoral joint: assessment of the changes in situ strain in the peripatellar retinaculum and the patellofemoral contact pressures and area, *J Rehabil Res Dev* 38(5):463-469, 2001.

82. Lee TQ, Morris G, Csintalan RP: The influence of tibial and femoral rotation on patellofemoral contact area and pressure, *J Orthop Sports Phys Ther* 33(11):686-693, 2003.

83. Hefzy MS, Jackson WT, Saddemi SR, et al: Effects of tibial rotations on patellar tracking and patello-femoral contact areas, *J Biomed Eng* 14(4):329-343, 1991.

84. Salsich GB, Perman WH. Patellofemoral joint contact area is influenced by tibiofemoral rotation alignment in individuals who have patellofemoral pain, *J Orthop Sports Phys Ther* 37(9):521-528, 2007.

85. Myer GD, Ford KR, Brent JL, et al: Differential neuromuscular training effects on ACL injury risk factors in "high-risk" versus "low-risk" athletes, *BMC Musculoskeletal Disord* 8:39, 2007.

86. Cowan SM, Bennell KL, Crossley KM, et al: Physical therapy alters recruitment of the vasti in patellofemoral pain syndrome, *Med Sci Sports Exerc* 34(12):1879-1885, 2002.

87. McConnell J: The management of chondromalacia patellae: a long term solution, *Aust J Physiother* 32:215-223, 1986.

88. Van Dillen LR, McDonnell MK, Fleming DA, et al: Effect of knee and hip position on hip extension range of motion in individuals with and without low back pain, *J Orthop Sports Phys Ther* 30(6):307-316, 2000.

89. Harris-Hayes M, Wendl PM, Sahrmann SA, et al: Does stabilization of the tibiofemoral joint affect passive prone hip rotation range of motion measures in unimpaired individuals? A preliminary report, *Physiother Theory Pract* 23(6):315-323, 2007.

90. Winslow J, Yoder E: Patellofemoral pain in female ballet dancers: correlation with iliotibial band tightness and tibial external rotation, *J Orthop Sports Phys Ther* 22(1):18-21, 1995.

91. Cichanowski HR, Schmitt JS, Johnson RJ, et al: Hip strength in collegiate female athletes with patellofemoral pain, *Med Sci Sports Exerc* 39(8):1227-1232, 2007.

92. Fredericson M, White JJ, Macmahon JM, et al: Quantitative analysis of the relative effectiveness of 3 iliotibial band stretches, *Arch Phys Med Rehabil* 83(5):589-592, 2002.

93. Willson JD, Ireland ML, Davis I: Core strength and lower extremity alignment during single leg squats, *Med Sci Sports Exerc* 38(5):945-952, 2006.

94. Willson JD, Binder-Macleod S, Davis IS: Lower extremity jumping mechanics of female athletes with and without patellofemoral pain before and after exertion, *Am J Sports Med* 36(8):1587-1596, 2008.

95. Chan GN, Smith AW, Kirtley C, et al: Changes in knee moments with contralateral versus ipsilateral cane usage in females with knee osteoarthritis, *Clin Biomech* 20(4):396-404, 2005.

96. Farrokhi S, Pollard CD, Souza RB, et al: Trunk position influences the kinematics, kinetics, and muscle activity of the lead lower extremity during the forward lunge exercise, *J Orthop Sports Phys Ther* 38(7):403-409, 2008.

97. Olivier N, Legrand R, Rogez J, et al: One-leg cycling versus arm cranking: which is most appropriate for physical conditioning after knee surgery? *Arch Phys Med Rehabil* 89(3):508-512, 2008.

98. Butler RJ, Barrios JA, Royer T, et al: Effect of laterally wedged foot orthoses on rearfoot and hip mechanics in patients with medial knee osteoarthritis, *Prosthet Orthot Int* 33(2):107-116, 2009.

99. Gelis A, Coudeyre E, Hudry C, et al: Is there an evidence-based efficacy for the use of foot orthotics in knee and hip osteoarthritis? Elaboration of French clinical practice guidelines, *Joint Bone Spine* 75(6):714-720, 2008.

100. Collins N, Crossley K, Beller E, et al: Foot orthoses and physiotherapy in the treatment of patellofemoral pain syndrome: randomised clinical trial, *BMJ* 337:a1735, 2008.

101. Franz JR, Dicharry J, Riley PO, et al: The influence of arch supports on knee torques relevant to knee osteoarthritis. *Med Sci Sports Exerc* 40(5):913-917, 2006.

102. Bizzini M, Childs JD, Piva SR, et al: Systematic review of the quality of randomized controlled trials for patello-femoral pain syndrome, *J Orthop Sports Phys Ther* 33(1):4-20, 2003.

103. Gross MT, Foxworth JL: The role of foot orthoses as an intervention for patellofemoral pain, *J Orthop Sports Phys Ther* 33(11):661-670, 2003.

104. Fitzgerald GK, Childs JD, Ridge TM, et al: Agility and perturbation training for a physically active individual with knee osteoarthritis, *Phys Ther* 82(4):372-382, 2002.

105. Fitzgerald GK, Axe MJ, Snyder-Mackler L: The efficacy of perturbation training in nonoperative anterior cruciate ligament rehabilitation programs for physical active individuals, *Phys Ther* 80(2):128-140, 2000.

106. Hewett TE, Paterno MV, Myer GD: Strategies for enhancing proprioception and neuromuscular control of the knee, *Clin Orthop* 1(402):76-94, 2002.

107. Blanpied P, Carroll R, Douglas T, et al: Effectiveness of lateral slide exercise in an anterior cruciate ligament reconstruction rehabilitation home exercise program, *Phys Ther* 30(10):609-611, 2000.

108. Louw Q, Grimmer K, Vaughan CL: Biomechanical outcomes of a knee neuromuscular exercise programme among adolescent basketball players: a pilot study, *Phys Ther Sport* 7(2):65-73, 2006.

109. Fitzgerald GK, Axe MJ, Snyder-Mackler L: A decision-making scheme for returning patients to high-level activity with nonoperative treatment after anterior cruciate ligament rupture, *Knee Surg Sports Traumatol Arthrosc* 8(2):76-82, 2000.

110. Foroughi N, Smith R, Vanwanseele B: The association of external knee adduction moment with biomechanical variables in osteoarthritis: a systematic review, *Knee* 16(5):303-309, 2009.

111. Miyazaki T, Wada M, Kawahara H, et al: Dynamic load at baseline can predict radiographic disease progression in medial compartment knee OA, *Ann Rheum Dis* 61:617-622, 2006.

112. Guo M, Axe MJ, Manal K: The influence of foot progression angle on the knee adduction moment during walking and stair climbing in pain free individuals with knee osteoarthritis, *Gait Posture* 26(3):436-441, 2007.

113. Jenkyn TR, Hunt MA, Jones IC, et al: Toe-out gait in patients with knee osteoarthritis partially transforms external knee adduction moment into flexion moment during early stance phase of gait: a tri-planar kinetic mechanism, *J Biomech* 16(5):591-599, 2008.

114. Lynn SK, Costigan PA: Effect of foot rotation on knee kinetics and hamstring activation in older adults with and without signs of knee osteoarthritis, *Clin Biomech* 23(6):779-786, 2008.

115. Chang A, Hurwitz D, Dunlop D, et al: The relationship between toe-out angle during gait and progression of medial tibiofemoral osteoarthritis, *Ann Rheum Dis* 66(10):1271-1275, 2007.

116. Wang JW, Kuo KN, Andriacchi TP, et al: The influence of walking mechanics and time on the results of proximal tibial osteotomy, *J Bone Joint Surg Am* 72(6):905-909, 1990.

117. Lindenfeld TN, Hewett TE, Andriacchi TP: Joint loading with valgus bracing in patients with varus gonarthrosis, *Clin Orthop Relat Res* 344:290-297, 1997.

118. Draper ER, Cable JM, Sanchez-Ballester J, et al: Improvement in function after valgus bracing of the knee. An analysis of gait symmetry, *J Bone Joint Surg Br* 82(7):1001-1005, 2000.

119. Irrgang JJ, Snyder-Mackler L, Wainner RS, et al: Development of a patient-reported measure of function of the knee, *J Bone Joint Surg Am* 80(8):1132-1145, 1998.

120. Magee DJ: *Orthopedic physical assessment*, ed 4, Philadelphia, 2002, Saunders.

121. Hardcastle P, Nade S: The significance of the Trendelenburg test, *J Bone Joint Surg Br* 67(5):741-746, 1985.

122. Cyriax J: *Textbook of orthopaedic medicine I: diagnosis of soft tissue lesions*, ed 8, London, 1982, Bailliere Tindall.

123. Bijl D, Dekker J, van Baar ME et al: Validity of Cyriax's concept capsular pattern for the diagnosis of osteoarthritis of hip and/or knee, *Scand J Rheumatol* 27(5):347-351, 1998.

124. Hayes KW, Petersen C, Falconer J: An examination of Cyriax's passive motion tests with patients having osteoarthritis of the knee, *Phys Ther* 74(8):697-707, 1994.

125. Lewek MD, Rudolph KS, Snyder-Mackler L: Control of frontal plane knee laxity during gait in patients with medial compartment knee osteoarthritis, *Osteoarthritis Cartilage* 12(9):745-751, 2004.

126. Lewek MD, Ramsey DK, Snyder-Mackler L, et al: Knee stabilization in patients with medial compartment knee osteoarthritis, *Arthritis Rheum* 52(9):2845-2853. 2005.

127. Childs JD, Sparto PJ, Fitzgerald GK, et al: Alterations in lower extremity movement and muscle activation patterns in individuals with knee osteoarthritis, *Clin Biomech* 19(1):44-49. 2004.

128. Jenkinson CM, Doherty M, Avery AJ, et al: Effects of dietary intervention and quadriceps strengthening exercises on pain and function in overweight people with knee pain: randomised controlled trial, *BMJ* 339:b3170, 2009.

129. Neyret P, Robinson AH, Le CB, et al: Patellar tendon length: the factor in patellar instability? *Knee* 9(1):3-6, 2002.

130. Escala J, Mellado J, Olona M, et al: Objective patellar instability: MR-based quantitative assessment of potentially associated anatomical features, *Knee Surg Sports Traumatol Arthrosc* 14(3):264-272, 2006.

131. Simmons E Jr, Cameron JC: Patella alta and recurrent dislocation of the patella, *Clin Orthop Relat Res* (274):265-269, 1992.

132. Leung YF, Wai YL, Leung YC: Patella alta in southern China. A new method of measurement, *Int Orthop* 20(5):305-310, 1996.

133. Lancourt JE, Cristini JA: Patella alta and patella infera. Their etiological role in patellar dislocation, chondromalacia, and apophysitis of the tibial tubercle, *J Bone Joint Surg Am* 57(8):1112-1115, 1975.

134. Brattstrom H: Patella alta in non-dislocating knee joints, *Acta Orthop Scand* 41(5):578-588, 1970.

135. Ahlback S, Mattsson S: Patella alta and gonarthrosis, *Acta Radiol Diagn* 19(4):578-584, 1978.

136. Al-Sayyad MJ, Cameron JC: Functional outcome after tibial tubercle transfer for the painful patella alta, *Clin Orthop Relat Res* (396):152-162, 2002.

137. Ward SR, Terk MR, Powers CM: Patella alta: association with patellofemoral alignment and changes in contact area during weight-bearing, *J Bone Joint Surg Am* 89(8):1749-1755, 2007.

138. Ward SR, Powers CM: The influence of patella alta on patellofemoral joint stress during normal and fast walking, *Clin Biomech* 19(10):1040-1047, 2004.

139. Mulligan BR: *Manual therapy: "NAGS", "SNAGS", "MWMs" etc*, ed 3, Wellington, New Zealand, 1995, Plane View Press.

140. Metheny JA, Mayor MB: Hoffa disease: chronic impingement of the infrapatellar fat pad, *Am J Knee Surg* 1(2):134-139, 1988.

141. Jacobson JA, Lenchik L, Ruhoy MK, et al: MR imaging of the infrapatellar fat pad of Hoffa, *Radiographics* 17:675-691, 1997.

142. Myer GD, Ford KR, Paterno MV, et al: The effects of generalized joint laxity on risk of anterior cruciate ligament injury in young female athletes, *Am J Sports Med* 36(6):1073-1080, 2008.

143. Loudon JK, Jenkins W, Loudon KL: The relationship between static posture and ACL injury in female athletes, *J Orthop Sports Phys Ther* 24(2):91-97, 1996.

144. Loudon JK: Measurement of knee-joint-position sense in women with genu recurvatum, *J Sport Rehabil* 9(1):15-25, 2000.

145. Ramesh R, Von Arx O, Azzopardi T, et al: The risk of anterior cruciate ligament rupture with generalised joint laxity, *J Bone Joint Surg Br* 87(6):800-803, 2005.

146. Noyes FR, Dunworth LA, Andriacchi TP, et al: Knee hyperextension gait abnormalities in unstable knees: recognition and preoperative gait retraining, *Am J Sports Med* 24(1):35-45, 1996.

147. Cowan SM, Hodges PW, Bennell KL, et al: Altered vasti recruitment when people with patellofemoral pain syndrome complete a postural task, *Arch Phys Med Rehabil* 83(7):989-995, 2002.

148. Cowan SM, Bennell KL, Hodges PW, et al: Delayed onset of electromyographic activity of vastus medialis obliquus relative to vastus lateralis in subjects with patellofemoral pain syndrome, *Arch Phys Med Rehabil* 82(2):183-189, 2001.

149. Callaghan MJ, McCarthy CJ, Oldham JA: Electromyographic fatigue characteristics of the quadriceps in patellofemoral pain syndrome, *Man Ther* 6(1):27-33, 2001.

150. Cesarelli M, Bifulco P, Bracale M: Study of the control strategy of the quadriceps muscle in anterior knee pain, *IEEE Trans Rehab Eng* 8(3):330-341, 2000.

151. Owings TM, Grabiner MD: Motor control of the vastus medialis oblique and vastus lateralis muscles is disrupted during eccentric contractions in subjects with patellofemoral pain, *Am J Sports Med* 30(4):483-487, 2002.

152. Karst GM, Willet GM: Onset timing of electromyographic activity in the vastus medialis oblique and vastus lateralis muscle in subjects with and without patellofemoral pain syndrome, *Phys Ther* 75(9):813-823, 1995.

153. Powers CM, Landel R, Perry J: Timing and intensity of vastus muscle activity during functional activities in subjects with and without patellofemoral pain, *Phys Ther* 76(9):946-955, 1996.

154. Sheehy P, Burdett RG, Irrgang JJ, et al: An electromyographic study of vastus medialis oblique and vastus lateralis activity while ascending and descending steps, *J Orthop Sports Phys Ther* 27(6):423-429, 1998.

155. Mohr KJ, Kvitne RS, Pink MM, et al: Electromyography of the quadriceps in patellofemoral pain with patellar subluxation, *Clin Orthop Relat Res* (415):261-271, 2003.

156. Elias JJ, Kilambi S, Goerke DR, et al: Improving vastus medialis obliquus function reduces pressure applied to lateral patellofemoral cartilage, *J Orthop Res* 27(5):578-583, 2009.

157. Ekstrom RA, Donatelli RA, Carp KC: Electromyographic analysis of core trunk, hip, and thigh muscles during 9 rehabilitation exercises, *J Orthop Sports Phys Ther* 37(12):754-762, 2007.

158. Yip SL, Ng GY: Biofeedback supplementation to physiotherapy exercise programme for rehabilitation of patellofemoral pain syndrome: a randomized controlled pilot study, *Clin Rehabil* 20(12):1050-1057, 2006.

159. Kirnap M, Calis M, Turgut AO, et al: The efficacy of EMG-biofeedback training on quadriceps muscle strength in patients after arthroscopic meniscectomy, *N Z Med J* 118(1224):U1704, 2005.

160. Steinkamp LA, Dillingham MF, Markel MD, et al: Biomechanical considerations in patellofemoral joint rehabilitation, *Am J Sports Med* 21(3):438-444, 1993.

161. Bockrath K, Wooden C, Worrell T, et al: Effects of patella taping on patella position and perceived pain, *Med Sci Sports Exerc* 25(9):989-992, 1993.

162. Salsich GB, Brechter JH, Farwell D, et al: The effects of patellar taping on knee kinetics, kinematics, and vastus lateralis muscle activity during stair ambulation in individuals with patellofemoral pain, *J Orthop Sports Phys Ther* 32(1):3-10, 2002.

163. Gilleard W, McConnell J, Parson D: The effect of patellar taping of vastus medialis obliquus and vastus lateralis muscle activity in persons with patellofemoral pain, *Phys Ther* 78(1):25-32, 1998.

164. Powers CM, Landel R, Sosnick T, et al: The effects of patellar taping on stride characteristics and joint motion in subjects with patellofemoral pain, *J Orthop Sports Phys Ther* 26(6):286-291, 1997.

165. Warden SJ, Hinman RS, Watson MA Jr, et al: Patellar taping and bracing for the treatment of chronic knee pain: a systematic review and meta-analysis, *Arthritis Rheum* 59(1):73-83, 2008.

166. Crossley K, Cowan SM, Bennell KL, et al: Patellar taping: is clinical success supported by scientific evidence? *Man Ther* 5(3):142-150, 2000.

167. Ryan CG, Rowe PJ: An electromyographic study to investigate the effects of patellar taping on the vastus medialis/vastus lateralis ratio in asymptomatic participants, *Physiother Theory Pract* 22(6):309-315, 2006.

168. Bennell K, Duncan M, Cowan S: Effect of patellar taping on vasti onset timing, knee kinematics, and kinetics in asymptomatic individuals with a delayed onset of vastus medialis oblique, *J Orthop Res* 24(9):1854-1860, 2006.

169. Cowan SM, Hodges PW, Crossley KM, et al: Patellar taping does not change the amplitude of electromyographic activity of the vasti in a stair stepping task, *Br J Sports Med* 40(1):30-34, 2006.

170. Christou EA: Patellar taping increases vastus medialis oblique activity in the presence of patellofemoral pain, *J Electromyogr Kinesiol* 14(4):495-504, 2004.

171. Pfeiffer RP, DeBeliso M, Shea KG, et al: Kinematic MRI assessment of McConnell taping before and after exercise, *Am J Sports Med* 32(3):621-628, 2004.

172. MacGregor K, Gerlach S, Mellor R, et al: Cutaneous stimulation from patella tape causes a differential increase in vasti muscle activity in people with patellofemoral pain, *J Orthop Res* 23(2):351-358, 2005.

173. Maxey L, Magnusson J: *Rehabilitation for the postsurgical orthopedic patient*, ed 2, St Louis, Mosby, 2007.

174. Cioppa-Mosca J, Cahill JB, Cavanaugh JT, et al: Postsurgical rehabilitation guidelines for the orthopedic clinician, St Louis, Mosby, 2006.

CHAPTER **7**

APPENDIX

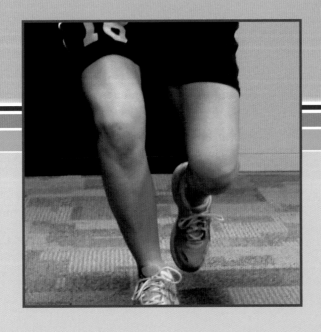

Tibiofemoral Rotation Syndrome

The principal movement impairment in tibiofemoral rotation (TFR) syndrome is knee joint pain associated with impaired rotation of the tibiofemoral joint (lateral rotation of the tibia and/or medial rotation of the femur). Correction of impairment often decreases symptoms. The subcategories of TFR syndrome are TFR with valgus (TFRVal) syndrome: Valgus knee during static/dynamic activities and TFR with varus (TFRVar) syndrome: Varus knee during static/dynamic activities.

Symptoms and History

- Pain along knee joint line or peripatellar pain
- Pain associated with weight-bearing activities (running) or non–weight-bearing activities (sitting)
- History of early stages of OA/DJD
- Often seen in individuals participating in activities requiring LR of the tibia such as ballet dancers, soccer players, equestrians, skaters, and swimmers (breast stroke)
- In ITB friction syndrome, diffuse pain is located over region of the lateral epicondyle of femur. Often aggravated with running downhill or cycling

Common Referring Diagnoses

- MCL sprain (acute, grade 1, or chronic)
- Patellofemoral joint dysfunction
- Hamstring tendinopathy or strain
- ITB friction syndrome
- Popliteus tendinopathy or muscle strain
- Pes anserine bursitis or tendinopathy
- Meniscal injury

Key Tests and Signs for Movement Impairment

Alignment Analysis

Standing

- LR of tibia or MR of femur
  - TFRVar: Varus knee, supinated foot; knee hyperextension may be present
  - TFRVal: Valgus knee, pronated foot, oblique popliteal crease

Movement Impairment Analysis

- Step-down, squat, or single-leg hop: TFR or knee valgus
  - If painful, correction decreases symptoms
- Gait: Observe MR of femur on stance or LR of tibia during swing
  - Varus: May demonstrate a varus thrust
- Single-leg stance: Observe MR of femur on stance leg on involved side Observe LR of tibia during knee flexion of non–weight-bearing leg on involved side
- Prone knee flexion: Observe LR of tibia
- Prone hip rotation: Excessive rotation or gliding of tibia relative to femur

Aggravating or Frequent Functional Activity

- Observe MR of femur or LR of tibia during activity
  - If painful, correction decreases symptoms

Muscle Length

- Hip flexor length test: Short TFL-ITB.
  - May observe rotation of tibia as hip is extended in midline
  - May have pain in neutral hip position
  - Decreased pain with manual correction of tibial rotation

Muscle Strength/Performance Impairments

- Weak posterior gluteus medius
- Weak intrinsic hip LR. Observe LR of tibia with performance
- Weak TFL

ACL, Anterior cruciate ligament; *AVN,* avascular necrosis; *DJD,* degenerative joint disease; *FCL,* fibular collateral ligament; *ITB,* iliotibial band; *LCL,* lateral collateral ligament; *LR,* lateral rotation; *MCL,* medial collateral ligament; *MR,* medial rotation; *OA,* osteoarthritis; *PCL,* posterior cruciate ligament; *RA,* rheumatoid arthritis; *ROM,* range of motion; *SCFE,* slipped capital femoral epiphysis; *TCL,* tibial collateral ligament; *TFL,* tensor fascia latae; *TFL-ITB,* tensor fascia latae-iliotibial band.

Source of Signs and Symptoms

Tibiofemoral Joint Involvement
- Palpation: Positive pain along joint line
- Meniscal tests: May experience mild tenderness with meniscal tests that involve rotation

Patellofemoral Pain
- Palpation: Positive pain along facets of patella and femoral condyles

ITB Friction Syndrome (ITB FS)
- Palpation: Positive pain along the insertion of ITB over the lateral epicondyle
- Hip flexor length test: Resisted knee extension may increase lateral knee pain
- Noble test: Positive

Meniscus
- Suggestive history
- Locking of knee
- Two positive provocative tests[1]
  - McMurray's
  - Joint line palpation (significant pain)
  - Apley's
  - Bohler's
  - Steinman's
  - Payr's

ACL
- Suggestive history
- Positive anterior drawer test
- Positive Lachman's test

PCL
- Suggestive history
- Positive sag sign
- Positive posterior drawer

TCL (MCL)
- Suggestive history
- Positive valgus test

FCL (LCL)
- Suggestive history
- Positive varus test

Associated Signs or Contributing Factors

Joint Integrity
- May have excessive tibiofemoral rotation ROM

Muscle Length
- Short gastrocnemius
- Active or passive dorsiflexion with the knee extended
- May be painful and may observe tibial LR

Muscle Strength/Performance Impairments
- Poor functional performance of quads in stairs and sit-to-stand
- May have poor abdominal control

Structural Variations
- Femoral antetorsion
- Genu recurvatum
- Genu valgus
- Tibial torsion
- Tibial varum in frontal or sagittal plane
- "Hypermobility syndrome" = increased general laxity

Differential Diagnosis

Movement Diagnosis
- Patellar lateral glide
- Tibiofemoral accessory hypermobility
- Low back syndrome
- Femoral syndrome
- Hip extension/knee extension

Potential Diagnoses Requiring Referral Suggested by Signs and Symptoms

Musculoskeletal
- Meniscal injury
- Internal derangement
- OA/DJD
- MCL sprain (grade 2 or 3)
- LCL sprain
- Posterolateral corner injury
- Acute or recurrent patellar dislocation or subluxation
- Fracture
- Sinding-Larsen-Johansson disease
- AVN of knee
- Osteochondritis dissecans: Baker's cyst
- SCFE
- AVN of hip
- Legg-Calvé-Perthes disease
- L3-L5 radiculopathy

Other
- RA
- Gout
- Lyme disease
- Neoplasm

Treatment

Emphasis of treatment is decreasing excessive rotation between the tibia on the femur.

Patient Education

The goal of patient education is correction of impaired postural habits and movements.

I. Alignment
    A. Improve alignment between femur and tibia.
        1. Relax/unlock knees to reduce knee hyperextension if present.
        2. Ideally, align knees over feet with neutral rotation of hips and tibias by decreasing MR of femur and LR of tibia.
        3. NOTE: If structural tibial torsion or femoral anteversion or retroversion is present, ideal alignment will not be possible. Instruct patient in proper alignment that accommodates these structural impairments. For example, if the person has the following:
            a. Tibial torsion: Allow appearance lateral deviation of the foot or "turn out" of the tibia and the foot.
            b. Femoral anteversion (torsion): Allow the appearance of MR of femur.
    B. Valgus: Individuals often stand with foot aligned laterally to the hip. The individual may or may not be able to correct entirely. Must accommodate for structural variations such as structural valgus, excessive soft tissue of thigh.
II. Functional activities that contribute to the movement impairment must be addressed.
    A. Gait
        1. Avoid hip MR and knee hyperextension during stance phase of gait cycle.
        2. Encourage proper heel-to-toe gait pattern (common fault is decreased push-off).
            a. If patient has the impairment of hyperextension, cue the patient to "lift the heel" to discourage recruitment of the hamstrings.
            b. If patient demonstrates MR of the femur without hyperextension, cue the patient to contract the gluteal muscles to control femoral MR. If the patient has difficulty contracting the gluteals on command an exercise such as weight shifting may be useful to teach proper contraction. Gait can then be attempted to see if contraction ability improves.
            c. TFRVar: In severe cases, the patient may be instructed to walk with a slight toe-out gait. Instruct the patient to rotate laterally at the hip and avoid lateral rotation at the tibiofemoral joint.
            d. Patient may require an assistive device to decrease the forces through the affected knee.
                (1) Cane is used in the opposite hand of the impaired lower extremity.
                (2) EXCEPTION: If patient has a varus alignment and using the cane in the opposite hand does not reduce symptoms, the cane may be placed on the same side of the affected knee. Observe gait to determine if desired effect of reducing varus alignment is being achieved. Also use the patient's pain response to determine the proper side of cane placement.
    B. Sit-to-stand; stand-to-sit
        1. Slide forward in chair.
        2. Feet hip-width apart and aligned behind knees.
        3. Use quadriceps and gluteus maximus muscles to lift body up and forward out of chair.
            a. Ensure that the tibia advances over the foot with performance (shifts weight forward).
            b. Avoid hip MR.
            c. Avoid pulling knees back to meet body.
    C. Stairs
        1. Instruct in use of rail to decrease weight bearing on the involved limb.
        2. Ascending stairs.
            a. Use quadriceps and gluteus maximus muscles to lift body up and forward.
                (1) Ensure that the tibia advances over the foot with performance (shifts weight forward).
            b. Avoid hip MR.
            c. Avoid pulling knee back to meet body.
        3. Descending stairs.
            a. Avoid hip MR.
            b. If difficult to perform without pain during initial visit, may need to instruct in step-to pattern leading with the involved extremity.
            c. If significantly limited, patient may need to descend stairs backward.
    D. Personal activities (work, school, leisure activities)
        1. Address activities that patients are performing throughout the day that may contribute to the movement impairment. These may include prolonged sitting, driving, and getting in and out of a car.
        2. Address fitness activities early to maintain patient's routine. Modifications or alternative activities may need to be provided. Modify intensity of activities to decrease stress to injured tissues.
            a. Running
                (1) Interval training is recommended.
                    (a) Begin with walking program and gradually mix in short bouts of running. Gradually increase the

time running and decrease the time walking.

(2) Modify surface of training if indicated.

(a) Instruct patient to initiate running with surfaces that reduce the ground reaction force on the lower extremities. A track or chip trail is better than asphalt, and asphalt is better than concrete. Concrete should be avoided if possible.

(b) Running on a street with a camber may contribute to common knee problems such as ITB friction syndrome. Runners should be encouraged to either avoid the camber or alternate the direction of their run.

(3) Modify activities that may encourage TFL-ITB recruitment over gluteus medius/maximus recruitment.

(a) Biking: Use of toe clips can encourage overrecruitment of the TFL-ITB. Patient should be encouraged to focus more on the pushing phase of the cycle and less on the pulling phase.

(b) Running: Patients often run with their body weight shifted posteriorly (referred to as *chasing their center of gravity*). Cue the patient to shift body weight slightly forward to encourage better recruitment of the gluteal muscles. Sometimes, use of a small incline will assist patients in shifting the weight forward.

Home Exercise Program

Patients should be instructed that they should not feel an increase in their symptoms during the performance of their exercises. In addition to monitoring for symptoms, they should not experience a "pressure" in the knee during exercises. If either pain or pressure occurs, they should review the instructions to the exercise to be sure that they are performing it correctly and try again. If they still experience pain or pressure, they should discontinue this exercise until they return for their next visit.

I.   Improve muscle performance

A. Intrinsic hip lateral rotators and posterior gluteus medius muscles

1. Strengthening: Progressing from easiest to most difficult.

a. Prone hip lateral rotation isometrics (prone foot pushes).

b. Prone hip abduction.

c. Sidelying hip abduction with lateral rotation (level 1, 2, or 3).

(1) Monitor to be sure patient feels the contraction in the "seat" region; the

therapist must palpate to be sure that the patient is recruiting the correct muscles. Common cues for improve performance of the hip lateral rotators include the following:

(a) Positioning: The pelvis may be rotated posteriorly too far. Ask the patient to roll the pelvis anteriorly.

(b) Positioning: Place a pillow between the knees.

(c) Spin the thigh around an axis longitudinally through the femur.

(d) CAUTION: Do not use foot as a guide for lateral rotation of the hip.

d. Hip lateral rotation against resistance.

(1) Sitting: Ligaments of the knee are most lax when the knee is in 90 degrees of flexion. This exercise should be monitored closely to be sure the patient is able to stabilize the tibia while performing this exercise.

(2) Standing.

e. Lunges.

(1) Perform with lower extremity in good alignment; initially without weight or resistance.

(2) Progression.

(a) Resisted: Using an elastic band around proximal thigh, the therapist pulls in the direction of MR and adduction.

(b) Patients can hold weights in their hands.

2. Recruitment.

a. Weight shifting with gluteal squeeze on the stance lower extremity.

(1) Progress to standing on one leg with correct alignment.

(2) Progress to resisted activities of the opposite leg while standing on the affected leg.

B. Gluteus maximus muscles

1. Prone hip extension with the knee flexed.

a. Positioning: Patient's that have short hip flexors with require a pillow under the pelvis.

b. Patient must be able to control the tibial positioning during prone knee flexion to begin this exercise.

2. Lunges, squats.

C. Abdominal muscles (if appropriate)

1. Strengthening: Lower abdominal progression as described by Sahrmann.[2]

2. Recruitment: Encourage patient to pull in abdominals with functional activities.

D. Quadriceps muscle

1. Functional activities.

a. Sit to stand, stand to sit, step-ups/step-downs as tolerated.

b. Lunges, wall sits as tolerated.

SPECIAL NOTE: *Knees with Malalignment or Excessive Varus or Valgus*

It is thought that the quadriceps muscles provide some shock absorption to the knee; however, recent studies show that increased quadriceps activity can actually increase the progression of OA in knees with malalignment. One must consider the compression forces that the quadriceps can add to a joint before administering quadriceps strengthening activities. Quadriceps performance should be enhanced only through the proper performance of functional activities, and therapeutic exercises to hypertrophy the quadriceps should be avoided in patients with malalignment of the knees.

II. Improve extensibility

A. TFL-ITB and rectus femoris muscles (listed in the order of least aggressive to most aggressive)

1. During all stretching exercises, be sure that the patient has good abdominal support to avoid pelvic anterior tilt or rotation.

   a. Prone bilateral knee flexion: With knees and feet together, flex both knees at the same time, monitor tibial position and avoid LR of tibia.

2. May need to begin with femurs in an abducted position and gradually adduct the hips as the patient improves.

3. Prone hip lateral rotation: Monitor tibial position and avoid LR of tibia.

4. Hip flexor length test position: Allow the hip to abduct as it extends, then actively adduct with the tibia in neutral (foot pointing forward or slightly inward).

5. Ober test position: Hip in LR and tibia in neutral to slight MR (level 3 of posterior gluteus medius progression).

B. Gastrocnemius and hamstring muscles

1. Active sitting knee extension with dorsiflexion in neutral hip rotation.

2. Hamstring muscles: Prolonged passive stretches in supine.

3. Gastrocnemius muscles: Standing runners stretch.

a. Patients with excessive pronation must have their arch supported during this stretch (shoes on).

III. Other

A. Taping

1. Posterior knee X taping may be helpful.

   a. To control rotation during taping, the patient should be positioned so that the lower extremity is in the desired position before applying the tape. The patient is asked to contract the gluteal muscles to laterally rotate the thigh.

   b. ITB friction syndrome: Tape placed along the ITB to support the tissue.

B. Bracing

1. Although bracing may not be the first choice in treatment for this patient population, it may be an option for patients who are not achieving adequate pain control with their activities.

   a. One theoretical benefit of bracing is that it can increase proprioception of the knee.[3-5]

   b. Unloader bracing has seemed to be beneficial in patients with OA and malalignment.[6,7] Must consider patient goals, motivation, and anthropomorphics.

C. Orthotics

1. Temporary orthotics may be tried to determine if they will be helpful; then custom orthotics may be ordered if indicated.

   a. Valgus.

      (1) For pronation that is flexible: Orthotics to assist in controlling motion at the foot.

   b. Varus.

      (1) For a rigid supinated foot: Cushioned insert to improve shock absorption.

D. Pain control

1. Modalities.

   a. Ice as often as needed.

2. Modify activities to reduce stress to injured tissues.

   a. Daily activities.

   b. Fitness activities.

E. Neuromuscular training (see Box 7-2)

NOTES

Tibiofemoral Hypomobility Syndrome

The principal movement impairment in tibiofemoral hypomobility (TFHypo) syndrome is associated with a limitation in the physiological motion of the knee. This limitation may result from degenerative changes in the joint or the effects of prolonged immobilization. In type I TFHypo syndrome, the potential for recovery of ROM is good; whereas the potential for recovery in type II TFHypo syndrome is poor.

Symptoms and History

- Pain with weight bearing (gait, standing, stairs), that decreases with rest
- Pain deep in joint and often described as vague
- Gradual onset

Degeneration

- May complain of stiffness, especially after periods of rest
- History of remote trauma or surgery to the knee
- Narrowing of joint space seen on standing radiographs
- Typically seen in older adults >55 years old

Immobilization

- History of recent trauma or surgery
- Knee ROM has not progressed as expected (slow recovery)

Common Referring Diagnosis

- OA/DJD
- Knee pain
- Patellofemoral joint dysfunction
- Knee contracture

Key Tests and Signs for Movement Impairment

Alignment Analysis

- *Both conditions* may have enlarged joint or signs of mild inflammation.

Movement Impairment Analysis

- Step-down test: Includes pain and impaired movement associated with lack of knee flexion.
- Gait: Antalgic gait. Ambulates with a flexed knee; decreased stride length.

Aggravating or Frequent Functional Activity

- Observe limitation of knee ROM during activity.

Joint Integrity

- ROM: Decreased PROM flexion and/or extension. Includes pain at end ROM tested passively.

Degeneration

- Repeated passive end-range flexion and extension should decrease pain or improve symptoms.
- May have PROM loss in capsular pattern (flexion greater than extension).

Source of Signs and Symptoms

Joint Involvement

- Palpation: Positive pain along joint line

Meniscal Tests

- May experience mild tenderness with meniscal tests that involve rotation

Associated Signs or Contributing Factors

- *Both conditions* may stand in knee flexion.

Muscle Length

- Short gastrocnemius
- Short hip flexors
- Short hamstrings

Muscle Strength/Performance Impairments

- Manual muscle test: Weakness
  - Gluteus maximus
  - Gastrocnemius
  - Gluteus medius/hip intrinsic LRs
- Poor functional performance of quadriceps in stairs and sit-to-stand

Structural Variations

- May have genu varus or genu valgus deformity

Movement Impairments

- Gait: Decreased use of plantarflexors from loading response to preswing to control/advance tibia
- Visible quadriceps atrophy

Differential Diagnosis

Movement Diagnosis

- Tibiofemoral rotation

Potential Diagnosis Requiring Referral Suggested by Signs and Symptoms

Musculoskeletal

- Fracture
- AVN of knee
- Meniscal dysfunction
- Ligamentous injury (grades 2 and 3)
- Rapidly increasing varus deformity
- AVN of hip
- OA of hip
- L3-L5 radiculopathy
- Spinal stenosis

Other

- Baker's cyst
- Neoplasm
- RA
- Gout
- Lyme disease
- Peripheral vascular disease
- Popliteal artery occlusion

Treatment

Type I Tibiofemoral Hypomobility Syndrome

The potential for recovery of ROM is good in patients with type I TFHypo syndrome. These individuals demonstrate a limitation in ROM; however, duration of limitation is not long. End-feel to PROM may be stiff: however, some extensibility is noted. The therapist should monitor progression of ROM over time to determine if the classification of type I is appropriate. If ROM does not improve in 3 to 4 weeks and all treatment strategies have been investigated, type II should be considered.

Treatment emphasis is on improving ROM, strength, and conditioning, without increasing pain and swelling. In the treatment of the knee with degeneration, consider that rotation may be contributing to the symptoms.

Patient Education

The goal of patient education is correction of impaired postural habits and movements.

I. Alignment
  A. Correct standing alignment as appropriate.
  B. If structural impairment is present, ideal alignment may not be possible.
II. Functional activities that contribute to the movement impairment must be addressed.
  A. Gait
    1. Avoid hip MR during stance phase of gait cycle.
    2. Encourage a "rolling" heel-to-toe gait pattern (common fault is decreased push-off).
      a. This is to improve the shock absorption value of the foot, as well as encourage proper gait pattern.
      b. Patient may require an assistive device to decrease the forces through the affected knee.
        (1) Cane is used in the opposite hand of the impaired lower extremity.
        (2) EXCEPTION: If patient has a varus alignment and using the cane in the opposite hand does not reduce symptoms, the cane may be placed on the same side of the affected knee. Observe gait to determine if the desired effect of reducing varus alignment is being achieved. Also, use the patient's pain response to determine the proper side of cane placement.
  B. Sit-to-stand; stand-to-sit
    1. Slide forward in chair.
    2. Feet hip-width apart and aligned behind knees.
    3. Use quadriceps and gluteus maximus muscles to lift body up and forward out of chair.
      a. Ensure that the tibia advances over the foot with performance (shifts weight forward).

4. Avoid hip MR.
    5. Avoid pulling knees back to push against chair behind them.
  C. Stairs
    1. Instruct in use of rail to decrease weight bearing on the involved limb.
    2. Ascending stairs.
      a. Use quadriceps and gluteus maximus muscles to lift body up and forward.
        (1) Ensure that the tibia advances over the foot with performance (shifts weight forward).
      b. Avoid hip MR.
      c. Avoid pulling knee back to meet body.
    3. Descending stairs.
      a. Avoid hip MR.
      b. If difficult to perform without pain during initial visit, may need to instruct in step-to pattern leading with the involved extremity.
      c. If significantly limited, patient may need to descend stairs backward.
  D. Personal activities (work, school, leisure activities)
    1. Address activities that patients are performing throughout the day that may contribute to the movement impairment, including prolonged sitting, driving, and getting in and out of a car.
    2. Fitness activities.
      a. Address fitness early to maintain patient's routine. Modifications or alternative activities may need to be provided.
        (a) Degeneration: While initiating exercises, it is safer to begin with high repetitions of relatively low weight.
      b. Modify intensity of activities to decrease stress to injured tissues.
        (a) Reduce weight bearing during initial phases and gradually increase weight bearing as tolerated by the patient.
          (i) Swimming, stationary biking
          (ii) Stair master, elliptical
          (iii) Treadmill
III. Education
  A. Degeneration: Arthritis and joint protection education
    1. Risk factors for progression of OA.
      a. Previous injury to the meniscus or ligament.
      b. Manual labor with prolonged positioning of knee flexion.
      c. Obesity.
      d. Laxity of the knee.
      e. Malalignment of the knee.

Home Exercise Program
Degeneration
Patients should be instructed that they should not feel an increase in their symptoms during the performance of their exercises. In addition to monitoring for their symptoms, they should not experience a "pressure" in their knee during their exercises. If either pain or pressure occurs, they should review the instructions to the exercise to be sure that they are performing it correctly and try again. If they still experience pain or pressure, they should discontinue this exercise until they return for their next visit.

Immobilization
Patients should be instructed that they will experience some discomfort (often described as pain or pressure) with their exercises to improve ROM. Patients should be encouraged to continue with the exercises as tolerated. Pain medications should be timed so that they are at maximum level during exercises.

I. Improve muscle performance
  A. Intrinsic hip lateral rotators and posterior gluteus medius muscle
    1. Strengthening
      a. Prone hip lateral rotation isometrics (prone foot pushes).
      b. Prone hip abduction.
      c. Sidelying hip abduction with lateral rotation (level 1, 2, or 3).
        (1) Monitor to be sure patient feels the contraction in the "seat" region; the therapist must palpate to be sure that the patient is recruiting the correct muscles. Common cues for improve performance of the hip lateral rotators include the following:
          (a) Positioning: The pelvis may be rotated posteriorly too far. Ask the patient to roll the pelvis anteriorly.
          (b) Positioning: Place a pillow between the knees.
          (c) Spin the thigh around an axis longitudinally through the femur.
          (d) CAUTION: Do not use foot as a guide for lateral rotation of the hip.
      d. Lunges.
        (1) Perform with lower extremity is good alignment; initially without weight or resistance.
        (2) Progression.
          (a) Resisted: Using an elastic band around proximal thigh, the therapist pulls in the direction of medial rotation and adduction.
          (b) Patients can hold weights in their hands.

    2. Recruitment
      a. Weight shifting with gluteal squeeze on the stance lower extremity
        (1) Progress to standing on 1 leg with correct alignment
        (2) Progress to resisted activities of the opposite leg while standing on the affected leg
  B. Gluteus maximus muscle
    1. Prone hip extension with the knee flexed
      a. Positioning: Patient's that have short hip flexors with require a pillow under the pelvis.
      b. Patient must be able to control the tibial positioning during prone knee flexion in order to begin this exercise.
    2. Lunges, squats
      a. CAUTION: Aggressive exercise. Must be sure patient is able to perform without difficulty
  C. Gastrocnemius muscle
    1. Elastic band resistance
    2. Standing heel raises, bilateral to unilateral
  D. Abdominal muscles (if appropriate)
    1. Strengthening: Lower abdominal progression as described by Sahrmann[2]
    2. Recruitment: Encourage patient to pull in abdominals with functional activities
  E. Quadriceps muscle
    1. Strengthen with functional activities only
      a. Sit to stand, stand to sit, step-ups/step-downs as tolerated.

Knees with Degenerative Changes and Malalignment, Excessive Varus or Valgus
It is thought that the quadriceps muscles provide some shock absorption to the knee; however, recent studies show that increased quadriceps strength can actually increase the progression of OA in knees that have malalignment. One must consider the compression forces that the quadriceps can add to a joint before administering quadriceps strengthening activities. The quadriceps performance should be enhanced only through the proper performance of functional activities, and therapeutic exercises to hypertrophy the quadriceps should be avoided in patients with malalignment of the knees.

II. Improve extensibility
  A. Hip flexors (listed in the order of least aggressive to most aggressive)
    1. During all stretching exercises, be sure that the patient has good abdominal support to avoid pelvic anterior tilt or rotation.
    2. Supine hip and knee extension (heel slide).
    3. Prone bilateral knee flexion: With knees and feet together, flex both knees at the same time; monitor tibial position, avoid LR of tibia.

a. May need to begin with femurs in and abducted position and gradually adduct the hips as the patient improves.

4. Prone hip lateral rotation: Monitor tibial position, avoid LR of tibia.

B. Gastrocnemius and hamstrings muscles

1. Active sitting knee extension with dorsiflexion in neutral hip rotation.

III. Other

A. Mobilization

1. Accessory mobilization

a. If patient is having pain at rest (e.g., in non–weight-bearing positions such as supine), distraction mobilization can be taught to the patient. A trial of gentle distraction should be performed to determine if this technique will be appropriate.

(1) Home program: Patient in sitting position with the foot dangling (a towel may be placed under the distal thigh to raise the thigh). A lightweight shoe may be applied (1 lb). Patient allows the leg to dangle up to 10 minutes to help relieve discomfort. This may be performed as often as needed to relieve pain.

(2) CAUTION: This activity is used only to relieve pain at rest.

b. Joint mobilization.

(1) Pain relief: Oscillatory I, II; sustained I, II.

(2) Increasing ROM: Oscillatory III, IV; sustained III.

2. Physiological mobilization

a. Assisted active ROM.

(1) Supine hip and knee flexion (heel slides).

(a) A towel or sheet may used by the patient to provide gentle overpressure.

(2) Sitting knee flexion/extension.

(3) Prone knee flexion as previously described.

(4) Stationary biking.

b. Passive ROM.

(1) Knee extension: Supine or prone.

(2) Proprioceptive neuromuscular facilitation (PNF) techniques, such as contract/relax and hold/relax, may be useful.

B. Edema and pain control

1. Modalities

a. Ice (if tolerated)

b. Compression wrap for swelling

c. Ultrasound

d. Moist heat pack

e. Electrical stimulation

C. Bracing

1. Degeneration

a. Bracing should be considered for patients who continue to have symptoms that are functionally limiting.

b. Unloader bracing has seemed to be beneficial in patients with OA and malalignment.[6,7] Must consider patient goals, motivation, and anthropomorphics.

2. Immobilization

a. Dynamic splinting/bracing may used to provide a low load, long duration stretch.

D. Neuromuscular training (see Box 7-2)

Type II Tibiofemoral Hypomobility Syndrome

The potential for recovery of ROM is poor in patients with type II TFHypo syndrome. These individuals may report a long duration of loss of ROM, either through immobilization or long-standing OA. End-feel to PROM to the joint are very stiff, with the soft tissues demonstrating very little extensibility. When in doubt, it is best to classify the individual with type I for a trial period and assess the patient's progress appropriately. Emphasis is on educating the patient in modifications of functional activities to accommodate for loss of ROM.

I. Treatment concepts are similar to the treatment of type I TFHypo syndrome; however, modifications must be made for the limited ROM of the knee.

A. Emphasis of treatment should be placed on functional activities specific to the patient. See treatment suggestions for type I TFHypo syndrome for specifics.

B. Proper footwear to provide shock absorption and proper support to the foot.

C. Independence in home exercise program to maintain current ROM of the knee.

D. Independence in home exercise program to maintain proper movement/alignment of the adjacent joints such as the hip, back, and ankle/foot.

E. If limitation significantly affects functional activities, an occupational therapy consult may be advised to address more specific modifications.

NOTES

Knee Extension Syndrome and Knee Extension with Patellar Superior Glide Syndrome

The principal movement impairment in knee extension (Kext) syndrome is knee pain associated with dominance of quadriceps muscles that results in excessive pull on the patella, patellar tendon/ligament, or tibial tubercle. The Kext syndrome has a subcategory of patellar superior glide (KextSG).

Symptoms and History

- Pain with activities that require repeated knee extension
- Associated with large quadriceps musculature
- Often present in runners, football linemen, and volleyball players
  - Kext: Pain located in suprapatellar region
  - KextSG: Pain located in infrapatellar or peripatellar region

Common Referring Diagnoses

- Jumper's knee
- Osgood-Schlatter disease
- Patellofemoral joint dysfunction
- Patellar tendonitis
- Anterior knee pain
- Chondromalacia patella
- Plica syndrome
- Quadriceps strain

Key Tests and Signs for Movement Impairment

Alignment Analysis

Standing

- Swayback, posterior pelvic tilt
- KextSG: Patella alta

Movement Impairment Analysis

- Step-up: May increase peripatellar pain
  - Observe: Does not shift body weight over the foot
  - Kext: Pain decreases when shifts body weight anteriorly (allows the tibia to move anteriorly over the foot)
  - KextSG: Pain decreases with inferior glide provided manually on the patella

Aggravating or Frequent Functional Activity

- Observe limited knee flexion excursion during activity, even though PROM is not limited (landing from a jump), demonstrates reduced knee flexion excursion

Muscle Length

- Short and/or stiff quadriceps

Muscle Strength/Performance Impairments

- Weak gluteus maximus

Source of Signs and Symptoms

Kext
- Quadriceps strain
  - Resisted tests: Quads will be painful with resistance, however may test strong
  - Palpation: Tenderness of quadriceps tendon or superior patellar facet

KextSG
- Patellofemoral pain
  - Palpation: Positive pain along patellar facets and/or femoral condyles
- Patellar tendinopathy
  - Palpation: Tenderness of infrapatellar tendon, fat pad, or peripatellar region
- Tibial tuberosity
  - Appearance: Enlarged

Associated Signs or Contributing Factors

Muscle Performance
- Poor muscle performance of gluteus maximus
- Overuse of quadriceps

Structural Variations
- Enlarged tibial tubercle

Differential Diagnosis

Movement Diagnosis
- Tibiofemoral rotation
- Patellar lateral glide

Potential Diagnosis Requiring Referral Suggested by Signs and Symptoms

Musculoskeletal
- Fracture
- Osgood-Schlatter disease
- Sinding-Larsen-Johansson disease
- AVN of knee
- Osteochondritis dissecans
- SCFE
- AVN of Hip
- Legg-Calvé-Perthes disease
- L3-L5 radiculopathy
- Baker's cyst

Other
- RA
- Gout
- Lyme disease
- Neoplasm

Treatment

Treatment emphasis in Kext syndrome is on decreasing the activity of the quadriceps while improving the performance of the hip extensors. In KextSG syndrome, treatment emphasis is similar to Kext syndrome; however, methods to stabilize the patellar glide may need to be implemented.

Patient Education

The following treatment is appropriate for both Kext and KextSG syndromes unless otherwise noted. The goal of patient education is correction of impaired postural habits and movements.

I. Alignment
    A. Correct alignment as appropriate
II. Functional activities that contribute to the movement impairment must be addressed.
    A. Gait
        1. Encourage proper heel-to-toe gait pattern (common fault is decreased push-off).
        2. Cue the patient to push off with the toes. Patient may also benefit from cues to shift weight slightly forward.
    B. Sit-to-stand; stand-to-sit
        1. Slide forward in chair.
        2. Feet hip-width apart and aligned behind knees.
        3. Use quadriceps and gluteus maximus muscles to lift body up and forward out of chair.
            a. Ensure that the tibia advances over the foot with performance (shifts weight forward).
    C. Sitting
        1. Patient should avoid prolonged periods of increased knee flexion ($\geq$90 degrees).
            a. Take standing/walking breaks every 30 minutes.
            b. When unable to take breaks, use sitting knee extension to decrease time spent in knee flexion.
            c. Patients with short rectus femoris muscles may need to sit with the knee in relatively less flexion initially. As symptoms improve, they should be instructed to gradually flex the knee until they are at a normal position.
    D. Stairs
        1. Instruct in use of rail to decrease weight bearing on the involved limb.
        2. Ascending stairs.
            a. Emphasize the use of the gluteus maximus muscle to lift body up and forward.
                (1) Ensure that the tibia advances over the foot with performance (shifts weight forward).
        3. Descending stairs.
            (1) If difficult to perform without pain during initial visit, may need to instruct in step-to pattern, leading with the involved extremity.
            b. If significantly limited, patient may need to descend stairs backward.
    E. Personal activities (work, school, leisure activities)
        1. Address activities that patients perform throughout the day that may contribute to the movement impairment. These may include prolonged standing or sitting.
        2. Fitness activities.
            a. Address fitness early to maintain patient's routine. Modifications or alternative activities may need to be provided.
            b. Modify intensity of activities to decrease stress to injured tissues.
                (1) Running
                    (a) Interval training is recommended.
                        i. Begin with walking program and gradually mix in short bouts of running. Gradually increase the time running and decrease the time walking.
                    (b) Modify surface of training if indicated.
                        ii. Instruct patient to initiate running with surfaces that reduce the ground reaction force on the lower extremities. A track or chip trail is better than asphalt and asphalt is better than concrete. Concrete should be avoided if possible.
                    (c) Modify strength training.
                        i. Patients should be discouraged from performing resistance activities to increase the hypertrophy of the quadriceps muscles.
                    (d) Modify activities to encourage gluteus medius/maximus muscle recruitment.
                        i. Biking: Patient should be encouraged to focus more on the pushing phase of the cycle (extension of hip = gluts) and less on the pulling phase (knee flexion = hams).
                        ii. Running: Patients often run with their body weight shifted posteriorly (referred to as *chasing their center of gravity* in Sahrmann[2]). Cue the patient to shift body weight slightly forward to encourage better recruitment of the gluteal muscles. Sometimes, use of a small incline will assist the patient in shifting the weight forward.

Home Exercise Program

The patient should be instructed that they should not feel an increase in their symptoms during the performance of their exercises. If this occurs, they should review the instructions to the exercise to be sure that they are performing it correctly and try again. If they still experience pain, they should discontinue this exercise until they return for their next visit.

I. Improve muscle performance
  A. Gluteus maximus muscle
    1. Prone hip extension with the knee flexed.
      a. Patient may require a pillow under the pelvis if short hip flexors.
    2. Weight shifting with gluteal squeeze on the stance lower extremity.
      a. Progress to standing on 1 leg with correct alignment.
      b. Progress to resisted activities of the opposite leg while standing on the affected leg.
    3. Lunges, squats.
      a. CAUTION: In patients who have knee extension, the quadriceps muscles place excessive pull on the patellar tendon and tibial tubercle. Quadriceps strengthening would be contraindicated in these patients.
II. Improve extensibility
  A. Quadriceps muscles (listed in the order of least aggressive to most aggressive)
    1. During all stretching exercises, be sure that the patient has good abdominal support to avoid pelvic anterior tilt or rotation.
      a. KextSG: During performance of exercises that stretch the quadriceps, patellar taping to reduce patellar glide may be required if the patient cannot perform the exercises without an increase in symptoms.
    b. Prone knee flexion.
      (1) May need to begin with pillows under pelvis if patient also has short hip flexors.
      (2) Perform within range that does not increase symptoms.
    c. Prone hip lateral rotation.
    d. Hip flexor length test position: Instruct the patient to flex the knee while the hip is in neutral rotation and neutral hip abduction/adduction.
III. Other
  A. Taping or bracing
    1. KextSG
      a. Horseshoe taping to discourage superior glide.
      b. Cho-pat strap across the patellar tendon.
    2. Patellar joint mobilization
      a. KextSG
        (1) Inferior glides to patella.
          a. Initially may need to perform least aggressive grades (I and II) but should be able to progress to more aggressive grades quickly. Grades III and IV are usually tolerated well. Patient may be instructed in proper performance for home exercise program.
        (2) Mobilization with movement.
      b. Sitting knee flexion: The patient allows the knee to flex from the fully extended position. As the knee flexes, the patient performs an inferior glide of the patella.
    3. Pain control
      a. Modalities.
        (1) Ice as often as needed.
    4. Neuromuscular training (see Box 7-2)

Knee Hyperextension Syndrome

The principal movement impairment in knee hyperextension (Khext) syndrome is knee pain associated with impaired knee extensor mechanism. Dominance of hamstrings and poor functional performance of gluteus maximus and quadriceps muscles result in hyperextension of the knee placing excessive stresses on the structures of the knee.

Symptoms and History

- Pain located peripatellar, joint line, or posterior knee pain; especially with activities that require repetitive knee extension
- Often present in activities that require rapid knee extension: Swimming (freestyle or breaststroke), kickboxing, martial arts
- Race walkers (prolonged foot flat)
- Increased pain at end-range extension positioning such as standing

Common Referring Diagnoses

- Patellofemoral joint dysfunction
- Fat pad syndrome
- Anterior knee pain
- Chondromalacia patella
- Plica syndrome
- Baker's cyst

Key Tests and Signs for Movement Impairment

Alignment Analysis

Standing

- Knee extension >5 degrees
- Posterior pelvic tilt
- Ankle plantarflexion

Movement Impairment Analysis

- Single-leg stance: Hyperextension of the knee on the stance limb
- Step-up: May increase pain
  - Observe: Does not shift body weight over the foot and demonstrates faulty movement of knee back to body
  - Hyperextension of knee may occur at final phase of step-up

Aggravating or Frequent Functional Activity

- Observe hyperextension of the knee during activity
  - If painful, correction decreases symptoms

Gait

- Excessive knee hyperextension during gait; may occur at heel strike through just prior to heel off; may have hard heel strike

Joint Integrity

- PROM: Knee extension >10 degrees; however, acute flare-ups of pain may demonstrate reduced knee extension

Muscle Strength

- Prone hip extension
  - Poor muscle performance of gluteus maximus
  - Overuse of hamstrings

Source of Signs and Symptoms

- Fat pad
  - Palpation: Tenderness of fat pad.
- Patellofemoral pain
  - Palpation: Positive pain along facets of patella and femoral condyles.
- Posterior structures of the knee
  - Palpation: Tenderness posterior knee

Associated Signs or Contributing Factors

Muscle Performance
- Poor performance of quadriceps
- Poor performance of abdominals

Muscle Length/Joint ROM
- Short gastrocnemius

Structural Variations
- "Hypermobility syndrome" = increased general laxity
- 6/9 positive on Beighton's scale[8]

Differential Diagnosis

Movement Diagnosis
- Tibiofemoral rotation
- Patellar lateral glide

Potential Diagnosis Requiring Referral Suggested by Signs and Symptoms

Musculoskeletal
- Fracture
- Jumper's knee
- Osgood-Schlatter disease
- Sinding-Larsen-Johansson disease
- AVN of knee
- Osteochondritis dissecans
- SCFE
- AVN of Hip
- Legg-Calvé-Perthes disease
- L3-L5 radiculopathy

Other
- RA
- Gout
- Lyme disease
- Neoplasm
- Baker's cyst

Treatment

Treatment emphasis in knee hyperextension syndrome is to decrease hyperextension of the knee.

Patient Education

The goal of patient education is correction of impaired postural habits and movements.

I. Alignment
   A. Improve alignment between femur and tibia.
      1. Relax/unlock knees to reduce hyperextension of knee.
         a. Improve alignment of pelvis if applicable.

II. Functional activities that contribute to the movement impairment must be addressed
   A. Gait
      1. Encourage proper heel-to-toe gait pattern.
         a. Knee hyperextension.
            (1) Avoid knee hyperextension during stance phase of gait cycle.
            (2) Cue the patient to "lift the heel" to discourage overrecruitment of the hamstrings.
            (3) Cue to land softly on the heel at heel strike.
   B. Sit-to-stand; stand-to-sit
      1. Slide forward in chair.
      2. Feet hip-width apart and aligned behind knees.
      3. Use quadriceps and gluteus maximus muscles to lift body up and forward out of chair.
         a. Ensure that the tibia advances over the foot with performance.
      4. Avoid pulling knees back to meet body; final position of knee should be relaxed knee (not hyperextension).
   C. Stairs
      1. Instruct in use of rail to decrease weight bearing on the involved limb.
      2. Ascending stairs.
         a. Use quadriceps and gluteus maximus muscles to lift body up and forward.
            (1) Ensure that the tibia advances over the foot with performance.
         b. Avoid pulling knee back to meet body.
      3. Descending stairs.
         a. If patient is unable to perform without pain during initial visit, may need to instruct in step-to pattern leading with the involved extremity.
         b. If significantly limited, patient may need to descend stairs backward.
   D. Personal activities (work, school, leisure activities)
      1. Address activities that patients perform throughout the day that may contribute to the movement impairment. These may include prolonged standing.

2. Fitness activities.
   a. Address fitness early to maintain patient's routine. Modifications or alternative activities may need to be provided.
   b. Modify intensity of activities to decrease stress to injured tissues.
      (1) Running
         (a) Interval training is recommended.
            i. Begin with walking program and gradually mix in short bouts of running. Gradually increase the time running and decrease the time walking.
         (b) Modify surface of training if indicated.
            i. Instruct patient to initiate running with surfaces that reduce the ground reaction force on the lower extremities. A track or chip trail is better than asphalt and asphalt is better than concrete. Concrete should be avoided if possible.
            ii. Running on a street with a camber may contribute to common knee problems such as ITB friction syndrome. Runners should be encouraged to either avoid the camber or alternate the direction of their run.
   c. Modify activities to encourage gluteus medius/maximus muscle recruitment.
      (1) Biking: Patients should be encouraged to focus more on the pushing phase of the cycle (extension of hip = gluts) and less on the pulling phase (knee flexion = hams).
      (2) Running: Patients often run with their body weight shifted posteriorly (referred to as *chasing the center of gravity* in Sahrmann[2]). Cue the patient to shift body weight slightly forward to encourage better recruitment of the gluteal muscles. Sometimes, use of a small incline will assist the patient in shifting the weight forward.
   d. Kickboxing: Educate patients to decrease speed of kicks to improve control of limb.
   e. Swimming: Educate patients to decrease intensity of wall push-off with turning.

Home Exercise Program

Patients should be instructed that they should not feel an increase in their symptoms during the performance of their exercises. If this occurs, they should review the instructions to the exercise to be sure that they are performing it correctly and try again. If they still experience pain, they should discontinue this exercise until they return for their next visit.

I. Improve muscle performance
  A. Gluteus maximus
    1. Prone hip extension with the knee flexed.
      a. Patient may require a pillow under the pelvis if short hip flexors.
    2. Weight shifting with gluteal squeeze on the stance lower extremity.
      a. Progress to standing on 1 leg with correct alignment
      b. Progress to resisted activities of the opposite leg while standing on the affected leg
    3. Lunges, squats.
  B. Abdominals (if appropriate)
    1. Strengthening: Lower abdominal progression as described by Sahrmann.[2]
    2. Recruitment: Encourage patient to pull in abdominals with functional activities.
  C. Quadriceps
    1. Progress quadriceps strengthening according to pain and results of resisted testing and functional testing such as stairs.
    2. Quadriceps: Sit to stand, wall sits, step-ups/step downs, lunges (emphasize correct hip and tibial alignment).
II. Improve extensibility
  A. Gastrocnemius muscles
    1. Active sitting knee extension with dorsiflexion in neutral hip rotation.
    2. Standing runners stretch.
  B. Hamstrings
    1. Prolonged hamstring stretch, maintain proper spinal alignment.
III. Other
  A. Taping or bracing
    1. Knee hyperextension.
      a. Posterior knee X taping to decrease hyperextension of the knee
      b. Unloader V taping to unload the fat pad
  B. Pain control
    1. Modalities.
      a. Ice as often as needed.
  C. Neuromuscular training (see Box 7-2)

Patellar Lateral Glide Syndrome

The principal movement impairment in patellar lateral glide syndrome is knee pain as a result of an impaired patellar relationship within the trochlear groove. Often a secondary diagnosis and therefore the movement impairments of tibiofemoral rotation (TFR) or knee hyperextension (Khext) should be considered. Correction of impairment often decreases symptoms.

Symptoms and History

- Peripatellar or retropatellar pain with any activity that requires loaded knee flexion/extension (stairs, running hills, squatting)
- Increased pain with sustained knee flexion in sitting (*movie goers syndrome*)
- Often associated with tibiofemoral rotation

Common Referring Diagnoses

- Patellofemoral joint dysfunction
- Chondromalacia patella
- Anterior knee pain
- Patellar dislocation
- Plica syndrome

Key Tests and Signs for Movement Impairment

Alignment Analysis

- Structural: Patella alta or infera
- Nonstructural: Lateral, rotated, tilted

Movement Impairment Analysis

- Squat test, step-down: Increased peripatellar pain
  - Decreased pain with manual correction of patellar positioning
- Prone knee flexion: May have pain with performance
  - Decreased pain with manual correction of patellar positioning
- Isometric quadriceps contraction: In long sitting, patella tracks laterally
- Sitting knee extension: Excessive lateral glide of the patella

Aggravating or Frequent Functional Activity

- Increased pain during activity
  - If painful, correction of patellar positioning decreases symptoms

Muscle Length

- Hip flexor length test: Short TFL-ITB. May have pain in neutral hip position
  - Decreased pain with manual correction of patellar positioning

Muscle Strength/Performance Impairments

- Possible poor performance of quadriceps, particularly the vastus medialis oblique (VMO)

Source of Signs and Symptoms

- Patellofemoral pain
  - Palpation: Positive pain along patellar facets and/or femoral condyle
  - Positive McConnell test

Associated Signs or Contributing Factors

Muscle Length

- Short/stiff lateral patellar retinacula
- Short/stiff gluteus maximus/ITB

Muscle Strength/Performance Impairments

- Manual muscle test: Weakness in posterior gluteus medius and hip LRs

Structural Variations

- Small patellae: May be associated with dislocation or subluxation
- Flat lateral femoral condyle
- Often associated with other movement diagnosis
  - Tibiofemoral rotation
  - Knee hyperextension

Differential Diagnosis

Movement Diagnosis

- Tibiofemoral rotation
- Knee extension with patellar superior glide
- Knee hyperextension

Potential Diagnosis Requiring Referral Suggested by Signs and Symptoms

Musculoskeletal

- OA/DJD
- Acute or recurrent patellar dislocation/subluxation
- Fracture
- Sinding-Larsen-Johansson disease
- AVN of knee
- Osteochondritis dissecans
- SCFE
- AVN of hip
- Legg-Calvé-Perthes disease
- L3-L5 radiculopathy

Other

- RA
- Gout
- Lyme disease
- Neoplasm
- Baker's cyst

Treatment

Treatment emphasis in patellar lateral glide syndrome is to address the impairment of patellar tracking. If patellar lateral glide syndrome is given as a secondary diagnosis, please refer to the treatment described for the primary diagnosis (tibiofemoral rotation or knee hyperextension) in addition to the treatment described below.

Patient Education

The goal of patient education is correction of impaired postural habits and movements.

I. Alignment
    A. Correct alignment as appropriate
II. Functional activities that contribute to the movement impairment must be addressed
    A. If a primary diagnosis of tibiofemoral rotation or knee hyperextension is determined, see treatment for the primary diagnosis.
    B. Stairs
        1. Instruct in use of rail to decrease weight bearing on the involved limb.
        2. Ascending stairs.
            a. Use quadriceps and gluteus maximus to lift body up and forward.
        3. Descending stairs.
            a. If difficult to perform without pain during initial visit, may need to instruct in step-to pattern leading with the involved extremity.
            b. If significantly limited, patient may need to descend stairs backwards.
    C. Sitting
        1. Patient should avoid prolonged periods of increased knee flexion (≥90 degrees).
            a. Take standing/walking breaks every 30 minutes.
            b. When unable to take breaks, use sitting knee extension to decrease time spent in knee flexion.
            c. In patients with short TFL-ITB, they may need to sit with the thighs slightly abducted initially. As symptoms improve, they should be instructed to gradually adduct the thigh until they are at a normal position.
    D. Personal activities (work, school, leisure activities)
        1. Address activities that patients are performing throughout the day which are pain provoking for the patient.
        2. Fitness activities.

Home Exercise Program

The patient should be instructed that they should not feel an increase in their symptoms during the performance of their exercises. In addition to monitoring for their symptoms, they should not experience a "pressure" in their knee during their exercises. If either pain or pressure occurs, they should review the instructions to the exercise to be sure that they are performing it correctly and try again. If they still experience pain or pressure, they should discontinue this exercise until they return for their next visit.

I. Improve muscle performance
    A. If a primary diagnosis of tibiofemoral rotation or hyperextension is determined, see treatment for the primary diagnosis.
        1. Quadriceps
            a. Recommend use of functional activities to improve quadriceps performance (listed in order of difficulty beginning with least aggressive)
                (1) Sit to stand transfers
                (2) Step-ups may progress to step downs as patient's symptoms improve
                (3) Lunges
                (4) Squats
                (5) Biofeedback may be beneficial for improving possible timing or recruitment of the vastus medialis oblique (VMO) muscle
II. Improve extensibility
    A. TFL-ITB
        1. Listed in the order of least aggressive to most aggressive.
        2. During all stretching exercises, be sure that the patient has good abdominal support to avoid pelvic anterior tilt or rotation.
        3. During performance of exercises that stretch the TFL-ITB, patellar taping to reduce patellar glide may be required if the patient cannot perform the exercises without an increase in symptoms.
            a. Prone knee flexion
                (1) May need to begin with femurs in an abducted position and gradually adduct the hips as the patient improves.
            b. Prone hip lateral rotation
            c. Hip flexor length test position: Allow the hip to abduct as it extends then actively adduct with the tibia in neutral
            d. Ober test position: Hip in lateral rotation and tibia in neutral to slight medial rotation (level 3 of post. glut. med. progression)
    B. Other muscles (as needed)
        1. Lateral patellar retinaculum
        2. Gluteus maximus/ITB
    C. Other
        1. Patellar taping/bracing
            a. McConnell taping for medial glide
        2. Patellar joint mobilization
            a. Medial glide to patella

b. Initially may need to perform least aggressive grades (I, II), but should be able to progress to more aggressive grades quickly. Grades III, IVs are usually tolerated well. Patient may be instructed in proper performance for home exercise program.

3. Pain control
    a. Modalities
        (1) Ice as often as needed
4. Neuromuscular training (see Box 7-2)

Knee Impairment

Knee impairment is the classification given in the absence of a specific movement impairment diagnosis or when a diagnosis cannot not be determined because of pain, physician-imposed restrictions, or both. If possible, the physical therapist should determine the pathoanatomical structure involved, as identified by the physician; the procedure performed, if any; and the stage for rehabilitation.

Factors that affect the physical stress of tissue and/or thresholds of tissue adaptation and injury[10] include the following:

I. Physiological factors
   A. Tissue factors specific to the knee
      1. Bone
         a. Tibial plateau
            (1) Cancellous bone and poor vascular supply.
            (2) Often non–weight-bearing for 2 to 3 months.
         b. Patella fracture: Quad contraction often contraindicated
      2. Cartilage
         a. Meniscus
            (1) Red zone: Peripheral one-third vascular, with good healing potential.
            (2) Pink zone: Middle one-third vascularity, with variable healing potential.
            (3) White zone: Inner one-third avascular, with poor healing.
            (4) Increased compression of meniscus at 90 degrees of knee flexion.
            (5) Aggressive hamstring exercise is contraindicated, especially if injury to posterior horn.
            (6) Change in weight-bearing surfaces with removal of meniscus.
      3. Muscle
         a. Quad atrophy common postsurgery or trauma to knee
      4. Tendon
         a. Quad tendon rupture
            (1) Quad contraction contraindicated.
            (2) May have flexion ROM restrictions.
      5. Ligament
         a. ACL
            (1) New graft is weakest from 4 to 12 weeks.
            (2) Avoid anterior tibial translation.
            (3) Avoid open-chain resisted knee extension in early rehabilitation phase.
         b. PCL
            (1) Avoid posterior tibial translation.
            (2) Avoid active hamstring contraction.
         c. MCL
            (1) Adolescent: Separation of distal femoral epiphysis can mimic MCL sprain. Radiographs must be performed.
         d. Patellar ligament rupture
            (1) Quad contraction contraindicated.
            (2) May have flexion ROM restrictions.
      6. Skin
      7. Nerve
         a. Fibular (peroneal) nerve injury possible with surgery or trauma to knee
   B. Types of surgeries (indications)
      1. Stabilization
      2. Osteotomy (malalignment or osteosarcoma)
         a. Femoral
         b. Tibial
      3. Arthroplasty (DJD, arthritis, joint destruction)
         a. Total/unicompartment
            (1) Cemented/uncemented
      4. Debridement (tear, degeneration)
         a. Meniscal
         b. Patellar ligament
         c. Patella
      5. Repair
         a. Ligament reconstruction (ACL, PCL)
         b. Meniscal repair
         c. Cartilage repair
            (1) Microfracture
            (2) Mosaicplasty, osteochondral autograft transplant (OATS)
      6. Meniscal transplant
      7. Soft tissue release (short tissues or spastic muscles)
            (1) ITB
            (2) Hamstrings
            (3) Hip adductors
   C. Medical complications
      1. Baker's cyst
      2. Peroneal nerve neurapraxia
      3. Leg length changes (total knee replacement)
II. Movement and alignment factors
   A. Variations
   B. Standing alignment
      1. May demonstrate protective stance or rotational impairments
   C. Underlying movement impairment syndromes
      1. TFR syndrome
         a. TFR syndrome with valgus
         b. TFR syndrome with varus
      2. TFhypo syndrome
      3. Kext syndrome
         a. Kext syndrome with patellar superior glide
      4. Khext syndrome
      5. PLG syndrome
      6. TFAH syndrome

Treatment for Knee Impairment

Emphasis of treatment is to restore ROM of the knee and strength of the lower extremity without adding excessive stresses to the injured tissues. Underlying movement impairments should be addressed during rehabilitation and functional activities to ensure optimal stresses to the healing tissues.

Impairments (Body Functions and Structures)
Pain
Be sure to clarify the location, quality, and intensity.
Stage 1
Surgical: Within the first 2 weeks of the postoperative period, some pain will be associated with exercises. Gradually, over the next few weeks, pain associated with the exercise should lessen. Sharp, stabbing pain should be avoided. Mild aching is expected after exercises but should be tolerable for the patient. This postexercise discomfort should decrease within 1 to 2 hours of the rehabilitation. Complaints of increasing pain, pain that is not decreasing with treatment, or burning pain are all "red flag" indicators that treatment is too aggressive or there is a disruption in the usual course of healing. Coordinating the use of analgesics with exercise sessions is important. Splinting, bracing, and/or assistive devices may be used during this period to protect the injured tissue.

Acute Injury: Despite discomfort, tests may need to be performed to rule out serious injury. Modalities and taping/bracing may be helpful to decrease pain. The patient may also require the use of an assistive device in the early phases of healing.
Stage 2 to 3
Surgical/Acute Injury: Pain associated with the specific tissue that was involved in the surgery should be significantly decreased by weeks 4 to 6. Precautions may be lifted during or by postoperative weeks 4 to 6. As activity level of the patient is progressed, the patient may report increased pain/discomfort with new activities such as returning to daily activities and fitness. Pain/discomfort location should be monitored closely. Muscle soreness is expected, similar to the response of muscle to overload stimulus (e.g., weight training). General muscle soreness should be allowed to resolve, usually 1 to 2 days before repeating the bout of activity. Pain described as stabbing should always be avoided.

Edema
Stage 1
Surgical/Acute Injury: Edema is quite common in the knee s/p surgery or injury. Edema has also been implicated in the inhibition of the quadriceps and therefore should be treated aggressively.[11-13] The patient should be educated in use of edema controlling techniques:
- Active ROM (AROM)
- Ice[14]
- Elevation
- Compression: Ace wraps, stockings

Patients should be encouraged to keep the lower extremity elevated as much as possible particularly in the early phases (1 to 3 weeks), without keeping the knee in a flexed position. Application of ice after exercise is recommended. Other methods to control edema in the knee include electrical stimulation or compression pumps. Edema should be measured at each visit. A sudden increase in edema may indicate that the rehabilitation program is too aggressive or a possible infection.
Stage 2 to 3
Surgical/Acute Injury: Time until swelling is resolved is variable among patients and surgical procedures. As patients increase the time spent on their feet, in regular daily activities, or doing more weight-bearing exercises, the patient may experience a slight increase in edema. This is to be expected; however, the patient should be further encouraged to use techniques stated previously to manage the edema.

Appearance
Stage 1
Surgical: Infection should be suspected if the area around the incision or the involved joint appears to be red, hot, and swollen. The physician should be consulted immediately if infection is suspected. It is common to observe bruising after surgery. This should be monitored continuously for any changes; an increase in bruising during the rehabilitation phases may indicate infection. Changes in hair growth, perspiration, or color may indicate some disturbance to the sympathetic nervous function, especially if in combination with the complaint of excessive pain. Stitches are typically removed in 7 to 14 days.
Stage 2 to 3
Surgical: Incision should be well healed. Bruising may still be present as far as 3 to 4 weeks after surgery but should be diminishing. Signs of increased bruising are a red flag and should be immediately referred to their physician.

Range of Motion
Stage 1
Surgical/Acute Injury: Refer to physician's precautions and specific protocols for guidelines regarding progression of the exercises. The most conservative, common ROM precautions include the following:
- ACL reconstruction: Flexion <120 degrees.
- Meniscal repair: Flexion <90 degrees.
- Collateral ligament repair: Avoid full extension.
- Patellar fractures and quadriceps tendon repairs: Restrictions can be varied for the amount of knee flexion allowed and/or when ROM exercises can begin.
- Mobilizations to the joint may be contraindicated.

Patellar mobilizations should begin as soon as possible after surgery. Common time frames to begin patellar mobilizations include the following:

- ACL reconstruction: Immediately after surgery.
- Meniscal repair: Immediately after surgery.
- Patellar fractures and quad tendon repairs: Within 1 week, however, consult with physician before initiation.

Tibiofemoral mobilizations after ACL reconstruction, meniscal repair or debridement, collateral ligament repair:

- There is little information in the literature that describes the "safe time" that mobilizations can begin. These mobilizations are not recommended until the initial healing phases are complete. If mobilizations are indicated, consult with physician before initiating.
- For mobilizations after meniscal debridement, it is recommended that distraction be added before performing glides to reduce shear to the meniscus.

Stage 2 to 3

Surgical/Acute Injury: Precautions are typically lifted by the time the patient reaches this stage. ROM should be approaching normal. Exercises may need to be progressed using passive force. To increase knee extension, prone knee extension, patients can be instructed to hang the limb off the edge of mat with weight on ankle. Patients should be advised to build up tolerance gradually and break up prolonged hang with knee flexion. For knee flexion the patient may raise knee toward the chest and use hands to add overpressure. Patient should be instructed that a stretching discomfort is expected; however, sharp pain should be avoided.

Mobilizations to the tibiofemoral joint may be indicated in later stages of rehabilitation to improve ROM. Consult with the physician before initiating joint mobilization after surgery of the knee.

Strength
Stage 1

Surgical/Acute Injury: Strengthening with overload often begins after the initial phase of healing (4 to 6 weeks). Isometrics and active movement within precautions may be started sooner. At times less than 4 weeks, emphasis should be placed on proper movement patterns in preparation for strengthening activities. After 4 weeks, strengthening may be gradually incorporated. Progression to resistive exercise is based on the patient's ability to perform ROM with a good movement pattern and without significant increase in pain.

Quadriceps muscles are most commonly affected with surgery or injury to the knee; however, others may be involved such as the hamstrings or gastrocnemius muscles. If the patient is having difficulty recruiting the quadriceps, the following cues are helpful:

- Have patient try to pull the knee cap up toward the hip.
- Have patient perform an isometric on the uninvolved side first.

- With the patient in short sitting, the clinician raises the knee passively into extension. Then the patient attempts to hold the leg straight as you gradually remove the support of your hands. Be careful not to "drop" the limb. Only remove the amount of assistance that allows the patient to perform successfully.
- Light tapping of the fingers on the quadriceps: Be careful of incisions.
- When performing quadriceps isometrics in long sitting, monitor for compensation of the hamstrings. Patients actually use hamstrings to pull the tibia posteriorly to extend the knee. Be sure you see the quadriceps change shape. If these cues do not work, ask patients to reduce their effort. Often, they pull harder trying to recruit the quadriceps, but it only increases the activity of the hamstrings.

Electrical stimulation or biofeedback may be used to improve strengthening (see the following "Medications/Modalities" section).

The patient may also have strengthening precautions per the physician. Common examples of these precautions include the following:

- ACL reconstruction: No resisted extension during open-chain exercises.
- Meniscus repair: Restrictions of hamstring strengthening.
- Patellar fractures and quadriceps tendon repairs: Restrictions of quadriceps strengthening.

NOTE: Caution should be used in single-leg raise in patients >55 years of age and patients with history of low back pain.

Stage 2 to 3

Surgical/Acute Injury: At this stage, precautions are typically lifted; however, with surgical procedures, such as ACL reconstruction/injury, some restrictions on open-chain resisted extension may still be in place. Strength activities can be progressed as tolerated by the patient. Common functional activities that can be considered strengthening activities include wall slides, lunges, and step-downs/step-ups. A common compensation is to shift weight away from the involved limb. Be sure that the patient maintains the appropriate amount of weight bearing during closed-chain activities.

Proprioception/Balance[15]
Stage 1

Surgical/Acute Injury: Activities to improve proprioception of the knee joint should be incorporated as soon as possible. Early in treatment, these activities include weight shifting, progressive increases in weight bearing on the involved lower extremity, and eventually unilateral stance. As the patient can take full weight on the involved knee, activities are progressed to use of a balance board and closed-chained activities such as wall sits, lunges, and single-leg stance.

Stage 2 to 3

Surgical/Acute Injury: In this stage, precautions are typically lifted. Activities should be progressed to prepare patient to return to daily activities, fitness routines, and work or sporting activities. As the patient progresses, proprioception can be challenged by asking the patient to stand on unstable surfaces (pillows, trampoline, or BOSU ball), perturbations can be applied through having the patient catch a ball being thrown to him or her while standing on one leg. Sliding board activities have been shown to be beneficial to patients after surgery.[16] See Box 7-2 for higher level neuromuscular training (Stage 3).

Cardiovascular and Muscular Endurance
Stage 1

Surgical/Acute Injury: Early in rehabilitation, if the patient does not have adequate knee ROM to complete a full revolution on a stationary bike, unilateral cycling can be performed with the uninvolved extremity. The involved extremity is supported on a stationary surface, while the patient pedals with the uninvolved extremity. Water walking and swimming are good substitutes for full weight-bearing activities. For swimming, if kicking against the resistance is contraindicated, the patient may participate in swim drills that mainly challenge the upper extremities for conditioning. Low resistance stationary cycling can begin when knee flexion ROM is approximately 110 degrees. As strength improves, resistance may be increased.

Stage 2 to 3

Surgical/Acute Injury: The patient may then be progressed to activities such as water walking → walking on the treadmill → elliptical machine → Nordic ski machine → StairMaster → running when appropriate. The patient should be given specific instruction in gradual progression of these activities. See Box 7-1 for progression of running.

Patient Education
Stages 1 to 3

Surgical/Acute Injury: Educate the patient in the structures and tissues involved and the specific medical precautions when indicated. Patients should also be taught schedule for use, and how to don and doff their brace/splint. Educate the patient in the timeline to return to activity, often driven by physician's guidelines and educate the patient in maintaining precautions during various functional activities such as ambulation, stairs, and transfers.

Scarring
Stage 1

Surgical: Scarring, although a normal process of healing, must be managed well. Exercise, massage, compression, silicone gel sheets, and vibration are used to manage scars. The use of silicone gel is best supported by evidence in the literature. However, clinical experts also commonly use the other methods of scar management. Further research is needed to determine the efficacy of these other methods. The gradual application of stress to the scar/incision helps the scar remodel so that it allows the necessary gliding between structures. A dry incision that has been closed and reopens because of the stresses applied with scar massage indicates that the scar massage is too aggressive. Scars may be classified according to type. Linear scars that are immature are confined to the area of the incision. They may be raised and pink or reddish in the remodeling phase. As they mature they become whitish and flatten. A hypersensitive scar requires desensitization. See Chapter 5 for the examination of the hand and general treatment guidelines and Box 5-3 for more treatment suggestions on managing scar.

Stage 2 to 3

A scar may continue to remodel for up to 2 years. Scar management techniques may be effective until the scar matures, although they are probably most effective early in the healing process.

Changes in Status
Stages 1 to 3

Surgical/Acute Injury: Consider carefully patient reports of increased pain or edema, decreased strength, or significant change in ROM, especially in combination. The patient should be questioned regarding precipitating events such as time of onset, or the activity. If the integrity of the surgery is in doubt, contact the physician promptly. If the patient has fever and erythema spreading from the incision, the physician should be contacted because of the possibility of an infection.

Function (Activity Limitations/Participation Restrictions)
Mobility
Stage 1

Surgical/Acute Injury: While following medical precautions, patients should be instructed in mobility, as follows:

- Sit-to-stand: The patient should be instructed in the proper use of an assistive device if a device is indicated.
- Ambulation: The patient may have weight-bearing precautions. The patient should be instructed in the proper use of an assistive device and proper gait pattern. Emphasis should be placed on normalizing the patient's gait pattern. If the patient is given partial or toe-touch weight-bearing restrictions, the patient should be instructed in using a heel-to-toe pattern while restricting the amount of weight that is accepted by the lower extremity. The patient should not place his or her weight on the ball of the foot only.
- Stairs: The patient should be instructed in the proper stair ambulation with use of an assistive device (if indicated). In the early phases of healing (after surgery or acute injury) the patient should be instructed to use a step to cadence, lead with the

involved lower extremity when descending stairs and lead with the uninvolved lower extremity when ascending stairs.

Stage 2 to 3

Surgical/Acute Injury: Instructions in mobility should be continued while following medical precautions.

All Mobility: As weight-bearing precautions are lifted, the patient should be instructed to gradually reduce the level or type of assistive device required. Progression away from the device depends on the ability of the patient to achieve a normal gait pattern. If the patient demonstrates a significant gait deviation secondary to pain or weakness, the patient should continue to use the device. This may prevent the adaptation of movement impairment and other pain problems in the future. A progression may be: walker → crutches → one crutch → cane → no assistive device.

Stairs: As the patient progresses through the healing stages and can accept more weight onto the involved leg, he or she should be instructed in normal stair ambulation.

Work/School/Higher Level Activities

Stage 1

Surgical/Acute Injury: The patient may be off work or school in the immediate postoperative period or after acute injury. When they are cleared to return to work or school, patients should be instructed in gradual resumption of activities. Emphasis should also be placed on edema control, particularly elevation and compression.

Stage 2 to 3

Surgical/Acute Injury: The patient should be prepared to return to their previous activities. Suggestions for improving proprioception and balance are provided in the preceding "Proprioception/Balance" section. In preparation to return to sports, sport-specific activities should be added. The initial phases of these activities will include straight plane activities at a slow pace and then gradually increase the level of difficulty. See Box 7-2 for more detail.

Sleeping

Stage 1 to 3

Surgical/Acute Injury: Sleeping is often disrupted in the immediate postoperative period or after acute injury. The lower extremity should be slightly elevated (foot higher than the knee and knee higher than the hip) to minimize edema. Avoid placing pillows so that the knee is held in the flexed position throughout the night.

Support

Stage 1

Surgical: A brace may be used to protect the surgical site, depending on the procedure or type of fracture. The brace should fit comfortably. The patient should be educated in the timeline for wearing the brace. Consult with physician if the wearing time is not clear.

It is common for a patient to complain of patellofemoral pain with rehabilitation after surgery. Taping can be helpful in the postoperative period. When applying tape, consider the underlying movement impairment (e.g., tibiofemoral rotation, patellar glide).

Acute injury: Taping may help decrease symptoms in a patient with acute knee injury. When applying tape, consider the underlying movement impairment (e.g., tibiofemoral rotation, knee hyperextension).

Stage 2 to 3

Surgical: The recommendations concerning the need for bracing long term are varied. Communication among the team (patient, physician, and physical therapist) is necessary. Functional bracing is recommended if the patient wishes to return to high level sporting activities and demonstrates either of the following:

1. Laxity in the joint
2. Performs poorly on functional tests[17]

Acute Injury: For injuries to the ACL that are not repaired or reconstructed, if the patient returns to sport, functional bracing is recommended.[18]

Medications/Modalities

Medications

Surgical: During the acute stage, physical therapy treatments should be timed with analgesics, typically 30 minutes after administration of oral medication. If medication is given intravenously, therapy often can occur immediately after administration. Communication with nurses and physicians is critical to provide optimal pain relief for the patient.

Acute injury: The patient's medications should be reviewed to ensure that they are taking the medications appropriately.

Aquatic Therapy

Surgical/Acute Injury: Aquatic therapy to decrease weight bearing during ambulation may be helpful in the rehabilitation of patients after fracture or surgical procedures. Often, this medium is not available but should be considered if the patient's progress is slowed secondary to pain or difficulty maintaining weight-bearing precautions. Incisions should be healed before aquatic therapy is initiated; however, materials to cover the incision may be used to allow patients to get into the water sooner.

Thermal Modalities

Surgical/Acute Injury: Instruct the patient in proper home use of thermal modalities to decrease pain. Ice has been shown to be beneficial, particularly in the immediate postoperative phases.[14]

Electrical Stimulation

Stage 1/Progression

Surgical/Acute Injury: Electrical stimulation can be used for three purposes: Pain relief, edema control, and strengthening. Interferential current has been shown to be helpful in decreasing pain and edema.[19-21] Sensory level transcutaneous electrical nerve stimulation (TENS) can assist in decreasing pain. Currently, no definitive answer exists for electrical stimulation for quadriceps strengthening. It was once believed that electrical stimulation did not provide a distinct advantage over high-intensity exercise training.[22-23] However, more recent studies support the use of stimulation to improve motor recruitment and strength.[23-26] Be sure to check for contraindications. Avoid areas where metal is in close approximation to the skin (e.g., wires/screws to fix patellar fracture). Electrical stimulation for quadriceps strengthening can be used in patients with total knee arthroplasty once staples have been removed.[25]

Biofeedback
Stage 1/Progression
Surgical/Acute Injury: Biofeedback has been shown to be an effective adjunct to exercise for strengthening the quadriceps in early postoperative phases.[27]

Discharge Planning
Stage 1
Surgical: Equipment, such as the following, may be needed, depending on the patient's abilities, precautions, and home environment.
- Assistive devices: Walker, crutches, cane
- Reacher
- Tub bench and hand-held shower

Therapy: Assess the need for physical therapy after discharge from the acute phase of recovery or from the following:
- Skilled nursing facility
- Rehabilitation facility
- Home health
- Outpatient physical therapy

After the acute phase of recovery, the patient should be reassessed to determine whether a movement impairment diagnosis exists. Supply the patient with documentation for consistency of care. Documentation should include the following:
- Physician protocol along with precautions and progression of activities
- Progress of patient during physical therapy
- Expected outcomes

REFERENCES
1. Muellner T, Weinstabl R, Schabus R, et al: The diagnosis of meniscal tears in athletes: a comparison of clinical and magnetic resonance imaging investigations, *Am J Sports Med* 25(1):7-12, 1997.
2. Sahrmann SA: *Diagnosis and treatment of movement impairment syndromes,* St Louis, 2002, Mosby.
3. Birmingham TB, Kramer JF, Kirkley A, et al: Knee bracing after ACL reconstruction: effects on postural control and proprioception, *Med Sci Sports Exerc* 33(8):1253-1258, 2001.
4. Birmingham TB, Kramer JF, Kirkley A, et al: Knee bracing for medial compartment osteoarthritis: effects on proprioception and postural control, *Rheumatology* 40(3):285-289, 2001.
5. Wu GK, Ng GY, Mak AF: Effects of knee bracing on the sensorimotor function of subjects with anterior cruciate ligament reconstruction, *Am J Sports Med* 29(5):641-645, 2001.
6. Lindenfeld TN, Hewett TE, Andriacchi TP: Joint loading with valgus bracing in patients with varus gonarthrosis, *Clin Orthop Relat Res* 344:290-297, 1997.
7. Draper ER, Cable JM, Sanchez-Ballester J, et al: Improvement in function after valgus bracing of the knee. An analysis of gait symmetry, *J Bone Joint Surg Br* 82(7):1001-1005, 2000.
8. Ramesh R, Von Arx O, Azzopardi T, et al: The risk of anterior cruciate ligament rupture with generalised joint laxity, *J Bone Joint Surg Br* 87(6):800-803, 2005.
9. Perry M, Morrissey M, Morrissey D, et al: Knee extensors kinetic chain training in anterior cruciate ligament deficiency, *Knee Surg Sports Traumatol Arthrosc* 13(8):638-648, 2005.
10. Mueller MJ, Maluf KS: Tissue adaptations to physical stress: a proposed "Physical Stress Theory" to guide physical therapist practice, education and research, *Phys Ther* 82(4):383-403, 2002.
11. Young A, Stokes M, Iles JF: Effects of joint pathology on muscle, *Clin Orthop* 219:21-27, 1987.
12. Delitto A, Lehman RC: Rehabilitation of the athlete with a knee injury, *Clin Sports Med* 8(4):805-839, 1989.
13. DeAndrade JR, Grant C, Dixon SJ: Joint distention an reflex muscle inhibition in the knee, *J Bone Joint Surg Am* 47:313-322, 1965.
14. Lessard L, Scudds R, Amendola A, et al: The efficacy of cryotherapy following arthroscopic knee surgery, *J Orthop Sports Phys Ther* 26(1):14-22, 1997.
15. Hewett TE, Paterno MV, Myer GD: Strategies for enhancing proprioception and neuromuscular control of the knee, *Clin Orthop* 1(402):76-94, 2002.
16. Blanpied P, Carroll R, Douglas T, et al: Effectiveness of lateral slide exercise in an anterior cruciate ligament reconstruction rehabilitation home exercise program, *Phys Ther* 30(10):609-611, 2000.
17. Fitzgerald GK, Axe MJ, Snyder-Mackler L: A decision-making scheme for returning patients to high-level activity with nonoperative treatment after anterior cruciate ligament rupture, *Knee Surg Sports Traumatol Arthrosc* 8(2):76-82, 2000.
18. Fitzgerald GK, Axe MJ, Snyder-Mackler L: Proposed practice guidelines for nonoperative anterior cruciate ligament rehabilitation of physically active individuals, *J Orthop Sports Phys Ther* 30(4):194-203, 2000.
19. Christie AD, Willoughby GL: The effect of interferential therapy on swelling following open reduction and internal fixation of ankle fractures, *Physiother Theory Pract* 6:3-7, 1990.
20. Johnson MI, Wilson H: The analgesic effects of different swing patterns of interferential currents of cold-induced pain, *Physiotherapy* 83:461-467, 1997.
21. Young SL, Woodbury MG, Fryday-Field K: Efficacy of interferential current stimulation alone for pain reduction

in patients with osteoarthritis of the knee: a randomized placebo control clinical trial, *Phys Ther* 71:252, 1991.

22. Lieber RL, Silva PD, Daniel DM: Equal effectiveness of electrical and volitional strength training for quadriceps femoris muscles after anterior cruciate ligament surgery, *J Orthop Res* 14(1):131-138, 1996.

23. Van Swearingen J: Electrical stimulation for improving muscle performance. In Nelson RM, Hayes KW, Currier DP, eds: *Clinical electrotherapy*, ed 3, Stamford, CT, 1999, Appleton & Lange.

24. Delitto A, Rose SJ, Lehman RC, et al: Electrical stimulation versus voluntary exercise in strengthening the thigh musculature after anterior cruciate ligament surgery, *Phys Ther* 68:660-663, 1988.

25. Stevens JE, Mizner RL, Snyder-Mackler L: Neuromuscular electrical stimulation for quadriceps muscle strengthening after bilateral total knee arthroplasty: a case series, *J Orthop Sports Phys Ther* 34(1):21-29, 2004.

26. Fitzgerald GK, Piva SR, Irrgang JJ: A modified neuromuscular electrical stimulation protocol for quadriceps strength training following anterior cruciate ligament reconstruction 1, *J Orthop Sports Phys Ther* 33(9):492-501, 2003.

27. Krebs DE: Clinical electromyographic feedback following menisectomy. A multiple regression experimental analysis, *Phys Ther* 61:1017-1021, 1983.

CHAPTER 8

Movement System Syndromes of the Foot and Ankle

Mary K. Hastings

INTRODUCTION

Use of the movement system classification in the examination and treatment of musculoskeletal pain problems of the foot and ankle starts with the basic premise that a large component of the stress that causes tissue injury is the result of movement. Movement results in injury and pain because the motion is completed in an imprecise manner (excursion is excessive, insufficient, and/or asynchronous with the functional requirements) and/or the repetitions of the motion or the duration the posture is maintained exceeds the tissue's capabilities. The physical therapist examines muscle length and performance, structural variations, and the ease and excursion through which the foot, ankle, knee, hip, and spine move. The physical therapist determines the component impairments contributing to injurious motions and/or forces at unsuitable distal or proximal anatomical sites within the foot and entire lower extremity. Daily activities and habits of the patient are also assessed. Additionally, the physical therapist considers the impact of body weight, age, foot size, and disease on the foot and ankle.

The foot and ankle have very complex and often opposing functional responsibilities during weight-bearing activities. The foot and ankle must be flexible to adapt to uneven surfaces, transfer high forces, and allow motion of the body in multiple directions around a planted foot. During weight-bearing activities, the foot must quickly transform into a rigid lever that allows muscular contractions to propel the body forward, upward, sideways, or any combination of these motions. The foot also has an important role in balance; sensing body location and maintaining an upright posture.

The most common movement system syndromes of the foot and ankle injury are related to the inability of the foot to function equally well as a flexible adapter (requiring motion in the direction of pronation) and a rigid lever (requiring motion in the direction of supination). The injured foot often falls toward an extreme of one of these two roles (either a great flexible adapter with poor ability to transform to a rigid lever or a rigid lever

with limited flexibility). The movement impairment often presents as excessive or incorrect timing of the normal motions of pronation and/or supination.

This chapter outlines key principles involved in the assessment of alignment, structural variations, movement, and tests of muscle length and strength. The syndromes are described, and suggestions for associated impairments in the hip and knee are mentioned. Additionally, treatment for restoring precise motion through limiting hypermobility, addressing limitations in joint and muscle extensibility, and training for the change in movement in daily activities and habits is provided.

ALIGNMENT OF THE ANKLE AND FOOT

Ankle

The joints of the ankle include the proximal tibiofibular joint, distal tibiofibular joint, and the talocrural joint. The fibula has a limited weight-bearing function but serves as the attachment of the biceps femoris and fibular collateral ligament (lateral collateral ligament). Additionally, the fibula has a role in increasing torsional stiffness (rotational stability) of the lower limb.[1] The alignment of the fibula at the proximal and distal tibia is challenging to assess. The determination of normal or impaired alignment is generally by comparison to the other side.

Foot progression angle (toe-out angle) during gait is an important alignment factor to consider in the assessment (Figure 8-1). The normal values for foot progression angle are between 7 to 13 degrees.[2] The foot progression angle is the result of rotation at the hip joint, rotation at the tibiofemoral joint, femoral torsion, and/or tibial torsion. The contribution of rotation at the hip or tibiofemoral joints is determined by assessing joint alignment. Femoral and tibial torsion can be more difficult to determine. The assessment of femoral torsion, the twist of the femur in the transverse plane, is discussed in detail in the chapter on the hip in Sahrmann.[3]

Tibial torsion, the twist of the bones of the tibia and fibula in the transverse plane, is often implicated in the

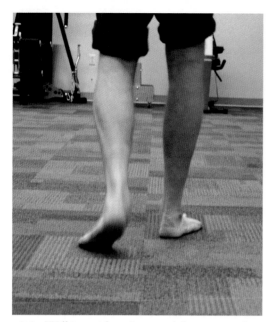

Figure 8-1. Walking with an increased foot progression angle.

predisposition of the lower extremity to injury. The normative data describe tibial torsion as usually between 20 to 40 degrees of lateral rotation.[4-6] The measurement techniques to collect normative data have generally used radiological images or cadaveric analysis. The external landmarks available for use by clinicians in determining torsion are generally poor. Use of femoral landmarks for the proximal alignment of the tibia and fibula compared to the medial and lateral malleoli[7] does not allow differentiation of lateral rotation at the tibiofemoral joint from torsion of the bones of the lower leg. Use of the tibial tuberosity and attempts to palpate the tibial condyles to determine proximal alignment is limited by variances in anatomy and difficulty in finding the tibial condyles. Because of the limitations in the nonradiological determination of tibial torsion, the clinically measured value should not be relied on, but general approach should be taken that considers the overall impact of foot progression angle on the function of the foot.

An increase in the foot progression angle rotates the foot away from the sagittal plane, into greater abduction and toward the frontal plane. During walking, the body moves forward in the sagittal plane, and rotation of the foot out of the plane of primary movement can contribute to injury. Body weight is now transferred to the medial side of the foot earlier, increasing the stress on the medial foot structures (talonavicular and first metatarsophalangeal [MTP] joint, as well as posterior tibialis muscle and tendon and the plantar fascia). The primary foot and ankle muscles involved in ambulation (the anterior tibialis and gastrocnemius/soleus muscles) are rotated out of their plane of primary importance. The fibularis (peroneus) longus and brevis become biased to aid in propelling the body forward, and the anterior tibialis has a decreased role in talocrural dorsiflexion or control of

plantar flexion and an increase in its function in inversion and control of eversion. Finally, less talocrural dorsiflexion is needed during walking, which can either contribute to a gradual reduction in dorsiflexion or can be a compensation for already reduced dorsiflexion. In summary, foot progression angle with walking can contribute to excessive stress that increases the risk of injury.

Foot

Hindfoot

The hindfoot includes the talus, calcaneus, and the subtalar joint (joint between the talus and calcaneus). Inclusion of the talus in both the ankle and the foot indicates the importance of the talus to the function of the foot, as well as the function of the leg. The talus is responsible for absorbing and transmitting rotatory forces that have come from the hip and/or knee but also transmits rotatory forces up to the knee and hip that originated in the foot. The interconnectedness of the leg to the foot by way of the talus has led many to consider alignment of the hindfoot key in understanding the mechanics of the foot. In assessing alignment of the hindfoot, one can begin by assessing standing calcaneal alignment. The calcaneal alignment is generally classified as valgus, varus, or neutral and generally rests in slight valgus (3.5 degrees).[8] The standing alignment of the calcaneus is then compared to the position of the calcaneus in subtalar joint neutral.

Assessment of subtalar joint neutral is the only clinical method available to determine structural variation in the hindfoot. Subtalar joint neutral is difficult to determine and measure in a reliable manner. However, the neutral alignment is a useful tool in interpreting standing alignment and providing a general reference for understanding the function of the foot. The determination of subtalar joint neutral occurs in prone. The examiner grasps the head of the talus with the thumb and index finger of one hand and the fifth metatarsal head with the other hand (Figure 8-2). The examiner uses the grasp on the fifth metatarsal head to move the forefoot and hindfoot into abduction and adduction until the fingers on the head of the talus palpate an equal proportion of the head of the talus on the medial and lateral side (under the thumb and index finger). The foot is held in this position to assess alignment. The alignment of the vertical bisection of the calcaneus is compared to the bisection of the lower leg.

The hindfoot is determined to be in varus alignment if the calcaneus is inverted relative to the lower leg, in valgus alignment if the calcaneus is everted relative to the lower leg, and neutral if the calcaneus is aligned with the lower leg (Figure 8-3, A). The forefoot alignment is determined to be in subtalar joint neutral by comparing the plane of the hindfoot to the plane of the forefoot. If the forefoot is inverted on the hindfoot, the forefoot is considered to have a varus alignment. If the forefoot is everted on the hindfoot, the forefoot has a valgus alignment, and if the

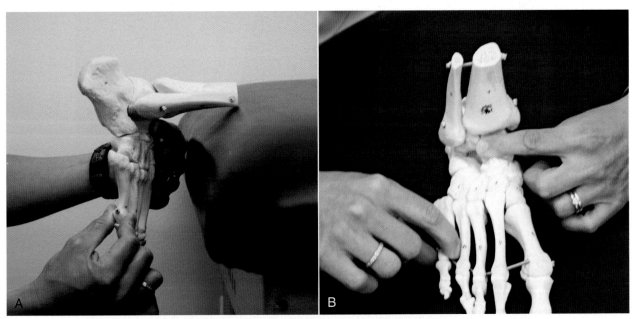

Figure 8-2. Subtalar joint neutral hand placement on skeleton: Outside hand at fifth metatarsal head and inside hand on head and neck of talus in standard position **(A)** and dorsal view **(B)**.

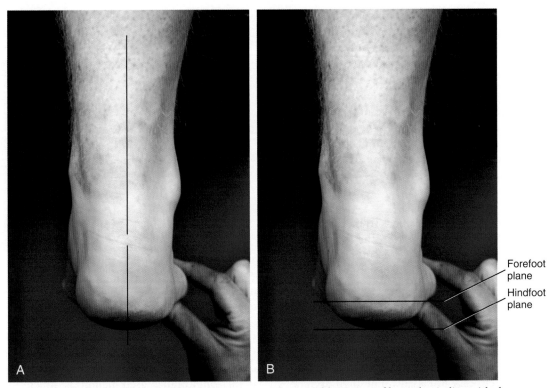

Forefoot plane

Hindfoot plane

Figure 8-3. **A,** Neutral hindfoot alignment with vertical bisection of lower leg in line with the vertical bisection of the calcaneus. **B,** Neutral forefoot to hindfoot alignment with the plane of the hindfoot parallel to the forefoot.

hindfoot and forefoot planes are parallel, the forefoot has a neutral alignment (Figure 8-3, *B*).

The alignment of the metatarsal heads can also be assessed at this time. The metatarsal heads should be aligned along the same plane. Often the first metatarsal head will be located in a more plantar position than the remaining metatarsal heads. This is called a *plantarflexed* (dropped) first ray, which is a forefoot compensation for structural variations of varus at the hindfoot or forefoot (Figure 8-4).

The non–weight-bearing subtalar joint neutral alignment, providing insight into structure variability, is the

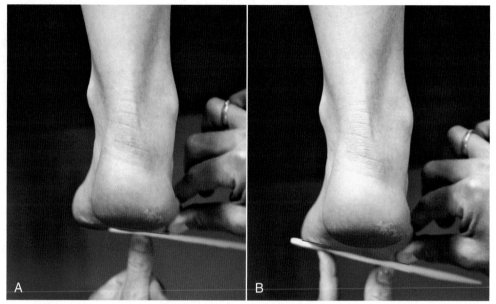

Figure 8-4. A, First metatarsal head is plantarflexed (dropped) below the plane of second to fourth metatarsal heads. **B,** Correction of the dropped first ray. The forefoot varus alignment relative to the hindfoot is now apparent.

backdrop for interpreting standing alignment and function. For example, suppose during prone subtalar joint assessment the neutral subtalar joint position was with the calcaneus inverted relative to the lower leg (hindfoot varus). During the standing alignment assessment, the calcaneus is vertical. The hindfoot is assessed as being able to compensate for the varus structural deviation (hindfoot alignment is termed *compensated hindfoot varus*); however, the standing calcaneal alignment is now understood as potentially harmful as the subtalar joint is being maintained near an end-range position.

Arches
Standing alignment assessment proceeds to the arches of the foot. There is truly only one arch in the foot that is continuous from anterior to posterior and medial to lateral, but the arch is usually described as three arches: the medial longitudinal arch, the lateral longitudinal arch, and the transverse arch. Much of the research on foot type, function, and injury has used the standing alignment of the medial longitudinal arch as the primary method of determining foot type.[9-11] The height of the arch is often a key element. Extremes of high arch and low arch are relatively easy to classify. The high arch, a supinated foot type, is often accompanied by calcaneal inversion and an adducted forefoot, and the head of the talus and navicular are more prominent on the dorsal surface of the foot. The low-arch foot, a pronated foot type, is often accompanied by calcaneal eversion and a splayed and abducted forefoot, and the head of the talus and the navicular are more prominent in the middle of the arch (medial bulge).

The lateral longitudinal arch has greater inherent bony stability than the medial longitudinal arch. The

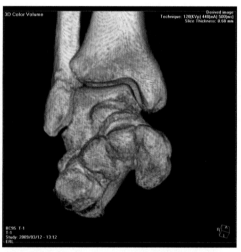

Figure 8-5. Non–weight-bearing computed tomography image of the foot in the frontal plane with the metatarsals and phalanges removed. Note the wedged shape of cuneiforms 1 to 3 contributing to the formation of the arch.

joint surfaces of the calcaneus and cuboid are concavo-convex, providing some restriction to movement.[12] The lateral longitudinal arch height is much lower, often appearing flat in visual assessment.

The transverse arch is formed in part by the wedge shape of the cuneiforms[12] (Figure 8-5). As the transverse arch is assessed more distally on the foot, the height of the arch decreases until all metatarsal heads are in a level plane and capable of bearing weight.

Forefoot
The forefoot includes the metatarsals and phalanges. The normal alignment of the forefoot includes metatarsal and

phalanges all aligned straight on one another. The toes should be relatively flat on the ground.

The common alignment impairment at the first MTP joint is hallux valgus. This alignment presents as angulation of the first metatarsal into abduction and the phalanx into adduction. The toes will also present with alignment faults that usually include a component of metatarsalphalangeal hyperextension with flexion at the all interphalangeal joints (claw toes) or flexion at the proximal interphalangeal joint and extension at the distal interphalangeal joint (hammer toes).

MOTIONS OF THE ANKLE AND FOOT

Static alignment determined in subtalar joint neutral and standing are only a small part of understanding how the foot functions. Examination of how the joints of the foot and ankle move and function during walking, running, hopping, squatting, and various daily activities provides the bulk of the information that directs the diagnosis and treatment.

Ankle

Proximal and Distal Tibiofibular Joints
The proximal tibiofibular joint has very little motion, and individual variability in the shape of the joint surfaces has resulted in a wide variety of associated fibular motions reported with dorsiflexion and plantarflexion.[13] The fibula at the proximal tibiofibular joint has been reported to glide anterior, lateral, and superior with talocrural dorsiflexion and to glide posterior, medial, and inferior with talocrural plantarflexion.[13] The distal tibiofibular joint consists of a convex fibula and a concave tibia.[12] During talocrural joint motion from neutral to dorsiflexion, the fibula at the distal tibiofibular joint has been found to have motions of internal rotation, lateral displacement (widens), and posterior and superior glide.[14] During talocrural motion from dorsiflexion to plantarflexion, the fibula at the distal tibiofibular joint has been found to be medially displaced.[15]

Talocrural Joint
The axis of motion at the talocrural joint is not uniplanar but triplanar, crossing all three planes of motion. The motions about the axis are termed *pronation* and *supination*. Table 8-1 shows component motion description. The axis at the talocrural joint, although it crosses all three planes, lies primarily in the transverse plane in a medial-to-lateral direction. Thus plantarflexion and dorsiflexion are the primary motions.

Dorsiflexion. Adequate dorsiflexion motion at the talocrural joint is crucial in advancing the tibia over the foot in walking, running, jumping, squatting, and many other weight-bearing activities. A minimum of 10 degrees of dorsiflexion (with the knee extended) is needed for walking and 30 degrees for running.[16] Dorsiflexion motion requires adequate length of the gastrocnemius

muscle, soleus muscle, and calcaneal (Achilles) tendon, as well as ligaments and joint structures of the talocrural joint. Because the head of the talus is wider anteriorly than posteriorly, a small amount of motion is required at the tibiofibular joint to fully accept the dome of the talus.[13] If dorsiflexion is found to be limited, the source of limited talocrural motion can be assessed by measuring talocrural dorsiflexion with the knee extended and flexed and assessing talocrural joint accessory motion. Additionally, dorsiflexion should be isolated to the talocrural joint, and compensations at the foot (e.g., eversion, midtarsal dorsiflexion, and pronation) should not be allowed during dorsiflexion. The following information is gleaned from this test:

- Gastrocnemius muscle/calcaneal (Achilles) tendon short if dorsiflexion is ≤10 degrees with the knee extended but ≥10 degrees with knee flexed.
- Soleus muscle short if dorsiflexion is ≤10 degrees regardless of knee position and accessory talocrural motion is normal.
- Talocrural joint limitation if dorsiflexion is ≤10 degrees regardless of knee position and accessory talocrural joint motion is limited (cannot rule out soleus muscle limitation in this case).

Without adequate motion at the talocrural joint, the body can employ a number of strategies for compensating. The patient can increase the foot progression angle, demonstrate an early heel rise, or use a forefoot strike pattern (only the forefoot is in contact with the ground) during walking and running to compensate for the lack of dorsiflexion. Additionally, the failure to dorsiflex at the talocrural joint during stance phase can be compensated for by hyperextending the knee and/or increasing the dorsiflexion that occurs at the more distal joints of the foot: talonavicular, naviculocuneiform, calcaneocuboid, and/or cuboid-metatarsal joints (Figure 8-6).

Plantarflexion. Plantarflexion at the talocrural joint plays an important role in propelling the body during walking, running, and jumping. Normal plantarflexion motion during gait is approximately 30 degrees. Plantarflexion at the talocrural joint alone, however, is relatively ineffective in propelling the body forward. The foot (calcaneus to metatarsal heads) must become a rigid

---

TABLE **8-1**

Motions at the Hindfoot Associated with Open- and Closed-Chain Pronation and Supination

	Open Chain	**Closed Chain**
Pronation	Calcaneal eversion	Calcaneal eversion
	Calcaneal dorsiflexion	Talar plantarflexion
	Calcaneal abduction	Talar adduction
Supination	Calcaneal inversion	Calcaneal inversion
	Calcaneal plantarflexion	Talar dorsiflexion
	Calcaneal adduction	Talar abduction

lever to transfer the plantarflexion force through the foot, raising the body over the toes. The foot becomes more rigid in a number of ways. First, the foot becomes rigid through maximizing bony alignment. The contraction of the plantarflexors has a supination component. Supination of the subtalar joint and transtarsal joint helps place the joints in their closed pack, which is a more stable position providing some stability to the foot.

The second way the foot becomes rigid is by the passive tensioning function of the plantar aponeurosis. The plantar aponeurosis is a thick fascial sheath originating at the calcaneal tubercle and inserting into multiple locations but primarily into the flexor tendons of the foot and the base of the fifth metatarsal. As the heel begins to rise at the end of the stance phase, the MTP joints dorsiflex and the plantar aponeurosis becomes taut. The joints of the foot are approximated, the arch rises, and the foot becomes more rigid (windlass mechanism). Third, the foot is rigid because of the muscular forces

that directly impact joint stability. The posterior tibialis muscle/tendon is aligned to provide not only a force that produces plantarflexion with supination but also a force directed along the long axis of the foot. The posterior tibialis tendon inserts into all the tarsal bones, except the talus, as well as the bases of second to fourth metatarsals. The posteriorly directed force along the long axis of the foot is critical to the function of the foot. The force provides muscular "cinching" of the foot bones, increasing foot rigidity and the effectiveness of the ankle plantarflexor muscles.[17] An extreme example of failure of the mechanisms that provide rigidity to the midfoot allowing plantar flexion at the midfoot is seen in Figure 8-7. (Contraction of the gastrocnemius in subject *B* of Figure 8-7 would result in isolated plantarflexion of the calcaneus without a forceful transfer of plantarflexion to propel the body.) The intrinsic muscles of the foot also function to support the arch of the foot and provide rigidity to the foot during plantarflexion.

Foot

Subtalar Joint

The axis of motion at the subtalar joint is also triplanar. The axis, although it crosses all planes, lies primarily between the sagittal and transverse plane, allowing more inversion and eversion and abduction and adduction than plantarflexion and dorsiflexion.

Inversion and eversion. Motion at the subtalar joint is fairly limited because of the lack of symmetry in shape of the three talar facets (the posterior talar facet is concave, whereas the middle and anterior talar facets are flat to convex). Subtalar joint range of motion (ROM) is reported to be between 5 to 10 degrees of calcaneal eversion and 20 to 30 degrees of calcaneal inversion.[18-20]

The triplanar motion of the subtalar joint is difficult to capture during weight-bearing activities using standard kinematic techniques. Passive calcaneal motion of inversion and eversion are easily measured goniometrically and often used to provide some indication of the movement at the subtalar joint. During walking the calcaneus contacts the ground in slight inversion

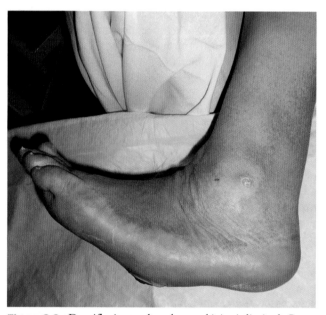

Figure 8-6. Dorsiflexion at the talocrural joint is limited. Compensation has occurred with dorsiflexion at the midtarsal joint.

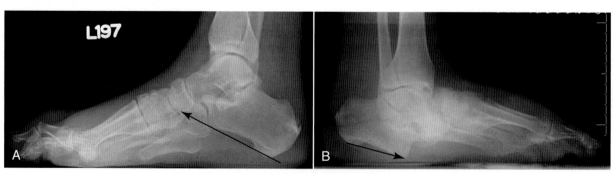

Figure 8-7. A, An individual with diabetes and peripheral neuropathy. Note the normal upward inclination of the calcaneus. **B,** The foot of an individual with diabetes, peripheral neuropathy, and Charcot's osteoarthropathy. This individual has lost the necessary rigidity of the foot and the pull of the gastrocnemius/soleus muscle through the calcaneal (Achilles) tendon resulted in calcaneal plantarflexion.

(approximately 2.5 degrees from standing calcaneal position). The calcaneus moves into slight eversion through heel-off and then begins the return to inversion (approximately 6 degrees from the standing calcaneal position) right before toe-off.[21]

In the weight-bearing foot, the intimate connection of the talus to the lower leg through the talocrural joint links medial rotation of the lower leg to subtalar joint pronation (talar adduction and calcaneal eversion) and vice versa, subtalar joint pronation to lower leg medial rotation. The same is true for the linking of lateral rotation of the lower leg to supination and supination to lateral rotation of the leg. The linking of foot and leg motion through the subtalar joint illuminates why many have worked to assess and understand subtalar alignment, motion, and function.

Transverse Tarsal or Midtarsal Joints

The transverse tarsal joint is comprised of the talonavicular and calcaneocuboid joints. The axes of motion at the transverse tarsal joints are triplanar, allowing pronation and supination. In most feet, motion at the subtalar joint is intimately connected to the motions that occur at the talonavicular and calcaneocuboid joints. As the subtalar joint supinates, it draws the transverse tarsal joint into supination, a more stable joint position of the transverse tarsal joint (locked position), converting the midfoot into a more rigid lever. As the subtalar joint pronates the transverse tarsal joint pronates, which creates a more loose position of the joints and a more flexible midfoot.[22,23]

The transverse tarsal joints are the intermediate joints between the hindfoot and the forefoot. One of the functions of the transverse tarsal joint is to position the forefoot for ground contact during push-off. In performing this function, the transverse tarsal joint becomes a frequent site of compensation for structural variances and movement impairments of both the hindfoot and forefoot. The transverse tarsal joint can become hyperflexible, limiting the ability of the foot to transform into a rigid lever and decreasing the stability of the longitudinal arches, which contributes to flat-foot deformities.

In the high arched or more rigid foot type, the subtalar joint and the transverse tarsal joints are maintained in the closed pack or locked position. The lack of mobility is thought to contribute to injuries at the foot and lower extremity as a result the inability of the rigid foot to dissipate the high forces occurring during weight-bearing activities.

Tarsometatarsal Joints

The tarsometatarsal joints generally have very little motion and are critical in providing the structure for the transverse arch. Motion that occurs at the tarsometatarsal joints is generally with the focus of positioning the forefoot flat on the ground for push-off. If the motion that has proceeded from the hindfoot to the midfoot during gait has inadequately prepared the forefoot for weight-bearing, the tarsometatarsal joints may assist. For example, insufficient pronation of the hindfoot and midfoot from heel strike through midstance might result in the medial side of the forefoot being up off the weight-bearing surface. If there is motion available at the tarsometatarsal joints, a pronatory twist will occur at the tarsometatarsal joints to bring the forefoot flat.[23] A supinatory twist will occur in the tarsometatarsal joints if too much pronation has occurred at the hindfoot and midfoot during early stance phase. The site of compensatory motion often becomes the source of symptoms.

Metatarsophalangeal Joints

The MTP joints' primary direction of function is into dorsiflexion. Adequate MTP dorsiflexion allows the foot to roll over the toes as the plantarflexor muscles propel the body forward. Additionally, MTP dorsiflexion stretches the plantar aponeurosis, elevating the arch and assisting in making the foot rigid during push-off. First MTP joint dorsiflexion needed for walking is reported to be between 30 to 60 degrees.[24,25] Lack of first toe extension prevents the normal pattern of roll-over, and weight is transferred either medial or lateral of the first toe. Medial weight transfer increases the abduction force on the proximal phalanx, predisposing the individual to hallux valgus deformity. Lateral transfer of weight increases the force borne by the second and third metatarsal heads, often resulting in pain at the MTP joints.

First MTP joint dorsiflexion can be limited by the length of the flexor hallucis longus, plantar aponeurosis (fascia), or joint restrictions. Theoretically, the contribution of flexor hallucis longus muscle length to limited MTP joint dorsiflexion motion can be determined by comparing MTP dorsiflexion ROM with the talocrural joint dorsiflexed (flexor hallucis longus on stretch) to MTP dorsiflexion ROM with the talocrural joint plantarflexed (flexor hallucis longus on slack). First MTP dorsiflexion in full plantarflexion should measure ≥60 degrees. First MTP dorsiflexion in full talocrural dorsiflexion is rarely measured. Hopson et al[25] found on average 85 degrees of MTP dorsiflexion in 0 degrees of talocrural dorsiflexion. Nawoczenski et al[24] found 35 to 45 degrees of MTP dorsiflexion in a standing passive and active test. Clinically, MTP dorsiflexion measured in talocrural dorsiflexion is very limited, between 10 to 15 degrees (Figure 8-8). Decreased MTP dorsiflexion in full talocrural dorsiflexion can indicate flexor hallucis muscle length impairment. However, the plantar aponeurosis may also be limiting MTP motion in this position because the position of maximum MTP and ankle dorsiflexion has been found to place maximum stretch on the plantar aponeurosis.[26]

Functionally, there is rarely an occasion in which maximum MTP dorsiflexion is needed during maximum talocrural dorsiflexion. During gait, 30 to 60 degrees of first MTP dorsiflexion[24,25] is needed during push-off when the talocrural joint is in approximately 10 to 25 degrees of talocrural plantarflexion.[21,23] Thus the most functional assessment of first MTP dorsiflexion would be to assess MTP dorsiflexion motion in approximately 20

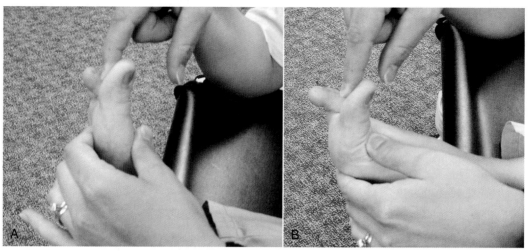

Figure 8-8. First metatarsophalangeal extension. **A,** In talocrural joint dorsiflexion. **B,** In talocrural joint plantarflexion.

degrees of talocrural plantarflexion. In summary, the following information can be gleaned from the test:

- Flexor hallucis longus short if <30 degrees of MTP joint dorsiflexion in talocrural dorsiflexion and ≥30 degrees of MTP joint dorsiflexion in talocrural plantarflexion. (Cannot determine the contribution of plantar aponeurosis length to test results.)
- First MTP joint limitation if first MTP joint dorsiflexion remains limited regardless of ankle position and accessory MTP joint motion is limited (cannot rule out flexor hallucis brevis or other one joint muscles crossing the MTP joint).

The contribution of MTP dorsiflexion to engage the windlass mechanism of the foot thus increasing foot rigidity during push-off is critical. Stretching into first MTP dorsiflexion should be approached with caution to avoid overlengthening of the foot structures critical for engaging the windlass mechanism of the foot.

Interphalangeal Joints

The interphalangeal joints have a critical role in increasing the area over which the weight-bearing force is distributed during push-off. To increase surface area during push-off, the toes must be flat on the ground. The intrinsic muscles of the foot are critical in stabilizing the MTP joints against excessive dorsiflexion (hyperextension) while extending the interphalangeal joints of the toes to provide a flat surface for force distribution. Without appropriate function of the intrinsic muscles of the foot, claw toe deformities develop as the extrinsic toe flexors and extensors act unopposed.

MUSCLE ACTIONS

Leg

The four muscular compartments of the leg are the superficial posterior compartment, the deep posterior compartment, the lateral compartment, and the anterior compartment. The compartments are separated by fascial encasements that are continuations from the tensor fascia latae of the thigh.[12] The fascial compartments assist the muscle by transferring the contractile force produced by the muscle to the bone (Figure 8-9). The fascial compartments also provide spatial constraints to edema and can compromise nerve and blood vessel function within a compartment when edema increases.

Posterior Compartments

The superficial and deep posterior compartments of the leg contain the primary plantarflexors of the ankle (the gastrocnemius, soleus, tibialis posterior, flexor hallucis longus, and flexor digitorum longus muscles), the posterior tibial artery and veins, tibial nerve, and fibular (peroneal) artery and veins. All posterior compartment muscles insert medial to the midline of the foot and therefore also assist in supination. Strong plantarflexion with supination is important in the muscular component that transforms the foot into the rigid lever for effective push off during gait. The posterior compartment also has a significant eccentric role during walking and running by controlling tibial progression over the foot and pronation of the foot from initial contact until the start of push-off.

The posterior tibialis, flexor hallucis longus, and flexor digitorum muscles and the posterior tibial artery and tibial nerve make a sharp turn around the medial malleolus and travel beneath the flexor retinaculum in the region posterior to the medial malleolus. The area in which this sharp turn occurs is a frequent site for tendon injury, as well as nerve compression.

Lateral Compartment

The lateral compartment contains the fibularis (peroneus) longus and brevis muscles and the superficial fibular (peroneal) nerve. The fibularis muscles are ankle evertors and weak ankle plantarflexors. Additionally, the fibularis

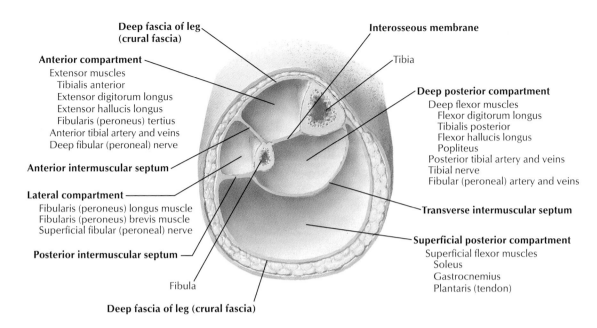

Cross section just above middle of leg

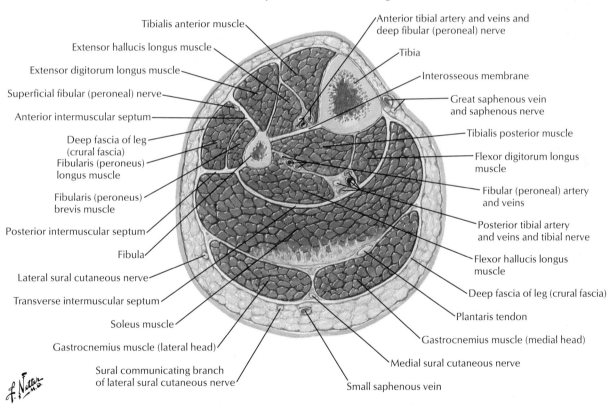

Figure 8-9. Fascial compartments and components. (From Greene WB: *Netter's orthopaedics*, Philadelphia, 2006, Saunders.)

longus muscle crosses the plantar surface of the foot and inserts on the base of the first metatarsal and medial cuneiform bone, providing a supportive sling for the foot and muscular control of the forefoot position. The fibularis brevis muscle inserts into the base of the fifth metatarsal, providing rigidity to the lateral column of the foot.

Anterior Compartment

The anterior compartment contains the tibialis anterior, extensor hallucis longus, and the extensor digitorum longus muscles; the anterior tibial artery and veins; and the deep fibular (peroneal) nerve. The muscles, the anterior tibial artery, and the deep fibular nerve pass under the superior and inferior extensor retinaculum. All muscles within the anterior compartment are ankle dorsiflexors. The insertions of the tibialis anterior and extensor hallucis longus are medial to the talocrural joint axis, inverting the foot during dorsiflexion. The insertion of the extensor digitorum longus is lateral to the talocrural joint axis and everts the foot during dorsiflexion. For balanced dorsiflexion that occurs primarily in the sagittal plane, the anterior tibialis and extensor hallucis longus inversion force must be countered by the eversion force produced by the extensor digitorum longus.

The anterior compartment muscles function concentrically during the swing phase of walking and running, dorsiflexing the foot, and clearing the toe. The anterior compartment muscles work eccentrically to control lowering of the foot from heel strike to foot flat in a heelstrike first pattern of walking and running.

Foot

The intrinsic muscles of the foot provide important stabilization of the arches and the MTP and interphalangeal joints of the foot, as well as help regulate tension and direction of force produced by the extrinsic muscles of the foot. The quadratus plantae muscle attaches from the calcaneus to the tendons of the flexor digitorum longus muscle to redirect the diagonal force of the flexor digitorum longus so that the toes flex in the sagittal plane (Figure 8-10). The lumbricals attach from the flexor digitorum longus tendon to the medial proximal phalanx and on to the dorsal expansion of the extensor digitorum longus. When the lumbricals contract, they flex the MTP joint, place the flexor digitorum longus tendons on slack, and pull on the extensor digitorum longus dorsal expansion to extend the interphalangeal joints. The interossei

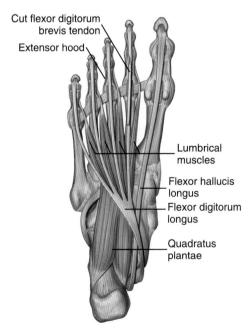

Figure 8-10. Quadratus plantae muscle. (From Drake R: *Gray's anatomy for students*, ed 2, Churchill Livingstone, 2009, London.)

attach to the shafts of the metatarsals and insert onto the base of the proximal phalanx, assisting in flexing the MTP joint, extending the interphalangeal joints, and providing a force to abduct and adduct the toes. Through the function of the interossei and lumbricals, hammer and claw toe deformities are prevented.[23]

The intrinsic muscles, in general, originate and insert along the longitudinal axis of the foot (they run proximal to distal). Through muscular contraction, the intrinsic muscles provide critical stabilization of the foot, assisting in the transformation of the foot from a flexible adaptor during initial phases of stance to a rigid lever during push off.[12]

An important function of the interossei and lumbricals is to stabilize the MTP joints during talocrural dorsiflexion. The extensor digitorum assists in producing balanced talocrural dorsiflexion but is also simultaneously acting to dorsiflex the MTP joints. MTP joint dorsiflexion during talocrural dorsiflexion is an unwanted action. First, the extensor digitorum tendon is shortened over both joints (the MTP and talocrural joints), decreasing the talocrural dorsiflexion torque production capability. Second, the plantar fascia is placed on maximum stretch, increasing the risk of injury. Finally, repetitive MTP extension contributes to hammer and claw toe deformities. The lumbricals and interossei muscles act to counter the action of the extensor digitorum longus and stabilize the MTP joints during talocrural dorsiflexion.

Interestingly, there are no intrinsic foot muscles that originate from the talus or calcaneus and attach to the navicular or cuboid. The stability of the transtarsal joint depends on bony shape, taut ligamentous restraints, and extrinsic muscles of the foot that cross this joint. The lack of intrinsic muscle joint restraints may contribute to the transtarsal joint becoming a frequent site of hypermobility.

Understanding the anatomy and kinesiology of the ankle and foot is the fundamental foundation necessary to critically examine functional activities of the foot and to determine the movement system diagnosis. The remainder of the chapter uses this knowledge of anatomy and kinesiology to assess movement and to determine when a movement impairment exists and what factors may be contributing to this movement impairment.

EXAMINATION OF THE ANKLE AND FOOT

History

A standard history should be collected by the physical therapist and should include the history of the injury, pain ratings (symptoms at their worst, best, and average) and frequency and the duration of the pain. The standard history also includes the effect of daily activities and positions on symptoms, and the physical therapist must become familiar with the patient's daily routine and requirements, as well as any changes in activity level that may have occurred around the onset of the symptoms.

The physical therapist must also ask additional questions regarding the patient's footwear. Detailed information about the type and age of the footwear and the frequency and duration that each type of footwear is worn should be obtained. The therapist should become familiar with previous inserts, orthoses, or lower extremity braces the patient has been prescribed and/or worn.

The systems review should include the patient's medical and surgical history and current medications. Musculoskeletal, neurovascular, and systemic sources of signs and symptoms must be examined and may require referral to a physician for additional management.

Potential Conditions Requiring Referral

Stress Fracture

Stress fractures are a common musculoskeletal source of undiagnosed foot and ankle symptoms that must be ruled out before completing a movement system examination and prescribing an intervention. Stress fracture pain generally is local and isolated to the bone, although symptom presentation can be diffuse and confusing. The six locations of stress fractures that are at high risk for serious sequelae if undertreated are anterior lateral tibial diaphysis, medial malleolus, talus, navicular, fifth metatarsal, and sesamoids.[27] Local or suspicious signs and symptoms in the high risk areas should be immediately referred to a physician because delayed treatment or undertreatment tends to result in progression to a complete fracture, a nonunion, the need for operative intervention, and/or recurrence or refracture.

Deep Vein Thromboses

Deep vein thromboses (DVT) can be the source of calf pain and edema. The strongest risk factors associated with development of a DVT include a fracture of the pelvis, femur, or tibia; hip or knee replacement; spinal cord injury; major general surgery; or major trauma. The Homans' sign[28-30] (calf squeeze) has been commonly used to assess the presence of DVTs. Unfortunately, Homans' sign has little diagnostic value.[31] The Clinical Decision Rule developed by Wells et al assesses signs and symptoms, assigning a score and a probability of the presence of a DVT and has been found reliable and valid.[32,33]

Diabetes Mellitus

The lower extremity is at risk for devastating consequences of diabetes mellitus. Peripheral neuropathy and small vessel vascular disease can lead to unperceived injury, deformity, and nonhealing ulcers. Lower extremity amputation is often the outcome. An aggressive and complete screening for sensation and blood flow (see the "Peripheral Vascular Disease" section) should be completed on all patients who have suspicious histories. Sensation should be tested with Semmes-Weinstein monofilaments. For the foot and ankle, individuals are considered to lack protective sensation, which is sensation capable of detecting injury, if they are unable to feel the 5.07/10-gm filament on any location on the foot.

For individuals with diabetes mellitus, the hemoglobin A1c level (HbA1c) measures the percentage of hemoglobin in the blood that has glucose attached, indicating blood glucose control over a 3 month period of time. Normally, this value should be ≤6%. A higher HbA1c value indicates poor glucose control and is correlated with an increase risk of developing complications related to diabetes.[34]

Peripheral Vascular Disease

Peripheral vascular disease can present as claudicating pain, which is pain in the lower leg that comes on with walking and decreases or resolves with rest. The clinician should look for loss of hair on the feet and legs, decreased capillary refill, nonpalpable pulses at the dorsalis pedis and/or posterior tibial arteries, and poor skin color. The patient may also report results from an ankle-arm index assessment that compares blood pressure in the arms to blood pressure in multiple sites in the lower extremity. Normal ankle-arm index values should be between 0.91 to 1.3.[35] There is and increased risk of a cardiovascular event with values <1.0 and ≥1.4.

Rheumatoid Arthritis

Although rare (16%), an initial presentation of rheumatoid arthritis (RA) occurs in the foot and ankle.[36] Specifically, individuals complain of forefoot pain. Hindfoot pain is often a later manifestation of RA.

Seronegative Spondyloarthropathies

Foot and ankle pain are also common complaints in ankylosing spondylitis, psoriatic arthritis, Reiter's syndrome, and inflammatory bowel arthritides. Foot and ankle complaints are generally accompanied by additional signs and symptoms specific to the disease.

Gout

Gout can present in an acute or chronic manner. The pain, redness, and swelling is generally localized to the first MTP.[37]

Potential Diagnoses and/or Conditions Requiring Referral

There are a number of undiagnosed conditions that should be suspected from the history and symptoms. If the conditions are not ruled out, they require a referral to a physician in addition to physical therapy or before physical therapy (see the Chapter 8 Appendix).

Movement System Syndromes
of the Ankle and Foot

A movement system diagnosis is useful because the treatment plan directly addresses the movement pattern causing excessive stress on a particular tissue and

TABLE **8-2**
Foot and Ankle Syndromes

Syndrome	Key Findings	Source of Symptoms
Pronation	Incorrect timing or amount of motion of the ankle/foot in the direction of pronation during weight-bearing activities (hindfoot, midfoot, and/or forefoot).	Plantar fascia, posterior and anterior tibialis muscle/tendon, metatarsal heads, interdigital or tibial nerves, medial column joints and ligaments (talocrural, subtalar, talonavicular, naviculocuneiform, tarsometatarsal, and MTP joints)
Supination	Incorrect timing or amount of motion of the ankle and foot in the direction of supination during weight-bearing activities (hindfoot, midfoot, and/or forefoot).	Plantar fascia, fibular muscle/tendon, gastrocnemius/soleus muscle, calcaneal tendon, metatarsal heads, lateral column joints and ligaments (talocrural, subtalar, calcaneocuboid, tarsometatarsal, and MTP joints)
Insufficient dorsiflexion	Insufficient dorsiflexion during weight-bearing activities that require the tibia to advance over the foot.	Plantar fascia, gastrocnemius/soleus muscle, calcaneal tendon, calcaneal bursa, anterior tibialis muscle/tendon, deep fibular nerve
Hypomobility	Limitation in physiological and accessory motion of the ankle/foot joint(s).	Individual ankle and foot joints
Foot/ankle impairment	Tissue injury from surgery or trauma that requires protection for repair.	Individual ankle and foot tissues (bone, cartilage, muscle, tendon, ligament, skin, nerve)
Proximal tibiofibular glide	Positional fault of the fibula on tibia or hypermobility of the tibiofibular joint during hamstring contraction.	Proximal tibiofibular joint

MTP, Metatarsophalangeal.

resulting in injury. The body structures that are stressed and injured with a particular movement system syndrome are numerous and those that are listed with each movement system syndrome are not meant to be exhaustive but reflect those most commonly seen by physical therapists (Table 8-2). The source of symptoms (the body structure injured) is not specific to the movement system syndromes and should not be used in determining the movement impairment diagnosis. In the foot and ankle, where almost all muscles cross more than one joint and produce multiplanar motions, a particular body structure can be overstressed and injured by more than one individual movement (Table 8-3).

PRONATION SYNDROME

The principal movement impairment associated with pronation syndrome is pronation at the foot/ankle during weight-bearing activities that is excessive for that individual and/or when there is insufficient movement of the foot in the direction of supination in later stance phase. The pronation impairment can occur in the hindfoot, midfoot, and/or forefoot. A foot with the pronation syndrome is a flexible foot that provides the path of least resistance to motion and the site of compensation for various structural and movement impairments within the foot, ankle, knee, and hip.

Symptoms and Pain

The stress of the pronation movement impairment results in tissue injury. The tissues at greatest risk of injury include those impacted by excessive tensile forces from overstretching or muscular efforts to resist the pronation movement and occasionally those tissues that experience compression as a result of the excessive joint position. The following section of possible structures involved in pronation syndrome is not complete but identifies the most common structures and the symptoms reported during the history component of the examination.

Plantar Aponeurosis (Fascia)
Involvement of the plantar aponeurosis is most often accompanied by patient complaints of heel pain that is worse with the first step out of bed in the morning and after a period of prolonged non–weight-bearing activities.

Posterior Tibialis Muscle and Tendon
The patient complains of pain localized to the muscle at distal one-third of the medial tibia or anywhere along the tendon as it follows its course around the medial malleolus to the primary insertion at the navicular bone. The symptoms are most apparent during the weight-bearing phase of activities as the muscle works eccentrically to control pronation and/or concentrically to supinate and plantarflex the foot and ankle.

Anterior Tibialis Muscle and Tendon
Pain is localized to the muscle at the proximal lateral tibia and/or the tendon as it inserts into the medial cuneiform and first metatarsal. The symptoms are often present at heel strike as the muscle works eccentrically to control

TABLE **8-3**

Differential Diagnoses for the Foot/Ankle

Symptom Location	Possible Diagnosis	Follow-up Tests and Questions	Referral Required: Discontinue Physical Therapy	Referral Required: Continue Examination and Treatment
LOCAL BONE PAIN				
Anterior lateral tibial diaphysis	Fracture (stress)	Palpation	×	—
Medial malleolus		Vibration of bone at location	×	—
Talus		away from site of symptoms	×	—
Navicular			×	—
Proximal (base) of the fifth metatarsal			×	—
Sesamoids			×	
Shaft or head of first through fifth metatarsals			—	×
Proximal lateral tibia			—	×
Distal medial tibia			—	×
Remaining tarsals and phalanges			—	×
Joint symptoms	DJD	Palpation	—	×
	Osteochondritis desiccans	Axial joint compression		
	RA	End-range joint motions		
Medial ankle and foot pain	Posterior tibial tendon insufficiency	Failure to complete a single-leg heel rise	—	×
	Tibial nerve compression at the tarsal tunnel	Tinel's distal to proximal along the nerve path	—	×
		Sustained provocative position		
		Tinel's in provocative position		
Calf pain	DVT	Well's Clinical Decision Rule	×	—
	Compartment syndrome	Palpation	×	—
		Pulses		
Dermatomal leg and foot pain	Low back referral (L4-S2)	Sensation tests	—	×
		Back movement tests		

X, Positive finding requiring referral.

DJD, Degenerative joint disease; *DVT,* deep vein thrombosis; *RA,* rheumatoid arthritis.

plantarflexion. Anterior tibialis muscle pain is often called *shin splints* and particularly apparent after running or long distance walking.

Tibial Nerve
Pain, tingling, and/or numbness is located on the posterior medial ankle and/or the plantar surface of the foot. Determining whether the tibial nerve is involved is critical but also difficult. Tinel's tapping test along the nerve pathway and if needed, Tinel's tapping test in the provocative positions of full dorsiflexion, calcaneal eversion, and toe extension can assist the physical therapist is determining the source of symptoms.[38]

Gastrocnemius/Soleus Muscles and Calcaneal (Achilles) Tendon
The patient complains of pain in the muscle belly or tendon, particularly during late stance, as the muscle is working eccentrically and the tendon is being placed on

stretch to control the tibia's progression over the foot and during the concentric contraction required during push-off.

Metatarsal Heads
For the movement impairment of pronation, metatarsal pain is localized to the head of the second and third metatarsals and increases during the late stance and the push-off phases of walking and running (Figure 8-11).

Interdigital Nerves
The interdigital nerves can become irritated, producing complaints of pain, tingling, or numbness between the metatarsals and into the corresponding toes. The most common location is between the third and fourth toes. The interdigital nerve often receives branches from both the medial plantar nerve and the lateral plantar nerve, increasing the size of the nerve and the risk of impingement during weight-bearing activities.

Medial Column Joints

The patient complains of generalized midfoot pain, often in the joints of the medial column (talus, calcaneus, navicular, three cuneiforms, or first, second, or third metatarsals). The pain can progress to joint degeneration and involve the joints of the lateral column.

Alignment: Structural Variations and Acquired Impairments

Standing foot alignment has been a primary method for determining foot type. The typical description of a pronated foot includes a combination of calcaneal eversion,

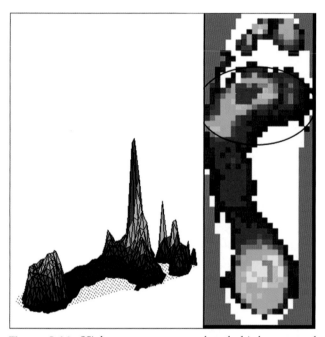

Figure 8-11. High pressure at second and third metatarsal heads in a subject with pronation during walking. Lateral midfoot pressure is related to cuboid subluxation.

medial bulge (prominence of the talonavicular joint medially), low medial longitudinal arch, forefoot abduction relative to the hindfoot at the transtarsal joint, and increased width of the forefoot (splayed forefoot) (Figure 8-12). Often, as the remainder of the lower extremity alignment is examined, there will be alignment impairments proximal to the foot that contribute to pronation at the foot. These include medial rotation at the hip, medial rotation at the knee, and structural variations of the femur and/or tibia that result in an increase in medially directed forces through the foot (e.g., femoral anteversion, medial tibial torsion, or genu valgus) (Figure 8-13).

There are a number of hindfoot and forefoot alignment variations that can contribute to the pronation syndrome. The most common structural variations are subtalar joint neutral alignment of hindfoot and/or forefoot varus. If adequate subtalar joint eversion motion is available, the calcaneus may evert to compensate for the varus alignment in an attempt to get the foot flat on the weight-bearing surface. If the midfoot and forefoot are flexible, they can also compensate for varus alignment faults contributing to a lowering of the medial longitudinal arch, forefoot abduction, and splaying (widening) of the forefoot (Figure 8-14). Valgus hindfoot and forefoot structural faults that persist with standing can also contribute to the pronated standing alignment.

Movement Impairments

Walking and Running

During walking and running, the pronation movement impairments can include excessive calcaneal eversion during the early and midstance phases, excessive arch flattening in the midstance phase, and/or insufficient movement of the foot in the direction of supination in the late stance phase (Figure 8-15). Often, there is poor contraction of the gastrocnemius muscle with very little

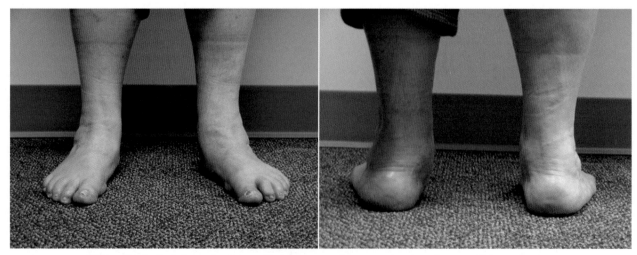

Figure 8-12. Left foot, classic standing alignment for pronation impairment: Calcaneal eversion, medial bulge, low medial longitudinal arch, forefoot abduction, and increased width of the forefoot.

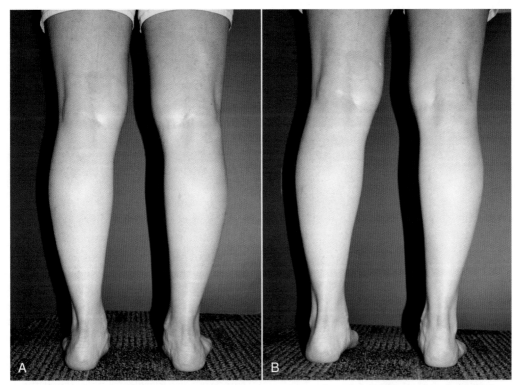

Figure 8-13. A, Individual with calcaneal valgus, dropped medial longitudinal arch, medial bulge, and abducted forefoot bilaterally. **B,** Same individual, is able to minimize foot pronation through correcting hip medial rotation and knee hyperextension.

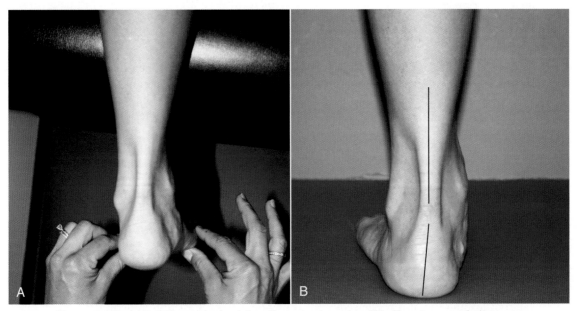

Figure 8-14. A, Left foot subtalar joint alignment in prone: Hindfoot in neutral alignment relative to the leg and a forefoot varus relative to the hindfoot. **B,** Left foot standing alignment includes slight calcaneal eversion, bulge in the medial longitudinal arch, and forefoot abduction. Calcaneal eversion indicates the ability of the hindfoot to assist in compensating for the forefoot varus structural variation.

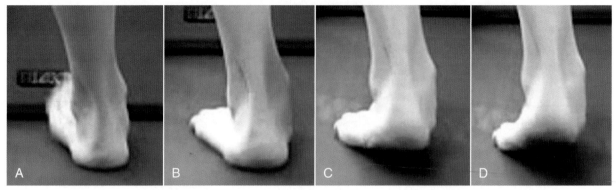

Figure 8-15. Instances in stance in an individual with pronation syndrome. **A,** Heel strike. **B,** Midstance. **C,** Heel off. **D,** Toe off.

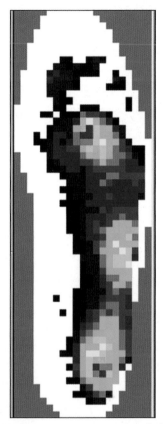

Figure 8-16. High pressure at second and third metatarsal heads in a subject with pronation during walking. Lateral midfoot pressure is related to cuboid subluxation

to control tibial advancement and assist with plantarflexion force. A running pattern that results in the midfoot or forefoot making the initial contact can contribute to pronation movement impairments. With a midfoot or forefoot initial contact, the force of body weight travels through the midtarsal joint and encourages dorsiflexion motion at the midtarsal joints. Additionally, the anterior compartment muscles are not recruited and the posterior compartment muscles remain active throughout stance, placing additional stress on the gastrocnemius and posterior tibialis muscles. The patient should be encouraged to run with a relatively frequent heel-strike–first pattern. In most cases, the patient does not need to make a complete shift to a heel-strike running pattern, but often a moderate decrease in the frequency or severity of the midfoot or forefoot strike pattern can result in a decrease in symptoms.

If symptoms are reproduced during walking and running and the pronation impairment is suspected, the secondary tests would be to provide cues to contract the gastrocnemius and posterior tibialis muscles, lifting from the heel and raising the medial longitudinal arch. If the patient is unable to control pronation during walking and running, external arch support (inserts, scaphoid pads, or arch taping) can be added, and movement and symptom reproduction is reassessed. If hip and knee medial rotation control appears to be an important factor, cues to contract the gluteal muscles and intrinsic hip lateral rotators can be used to assess the impact of the hip and knee movement impairment on foot function and symptom production.

Single-Leg Hopping

The patient is asked to repetitively hop on one leg. Individuals with the pronation syndrome demonstrate calcaneal eversion, dropping of the medial longitudinal arch, forefoot abduction, and/or knee and hip medial rotation. Poor contraction of the gastrocnemius is often very apparent during the single-leg hop test. The patient has a decreased jump height and compensates for the lack of plantarflexion strength with an increased swing of the upper extremities and increased reliance on the quadriceps and/or hip extensors to complete the jump. The

push-off noted. Medial rotation of the hip with an increase in medial foot loading can also be viewed.

Plantar pressure scans taken during barefoot walking show an increase in force distributed through the medial side of the foot, as well as high pressure through second and third metatarsal heads (Figure 8-16).

During running, the pattern used by most people is to contact the ground first with the heel of the foot. A heel-strike pattern of running recruits the anterior compartment muscles to absorb shock and lower the foot down. The posterior compartment muscles are then recruited contributing movement impairments of medial rotation at the hip and/or knee are also easily assessed during single-leg hop. If symptoms occur during single-leg hop, the secondary tests would be similar to those described for the walking and running test: Encourage gastrocnemius muscle contraction, add external arch support, and correct associated hip and knee movement impairments to assess movement and symptom production.

Step-Down and/or Small Knee Bend

The patient is asked to perform a step-down and/or a small knee bend. The physical therapist assesses the movement and symptom reproduction. Movement impairments consistent with pronation (calcaneal eversion, arch flattening, and weight transferred over the medial side of the foot and knee or hip medial rotation) and symptom reproduction support the movement system diagnosis of pronation. If symptoms are reproduced or the therapist suspects baseline symptoms could be reduced, the patient is cued to correct the movement impairment raising the arch, transferring weight slightly more lateral, and contracting the hip lateral rotators to control femoral medial rotation. A decrease in symptoms with the correction of the movement impairment supports the diagnosis of pronation syndrome.

Joint Integrity and Muscle Length

Talocrural Dorsiflexion

See the previous "Dorsiflexion/Talocrural Joint" section.

Passive First Metatarsophalangeal Dorsiflexion

Adequate dorsiflexion motion of the first MTP joint is required as the tibia advances over the foot and the heel begins to rise from the floor. MTP dorsiflexion is measured in full plantarflexion and in 20 degrees of plantar flexion.

Subtalar Joint Eversion

In the presence of adequate eversion ROM, varus structural variations of the hindfoot and/or forefoot often result in pronation syndrome at the hindfoot (calcaneal eversion) in weight bearing.

Muscle Strength/Performance Impairments

Determining the muscle performance impairments in the foot and ankle can be challenging. The forces experienced by the ankle and foot during walking, running, and hopping are often larger than the forces a physical therapist can generate during manual muscle testing (MMT). Additionally, the muscles of the foot and ankle often have an extremely large eccentric role that is not tested with standard MMT. Functional tests should be incorporated to determine true muscle performance.

Gastrocnemius/Posterior Tibialis Muscles

The gastrocnemius muscle is critical in producing powerful plantarflexion during walking and running. Along

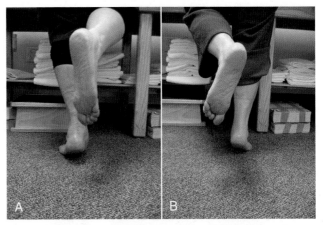

Figure 8-17. This patient has posterior tibialis dysfunction on the left. **A,** Note that on the left the calcaneus remains everted and the heel does not rise through full motion. **B,** Inversion of calcaneus during right heel raise.

with the posterior tibialis, flexor digitorum longus, and flexor hallucis longus, the gastrocnemius muscle contributes to supination of the foot during the late stance phase. To assess function, observe the calcaneus during single-leg heel rise. Together, the ankle plantarflexors should contract and result in calcaneal inversion and elevation of the calcaneus through the full available motion. The ability to complete 25 single-leg heel raises is considered normal.[39] Dysfunction of the posterior tibialis tendon and muscle is evident during a single-heel rise since the calcaneus does not invert, the individual is unable to complete a full heel raise, and often dorsiflexion is seen at the midfoot (Figure 8-17). During walking and running, a visible and strong contraction of the gastrocnemius muscle is expected. Weakness or poor recruitment of the plantarflexor muscles contributes to pronation that occurs past midstance.

Posterior Gluteus Medius, Gluteus Maximus, and Intrinsic Hip Lateral Rotation Muscles

Performance impairment of the hip lateral rotators results in excessive hip medial rotation. Hip medial rotation can cause pronation motion at the foot.

Intrinsic Muscles of the Foot

The intrinsic muscles of the foot are important in maintaining the arches of the foot during weight-bearing activities. The strength assessment is often indirect, observing the individual's ability to complete a towel crunch with the toes, lifting the arch, and flexing the MTP joints.

Plantar Callus Findings

Callus formation is an indication of high stress, either friction or force. In the patient with pronation syndrome the location of calluses are generally on the second metatarsal head, third metatarsal head, and/or medial side of the first toe. Callus formation at the second and third

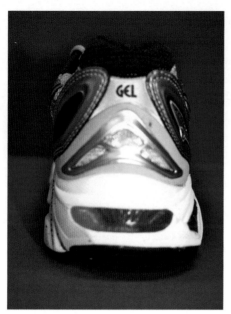

Figure 8-18. Right Asics Gel Foundation 8. Firm density material at the medial heel with less dense material laterally. Gel material is also dual density with firm gel medial and soft gel lateral.

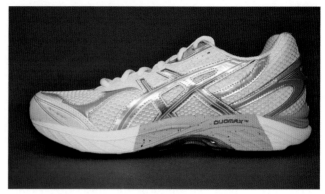

Figure 8-19. Right Asics GT-2150. Note multidensity arch material to increase support for the midfoot.

metatarsal heads indicates that the location of force during push-off remains in the center of the foot. The normal pattern of force during the final phase of push-off is through the first and second metatarsal heads. The medial toe callus represents late pronation (pronation at push-off).

Footwear Considerations

Heel Counter

The heel counter is the posterior component of the shoe that wraps around the heel and is attached to the sole of the shoe. The purpose of the heel counter is to cup the heel and control hindfoot motion. The heel counter should fit the heel snugly and should be made of firm material. If the material is flexible or absent (e.g., an open-back sandal) there is no external assistance to control the calcaneal motion of eversion that can contribute to pronation syndrome.

Shoe Sole Components

The density (firmness) of the material used in the sole of the shoe impacts the shoe's "resistance" to a particular motion. Shoes manufactured to control pronation often have a dual or multidensity sole. A material with increased firmness is added to the medial side of the shoe (a less dense or softer material remains lateral), discouraging motion in the direction of pronation (Figure 8-18).

The location of the firm material as it relates to the patient's specific movement impairment is very important. For a patient with a neutral calcaneus but increased pronation at the midfoot, the firm material should be located only at the medial midfoot (Figure 8-19). For this

particular patient, inclusion of firm material at the hindfoot may encourage a new movement impairment of calcaneal inversion and potentially result in new symptoms. If the pronation impairment occurs at the hindfoot and midfoot, the firm material should run from the heel through the midfoot.

The general flexibility of the sole should be assessed. The sole of the shoe should bend easily only at the toe break. Where the shoe breaks is in part determined by the location of the grooves in the sole material. The removal of sole material to form the grooves encourages bending at the specific location. The groove on the shoe should match the patient's MTP joint line from the first to the fifth toes (Figure 8-20). Footwear with little sole rigidity results in bending at the midfoot, which encourages dorsiflexion at the midtarsals and tarsometatarsal joints (Figure 8-21).

Heel-to-Toe Height

Limited dorsiflexion contributes to pronation as discussed previously in this chapter. Limited dorsiflexion can be compensated for by lifting the heel slightly above the toe. This can be accomplished through footwear and is often unnoticed by the individual wearing the shoe (Figure 8-22). The onset of foot symptoms related to a change in footwear may be associated with a change in the heel to forefoot height (the amount of heel lift). Even a small reduction of heel height can increase the stress on the foot and result in injury.

Arch Support

The amount of direct arch support material in the insole of the shoe is generally small and often made of very soft (compressible) materials. The location is also fixed and may fail to support the arch in the appropriate location. External arch pads (scaphoid/navicular pads) can be easily added to most any footwear.

Last Shape

The last of a shoe is the mold used to shape the shoe. The shape of shoes is generally straight, semi-curved, or

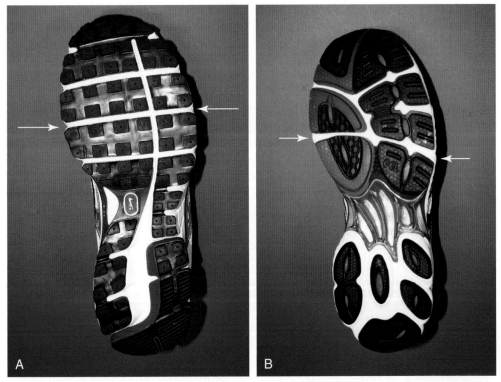

Figure 8-20. A, Left Air Pegasus+ 26. Note the white line of material at the metatarsal break is more distal lateral than medial. **B,** Left Asics Gel Nimbus 11. The white line of material is more proximal lateral than medial. The pattern of sole material removal at the forefoot should match the outline of the metatarsophalangeal joints where dorsiflexion occurs during walking and running.

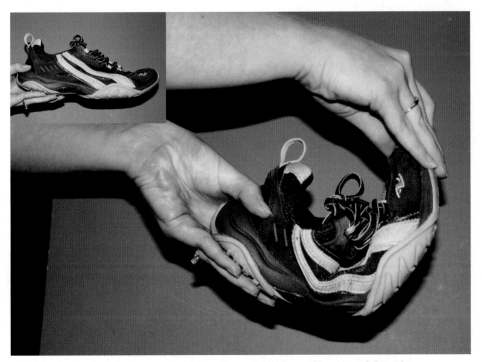

Figure 8-21. A shoe that bends easily at the midportion of the sole.

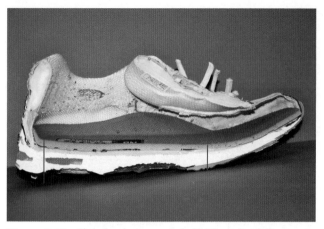

Figure 8-22. Shoe has been cut in half. Note the difference in height of the heel of the shoe compared to the toe of the shoe.

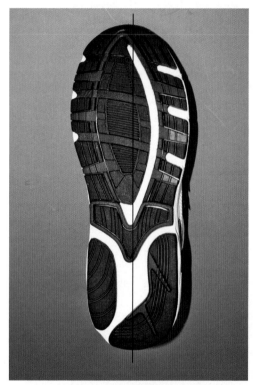

Figure 8-23. Left New Balance 883. Pronation control shoe with a straight last.

curved. To assess last shape, bisect the heel into equal amounts of sole material, medial and lateral. Continue the line that bisects the heel up to the forefoot of the shoe. A straight last will have equal amounts of forefoot sole material on the medial and lateral sides of the line that bisects the heel (Figure 8-23). Curved lasts will have more material on the medial side of the forefoot portion of the shoe compared to the lateral side. Individuals with pronation syndrome often have a straighter foot and would fit best into a straight or semi-curved last. The shape of the shoe should not be used to force a change in foot shape.

Summary

Pronation syndrome is characterized by pronation during weight-bearing activities that is excessive for that individual and/or is occurring past midstance during walking or running. The movement impairment will be observed during weight-bearing activities (walking, running, single-leg hop, small knee bends, and/or stepping down). The movement impairment of pronation occurs in the presence of a foot that is flexible and accommodates for limitations. The associated limitation can be limited dorsiflexion motion at the talocrural joint, weakness of the foot and ankle supinators and/or foot intrinsic muscles, and/or hip lateral rotators.

Treatment

Walking and Running

The patient is instructed to work on the specific cues that assisted in symptom reduction during the examination or the cues that the physical therapist believes, with practice, may result in symptom reduction. The following cues are among the possibilities that may assist the patient:

- Contract the gastrocnemius muscle by lifting from the heel.
- Raise the medial longitudinal arch.
- Contract the gluteal muscles (squeeze the buttock of the stance leg).
- Hit with the heel first.

Many of the changes being requested of the patient during walking and running are similar to a strengthening program. As such, encourage the patient to have focused practice time and gradual implementation to avoid injury.

Muscle Performance

Weakness of the supinators (gastrocnemius and posterior tibialis muscles) can be addressed with a progressive strengthening program, which includes elastic band resistance exercise into plantarflexion and plantarflexion/inversion, heel raises, and single-leg hopping. During the exercise, assess the contraction of the gastrocnemius muscle cueing the patient to raise the heel.

Intrinsic muscles of the foot can be strengthened by completing towel crunches using the toes to grab the towel and pull the towel under the foot. The movement must be accomplished by flexing at the MTP joints, raising the arch, and cupping the foot (Figure 8-24, *A*). The patient should not be allowed to complete the towel crunch with isolated motion of the flexor digitorum longus with flexion occurring only at the proximal and distal interphalangeal joints (Figure 8-24, *B*). Weight can be added to the towel to increase resistance.

Posterior hip muscle strengthening is described in detail in Chapter 7, "Corrective Exercises: Purposes and Special Considerations," in Sahrmann.[3] An appropriate strengthening progression activity includes sidelying hip lateral rotation progressing to lateral rotation with abduction and adding weight as appropriate.

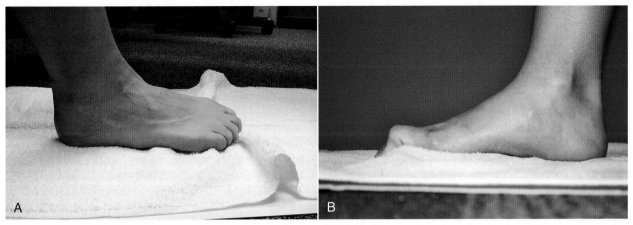

Figure 8-24. **A,** Towel crunch with toes using intrinsic muscles to flex the metatarsophalangeal joints. **B,** Toe intrinsic exercise done incorrectly using flexor digitorum longus and flexor hallucis longus to curl toes without flexing the metatarsophalangeal joint and raising the arch.

Muscle strengthening occurs when the muscle is overloaded. The general recommendations are that the exercise should be completed at 70% of the patient's maximum voluntary contraction for 10 repetitions, 3 sets, 3 to 5 times/week. In general, exercise or activity is permissible if pain remains ≤2/10 on a 0 to 10 scale.

Muscle Length and Joint Integrity
Decreased length of the gastrocnemius muscle and tendon can be addressed with a small lunge stretch at the wall, dropping the heel off a ledge, or long sitting dorsiflexion towel stretch; all stretches would be done with the knee extended. The soleus muscle and tendon can be stretched by bending the knee during the wall, heel hang, or towel stretch. Unique instructions for patients with pronation syndrome include preventing pronation during the stretch (this could include active patient correction of pronation and wearing good footwear during the stretch) and keeping the foot facing forward or in line with the femur and tibia. The heel should be kept on the ground during the stretch.

To address talocrural joint limitation, a posterior glide or a distraction technique of the talus on the ankle mortise is recommended in addition to the stretches described. Additionally, a prolonged stretch can be provided by a dorsiflexion splint. The splint is a non–weight-bearing brace and is generally recommended for night wear but could be used during the day if the individual could remain non–weight-bearing during splint use. Splint use in the foot and ankle is often reserved for patients whose symptoms do not respond to the traditional treatment plan to improve dorsiflexion. Splint wearing at night can be uncomfortable, disrupting sleep, which often results in poor patient compliance.

Limited talocrural dorsiflexion can be compensated for by adding a heel lift in the shoe. A heel lift used long term can contribute to loss of talocrural dorsiflexion and should be approached with caution.

Limited extensor digitorum longus muscle and tendon extensibility can be addressed by having the patient plantarflex the involved foot with the toes plantarflexed either in a sitting position or while on hands and knees and rocking back. Limited first MTP dorsiflexion related to decreased extensibility of the flexor hallucis longus can be addressed with a prolonged stretch into dorsiflexion with the ankle in dorsiflexion. To address limitations in first MTP joint dorsiflexion, an anterior glide of the proximal phalanx on the metatarsal can be performed.

Stretching should be held for 30 seconds, 2 to 3 repetitions, completed regularly throughout the day (5 to 8 times/day), and completed 5 to 7 days/week.

Activity Modification
Activity level should be modified to decrease forces on the foot. If the symptoms are severe, the therapist should consider the use of an assistive device or a period of immobilization to decrease tissue irritability.

As the tissue heals, a cautious and gradual increase in activity will assist in returning the patient to the previous level of activity. If appropriate for the patient's goals, activity should progress to dynamic activities such as jumping, hopping, shuttle run, cutting, and so on. A guide for progressing from walking to running begins with a run/walk program. Generally, a 1:4 ratio (1 minute run with a 4 minute walk) is a reasonable place to begin. The physical therapist should closely monitor symptoms. The symptoms guidelines used in clinical practice are that symptoms should remain ≤2 out of 10, and symptoms that come on with activity should resolve within a very short time after activity (no longer than 1 hour). As the tissue tolerance to activity improves, the number of run/walk cycles is increased and then duration of running is increased while walking duration is decreased.

The progression to high level agility sport activity includes starting with straight plane jogging and jumping on a smooth flat surface. The most effective strategy is to work on increasing distance before increasing speed because an increase in speed increases the peak forces through the foot and is more likely to result in tissue injury or reinjury. As the patient's tolerance of weight-bearing activities improves, the terrain should be varied, as well as the addition of hills, cutting, and progressing to unexpected turns. The equipment (balls, cleats, sticks, rackets, and so on) associated with the sport of interest should be introduced, as well as a plan to gradually introduce other players and to address the dynamics of the sport (player contact, single-leg balance activities, speed of the sport, or ball movement).

External Tissue Support

Footwear. The footwear prescription is specific to each individual, but some general guidelines for pronation syndrome can be provided. The last (shape) of the shoe should look like the patient's foot. Most often a straight or semi-curved last is appropriate. A firm heel counter to control hindfoot motion is advisable for most all individuals. If pronation occurs at the hindfoot, the shoe should include more rigid material at the medial heel and less rigid material at the lateral heel. The medial structure of the shoe should be made of firm materials, and the sole should be rigid from hindfoot through midfoot, bending only at the metatarsal heads. The shoe length, width, and height of the toe box should accommodate the size of the foot and any deformities present.

Orthoses. Orthoses are not recommended for all patients. Indications that orthoses may be appropriate include (1) the inability to correct the movement impairment through cueing, (2) significant structural variations, (3) the problem is recurrent, or (4) the foot alignment places the individual at risk for future problems. A temporary orthosis is a cheap and efficient method to assess the usefulness of an orthosis. Components can be easily added and removed to aid in determining what is most helpful for managing the patient's symptoms. The component most often added is arch support (scaphoid/navicular pad). Medial hindfoot and forefoot posts are additional options that can assist with limiting motion that results in symptoms (Figure 8-25). The goal of the orthosis is not to achieve a subtalar joint neutral position but to prevent excessive or end-range motion so that the symptoms resolve. For local metatarsal pain, a common orthoses component is a metatarsal pad (Figure 8-26). The pad should be located just proximal (0.5 to 1 cm proximal) to the metatarsal head to unload the metatarsal heads and limit MTP hyperextension.[40]

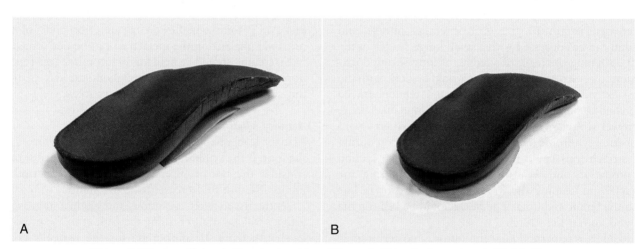

Figure 8-25. An off-the-shelf orthosis with a **(A)** scaphoid/navicular pad and **(B)** hindfoot medial post.

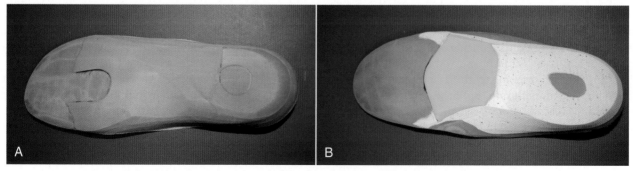

Figure 8-26. A, Total contact insert with local metatarsal relief. **B,** Global (all) metatarsal head relief.

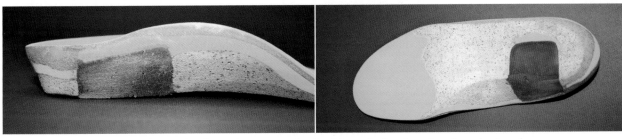

Figure 8-27. Example of a total contact orthosis with professional quality visco elastic polymer (Riecken's, Evansville, Ind.) at the medial heel.

An important orthoses modification for patients with tarsal tunnel nerve (tibial nerve) involvement is to avoid firm materials in the medial heel of the orthosis or sole of the shoe. Firm materials may contribute to nerve compression and irritation (Figure 8-27).

Taping. Taping to support the arch can assist in symptom management while additional treatment options are being implemented. There are a variety of techniques, but most have a common component of restraining longitudinal motion between the calcaneus and the metatarsal heads (Figure 8-28).

CASE PRESENTATION
Pronation Syndrome

Symptoms and History

An internist referred a 42-year-old female for evaluation and treatment of right "heel pain." Her heel pain began approximately 10 weeks ago when she returned to work full time as a floor salesperson at a local shopping center. The patient has had to decrease her working hours from 40 to 20 because she was unable to tolerate the heel pain. The patient's pain is located on the plantar surface of the heel. She states the pain occurs only during weight bearing and is much worse in the morning when she first gets out of bed (7/10) than later in the afternoon (4/10). She states her pain is worse when walking barefoot or in her work shoes, which are dress flats. She reports increasing pain with walking more than 15 minutes and has difficulty completing daily activities like grocery shopping and playing games with her children. She is 5 foot 6 inches and weighs 190 lb. Her Foot and Ankle Ability Measure score is 49% (100% indicates normal function).

Alignment Analysis

In standing, the foot alignment shows a vertical calcaneus and a normal-to-low arch bilaterally. The alignment of the hip and knee includes medial rotation of the femur and slight lateral rotation of the tibia bilaterally. Symptoms in standing were 3/10. In prone the assessment of subtalar joint neutral reveals a small hindfoot varus and neutral forefoot alignment.

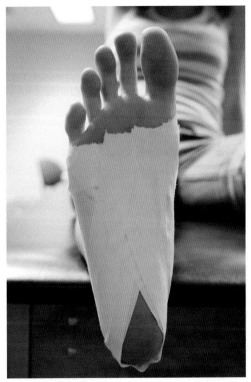

Figure 8-28. Arch taping to provide external arch support during weight-bearing activities.

Movement Analysis

Walking/running

During walking, the calcaneus hits in inversion, moves into eversion by midstance, and remains in the everted position through late stance (right foot greater than left). Symptoms during barefoot walking increased to 5/10. Secondary tests, including cues to raise her heel earlier in stance and to contract her gastrocnemius, decreased the amount of eversion during midstance to late stance and decrease her symptoms minimally (4/10).

Single-leg hopping

The patient demonstrated decreased use of plantarflexors during single-leg hopping. Symptoms were generally less (3/10) when remaining on her toes and avoiding weight bearing through the heel.

Small knee bend

An increase in calcaneal eversion and a lowering of the arch was noted (right greater than left) during a small knee bend. Symptoms remained at 3/10.

Muscle Length/Joint ROM Analysis

	Right	Left
Talocrural dorsiflexion (knee extended)	0 degrees	5 degrees
Talocrural dorsiflexion (knee flexed)	5 degrees	10 degrees
Calcaneal eversion	5 degrees	5 degrees
First MTP joint extension (30 degrees talocrural plantarflexion)	60 degrees*	60 degrees

*Increased symptoms at the calcaneal tubercle and into the arch.

Joint accessory motion assessment found no difference in mobility between the right and left talocrural joints during an anterior-to-posterior glide of the talus on the ankle mortise.

Muscle Performance Impairments

- Single-leg heel raise could be completed 10 times through full plantarflexion and inversion range with fatigue, resulting in a decreased height of the heel raise and incomplete inversion in subsequent repetitions.
- Sidelying gluteus medius strength was 3+/5 on the right and 4/5 on the left.

Towel crunch with toes: the toes flexed, the MTP joints extended. The patient was able to correct performance to lift arch and plantarflex the MTP joints, but the foot cramped after five toe crunches.

Footwear

Patient wore her work shoes, which were dress flats. The heel counter was flexible, and the sole was made of a flexible plastic.

Palpation

Symptoms were reproduced with palpation of the calcaneal tubercle on the right foot. Pain continued with palpation of the plantar aponeurosis into the arch of the foot.

Diagnosis

Pronation occurred past midstance with no motion in the direction of supination during late stance. The primary contributing factors to pronation syndrome were decreased talocrural dorsiflexion ROM from decreased length of the gastrocnemius and soleus muscles and weakness of the gluteus medius/hip lateral rotators and foot plantarflexors/supinators. There was also a slight structural variation (hindfoot varus in the presence of sufficient calcaneal eversion motion) that could contribute to pronation. Additionally, the footwear provided insufficient support and cushion for a job that requires prolonged standing. The stage for rehabilitation is 2. The pain rating was moderate to high, she was mobile but limited in her ability to complete activities that require longer weight bearing, and her Foot and Ankle Ability Measure indicates a moderate amount of disability. Source of the symptoms was the plantar aponeurosis. The patient was seen 1 time/week for 8 weeks to assess and modify the treatment plan.

Treatment and Outcomes

Table 8-4 includes pronation syndrome interventions and outcomes.

Activity education

- First-step pain
  - Gentle dorsiflexion stretch before stepping onto the foot after a prolonged period of non–weight-bearing activity (e.g., sleeping).
  - Step directly into her most supportive shoes as she gets out of bed and for as long in the morning as she is able to avoid the trauma associated with first-step pain and morning symptoms.
- Femoral medial rotation and pronation
  - Patient instructed to squeeze the buttock, keep the knee over the toe (not medial), and lift the arch during weight-bearing activities.
  - Gluteus medius strengthening.

Arch taping resulted in an immediate decrease in symptoms with weight bearing to a 2/10. First step morning pain decreased to a 4/10 within the first week after implementation of the suggested changes to her morning routine. The temporary addition of a heel lift and scaphoid pad to the shoe was needed to assist with initial symptom relief. The patient continued the home exercise program to strengthen the hip, ankle, and foot, increase talocrural dorsiflexion motion, and modify the medial femoral rotation and foot and ankle pronation for approximately 8 weeks before symptoms consistently remained at 0/10 with a full 40-hour week of work.

SUPINATION SYNDROME

The principal movement impairment associated with supination syndrome is supination of the foot and ankle that occurs at the wrong time (heel strike to midstance in the gait cycle) or that occurs in an amount that is excessive for that individual. The supination impairment can occur in the hindfoot, midfoot, and/or forefoot. The foot with the supination impairment is generally a rigid foot with little or no ability to absorb shock and compensate for structural or movement impairments within the foot and ankle, knee, or hip.

Symptoms and Pain

Plantar Aponeurosis (Fascia)

Involvement of the plantar aponeurosis is most often accompanied by patient complaints of heel pain that is worse with the first step out of bed in the morning and after a period of prolonged non–weight-bearing function.

TABLE 8-4
Pronation Syndrome: Interventions and Outcomes

Limitation/Initial Prescription	Progression Week 1	Progression Week 3	Progression Week 6
TALOCRURAL DORSIFLEXION			
Wall stretch	Progression of stretches to improve talocrural dorsiflexion may include changing from non–weight bearing to weight bearing exercises. All stretches should be held for a minimum of 30 seconds and repeated 3 to 5 repetitions and done frequently throughout the day (at least 5 times per day).		
Heel hang			
Towel stretch			
Instruction: Prevent foot pronation, hip medial rotation, and keep foot aligned with the fibula.			
PLANTARFLEXOR MUSCLE PERFORMANCE			
Elastic band plantar flexion/ inversion	Heel raises (Bilateral progressing to unilateral)	Bilateral hopping	Single-leg hopping
Eccentric strengthening: Bilateral heel rise, lowering on one foot	Eccentric strengthening: Add additional weight to a backpack, waist, or leg and increase repetitions as the patient is able tolerate the exercise. Pain is used as an indicator that the stress is excessive and the prescription is too aggressive.		
Instruction: Squeeze the calf and relax the toes.			
INTRINSIC FOOT MUSCLE PERFORMANCE			
Towel crunches with toes	—	Weight added to towel as tolerated	—
Instruction: The arch and MTP joints should lift during towel crunches.			
GLUTEUS MEDIUS MUSCLE PERFORMANCE			
Sidelying level 2	Sidelying Level 3	Bilateral hopping	Single-leg hopping
Instruction: Avoid hip medial rotation and flexion during abduction.			
EXTERNAL SUPPORT			
Arch taping	Heel lift and scaphoid pad. Reduce height of heel lift as talocrural dorsiflexion increases.		
Footwear	Firm heel counter, firm medial heel and midfoot components, increased heel-to-toe height ratio.		

MTP, Metatarsophalangeal.

Fibular (Peroneal) Muscles and Tendon

The patient complains of pain localized to the muscles (posterior to the fibula) or anywhere along the tendon as it follows its course around the lateral malleolus to the insertion at the base of the fifth metatarsal for the fibularis brevis or following the fibularis longus as it runs along the lateral border of the cuboid and to the plantar surface of the foot. The symptoms are most apparent during the weight-bearing phase of activities as the muscle works to eccentrically control supination and dorsiflexion and during push-off as the muscle acts concentrically to assist with plantarflexion.

Gastrocnemius/Soleus Muscles and Calcaneal (Achilles) Tendon

The patient complains of pain in the muscle belly or tendon, particularly during late stance, as the muscle is working eccentrically and the tendon is being placed on stretch to control the tibia's progression over the foot and during the concentric contraction required during push-off.

Metatarsal Heads

The patient complains of metatarsal pain localized to the head of the first and fifth metatarsals that becomes worse during late stance and the push-off phase of walking and running.

Lateral Column Joints

The patient complains of generalized pain along the joints of the lateral column of the foot (talus, calcaneus, cuboid, and fourth and fifth metatarsals).

Alignment: Structural Variations and Acquired Impairments

The description of a supinated foot type includes a combination of calcaneal inversion, lateral bulge (prominence of the talonavicular joint dorsal and lateral), high medial longitudinal arch, forefoot adduction relative to the hindfoot at the transtarsal joint, and narrow forefoot width (Figure 8-29). Lower extremity alignment impairments that contribute to a supination impairment at the foot include lateral rotation at the hip and/or knee or

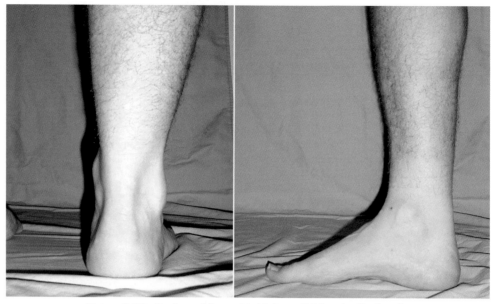

Figure 8-29. Supinated foot with high medial longitudinal arch.

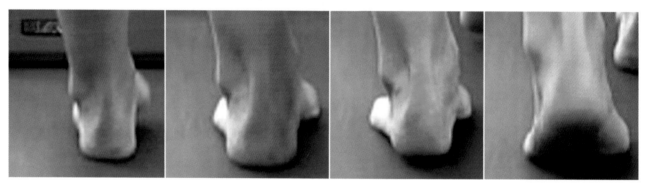

Figure 8-30. Calcaneus stays vertical and arch is high from heel strike through push-off.

structural variations of the femur or tibia that seem to be associated with a supinated foot (e.g., femoral retroversion, lateral tibial torsion).

The most common subtalar joint neutral alignment finding in individuals with supination syndrome includes a hindfoot and/or forefoot varus in which the joint mobility is limited and there is no ability to compensate with subtalar or midtarsal joint motion. Valgus hindfoot and forefoot structural variations that are compensated by inversion in standing can also contribute to the supinated standing alignment. In the prone position, an individual with supination syndrome may also have a first metatarsal head that is plantarflexed below the plane of the second to fifth metatarsal heads; this is called a *plantarflexed* or *dropped first ray* and is a common compensation for a forefoot varus (see Figure 8-4).

Movement Impairments

Walking and Running

During walking and running, the supination movement impairment usually includes calcaneal inversion at heel strike that remains through push-off. There is generally an absence of pronation during the initial portion of stance. The center of gravity during stance remains lateral on the weight-bearing surface of the foot (Figure 8-30). There is often a very late whip to the medial side of the foot during push-off. The foot is rigid, and there is very little shock absorption during walking and running, which can contribute to symptoms at the knee, hip, and back. The rigid foot can also produce varus motion at the knee that can contribute to knee symptoms.

The barefoot plantar pressure assessment in Figure 8-31 is common in individuals with the supination movement impairment. There is no loading of the midfoot, which reduces the surface area for force distribution (increases localized pressure). The metatarsal head pressure is high, particularly under the first metatarsal. In this individual, there is also very high medial great toe pressure, evidence of the late transfer of weight medially over the first toe.

If symptoms are reproduced during walking and running and the movement impairments previously

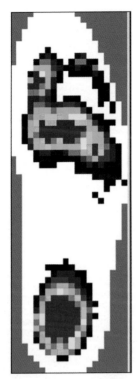

Figure 8-31. Barefoot pressure scan during walking of supinated individual. Note the lack of midfoot loading and the high forefoot pressure under the first metatarsal.

described are noted, the supination impairment is suspected. The secondary tests for supination impairment can be challenging to implement as the foot and the movement pattern are often fixed and unable to be volitionally corrected. Attempts can be made to control the offending motion (calcaneal inversion, late medial motion) with verbal cues to avoid extreme lateral loading through the foot, to soften the landing with knee flexion, and to roll medially sooner. Unfortunately, the rigidity of the foot often prevents the individual from changing the movement pattern. Attempts can be made to post the heel laterally to encourage eversion motion. Additionally, an arch support can be added to footwear to assess the effect of increasing the contact area over which the load is borne.

Single-Leg Hopping
The patient is asked to hop repetitively on one foot. The rigid foot associated with supination syndrome is an excellent lever for the plantarflexors, transferring the plantarflexor force easily and propelling the body up. Often, the patient with supination syndrome is able to jump fairly high and with what seems like little effort. The supination movement impairment at the foot is generally not apparent during the single-leg hop, since only the forefoot is striking the ground. Observation of the single-leg hop provides valuable information about plantarflexor muscle performance, as well as contributing movement impairments at the knee and hip. If symptoms occur during

single-leg hop, the secondary test would be cues to address hip and knee movement impairments (lateral rotation or varus motions) and soften the landing with knee flexion. Weakness of the gastrocnemius/soleus complex should also be assessed further through single-leg heel rises. The addition of arch support may not affect the symptoms during the test because the heel and midfoot do not touch the ground during single-leg hopping.

Step-Down and/or Small Knee Bend
During a step-down or small knee bend, the most common impairment noted is limited dorsiflexion. The compensation is often an early heel rise and the rigidity of the foot becomes apparent (no decrease in arch height during the motion). The lateral distribution of force through the foot can also be seen during the small knee bend. Symptom reproduction during low impact activities like step-downs or small knee bends is rare. However, if symptoms are reproduced or the therapist suspects baseline symptoms could be reduced, the patient is cued to correct the movement impairment keeping weight more central (away from the lateral aspect of the foot). A decrease in symptoms with the correction of the movement impairment supports the diagnosis of supination syndrome. Additionally, the physical therapist can assess the role of insufficient dorsiflexion in symptom reproduction by limiting dorsiflexion motion to avoid end-range or adding a small heel lift. If correction of the insufficient dorsiflexion results in symptom reduction, the therapist needs to consider insufficient dorsiflexion syndrome as a possible movement impairment diagnosis (see the following "Insufficient Dorsiflexion Syndrome" section).

Muscle Length/Joint Range of Motion Impairments
Talocrural Dorsiflexion and Passive First Metatarsophalangeal Dorsiflexion
Limitation in motion at the talocrural joint and the first MTP joint are also associated with the supination movement impairment. Decreased talocrural dorsiflexion during late stance results in either an early heel rise or transfer of weight lateral for the tibia to advance over the foot. Limited first MTP motion results in a transfer of force medial at late stance (push-off) or keeps the force lateral. The tests to determine source of limitation are described in the "Metatarsophalangeal Joints" section.

Subtalar Joint Eversion
Subtalar joint eversion is often limited (<0 degrees) in patients with supination syndrome.

Footwear Considerations
Heel Counter
In patients with supination syndrome the heel counter should have qualities similar to those recommended for pronation syndrome in that the counter should be made of firm material and hold the heel snugly. In the case of

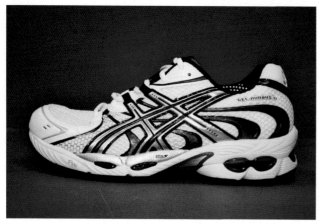

Figure 8-32. Asics GEL-Nimbus 11. Manufactured primarily for cushion and flexibility with the inclusion of gel and sole materials that attenuate shock.

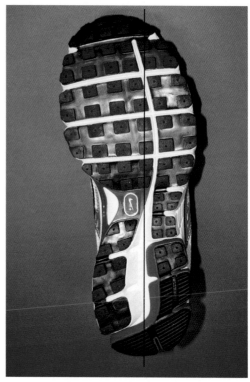

Figure 8-33. Left Nike Air Pegasus +26. Curved last with additional material on the medial forefoot compared to the lateral forefoot.

supination syndrome the heel counter will help to control inversion of the calcaneus.

Shoe Sole Components

The supinated foot has a decreased ability to absorb shock during early stance and may require additional attention to cushioning. Sole components, such as air and soft materials, are marketed to attenuate shock (Figure 8-32). Footwear manufacturers rarely add firm material components to the lateral side of the shoe to encourage pronation. However, the individual with supination syndrome should not wear a shoe designed for pronation syndrome because the shoe would have firm materials medially and would encourage the supination movement impairment.

As with pronation syndrome, the sole of the shoe should bend easily only at the MTP joint line. The groove on the forefoot of the shoe should match the patient's MTP joint line from the first to the fifth toes.

Heel-to-Toe Height

Limited dorsiflexion is also associated with supination syndrome and can be compensated for by lifting the heel slightly above the toe. A reduction in the heel-to-toe height ratio can contribute to symptom onset similar to that described with pronation syndrome.

Arch Support

The lack of contact area of the supinated foot during walking contributes to high pressure. Footwear should be assessed for the ability of the insoles to provide contact, support, and force distribution through the entire foot.

Last Shape

The most common shape of a supinated foot is forefoot adduction relative to the hindfoot. A curved last generally matches the shape of the supinated foot best (Figure 8-33). The shape of the shoe should not be used to force

a change in the shape of the foot or to attempt to alter motion of the foot.

Plantar Callus Findings

In the patient with supination syndrome, the location of calluses are generally on the first metatarsal head, fifth metatarsals, and/or medial side of the first toe. Callus formation at the first and fifth metatarsal heads indicates the late lateral loading under the fifth and often a rigid first ray that bears a large load. The medial toe callus is a result of the late pronation that occurs during push-off as a result of the prolonged lateral loading in the supinated foot.

Summary

Supination syndrome is characterized by a rigid, high-arched foot that has little ability to compensate for structural and movement impairments within the foot and ankle or up the leg to the hip. The high arch, calcaneal inversion, and forefoot adduction will be apparent with weight-bearing activities. There is generally poor shock absorption and little loading through the midfoot.

Treatment

Walking and Running

The patient is instructed to work on the tasks that use specific cues that assisted in symptom reduction during the examination or the cues that the physical therapist believes with practice may result in symptom reduction. Often, the cues are related to softening the landing, hitting more centrally on the heel, and concentrating on trying to limit lateral loading through the foot.

Range of Motion
The treatment plan for limited motion is similar to that described for pronation syndrome.

Activity Modification
The general guidelines for activity restriction and progression described in the "Pronation Syndrome" section apply here as well. For supination syndrome, specific suggestions include use of softer surfaces when shock absorption is a concern.

External Tissue Support
Footwear. Footwear for the patient with supination syndrome should include a last that looks like the patient's foot, most often a semi-curved or curved last. As with pronation syndrome, a firm heel counter to control hindfoot motion and a sole that resists bending from hindfoot to midfoot, bending only at the metatarsal heads, is advisable for most all individuals. Cushioning is important and should be included within the shoe. The cushioning component of the footwear may wear down quickly, and footwear may need to be replaced more frequently. Finally, for all individuals, shoe length and width and height of the toe box should accommodate the size of the foot and any deformities.

Orthoses. As with pronation syndrome, orthoses are not recommended for all patients and the indications for permanent orthoses include significant structural variations, a recurrent problem, or if the foot alignment places the individual at risk for future problems. The temporary orthosis components that may be appropriate for a patient with supination syndrome include arch support to

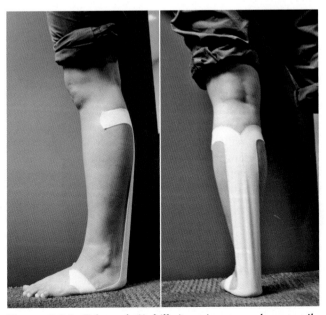

Figure 8-34. Calcaneal (Achilles) taping to reduce tensile forces at the calcaneal tendon.

distribute force more evenly but avoid increasing lateral forces and inversion ankle instability.

Taping. Taping to support the arch can be helpful in supination syndrome as well. The indications for taping are that providing support for the arch and assisting with force distribution (arch supports were helpful) decreased symptoms during the examination. Calcaneal (Achilles) tendon irritation can be assisted with a taping technique that provides support to the tissue (Figure 8-34).

CASE PRESENTATION
Supination Syndrome

Symptoms and History
A 35-year-old male, who stands 6 foot tall and weighs 175 lbs, was referred by an internist for evaluation and treatment of right foot pain. His foot pain began approximately 1 month ago during a 10-mile run in new shoes. He reports running approximately 30 miles/week, including 1 long run (10 to 15 miles) on the weekend.

The patient's pain is located on the plantar surface of the fifth metatarsal head. The patient reports limitation caused by pain during walking (5/10), running (7/10), as well as a very sharp pain (8/10) when he turns on a planted right foot. The pain is reproduced when he manually extends his fifth toe and is generally tender to the touch on the plantar surface. When he is standing, symptoms are minimal (2/10) and absent when sitting. His Foot and Ankle Ability Measure score was 54% (100% indicates normal function) and the Foot and Ankle Ability Measure Sport Scale was 32% (100% indicates normal function).

Alignment Analysis
In standing, the calcaneus is inverted and the arch is high bilaterally. The forefoot is slightly adducted on the hindfoot. There is an increase in lateral tibial torsion. In prone, the assessment of subtalar joint neutral finds hindfoot and forefoot varus alignment.

Movement Analysis
Standing/walking/running
During walking and running, the calcaneus hits in inversion and remains in an inverted position through late stance. Push-off occurs through the lateral side of the foot, symptoms are 5/10. Symptoms increased to 7/10 during running, and cues to roll through the middle of the foot (not as lateral) during walking and running decreased symptoms to 4/10.
Single-leg hopping
Lateral loading of the forefoot noted with single-leg hopping and patient reports increased pain (7/10). A cue to load the foot more centrally decreased symptoms to 4/10.
Small knee bend
During the small knee bend, the patient demonstrated limited talocrural dorsiflexion ROM and weight remained

on the lateral aspect of the foot. No symptoms were reproduced.

Muscle Length/Joint ROM Impairments

	Right	Left
Talocrural dorsiflexion (knee extended)	−5 degrees	0 degrees
Talocrural dorsiflexion (knee flexed)	0 degrees	10 degrees
First MTP joint extension (30 degrees talocrural plantarflexion)	25 degrees	25 degrees

Joint accessory motion assessment found limited mobility bilaterally during an anterior-to-posterior glide of the talus on the ankle mortise.

Footwear

Patient is wearing his old running shoes and brought his new running shoes with him. The new running shoes have a curved last, the metatarsal break is distal to the first metatarsal head and proximal to the fifth metatarsal head, and the sole is flexible, bending easily from the middle of the shoe to the toe.

Diagnosis

The patient's movement tests support a movement system syndrome of supination. The patient's foot is supinated throughout stance with lateral loading of the foot throughout. The likely source of symptoms is the fifth metatarsal head. The stage for rehabilitation is 2. Although the patient's symptoms are high during weight bearing, symptoms were easily reduced with modification to the walking pattern. The patient is completing daily activities, and the Foot and Ankle Ability Measure indicates moderate disability. The primary contributing factor to the movement impairment is a rigid foot that has little capacity for changing ROM. There is a varus structural variation of the hindfoot and forefoot in the presence of limited calcaneal eversion motion that contributes to supination. Additionally, the new footwear provided little support and encouraged additional lateral loading and hyperextension at the fifth metatarsal joint because the metatarsal head break in his new shoe is proximal to his joint line.

Prognosis

Prognosis is excellent for resolving symptoms with compensations that include modifying footwear with a temporary insert. The patient is relatively young with a short time since onset of symptoms. The severity of symptoms is fairly high but primarily occur with high impact activity. Clinical experience has found very little success in changing talocrural dorsiflexion and first MTP motion in individuals with very rigid and supinated feet.

Treatment

The primary goal of treatment is to decrease the load borne by the fifth metatarsal head. The patient works to avoid exaggerating the pattern of lateral loading that

his foot structure encourages. Cues to heel strike in less inversion and to roll more centrally through his foot do decrease his symptoms and should be implemented as part of the treatment plan. Additionally, a temporary orthosis can be fabricated that will include a metatarsal pad under the fifth metatarsal head to provide unloading of the bone during healing. A lateral post to encourage pronation can be added as well; however, the rigidity of the foot often prevents the lateral post from changing motion and symptoms. A stretching program to address the talocrural and first MTP motion will be implemented. The recommended footwear components for his running shoe include a last that is less curved (semi-curved), a firm heel counter, sole materials and design that allows the primary break in the shoe to occur at the location that matches his metatarsal joints, and an increased heel-to-toe ratio to compensate for limited dorsiflexion.

Outcome

The patient was seen 1 time/week for 8 weeks. The addition of the temporary orthosis with arch support and a metatarsal pad, change in footwear, stretching program, and cues for changing weight-bearing patterns reduced maximum symptoms to a 2/10 within 2 visits. Complete resolution of symptoms at the fifth metatarsal head required a 3 week rest from running. The patient continued with low-impact aerobic training (bicycling and swimming). As the symptoms improved to 0/10 with walking, running was gradually increased with a walk/run program in which the patient started with running 1 minute and walking 4 minutes for 5 bouts (total weight-bearing time was 20 minutes). Gradually, the amount of time spent running was increased, the amount of time walking was decreased, and the number of bouts were increased until the patient had returned to running 10 miles pain-free.

INSUFFICIENT DORSIFLEXION SYNDROME

The principal movement impairment associated with insufficient dorsiflexion syndrome is insufficient talocrural dorsiflexion. The impairment occurs during mid-stance to push-off or during swing phase and is not associated with excessive supination or pronation. Limited talocrural dorsiflexion is a common impairment that could be present in all other foot and ankle syndromes. A patient is given the diagnosis of insufficient dorsiflexion only after all other diagnoses have been ruled out (pronation syndrome, supination syndrome, and hypomobility syndrome).

Symptoms and Pain

Plantar Aponeurosis (Fascia)

Involvement of the plantar aponeurosis is most often accompanied by patient complaints of heel pain that are worse with the first step out of bed in the morning and after a period of prolonged non–weight-bearing activities.

Gastrocnemius/Soleus Muscle and Calcaneal (Achilles) Tendon

The patient complains of pain in the muscle belly or tendon, particularly during late stance, as the muscle is working eccentrically and the tendon is being placed on stretch to control the tibia's progression over the foot and during the concentric contraction required during push-off.

Bursa

Pain is reported at posterior calcaneus, most apparent with direct pressure. The pain provoking pressure can occur during midstance through push off, when squatting or when sitting in a position that applies direct pressure to the bursa.

Anterior Tibialis Muscle and Tendon

The patient complains of pain localized to the muscle at the anterior and lateral proximal fibula or anywhere along the tendon as it follows its course to insert on the medial cuneiform and base of the first metatarsal bone. The symptoms are most apparent from heel strike to foot flat as the anterior tibialis is working eccentrically to lower the foot to the ground or during swing phase as the anterior tibialis is working concentrically to clear the foot.

Deep Fibular Nerve

The patient reports achiness, tingling, and/or numbness on the dorsum of foot and can radiate into toes. Symptoms are most common when shoes are on (tied tightly on the dorsum of the foot) and/or during activities requiring maximum dorsiflexion (running up hills, squatting).

Talocrural Joint

The patient reports sharp pinching pain at the anterior joint line during end range dorsiflexion activities such as squatting and running up hills. The anterior talocrural joint is often point tender.

Metatarsal Heads

Metatarsal pain localized to the metatarsal head and worse during late stance and the push-off phase of walking and running.

Alignment: Structural Variations and Acquired Impairments

Patients with insufficient dorsiflexion syndrome often stand with knee hyperextension and the ankles in relative plantarflexion. There are no specific clinical tests that can be performed to evaluate the contribution of structural variations to limited talocrural dorsiflexion motion.

Movement Impairments

Walking and Running

During walking and running those with isolated insufficient talocrural dorsiflexion demonstrate a number of gait impairments during stance. The inability of the tibia to easily advance over the foot during late stance can be

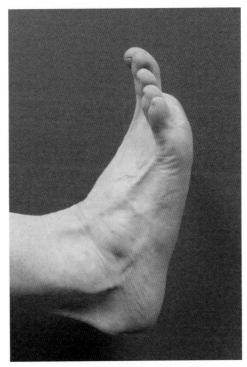

Figure 8-35. Individual with limited dorsiflexion using toe extension to compensate.

compensated for in a number of ways: (1) early heel rise, (2) knee hyperextension, and/or (3) increase in the foot progression angle (toe is pointed out). Limited talocrural dorsiflexion during swing phase is also visible, often with overuse of the extensor digitorum and poor stabilization of the metatarsal heads with the intrinsic muscles of the foot (Figure 8-35).

Individuals with insufficient talocrural dorsiflexion often rely on the passive tension of the gastrocnemius and soleus muscles and calcaneal tendon to control the advancement of the tibia over the foot during stance. There is often poor eccentric use of the gastrocnemius muscle in tibial control.

If symptoms are reproduced during stance phase of walking and running, a secondary test is adding a heel lift and assessing symptom reproduction. Cues to contract the gastrocnemius, lifting the heel actively, can be helpful in addressing the use of passive tension. The secondary test for symptoms produced during swing includes cues to relax the toes, avoiding toe hyperextension to see if symptoms are reduced.

Squat

The contribution of limited dorsiflexion to the patient's pain is often overlooked because active ROM (AROM) in non–weight-bearing activities often appears equal between sides. However, if the patient squats, the therapist will notice that on the involved side, the heel is higher or the tibia is more posterior and this end-range position with loading often reproduces the patient's complaints (Figure 8-36).

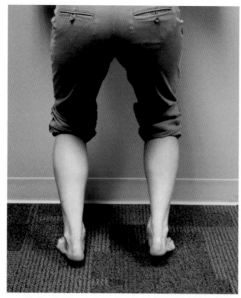

Figure 8-36. Squat test in an individual with limited talocrural dorsiflexion. Note the right heel is higher (less dorsiflexion) than the left.

The secondary test for symptoms produced during end-range squatting is to provide a posterior glide of the talus during squatting.

Step-Down and/or Small Knee Bend

During a step-down or small knee bend, an early heel rise is noted. A secondary test is to add a posterior glide at the talus during the small knee bend or step-down (Figure 8-37).

Muscle Length/Joint Range-of-Motion Impairments

Talocrural Dorsiflexion

The tests to determine the source of limitation are described in the "Pronation Syndrome" section.

Footwear Considerations

Recent Decrease in Heel-to-Toe Height

Limited talocrural dorsiflexion can be compensated for by lifting the heel slightly above the toe. A reduction in the heel-to-toe height ratio of the shoe can contribute to symptom onset similar to that described with pronation

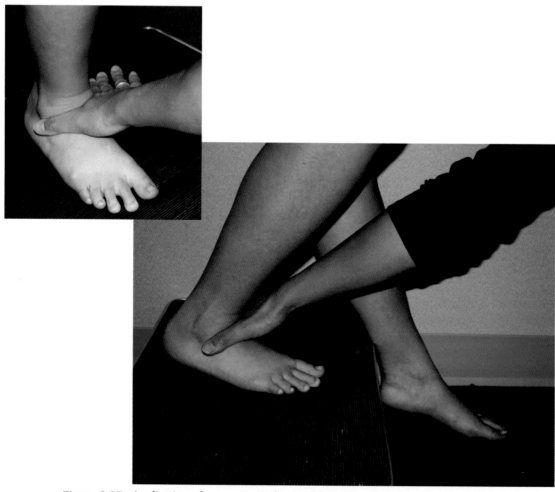

Figure 8-37. Application of a posterior/inferior glide on the talus during a step-down.

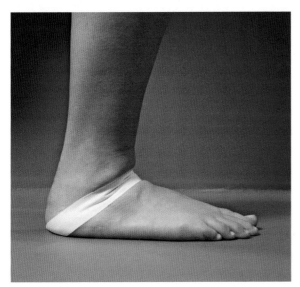

Figure 8-38. Use of tape from talus to calcaneus to stabilize the talus during tibial advancement when talocrural joint limitation is present.

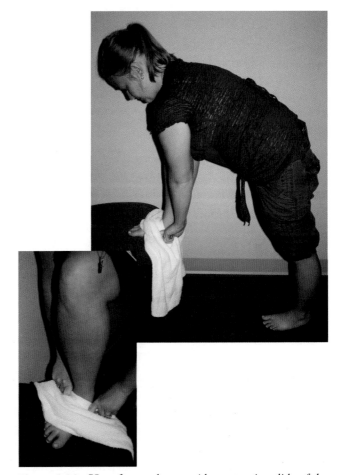

Figure 8-39. Use of a towel to provide a posterior glide of the talus during closed-chain dorsiflexion activities.

syndrome. Frequent use of shoes with high heels can contribute to insufficient dorsiflexion syndrome.

Summary

Insufficient dorsiflexion syndrome is characterized by limited talocrural dorsiflexion with the absence of other movement impairments of pronation, supination, or global limitation in motion (hypomobility). The impairment is noted in late stance, during swing, and/or during activities requiring maximum talocrural dorsiflexion (squatting, step-down, lunges, and so on).

Treatment

Walking and/or Running

Walking and running cues focus primarily on encouraging active contraction of the gastrocnemius muscle to reduce the reliance on the passive tension of the gastrocnemius and soleus muscle and calcaneal tendon unit. The specific cues are to have the patient actively lift the heel during late stance.

Decreased Range of Motion

The primary treatment focuses on addressing limited talocrural motion. The treatment options related to length of the gastrocnemius/soleus muscle and tendon are similar to those described for pronation syndrome. Joint mobilizations to increase dorsiflexion are also useful. A unique treatment option to provide a self-mobilization to the talocrural joint includes applying a piece of tape from the talus anterior progressing inferiorly and posteriorly on the medial and lateral side of the talus and attaching the tape to the plantar surface of the calcaneus (Figure 8-38). With the tape in place, the patient performs standing activities requiring tibial advancement over a fixed foot (lunges, squats). The tape can be used during functional

activities to assist with providing a stabilizing force for the talus as the tibia advances over the foot during closed chain activities. The tape can be substituted with a towel, and the patient can provide the posterior inferior glide of the talus with the edge of the towel while actively advancing the tibia over the fixed foot (Figure 8-39).

Activity Modification

The general guidelines for activity restriction and progression described in the "Pronation Syndrome" section apply here as well.

External Tissue Support

Footwear. The last of the shoe should match the patient's foot. Additionally, as with most individuals, a firm heel counter with a sole that bends at the metatarsal head break is generally appropriate. Shoe length and width and height of the toe box should accommodate the size of the foot and any deformities. An increase in the heel-to-toe ratio may be a reasonable compensation, particularly if the treatment to address talocrural dorsiflexion limitation is unsuccessful.

Orthoses. A heel lift may be indicated temporarily or permanently, depending on the ability of the stretching plan to improve talocrural dorsiflexion.

CASE PRESENTATION
Insufficient Dorsiflexion Syndrome

Symptoms and History

A 27-year-old male was referred to physical therapy by the orthopedist for treatment of right ankle pain, with an osteochondral defect of the talus and 1 year after microfracture repair.

The patient reports ankle joint pain (5/10) when performing squats during weight lifting. He has had to stop squats. He is also unable to complete some of his taekwondo kicks and positions because of ankle pain. The patient's pain is located on the anterior talocrural joint, primarily lateral. There is no pain with walking. He has minor pain (3/10) during running. Foot and Ankle Ability Measure score was 95% (100% indicates normal function), and the Foot and Ankle Ability Measure Sport Scale was 68% (100% indicates normal function).

Alignment Analysis

In standing, the calcaneus is vertical and the medial longitudinal arch height is normal. In prone, the assessment of subtalar joint neutral finds hindfoot and forefoot neutral alignment.

Movement Analysis

Standing/walking/running

During walking and running, the calcaneus hits in inversion and moves into eversion through midstance. The calcaneus moves toward inversion during push-off. The same movement pattern is noted during running. Anterior talocrural joint pain is reproduced during late stance phase. Cues to lift heel earlier in stance phase decreased anterior talocrural joint pain. No difference in dorsiflexion ROM is noted during gait assessment.

Single-leg hopping

No symptoms were reproduced, and no movement impairments noted.

Small knee bend

Small knee bend produced no symptoms, and no movement impairment was noted. A full squat was completed because of the patient's functional complaint. The heel on the right came off the ground earlier than the left. Symptoms (a pinching feeling) were reproduced at end-range. A posterior glide of the talus during the full squat relieved symptoms.

Muscle Length/Joint ROM Impairments

Talocrural dorsiflexion with the knee extended was 0 degrees on the right and 10 degrees on the left. With the knee flexed, talocrural dorsiflexion was 0 degrees on the right and 15 degrees on the left. Joint accessory mobility was limited with the anterior-to-posterior glide on the right. Subtalar joint motion is normal (10 degrees eversion, 20 degrees inversion), and first MTP motion was normal bilaterally.

	Right	Left
Talocrural dorsiflexion (knee extended)	0 degrees	10 degrees
Talocrural dorsiflexion (knee flexed)	0 degrees	15 degrees
Subtalar joint inversion	20 degrees	20 degrees
Subtalar joint eversion	10 degrees	10 degrees
First MTP joint extension (30 degrees talocrural plantarflexion)	60 degrees	60 degrees

Joint accessory motion assessment found limited mobility during an anterior-to-posterior glide of the talus on the ankle mortise on the right.

Footwear

Patient is wearing new running shoes. The last was semi-curved, and the heel counter is firm. The sole has gel pockets for cushion in the heel, increased density of the foam under the arch, and bends easily only at the metatarsal head break. The difference between the heel height and toe height of the shoe is 1 inch.

Diagnosis

The patient's movement tests support a movement system diagnosis of insufficient dorsiflexion. The patient's foot displays a normal movement pattern of pronation during early stance and supination during push-off. The likely source of symptoms is the anterior talocrural joint. The stage for rehabilitation is 3. Stage 3 is chosen because the patient has pain only with high level activities (pain is not limiting walking and running). The primary contributing factor to the movement impairment is limited talocrural dorsiflexion.

Prognosis

The prognosis for resolving symptoms so that high level activities can be performed with minimal pain is good. The patient is relatively young; however, the duration of limited motion is fairly long and the history of cartilage damage and surgical intervention leaves the status of the anatomy unknown.

Intervention

The patient was seen once/week for 4 weeks and then once every 2 weeks for 8 weeks to assist him in returning to his fitness and sport activities. The primary goal of intervention was to increase talocrural joint dorsiflexion. The home program included prolonged dorsiflexion stretches. The patient was instructed in a self-mobilization with movement using a towel at the talus during dorsiflexion in kneeling. Additionally, physical therapy treatment included anterior-to-posterior glides of the talus on the ankle mortise. The patient also experienced symptom relief with taping the talus to the calcaneus during weight-bearing activities, as well as during stretching. He was taught to tape himself for his daily fitness activities. No footwear changes were recommended, and no heel lift was added.

Outcome

The talus taping technique decreased squatting symptoms to 2/10. The patient progressed over the next 12 weeks to being able to complete all sport activities without symptoms. There were occasional days with ankle symptoms, generally a day or 2 after a vigorous workout. However, the symptoms resolved within 2 to 3 days with rest.

HYPOMOBILITY SYNDROME

The principal movement impairment in this syndrome is associated with a limitation in the physiological and accessory motions of the foot and ankle. This may result from degenerative changes in the joint or the effects of prolonged immobilization.

Symptoms and Pain

Degenerative Changes

The patient complains of pain with weight bearing (gait, standing, and stairs) that decreases with rest. However, the patient often reports stiffness in the morning or after prolonged periods of rest. The onset of pain is generally gradual, and the location and description of symptoms is often vague and deep within the joint. Osteoarthritis (OA) in the foot and ankle is often associated with a previous history of trauma and joint narrowing and irregular articular surfaces. Rheumatoid arthritis (RA) is associated with joint stiffness, destruction, and deformity.

Immobilization

The patient reports a relatively recent trauma or surgery to the foot and ankle that resulted in a period of immobilization. Foot and ankle motion is not progressing as expected.

Alignment: Structural Variations and Acquired Impairments

There are no common structural variations associated with hypomobility. Visually, the calf will appear atrophied. General enlargement of the foot and ankle from edema may be present, as well as localized enlargement from bone and joint changes as a result of the degeneration and/or surgery.

Movement Impairments

Walking and Running

The patient demonstrates a walking pattern that includes a decreased step length on the uninvolved side, decreased stance time on the involved side, an increase in the foot progression angle (toe out), little heel strike, and push-off. The knee may hyperextend to compensate for limited ankle motion. The patient is often dependent on an assistive device and reports limited tolerance of weight-bearing activities. The patient may be unable to run or hop.

Squat, Step-Down, and/or Small Knee Bend

The patient has limited mobility during the squat, step down, and/or small knee bend. Descending stairs is problematic, and the patient may need to turn sideways and/or descend the stairs in a nonreciprocal pattern.

Muscle Length/Joint Range-of-Motion Impairments

Hypomobility syndrome includes limitations in physiological and accessory joint motion. Hypomobility syndrome is differentiated from insufficient dorsiflexion syndrome because the limitations in motion are in more directions and include more than the talocrural joint. In most cases, talocrural dorsiflexion is limited in those with hypomobility syndrome, but plantarflexion will also be limited and additional joints can be involved (subtalar, intertarsal, intermetatarsal, and MTP joints). Decreased joint motion related to surgery, trauma, and/or immobilization requires additional research by the physical therapist. A copy of the operative report and/or clarification with the surgeon can assure joints were not purposely fused or that hardware is not traversing a joint. The physical therapist needs a clear understanding as to whether joint motion should be increased or if compensations should be implemented because increasing motion is contraindicated.

During the assessment, if joint limitations are associated with osteoarthritis, repetition of passive motion often improves motion and symptoms. Throughout the examination in an individual suspected of hypomobility, it is likely that the limited joint motion is being compensated for by proximal and distal joints that do not have limited mobility. The hip abduction, knee hyperextension, and midfoot joint dorsiflexion are especially common compensatory motions.

Muscle Strength/Performance Impairments

MMTs of the ankle and foot muscles find weakness throughout. Often the patient is unable to complete even one single-leg heel rise through the full ROM.

Balance and Proprioception Impairment

The ability to maintain single-leg stance on the involved side will be impaired (poor control and decreased duration). Lack of ability to balance on one foot is often evident with the eyes open, and performance will worsen when the patient is instructed to close the eyes, limiting visual input and isolating foot and ankle proprioception.

Summary

Hypomobility syndrome is primarily defined by physiological and accessory joint limitations. Multiple directions of motions and/or joints will be involved in the loss of motion. Associated with the limitation in motion and the history of immobilization is general foot and ankle weakness and impaired balance and proprioception.

Treatment

Decreased Range of Motion

Joint stiffness from injury, surgery, and/or immobilization often requires an aggressive ROM treatment plan. Prolonged stretching with braces, casting, or increasing the duration and frequency of home stretches is often indicated. In therapy, joint mobilization and manipulation are also indicated.

Decreased motion caused by OA and RA is addressed more gently to avoid joint irritation and worsening of symptoms. The limitation to motion often involves changes in bone and joint anatomy, and ROM exercises are often used before activity to improve function and prevent progressive loss of motion not to increase joint motion.

Muscle Performance Impairments

Plantarflexor muscle performance limitations impair function the most. Generally, resistance band strengthening is an appropriate place to start since weight bearing is often painful. Progression to heel raises with a leg-press machine, bilateral heel raises, and single-leg heel raises is important. Completion of heel raises does not always translate into enough strength for push-off with walking and running.

Control of ankle dorsiflexion when landing on the toes during hopping, running, sprinting, and descending stairs is the result of an eccentric contraction of the plantarflexors. Specific eccentric overloading of the plantarflexors is critical for patients with high level activity goals.[41-43] Finally, progression to dynamic bilateral and single-leg hopping, cutting, and sport specific exercises is required for full return of plantar flexor strength.

Balance and Proprioception Impairments

Impaired balance and proprioception is often a key contributor to falls and additional injuries. The treatment plan should include progression from eyes open to eyes closed and from solid surfaces to moving/uneven surfaces (mini-trampoline) and should progress to dynamic activities like high marching over objects, kicking balls, and walking backward. When participation in sport activities is a goal, balance and proprioception activities must include progression to quick stops and starts, maintaining balance during player contact, and gradual return to full game participation.

Activity Modification

The general guidelines for activity restriction and progression described in the section on Pronation Syndrome apply here as well. If the patient has OA and RA, continuing with weight bearing, high impact, high-repetition activities (walking or running for fitness) is often contraindicated. The patient often needs to be guided into lower impact activities, such as stationary bicycling, water aerobics, or StairMaster/elliptical, or activities, such as rowing, that involve aerobic fitness through the upper extremities. Weight loss can also significantly impact pain with weight-bearing activities and should be discussed if appropriate for the patient. Use of assistive devices may be temporarily or permanently indicated for patients with arthritis.

External Tissue Support

Footwear. For patients with hypomobility syndrome, shoe size and shape are particularly important. The involved foot and ankle is often larger, and edema fluctuates with weight-bearing activity. A shoe that has extra depth with laces is helpful to accommodate size and edema fluctuation. An increase in the heel-to-toe ratio may be a reasonable compensation, particularly if the treatment to address talocrural dorsiflexion limitation is unsuccessful.

For patients with OA or RA, there are a number of shoe modifications that can be made to assist with foot and ankle symptoms during weight bearing. A steel shank in the sole of the shoe (making the sole of the shoe rigid) with a rocker at the toe break allows the patient to more easily roll over the foot without needing as much talocrural dorsiflexion or MTP dorsiflexion.

Orthoses. For individuals with OA or RA, a total contact insert made of accommodative material is often indicated. Deformities of the foot should be considered in the design and materials chosen for the orthosis. A heel lift may be necessary to manage the loss of dorsiflexion ROM. Temporary orthoses or additional arch support are often indicated to manage foot pain that is often related to the new onset of a pronation impairment that results from the limited foot and ankle mobility.

CASE PRESENTATION
Hypomobility Syndrome

Symptoms and History

A 78-year-old male was referred by the orthopedist for evaluation and treatment of the right ankle, status/post (s/p) open reduction, internal fixation (ORIF). The patient states that 6 months ago he fell in his bathroom. His right foot was caught under the cabinet, and he heard a snap. The patient had surgery with pins and plates that provided internal fixation for a fractured tibia and fibula. He was casted for 8 weeks. He had physical therapy 3 times/week at home for the first 4 weeks. No additional physical therapy was ordered by his physician until his 6 month follow-up visit when the physician noted the continued limp and the patient complained of limited ability to complete many activities required by his daily life (taking care of his lawn, walking through the grocery store, and completing his daily walk for fitness). His Foot and Ankle Ability Measure score was 40% (100% indicates normal function).

Alignment Analysis

The ankle, foot, and toes are moderately swollen making assessment of alignment difficult.

Movement Analysis

Standing/walking/running

Patient has been using a walker since surgery and ambulates limited distances on all surfaces. There is decreased step length on the left and decreased stance time on the right. His right foot is pointed out. He reports inability to descend stairs or a curb leading with the left leg.

Muscle Performance Impairments

Patient is unable to tolerate full resistance to any motion. Approximate muscle strength of 2–/5 throughout ankle musculature.

Muscle Length/Joint ROM Impairments

	Right	Left
Ankle dorsiflexion (knee extended)	–10 degrees	6 degrees
Plantar flexion	10-30 degrees	0-48 degrees
Inversion	0-4 degrees	0-24 degrees
Eversion	0-2 degrees	0-8 degrees
First MTP dorsiflexion	0-20 degrees	0-60 degrees

Footwear

The patient is wearing a pair of old canvas slip on shoes because his old shoes have not fit since the surgery.

Diagnosis

The patient's movement tests support a movement system syndrome of hypomobility. The patient is 6 months postsurgery, the tissues have healed, but ROM continues to be limited and general foot function is compromised. The stage for rehabilitation is 2. Stage 2 is chosen because the patient is outside of the tissue protection phase and requires progression of activity, strengthening, and ROM. The primary contributing factor to the movement impairment is limited motion at the talocrural, subtalar, and MTP joints. Additionally, ankle and foot muscle performance is limited.

Prognosis

The prognosis for returning the patient to his full function is good. He is older and the duration since onset is long; however, little intervention has been attempted and activity expectations are reasonable.

Treatment

The patient was seen initially 3 times/week for 4 weeks. Treatment frequency decreased to 1 to 2 times/week for 8 additional weeks. The primary goals of intervention were to increase ROM, address muscle performance, and functional limitations. The patient was given a home and in-therapy stretching program to address the talocrural and first MTP motion and a therapist-assisted subtalar joint ROM program. The stretching program began gently, with minimal overpressure, 30-second duration hold, and 3 to 5 times/day frequency. Mobilizations were shy of end–range and were closely monitored for symptom response. Patient progress and tolerance was assessed with the gentle ROM program. The stretching and mobilization treatments were progressed over the first 2 weeks of physical therapy, and prolonged stretching was implemented with the use of a night splint (that can be used during the day) after 3 weeks of physical therapy. Lower extremity strengthening exercises focused on calf, anterior thigh (quadriceps), and hip muscles. Additionally, general fitness was addressed with the stationary bicycling initially, progressing to treadmill and outside walking as patient tolerance increased. Single-limb stance tolerance was addressed initially in the parallel bars, progressing to walking without an assistive device and adding surface variations as tolerated. The canvas shoe provided very little stability for his foot. With the assistance of a trained footwear specialist, he was able to find a shoe that accommodated his edematous foot yet provided support during weight-bearing activities. Edema management included a double thickness of Tubigrip (ConvaTec Inc., Stillman, NJ), extending from the tip of the toes to midcalf.

Outcome

ROM was slow to progress despite the aggressive program. Dorsiflexion at the talocrural joint progressed to 0 degrees, plantar flexion increased to 35 degrees, and first MTP motion increased to 35 degrees by the end of 12 weeks of physical therapy. Despite the lack of full motion, the patient's strength, balance and proprioception, and weight-bearing tolerance increased so that the patient could walk without a noticeable limp on all flat and uneven surfaces.

FOOT AND ANKLE IMPAIRMENT

A key criterion for placement into the foot and ankle impairment diagnostic category is the need to protect tissue. Usually, the tissue involved is stressed by a surgical procedure or trauma and may cause significant pain at rest and during movement. The patient is unable to tolerate a typical movement system examination. The limitation in movement is not primarily related to a chronic pain condition. These are general guidelines and not intended to stand alone. Consult the physician for specific precautions, protocols, and progressions. The physical therapist must be familiar with the tissues that were affected in the surgical procedure or injury.

The general diagnosis of foot and ankle impairment is used if the tissue injured and/or impacted by surgery is unknown. The tissue injured and/or impacted by surgery is used in the diagnosis when it is known, through the physician's referral or the patient's medical record. For example, the diagnosis might be tibia and fibula fracture s/p ORIF. For additional information regarding the tissue impairment diagnosis, see Chapter 2.

Unique Physiological Factors for the Foot and Ankle

In most cases, the bones, muscles, tendons, cartilage, and ligaments of the foot and ankle respond to stress and follow healing patterns similar to structures elsewhere in the body. There are some unique physiological factors that are specific to the foot/ankle that will help guide the physical therapist in decision making regarding the examination and in planning the treatment program.

Bone

Fractures of the base of the fifth metatarsal have a high probability of nonunion secondary to the pull of the fibularis brevis. Additionally, stress fractures of the anterior lateral tibial diaphysis, medial malleolus, talus, navicular, and sesamoids are high-risk areas that often fail to heal; re-fractures occur and operative intervention is needed.[28]

Muscle

It is common to loose dorsiflexion ROM and to experience gastrocnemius/soleus muscle atrophy with immobilization.

Tendon

Calcaneal (Achilles) tendon rupture can be treated conservatively with cast immobilization or be surgically repaired with a period of cast immobilization. During the healing process, strong gastrocnemius/soleus contractions and end-range dorsiflexion motions are restricted. After the period of immobilization, the physical therapist needs to cautiously strengthen the gastrocnemius/soleus muscle and tendon.

If severe, a posterior tibial tendon injury or insufficiency may result in significant deformity of the arch (flattening). If treated conservatively, this injury or insufficiency may require long periods of immobilization. Surgical repair with a tendon transfer is often required for resolution of the symptoms. Cast immobilization is typical after posterior tibial tendon repair and tendon transfer. Contraction of the posterior tibial muscle would be contraindicated until adequate healing has occurred.

Ligament

Lateral ankle sprains can be accompanied by fractures. The Ottawa Ankle Rules indicate that indications for additional imaging after ankle sprain include the inability to bear weight or tenderness at the base of the fifth metatarsal, navicular, or the posterior edge or tip of either malleolus.[44]

Syndesmotic ankle sprain ("high ankle sprain") is associated with greater discomfort during weight bearing and longer healing time and may require immobilization.[45]

Skin

Edema has the potential to limit mobility and compromise the space occupied by nerves and arteries. The areas where space is limited and nerves and arteries pass include

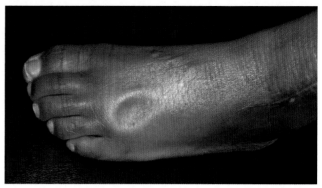

Figure 8-40. Patient 8 weeks after an open reduction internal fixation of a tibia/fibular fracture. Note dorsal pitting edema.

the compartments within the leg, the extensor retinaculum and the flexor retinaculum.

It is important to inspect the surgical incision. The therapist should note the location, appearance, mobility, sensitivity of the incision, and if the incision appears healed (approximately 10 days). Signs of infection (red, warm, drainage, patient fever, or lymph streaking) should be reported to the physician immediately.

Nerve

The common fibular (peroneal) nerve is superficial and easily injured as it wraps around the head of the fibula. The deep fibular (peroneal) nerve can be compromised as it runs through the anterior compartment of the leg and/or beneath the extensor retinaculum. The tibial nerve can be compressed as it runs through the posterior compartment and/or beneath the flexor retinaculum (tarsal tunnel). The interdigital nerve can be compromised between the metatarsals. The most common site of symptoms is between the third and fourth metatarsals. The interdigital nerve between the third and fourth metatarsals is often enlarged because it can receive nerve fibers from both the medial and lateral plantar nerves.

Unique Assessment and Treatment for the Foot and Ankle

A full and detailed list of items to assess and guidelines for test completion and interpretation are outline in Chapter 2. The items unique to the foot and ankle are highlighted here.

Edema

The foot and ankle are prone to edema after trauma and/or surgery, and this edema warrants close examination, documentation, treatment, and monitoring (Figure 8-40) Treatment often requires the use of compression garments, as well as basic techniques of ice and elevation.

Appearance

Loss of the gastrocnemius/soleus muscle bulk is the most apparent change after a prolonged period of lower extremity immobilization. However, all lower extremity muscles (hip, knee, and foot and ankle) on the involved side will be affected by a period of immobilization.

Proprioception/Balance

When appropriate, given weight-bearing precautions, the ability to maintain single-leg stance with eyes open and with eyes closed should be assessed. Treatment must include activities with the eyes closed to remove visual compensation. Additionally, progression to dynamic activities on variable surfaces is important, including uneven (grass, rocks) and moving (wobble board) surfaces. If interested in returning to sport activities, balance during cutting or rapid changes in direction and sport-specific activities must be assessed.

Functional Mobility

Lower extremity injuries often require the use of an assistive device. The patient's ability to complete all mobility tasks while maintaining weight-bearing precautions is critical (sit to and from stand, ambulation, stairs, and transfers in and out of a car).

Plantarflexion function during walking and running should be assessed, when allowed. Often, the patient is able to complete single-leg heel raises in standing; however, dynamic plantar flexion function during walking is impaired and the heel fails to rise appropriately during push-off. During running and sprinting the patient will complain of an inability to remain on their toes. Improving gastrocnemius/soleus muscle function can be challenging. A progressive overload program must be established and include the addition of hopping and running.

Summary

Foot and ankle impairment is a classification system that allows the therapist to clarify the tissue involved, as well as the surgery. The examination is guided by the therapist's assessment of the rehabilitation stage and his or her knowledge of the surgical procedure, precautions, and rehabilitation protocol. This classification is used when there is no apparent and contributing movement impairment, or symptoms are so severe that a full movement system examination cannot be completed.

CASE PRESENTATION
Ankle Impairment Stage 1

Symptoms and History

The patient is a 40-year-old female referred by the orthopedist for physical therapy 6 weeks s/p right ankle bimalleolar fracture, ORIF. The patient reports that 6 weeks ago she missed the last step going down to her basement and fractured her right tibia and fibula. The patient reports non–weight-bearing activity in a cast for 2 weeks after surgery and progressed to partial weight bearing in a walking cast for 4 weeks. The physician started her on full weight-bearing activity 3 days ago in a boot. She reports

she always has a bit of pain even when sitting or resting (3/10). Pain increases to 5/10 with attempts at full weight bearing activity. Her Foot and Ankle Ability Measure score was 10% (100% indicates normal function).

Alignment Analysis

Patient is obese with visible psoriatic patches noted on bilateral lower and upper extremities. The ankle, foot, and toes are moderately swollen with pitting edema of the right ankle and foot.

Girth measurements:
- Figure 8 at the ankle: 60 cm right and 58 cm left
- Calf: 42.8 cm right and 44.3 cm left

Scar: Incision closed, no redness, no warmth, no drainage. Scar is slightly adhered centrally with very mild hypersensitivity to touch.

Movement Analysis
Standing/walking

Assessed in boot only without assistive device. Patient walks with decreased stance time right, no push-off on right, and decreased step length on left.

Muscle Performance Impairments

Not assessed this visit.

Muscle Length/Joint ROM Impairments

	Right	Left
Ankle dorsiflexion (knee extended)	−16 degrees	−4 degrees
Ankle dorsiflexion (knee flexed)	−10 degrees	2 degrees
Plantar flexion	51 degrees	54 degrees
Inversion	40 degrees	43 degrees
Eversion	2 degrees	8 degrees

Diagnosis

The patient's evaluation supports a diagnosis of bimalleolar fracture, s/p open reduction internal fixation, Stage 1. The patient is 6 weeks postsurgery and just beginning to progress toward full weight-bearing activities and is still in an immobilization boot. The patient would likely progress to Stage 2 quickly once weight-bearing tolerance improves. The primary contributing factor to the foot and ankle impairment is the need to protect and gradually load tissue after surgical intervention. Weight-bearing tolerance is limited, talocrural dorsiflexion in decreased, and edema is present.

Prognosis

The prognosis for returning the patient to her full weight-bearing function is good. The patient's increased weight will likely delay tolerance of full weight-bearing activities.

Treatment

The patient was seen 3 times/week for 4 weeks and then 1 to treatment times/week for 8 additional weeks. The initial goals of treatment were to increase weight-bearing tolerance and wean her from wearing the boot. A home program was implemented to address decreased ROM and as appropriate, strength. The patient received education about edema management and scar mobilization.

Outcome

Initial attempts at weaning from the immobilization boot were met with an increase in irritation of the posterior tibialis tendon from increased pronation during weight bearing. The patient required the addition of a heel lift, scaphoid pad, and arch taping to manage the posterior tibialis tendon symptoms. Two weeks were required for the patient to wean from the boot to regular footwear for ambulation. Talocrural dorsiflexion ROM improved to −5 degrees but remained limited at 6 months after surgery. The patient was instructed to continue with talocrural dorsiflexion stretching, but she continued to need a small heel lift to avoid posterior tibialis tendon irritation.

PROXIMAL TIBIOFIBULAR GLIDE SYNDROME

The principal movement impairment is posterior and/or superior motion of the fibula on the tibia during active hamstring contraction (especially during running). The principal positional impairment is the fibula located anterior, posterior, superior, or inferior to the normal position on the tibia after trauma, particularly an ankle sprain.

Symptoms and Pain

Pain in posterolateral or lateral aspect of tibiofibular joint is often associated with running or general tibiofibular pain is associated with a history of lateral ankle sprains. Tingling or numbness can also be reported if the fibular head is compressing the common fibular (peroneal) nerve. The location of the tingling or numbness can be locally at the lateral knee or referred to the lateral distal leg and/or dorsum of the foot.

Alignment: Structural Variations and Acquired Impairments

Palpation of fibula location on tibia, relative to uninvolved side, reveals malalignment (anterior, posterior, and/or superior). A glide in the direction of the positional or movement impairment increases pain. A glide in the opposite direction of the positional or movement impairment will decrease symptoms.

Movement Impairments

Walking/Running

The movement impairment is very small and not visible during motions. Symptoms are localized to the fibular head, or referred to areas innervated by the common fibular (peroneal) nerve or its branches, during walking and running. If the symptoms are reduced or go away

with stabilization of the tibiofibular joint the diagnosis of proximal tibiofibular glide syndrome is supported.

Sitting

Resisted hamstring contraction can reproduce symptoms in an individual with proximal tibiofibular glide syndrome, and the symptoms are reduced with joint stabilization.

Talocrural dorsiflexion has associated tibiofibular motions and can reproduce symptoms. If symptoms are related to proximal tibiofibular glide syndrome, stabilization at the proximal tibiofibular joint will reduce symptoms.

Muscle Length/Joint Range-of-Motion Impairments

Hamstring length and talocrural dorsiflexion impairment are common with this diagnosis. Positions when the hamstring are stretched or when the talocrural joint is at end-range of motion can reproduce symptoms. Stabilization of the fibular head during the stretch decreases symptoms.

Summary

Proximal tibiofibular glide syndrome is either a positional fault generally occurring after ankle and foot trauma (ankle sprain) or a movement impairment as a result of hamstring contraction pulling the fibula posteriorly. The positional or movement impairments are difficult to see and palpate, but when correction of a suspected positional impairment or stabilization against a suspected motion decreases symptoms, the diagnosis is supported.

Treatment

Alignment Impairments

Positional impairments of the tibiofibular joint can be addressed by gliding the fibula on the tibia as indicated by evaluation findings.

Decreased Range of Motion

Hamstring and talocrural dorsiflexion limitations should be addressed with a home program.

External Tissue Support

Taping. Taping to immobilize or limit motion between the proximal tibia and fibula can help reduce symptoms (Figure 8-41). Caution should be taken to avoid compression of the common fibular nerve as it passes superficially around the fibular head. Taping of the fibula is a required precursor to hamstring and talocrural stretching exercises that assist in stabilizing the joint during the prescribed exercise. Taping of the fibula is also helpful after mobilization treatments correcting positional impairments.

CONCLUSIONS

The foot and ankle are a complex chain of joints that must convert quickly from a flexible adapter and shock

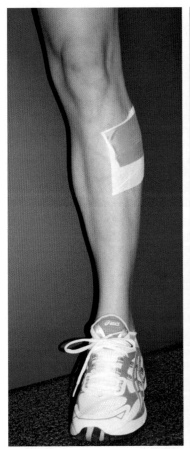
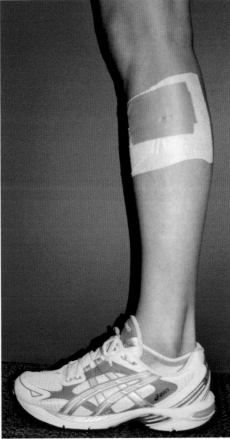
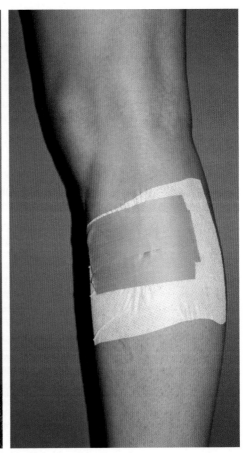

Figure 8-41. Example of fibular taping, avoiding the fibular (peroneal) nerve while providing resistance to posterior motion of the fibular head.

attenuator to a rigid lever capable of propelling the body in all different directions. The ability of the foot to perform these diverse and opposing functions and precisely time the function to the intended task is impacted by a number of factors. Joint stability, muscle function, and motor coordination are critical to the foot and ankle. However, function at the foot and ankle is intimately connected to the function and alignment of the knee and hip. The physical therapist is the most highly trained health professional with the ability to evaluate weight-bearing activities, understand the functional requirements of the lower extremity, recognize the movement impairment(s), assess the factors that contribute to the movement impairment, and develop a focused and effective treatment plan.

REFERENCES

1. Thambyah A, Pereira BP: Mechanical contribution of the fibula to torsion stiffness in the lower extremity, *Clin Anat* 19(7):615-620, 2006.
2. Lin CJ, Lai KA, Chou YL, et al: The effect of changing the foot progression angle on the knee adduction moment in normal teenagers, *Gait Posture* 14(2):85-91, 2001.
3. Sahrmann SA: *Diagnosis and treatment of movement impairment syndromes*, St Louis, 2002, Mosby.
4. Seber S, Hazer B, Kose N, et al: Rotational profile of the lower extremity and foot progression angle: computerized tomographic examination of 50 male adults, *Arch Orthop Trauma Surg* 120(5-6):255-258, 2000.
5. Schneider B, Laubenberger J, Jemlich S, et al: Measurement of femoral antetorsion and tibial torsion by magnetic resonance imaging, *Brit J Radiol* 70(834):575-579, 1997.
6. Yoshioka Y, Siu DW, Scudamore RA, et al: Tibial anatomy and functional axes, *J Orthop Res* 7(1):132-137, 1989.
7. Piva SR, Fitzgerald K, Irrgang JJ, et al: Reliability of measures of impairments associated with patellofemoral pain syndrome, *BMC Musculoskeletal Disord* 7, 2006.
8. McPoil T, Cornwall MW: Relationship between neutral subtalar joint position and pattern of rearfoot motion during walking, *Foot Ankle Int* 15(3):141-145, 1994.
9. Nigg BM, Cole GK, Nachbauer W: Effects of arch height of the foot on angular motion of the lower-extremities in running, *J Biomech* 26(8):909-916, 1993.
10. Williams DS, Mcclay IS, Hamill J, et al: Lower extremity kinematic and kinetic differences in runners with high and low arches, *J Appl Biomech* 17(2):153-163, 2001.
11. Hunt AE, Smith RM: Mechanics and control of the flat versus normal foot during the stance phase of walking, *Clin Biomech* 19(4):391-397, 2004.
12. *Gray's anatomy: the anatomical basis of medicine and surgery*, ed 38, Edinburgh, 1999, Churchill Livingstone.

13. Soavi R, Girolami M, Loreti I, et al: The mobility of the proximal tibio-fibular joint. A roentgen stereophotogrammetric analysis on six cadaver specimens, *Foot Ankle Int* 21(4):336-342, 2000.

14. Beumer A, Valstar ER, Garling EH, et al: Effects of ligament sectioning on the kinematics of the distal tibio-fibular syndesmosis. A radio stereometric study of 10 cadaveric specimens based on presumed trauma mechanisms with suggestions for treatment, *Acta Orthop* 77(3):531-540, 2006.

15. Bragonzoni L, Russo A, Girolami M, et al: The distal tibiofibular syndesmosis during passive foot flexion. RSA-based study on intact, ligament injured and screw fixed cadaver specimens, *Arch Orthop Trauma Surg* 126(5):304-308, 2006.

16. Novacheck TF: The biomechanics of running, *Gait Posture* 7(1):77-95, 1998.

17. Rattanaprasert U, Smith R, Sullivan M, et al: Three-dimensional kinematics of the forefoot, rearfoot, and leg without the function of tibialis posterior in comparison with normals during stance phase of walking, *Clin Biomech* 14(1):14-23, 1999.

18. Kaufman KR, Brodine SK, Shaffer RA, et al: The effect of foot structure and range of motion on musculoskeletal overuse injuries, *Am J Sports Med* 5:585-593, 1999.

19. Grimston SK, Nigg BM, Hanley DA, et al: Differences in ankle joint complex range of motion as a function of age, *Foot Ankle* 14(4):215-222, 1993.

20. Astrom M, Arvidson T: Alignment and joint motion in the normal foot, *J Orthop Sports Phys Ther* 22(5):216-222, 1995.

21. Cornwall MW, McPoil TG: Motion of the calcaneus, navicular, and first metatarsal during the stance phase of walking, *J Am Podiatr Med Assoc* 92(2):67-76. 2002;

22. Neumann DA: *Kinesiology of the musculoskeletal system: foundations for physical rehabilitation*, St Louis, 2002, Mosby.

23. Levangie PK, Norkin CC: *Joint structure & function: a comprehensive analysis*, ed 4, Philadelphia, 2005, FA Davis.

24. Nawoczenski DA, Baumhauer JF, Umberger BR: Relationship between clinical measurements and motion of the first metatarsophalangeal joint during gait, *J Bone Joint Surg Am* 81(3):370-376, 1999.

25. Hopson MM, McPoil TG, Cornwall MW: Motion of the first metatarsophalangeal joint—reliability and validity of 4 measurement techniques, *J Am Podiatr Med Assoc* 85(4):198-204, 1995.

26. Flanigan RM, Nawoczenski DA, Chen LL, et al: The influence of foot position on stretching of the plantar fascia, *Foot & Ankle Int* 28(7):815-822, 2007.

27. Kaeding CC, Yu JR, Wright R, et al: Management and return to play of stress fractures, *Clin J Sport Med* 15(6):442-447, 2005.

28. Hoppenfeld S: *Physical examination of the spine and extremities*, Norwalk, CT, 1976, Appleton-Century-Crofts.

29. Evans RC: Lower leg, ankle, and foot. In Evans RC: *Illustrated orthopedic physical assessment*, St Louis, 2001, Mosby.

30. Magee DJ: *Orthopedic physical assessment*, ed 4, Philadelphia, 2002, Saunders.

31. Goodacre S, Sutton AJ, Sampson FC: Meta-analysis: the value of clinical assessment in the diagnosis of deep venous thrombosis, *Ann Intern Med* 143(2):129-139, 2005.

32. Wells PS, Anderson DR, Bormanis J, et al: Value of assessment of pretest probability of deep-vein thrombosis in clinical management, *The Lancet* 350:1795-1798, 1997.

33. Riddle DL, Wells PS: Diagnosis of lower-extremity deep vein thrombosis in outpatients, *Phys Ther* 84(8):729-735, 2004.

34. Kumar V, Cotran RS, Robbins SL: *Basic pathology*, ed 5, Philadelphia, 1992, Saunders.

35. Sutton-Tyrrell K, Venkitachalam L, Kanaya AM, et al: Relationship of ankle blood pressures to cardiovascular events in older adults, *Stroke* 39(3):863-869, 2008.

36. Geppert MJ, Mizel MS: Management of heel pain in the inflammatory arthritides, *Clin Orthop* 349:93-99, 1998.

37. Huether SE, McCance KL: *Understanding pathophysiology (with media)*, ed 4, St Louis, 2007, Mosby.

38. Kinoshita, M, Okuda R, Morikawa J, et al: The Dorsiflexion-eversion test for diagnosis of tarsal tunnel syndrome, *J Bone Joint Surg Am* 83(12):1835-1839, 2001.

39. Lunsford BR, Perry J: The standing heel-rise test for ankle plantar flexion: criterion for normal, *Phys Ther* 75(8):694-698, 1995.

40. Hastings MK, Mueller, MJ, Pilgram TK, et al: Effect of metatarsal pad placement on plantar pressure in people with diabetes and peripheral neuropathy, *Ankle Foot Int* 28(1):84-88, 2007.

41. Roos EM, Engstrom M, Lagerquist A, et al: Clinical improvement after 6 weeks of eccentric exercise in patients with mid-portion Achilles tendinopathy—a randomized trial with 1-year follow-up, *Scand J Med Sci Sport* 14(5):286-295, 2004.

42. Alfredson H, Pietila T, Jonsson P, et al: Heavy-load eccentric calf muscle training for the treatment of chronic Achilles tendinosis, *Am J Sports Med* 26(3):360-366. 1998.

43. Sayana MK, Maffulli N: Eccentric calf muscle training in non-athletic patients with Achilles tendinopathy, *J Sci Med Sport* 10(1):52-58. 2007;

44. Stiell IG, Greenberg GH, McKnight RD, et al: Decision rules for the use of radiography in acute ankle injuries. Refinement and prospective validation, *JAMA* 269(9):1127-1132,1993.

45. Boytim MJ, Fischer DA, Neumann L: Syndesmotic ankle sprains, *Am J Sports Med* 19(3):294-298, 1991.

CHAPTER 8

APPENDIX

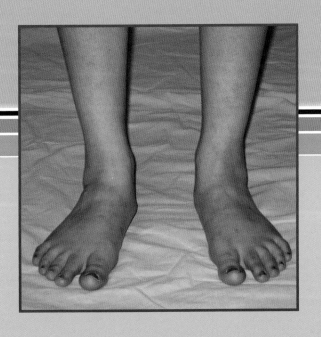

Pronation Syndrome

The principal movement impairment in pronation syndrome is pronation at the foot and ankle. Pronation is considered abnormal and an impairment when the amount of pronation during weight-bearing activities is excessive for that individual and/or when there is insufficient movement of the foot in the direction of supination in later stance phase. The pronation impairment can occur in the hindfoot, midfoot, and/or forefoot. A foot with a pronation movement impairment is a flexible foot that compensates for various structural and movement impairments within the foot and ankle, as well as those at the knee and hip.

Symptoms and History

- *Plantar fascia:* Heel pain with first step in morning or after prolonged non–weight-bearing function
- *Posterior and anterior tibialis muscle/tendon:* Pain in muscle or tendon, most apparent with weight bearing as the muscle works to control pronation
- *Tibial nerve:* Pain, tingling, and/or numbness on the posterior, medial ankle and/or into the plantar surface of the foot
- *Gastrocnemius/soleus muscle/calcaneal tendon:* Pain in muscle or tendon as tibial forward progression is controlled in stance and during propulsion phase of weight bearing
- *Metatarsal heads:* Pain localized to the second and third metatarsal heads
- Interdigital nerve: Pain, tingling, or numbness between metatarsal heads (most often third and fourth) radiating into corresponding toes
- *Medial column joints:* Generalized foot pain (often in the midfoot) in the medial column joints; pain can progress to joint degeneration and involvement of the joints of the lateral column

Common Referring Diagnoses

- Shin splints
- Stress fracture
  - Tibia
  - Metatarsals
- Posterior/anterior tendonitis
- Plantar fasciitis
- Foot pain
- Tarsal tunnel syndrome
- Metatarsalgia
- Digital neuroma

Key Tests and Signs for Movement Impairment

Alignment Analysis

- Hindfoot: Calcaneal eversion
- Midfoot: Talonavicular joint dropped down (medial bulge)
- Low medial longitudinal arch
- Forefoot: Abduction in relationship to the hindfoot at the transtarsal joint
- Increased width of forefoot
- Hip/knee medial rotation or compensation for hip/knee lateral rotation

Movement Impairment Analysis

Standing

Gait/running

- Excessive calcaneal eversion in stance phase
- Excessive arch flattening in stance phase
- Insufficient movement of the foot in the direction of supination in later stance phase
- Poor plantar flexor contraction and push-off
  - Support of the arch (supinator contraction, tape, scaphoid pad) decreases symptoms in the four impairments
- Hip/knee medial rotation
  - Gluteal muscle contraction decreases medial rotation and symptoms

Single-leg hopping

- Calcaneus everted
- Arch flattening
- Poor plantarflexor contraction (decreased jump height)
  - Plantarflexion contraction improves jump and decreases symptoms
  - Contraction of gluteal muscles decreases medial rotation and symptoms

Step-down or small knee bend

- Calcaneal eversion
- Arch flattening
- Knee/hip medial rotation
- Weight transferred over medial column of foot

Sitting

Active first MTP extension

- First MPT extension results in plantar flexion at the first metatarsocuneiform and prominence of the MTP on the plantar surface of the foot. Symptoms may be produced at the MTP and/or metatarsocuneiform joints
- MTP or metatarsocuneiform stabilization decreases symptoms

Source of Signs and Symptoms

Heel and/or Arch Symptoms

Plantar Fascia

- Special test: Toe extension increases symptoms with/without palpation along the fascia
- Palpation: Tender at the insertion of plantar fascia on medial calcaneal tubercle and can be tender along the fascia into the midfoot

Posterior and Anterior Tibialis Muscle/Tendon

- Special test: Soft tissue differential may be weak and painful or strong and painful with appropriate resisted contraction in neutral foot position ($\approx$10 degrees plantar flexion)

Palpation

- Posterior tibialis muscle and tendon: Tender distal, posterior, medial tibia to plantar navicular
- Anterior tibialis muscle and tendon: Tender at the proximal lateral tibia, dorsal/medial to first cuneiform and/or base of first metatarsal

Tibial Nerve

- Special test: Positive Tinel's, placement in provocative position (dorsiflexion, toes extended, and calcaneus everted) or Tinel's in provocative position

Hindfoot Symptoms

Gastrocnemius/Soleus Muscle/Calcaneal Tendon:

- Palpation: Tender posterior calf and tendon to calcaneus

Forefoot Symptoms

Metatarsal Heads

- Palpation: Tender at the second and third metatarsal heads

Interdigital Nerves

- Special test: Squeeze test positive (most common between third and fourth metatarsals)

DJD, Degenerative joint disease; *DVT,* deep vein thrombosis; *MTP,* metatarsophalangeal; *RA,* rheumatoid arthritis; *ROM,* range of motion.

Associated Signs or Contributing Factors

Structural Variations

Foot

- Subtalar joint neutral findings modified by weight bearing
- Uncompensated hindfoot valgus
- Uncompensated forefoot valgus
- Compensated hindfoot varus
- Compensated forefoot varus

Femur/Tibia

- Long leg on pronated side
- Femoral anteversion

Muscle Length/Joint ROM Impairments

Talocrural Dorsiflexion

- Limited if dorsiflexion <10 degrees with knee extended
  - Gastrocnemius short if dorsiflexion ≥10 degrees with knee flexed
  - Soleus short if dorsiflexion ≤10 degrees with knee flexed and normal accessory talocrural motion
  - Talocrural joint limitation if dorsiflexion ≤10 degrees, regardless of knee position and limited accessory talocrural joint motion (cannot rule out soleus limitation in this case)

Passive First MTP Extension

- Limited if <60 degrees in full plantar flexion without stabilizing MTP
- Limited if <30 degrees in 30 degrees of ankle plantar flexion
  - Flexor hallucis longus short if ≥30 degrees of first MTP extension in full plantar flexion compared to 30 degrees of plantar flexion
  - First MTP joint limitation if first MTP extension remains limited, regardless of ankle position, and accessory MTP motion is limited (cannot rule out flexor hallucis brevis or other 1-joint muscles crossing the MTP)

Subtalar Joint Eversion

- Hindfoot pronation-eversion ROM is available

Muscle Strength/Performance Impairments

- Gastrocnemius/soleus weakness
- Posterior gluteus medius, intrinsic hip lateral rotators
- Inadequate stabilization of MTP joints by the intrinsic muscles of the foot results in extension of the MTPs during active talocrural dorsiflexion
- Dominance of extensor digitorum longus results in dorsiflexion with eversion

Improper Footwear

- Flexible heel counter
- Shoe sole components
- Recent decrease in heel-to-toe height

Activity Level

- Recent increase in activity level

Plantar Callus Findings

- Second and third metatarsals
- Medial first toe

Differential Diagnosis

Movement Diagnosis

- Insufficient dorsiflexion
- Supination

Potential Diagnosis Requiring Referral Suggested by Signs and Symptoms

Musculoskeletal

- Stress fracture
- DJD
- Low back (L4-S2)
- Posterior tibialis tendon insufficiency

Neurovascular

- DVT
  - Well's Clinical Decision Rule
  - Homans' sign
- Compartment syndrome
- Tarsal tunnel syndrome

Systemic

- RA

Treatment
Inflammation and Pain Control
- Ice
- Iontophoresis
- Electrical stimulation

Walking and/or Running
The patient is instructed to work on the specific cues that assisted in symptom reduction during the examination or the cues that the physical therapist believes with practice may result in symptom reduction. The following cues are among the possibilities that may assist the patient:
- Contract the gastrocnemius muscle by lifting from the heel.
- Raise the medial longitudinal arch.
- Contract the gluteal muscles (squeeze the buttocks).
- Hit with the heel first.

Many of the changes being requested of the patient during walking and running are similar to a strengthening program. As such, the patient should be encouraged to have focused practice time and gradual implementation to avoid injury.

Muscle Performance
- Supinators (gastrocnemius, posterior tibialis)
  - Thera-Band resistance exercise into plantarflexion and plantarflexion inversion
  - Heel raises
  - Hopping
- Intrinsic muscles of the foot
  - Towel crunches: Towel placed on the floor, use toes to grab towel and pull it under the foot. Weight can be added to the towel to increase resistance. The arch should lift; do not allow the patient to only use the flexor digitorum longus.
- Posterior hip muscles
  - Sidelying hip lateral rotation progressing to lateral rotation with abduction adding weight as appropriate. Patient may need a pillow between knees for comfort.
  - Prone hip extension with the knee flexed. Patient should be over a pillow.
  - Posterior hip muscle strengthening must progress to weight-bearing dynamic activities to prepare the muscles for walking, running, and jumping activities.

After the injured tissue has been protected from excessive stresses and the inflammation has subsided, the involved muscle and tendon should undergo a progressive strengthening program and a progressive return to activity. In general, exercise or activity is permissible if pain remains at 2/10 on a 0 to 10 scale. The strengthening exercise should be completed at a minimum of 70% maximal voluntary contraction for 10 repetitions, 3 sets, 3 to 5 times/week.

Decrease Range of Motion
- Short gastrocnemius/soleus muscle/calcaneal (Achilles) tendon.
  - Wall stretch: The knee is extended for gastrocnemius muscle shortness and flexed for soleus muscle length deficits. The patient should prevent pronation (active patient correction and wearing good footwear). The patient should be instructed to keep the foot facing forward or in line with the femur and tibia. The heel should be kept on the ground during the stretch.
  - Heel hang stretch: The knee can be extended or flexed as described for the wall stretch. The patient should prevent pronation through active correction and by wearing good footwear.
  - Long sitting towel-assisted dorsiflexion: The patient should prevent pronation through active correction and by modifying the direction of force through the towel.
- Talocrural joint limitation: In addition to the standing stretches, joint limitations can be addressed with mobilization.
  - Mobilize the talocrural joint using a posterior glide of the talus on the ankle mortise.
  - Mobilize the talocrural joint using a distraction technique.
  - Heel lift in the shoe until length changes are apparent.
  - Night splint to maintain dorsiflexion position.
- Short extensor digitorum longus.
  - Patient plantar flexes the involved foot with the toes flexed. Can be completed in sitting or can be stretched in hands and knees rocking back.
- First MTP extension limitation:
  - Mobilize the MTP joint using an anterior glide of the proximal phalanx on the metatarsal.
  - Passive ROM (PROM) into first MTP extension (talocrural dorsiflexion with first MTP extension).

Stretching should be held for 30 seconds, 2 to 3 repetitions, completed regularly throughout the day (5 to 8 times/day), and completed 5 to 7 days/week.

Activity
- Modify activity level to decrease forces on the foot. May require use of an assistive device if symptoms are severe.
- If appropriate for the patient's goals, progress to dynamic activities such as jumping, hopping, shuttle run, cutting, and so on.
- Running progression rules:
  - Start with a run/walk program gradually progressing to all running.
  - Start with straight plane jogging and jumping on a smooth flat surface.
  - Work on distance tolerance first.
  - Increase speed as tolerated.

- Add varied terrain, hills, and cutting (these can include figure 8s).
- Finally, add cuts and turns that are unexpected. For example, have the patient run straight forward and call cut right. He or she is expected to change directions immediately. Mix the calls, including cut left, 180 degrees turn, 360 degrees turn, and bend down.

External Tissue Support
Footwear
- A last that looks like the foot. The most common last for a pronated foot is a straight or semi-curved last.
- Firm heel counter to control hindfoot motion. If pronation is occurring at the hindfoot, the shoe should include rigid material at the medial heel and less rigid material at the lateral heel.
- A sole that bends only at the metatarsal heads and rigid from hindfoot to midfoot.
- Adequate arch support with medial structures of the footwear generally made of firm, controlling materials.

- Appropriate width and depth to accommodate the foot
- Cushion indicated as needed for appropriate shock absorption.

Orthoses/Taping
- The orthosis should prevent pronation. Start with adding an arch support, then if necessary post at the hindfoot, then the forefoot. If the metatarsal heads are involved, the orthosis may also need to include a metatarsal pad.
- For calcaneal tendon involvement, hindfoot eversion must be correct with a medial hindfoot post to maximize tendon alignment.
- For tarsal tunnel involvement, hindfoot orthosis additions must be soft to avoid nerve compression.
- Arch taping: Used most frequently for involvement of the plantar fascia but is appropriate for any condition that would benefit from additional arch support and prevention of pronation.

Supination Syndrome

The principal movement impairment in supination syndrome is supination at the foot and ankle. Supination is considered abnormal and an impairment when the amount of supination during weight-bearing activities is excessive for that individual or when it occurs from heel strike to midstance in the gait cycle. The supination impairment can occur in the hindfoot, midfoot, and/or forefoot. The foot with a supination impairment is generally a rigid foot with little or no ability to absorb shock and compensate for structural or movement impairments within the foot and ankle, knee, or hip.

Symptoms and History

- *Plantar fascia:* Heel pain with first step in the morning or after prolonged non–weight-bearing function
- *Fibular muscles/tendon:* Pain in muscle or tendon, most apparent with weight bearing as the muscle works to control supination
- *Gastrocnemius/soleus muscles/calcaneal tendon:* Pain in muscle or tendon as tibial forward progression is controlled in stance and during propulsion phase of weight bearing
- *Metatarsal heads:* Pain localized to the first and fifth metatarsal heads
- *Lateral column joint:* Lateral column joint pain with weight bearing
- Generalized foot pain, knee, hip, or low back pain associated with a "rigid" foot

Common Referring Diagnoses

- Stress fracture
  - Tibia
  - First or fifth metatarsal
- Fibularis muscle strain or tendonitis
- Plantar fasciitis
- Foot pain
- Metatarsalgia

Key Tests and Signs for Movement Impairment

Alignment Analysis

- Hindfoot: Calcaneal inversion
- Midfoot: Talonavicular joint located more dorsal (lateral bulge)
- Forefoot: Adduction in relationship to the hindfoot at the transtarsal joint
- High medial longitudinal arch
- Femur and/or tibia excessive lateral rotation
- Decreased width of the forefoot

Movement Impairment Analysis

Standing

Gait/running

- Decreased calcaneal eversion
- Minimal flattening of the arch from heel strike through midstance
- Hip/knee lateral rotation
- Knee varus moment
- Late stance (heel off) foot moves into pronation

Single-leg hopping

- Efficient plantar flexor force (jump is high and well controlled)
- Hip/knee lateral rotation
- Knee varus moment

Step-down or small knee bend

- Limited dorsiflexion
- Arch moves very little from initial position
- Weight transferred over lateral column

Source of Signs and Symptoms

Heel and/or Arch Symptoms
Plantar Fascia

- Special test: Toe extension increases symptoms with/without palpation along the fascia
- Palpation: Tender at the insertion of plantar fascia on medial calcaneal tubercle and can be tender along the fascia into the midfoot

Lateral Ankle/Foot Symptoms
Fibularis Muscle/Tendon

- Special test: Soft tissue differential may be weak and painful or strong and painful with appropriate resisted contraction in neutral foot position (≈10 degrees plantar flexion)
- Palpation: Tender posterior and lateral to the fibula, posterior to the lateral malleolus, to the base of the fifth MTP or at the cuboid as the longus runs on the plantar surface of the foot

Hindfoot Symptoms
Gastrocnemius/Soleus Muscle/Calcaneal Tendon

- Special test: Soft tissue differential may be weak and painful or strong and painful with appropriate resisted contraction in neutral foot position (≈10 degrees plantar flexion)
- Palpation: Tender posterior calf and tendon to calcaneus

Forefoot Symptoms
Metatarsal Heads/Sesamoids

- Palpation: Tender at the first and fifth metatarsal heads

Associated Signs or Contributing Factors
Structural Variations
Foot
- Subtalar joint neutral findings modified by weight bearing
- Uncompensated hindfoot varus
- Uncompensated forefoot varus
- Compensated hindfoot valgus
- Compensated forefoot valgus
- Plantar flexed first ray

Femur/Tibia
- Short leg on supinated side
- Femoral retroversion
- Tibial torsion

Muscle Length/Joint ROM Impairments
Talocrural Dorsiflexion
- Limited if dorsiflexion <10 degrees with knee extended
  - Gastrocnemius short if dorsiflexion ≥10 degrees with knee flexed
  - Soleus muscle short if dorsiflexion ≤10 degrees with knee flexed and normal accessory talocrural motion
  - Talocrural joint limitation if dorsiflexion ≤10 degrees, regardless of knee position and limited accessory talocrural joint motion (cannot rule out soleus muscle limitation in this case)

Passive First MTP Extension
- Limited if <60 degrees in full plantar flexion without stabilizing MTP
- Limited if <30 degrees in 30 degrees of ankle plantarflexion
  - Flexor hallucis longus short if ≥30 degrees of first MTP extension in full plantarflexion compared 30 degrees of plantarflexion
  - First MTP joint limitation if first MTP extension remains limited, regardless of ankle position, and accessory MTP motion is limited (cannot rule out flexor hallucis brevis or other 1-joint muscles crossing the MTP)

Subtalar Joint Eversion
- Hindfoot eversion ROM is limited

Extensor Digitorum Longus
- Toe flexion ROM is decreased when the talocrural joint is plantarflexed compared to dorsiflexion

Improper Footwear
- Insufficient cushion
- Straight last
- Sole structure that encourages supination (lateral soft material in combination with medial rigid materials)

Activity Level
- Recent increase in activity level

Plantar Callus Findings
- First and fifth metatarsals
- Medial first toe

Differential Diagnosis
Movement Diagnosis
- Insufficient dorsiflexion
Potential Diagnosis Requiring Referral Suggested by Signs and Symptoms
- Stress fracture
- DJD
- Low back (L4-S2)
Neurovascular
- DVT
  - Well's Clinical Decision Rule
  - Homans' sign
- Compartment syndrome
Systemic
- RA

Treatment

Inflammation and Pain Control

- Ice
- Iontophoresis
- Electrical stimulation

Walking and/or Running

The patient is instructed to work on the specific cues that assist in symptom reduction during the examination or the cues that the physical therapist believes, with practice, may result in symptom reduction. Often, the cues are related to softening the landing, hitting more centrally on the heel, and concentrating on trying to limit lateral loading through the foot.

Muscle Performance

- Gastrocnemius/soleus muscle
  - Thera-Band resistance exercise into plantar flexion
  - Heel raises
  - Hopping
- Fibularis (peroneus) longus and brevis
  - Thera-Band resistance exercise into plantar flexion and plantarflexion eversion

After the tissue injury has been protected from excessive stresses and the inflammation has subsided, the involved muscle and tendon should undergo a progressive strengthening program and a progressive return to activity. In general, exercise or activity is permissible if pain remains at 2/10 on a 0 to 10 scale. The strengthening exercise should be completed at a minimum of 70% maximal voluntary contraction for 10 repetitions, 3 sets, 3 to 5 times/week.

Decreased Range of Motion

- Short gastrocnemius/soleus muscle length
  - Wall stretch: The knee is extended for gastrocnemius muscle shortness and flexed for soleus muscle length deficits. The patient should be instructed to keep the foot facing forward or in line with the femur and tibia. The heel should be kept on the ground during the stretch. The patient should prevent foot supination correction and by wearing good footwear. The stretch should be held for 30 seconds, complete 2 to 3 time/session, and done regularly throughout the day (5 to 8 times/day).
  - Heel hang stretch: The knee can be extended or flexed as described for the wall stretch. The patient should prevent subtalar joint supination through active correction and by wearing good footwear.
  - Long sitting towel-assisted dorsiflexion. The patient should prevent foot supination through active correction and by modifying the direction of force through the towel.

- A night splint to maintain dorsiflexion position is often helpful.
- Talocrural joint limitation
  - Mobilize the talocrural joint using a posterior glide of the talus on the ankle mortise
  - Mobilize the talocrural joint using a distraction technique
  - May need to include a heel lift in the shoe until length changes are apparent
  - Talocrural joint limitation
- Decreased length of extensor digitorum longus
  - Patient plantarflexes the involved foot with the toes flexed. Can be completed in sitting or if extremely short, can be stretched in hands and knees rocking back
- Decreased great toe extension
  - Mobilize the MTP joint using an anterior glide of the proximal phalanx on the metatarsal.
  - Passive ROM into great toe extension. Patient dorsiflexes the talocrural joint and then extends the great toe.

Stretching should be held for 30 seconds, 2 to 3 repetitions, completed regularly through out the day (5 to 8 times/day), and completed 5 to 7 days/week.

Activity

- Modify activity level to decrease forces on the foot. May require use of an assistive device if symptoms are severe.
- If appropriate for the patient's goals, progress to dynamic activities such as jumping, hopping, shuttle run, cutting, and so on.
- Running progression rules:
  - Start with straight plane jogging and jumping on a smooth flat surface.
  - Work on distance tolerance first.
  - Increase speed as tolerated.
  - Add varied terrain, hills, and cutting (these can include figure 8s).
  - Finally, add cuts and turns that are unexpected. For example, have the patient run straight forward and call cut right. He or she is expected to change directions immediately. Mix the calls, including cut left, 180 degrees turn, 360 degrees turn, or bend down.

Footwear

- A last that looks like the foot. The most common last for a supinated foot is a curved last.
- Firm heel counter to control hindfoot motion. The hindfoot sole material should NOT include a material density differential that would encourage calcaneal inversion.
- Cushioned, conforming insole is a key component in treating the supinated foot.
- Appropriate width and depth to accommodate the foot.
- Adequate arch support.

External Tissue Support

- Accommodative insert with soft materials. May need additional arch support to assist in distributing force through greater weight-bearing surface. If the metatarsal heads are involved, the orthotic may also need to include a metatarsal pad.

- Arch taping: Used most frequently for plantar fascia involvement but is appropriate for any condition that would benefit from additional arch support.
- Calcaneal (Achilles) tendon taping: Used to reduce stress on the calcaneal tendon.

Insufficient Dorsiflexion Syndrome

The principal movement impairment in insufficient dorsiflexion syndrome is insufficient dorsiflexion. The impairment can occur during midstance to push-off or during swing phase and is not associated with excessive supination or pronation.

Symptoms and History

- *Plantar fascia:* Heel pain with first step in the morning or after prolonged non–weight bearing
- *Gastrocnemius/soleus muscle/calcaneal (Achilles) tendon:* Pain in muscle/tendon
  - Symptoms most apparent from midstance through push-off
- *Bursa:* Pain at posterior calcaneus
  - Symptoms most apparent with direct pressure.
  - The pain-provoking pressure can occur during midstance through push-off or when squatting as the calcaneal tendon is pressing the bursa or when sitting with direct pressure is on the bursa
- *Anterior tibialis muscle/tendon:* Pain in muscle/tendon, most apparent during the swing phase of walking or jogging as the anterior tibialis attempts to dorsiflex the foot
- *Deep fibular nerve:* Achy, tingling, and numbness on the dorsum of foot and can radiate into toes; most common when shoes are on and activities requiring maximum dorsiflexion (running up hills, squatting)
- *Talocrural joint:* Sharp pinching pain at end-range dorsiflexion such as squatting and running up hills
  - The talocrural joint is often point tender
- *Metatarsal heads/sesamoids:* Pain localized to the metatarsal heads

Common Referring Diagnoses

- Achilles tendonitis
- Bursitis
- Shin splints

Key Tests and Signs for Movement Impairment

Alignment Analysis

- Knee hyperextension
- Ankle in relative plantar flexion

Movement Impairment Analysis

Standing

Gait/running

- Early heel rise after midstance as the tibia attempts to advance over the foot
- Knee hyperextension during stance
- Increase in foot progression angle
- Increase in knee flexion during stance phase
- Uses passive tension of gastrocnemius/soleus muscle/calcaneal tendon to control tibia position during stance
- Limited dorsiflexion during swing phase of gait

Full squat

- Limited dorsiflexion
- Heel is higher on involved side and/or tibia is more posterior

Step-down or small knee bend

- Early heel rise, inability to keep heel on the ground

Sitting

Active dorsiflexion

- Completes with toe extension. Poor stabilization of the MTP joints with the foot intrinsics

Muscle Length/Joint ROM Impairments

Talocrural Dorsiflexion

- Limited if dorsiflexion <10 degrees with knee extended
  - Gastrocnemius short if dorsiflexion ≥10 degrees with knee flexed
  - Soleus muscle short if dorsiflexion ≤10 degrees with knee flexed and normal accessory tal-crural motion
  - Talocrural joint limitation if dorsiflexion ≤10 degrees, regardless of knee position and limited accessory talocrural joint motion (cannot rule out soleus muscle length limitation in this case)

Source of Signs and Symptoms

Hindfoot Symptoms
Plantar Fascia
- Special test: Toe extension increases symptoms with or without palpation along the fascia
- Palpation: Tender at the insertion of plantar fascia on medial calcaneal tubercle and can be tender along the fascia into the midfoot

Gastrocnemius/Soleus Muscle/Calcaneal Tendon
- Special test: Soft tissue differential may be weak and painful or strong and painful with appropriate resisted contraction in neutral foot position (≈10 degrees plantarflexion)
- Palpation: Tender posterior calf and tendon to calcaneus

Bursa
- Symptoms reproduced with any motion that compresses the bursa (active or passive dorsiflexion, active plantar flexion)
- Palpation: Tender at posterior heel

Anterior Ankle/Foot Symptoms
Anterior Tibialis Muscle/Tendon
- Special test: Soft tissue differential may be weak and painful or strong and painful with appropriate resisted contraction in neutral foot position (≈10 degrees plantar flexion)
- Palpation: Anterior tibialis muscle and tendon: Tender at the proximal lateral tibia, dorsal/medial to first cuneiform and/or base of first metatarsal

Deep Fibular Nerve
- Special test: Positive Tinel's

Talocrural Joint
- Palpation: Tender at talocrural joint space

Forefoot Symptoms
Metatarsal Heads/Sesamoids
- Palpation: Tender at metatarsal heads

Associated Signs or Contributing Factors

Muscle Length/Joint ROM Impairments
Extensor Digitorum Longus
- Plantarflexion ROM decreases when toes are flexed compared to when toes are extended

Improper Footwear
- Recent change to a shoe with a lower heel
- Frequent wearing of high heels

Activity Level
- Recent increase in activity level

Visual Appraisal
- Local signs of inflammation may be present, including edema, redness, or increased temperature

Differential Diagnosis

Movement Diagnosis
- Pronation
- Supination
- Hypomobility

Potential Diagnosis Requiring Referral Suggested by Signs and Symptoms
Musculoskeletal
- Stress fracture
- DJD
- Low back (L4-S2)

Neurovascular
- DVT
  - Well's Clinical Decision Rule
  - Homans' sign
- Compartment syndrome

Systemic
- RA

Treatment
Inflammation and Pain Control
- Ice
- Iontophoresis
- Electrical stimulation

Walking and/or Running
- Walking and running cues focus primarily on encouraging active contraction of the gastrocnemius muscle to reduce the reliance on the passive tension of the gastrocnemius/soleus muscle/calcaneal tendon unit. The specific cues are to have the patient actively lift the heel during late stance.

Muscle Performance
- Weakness of the anterior tibialis:
  - Thera-Band resistance exercise into dorsiflexion inversion with toes curled.
- Weakness of the intrinsic muscles of the foot.
  - Towel crunches: Towel placed on the floor, use toes to grab towel and pull it under the foot. Weight can be added to the towel to increase resistance. The arch should lift; do not allow the patient to only use the flexor digitorum longus.

After the tissue injury has been protected from excessive stresses and the inflammation has subsided, the involved muscle and tendon should undergo a progressive strengthening program and a progressive return to activity. In general, exercise or activity is permissible if pain remains at 2/10 on a 0 to 10 scale. The strengthening exercise should be completed at a minimum of 70% maximum voluntary contraction for 10 repetitions, 3 sets, 3 to 5 times/week.

Decreased Dorsiflexion
- Short gastrocnemius/soleus muscle/calcaneal tendon
  - Wall stretch: The knee is extended for gastrocnemius muscle shortness and flexed for soleus muscle length deficits. The patient should be instructed to keep their foot facing forward or in line with the femur and tibia. The heel should be kept on the ground during the stretch. The patient should prevent subtalar joint pronation through active correction and by wearing good footwear. The stretch should be held for 30 seconds, completed 2 to 3 times/session, and done regularly throughout the day (5 to 8 times/day).
  - Heel hang stretch: The knee can be extended or flexed as described for the wall stretch. The patient should prevent subtalar joint pronation through active correction and by wearing good footwear.
  - Long sitting towel-assisted dorsiflexion: The patient should prevent subtalar joint pronation through active correction and by modifying the direction of force through the towel.
  - A night splint to maintain dorsiflexion position is often helpful.

- Stretches should be held for 30 seconds, 2 to 3 repetitions, completed regularly throughout the day (5 to 8 times/day), and done 5 to 7 days/week.
- Talocrural joint limitation
  - Mobilize the talocrural joint using a posterior glide of the talus on the ankle mortise.
  - Mobilize the talocrural joint using a distraction technique.
  - May need to include a heel lift in the shoe until length changes are apparent.

Activity
- Modify activity level to decrease forces on the foot until healed. May require use of an assistive device if symptoms are severe.
- If appropriate for the patient's goals, progress to dynamic activities such as jumping, hopping, shuttle run, cutting etc.
- Running progression rules:
  - Start with straight plane jogging and jumping on a smooth flat surface.
  - Work on distance tolerance first.
  - Increase speed as tolerated.
  - Add varied terrain, hills, and cutting.
  - Finally, add cuts and turns that are unexpected. For example, have the patient run straightforward and call cut right. He or she is expected to change directions immediately. Mix the calls, including cut left, 180 degrees turn, 360 degrees turn, and bend down.

External Tissue Support
Footwear
- Heel-to-toe height of the shoe that accommodates for the lack of dorsiflexion ROM. However, the goal would be to increase dorsiflexion ROM to avoid needing a shoe with a heel.
- Appropriate width and depth to accommodate the foot.
- A last that looks like the foot. May be curved, straight, or in between (midlast), depending on the shape of the individual's foot.
- Footwear should include the standard shoe components to provide the necessary support and cushion. This includes a firm heel counter, the appropriate amount of arch support, and cushion indicated as needed for shock absorption.
- The angle formed by the heel counter and the sole of the shoe at the posterior heel to the vertical line from the floor at the most-posterior portion of the sole of the shoe should be relatively small. A large angle increases the work demand on the anterior tibialis muscle and tendon.
- With involvement of the bursa, pain may occur with pressure from the heel of the shoe on the bursa. The patient may need to wear open-heeled shoes temporarily.

Orthoses/Taping
- Insert a heel lift into the shoe to relieve stress from decreased talocrural dorsiflexion motion. As the individual completes their home stretching program, the height of the heel lift can be reduced.

- Calcaneal tendon taping: Tape the ankle posteriorly to support the tendon, place the foot in plantarflexion, tape from the distal posterior calf to midarch of the foot.

Hypomobility Syndrome

The principal movement impairment in hypomobility syndrome is associated with a limitation in the physiological and accessory motion of the foot and ankle. This may result from degenerative changes in the joint or the effects of prolonged immobilization.

Symptoms and History

Degenerative Changes (OA, RA)
- Pain with weight bearing (gait, standing, stairs), that decreases with rest
- Pain location deep in joint and often described as vague
- Gradual onset
- May complain of stiffness, especially after periods of rest
- History of remote trauma or surgery to the ankle/foot
- Narrowing of joint space seen on standing x-rays
- Typically seen in older adults >55 years old

Immobilization
- History of recent trauma or surgery
- Ankle/foot ROM has not progressed as expected (slow recovery)

Common Referring Diagnoses
- ORIF of ankle and/or foot
- Fracture of ankle and/or foot
- Tendon or muscle rupture/repair
- Microfracture surgery (most often on talus)
- Osteochondritis dissecans
- OA
- RA

Key Tests and Signs for Movement Impairment

Alignment Analysis
- Atrophy of calf and foot muscles
- Edema
- Signs of inflammation in foot and ankle

Movement Impairment Analysis

Standing

Gait/running
- Antalgic gait: Decreased step length on uninvolved side or bilaterally secondary to joint pain and ROM limitation of ankle/foot
- Poor tolerance of full weight bearing
- Dependent on assistive device for ambulation

Step-down or small knee bend
- Limited ankle mobility
- Descending stairs forward is limited by ankle mobility; patient may need to turn sideways, backward, or avoid descending reciprocally

Single-Leg Stance
- The ability to maintain single-leg stance on the involve side will be impaired (poor control and decreased duration).
- Lack of ability to balance on one foot is often evident with the eyes open and performance worsens when the patient is instructed to close their eyes, limiting visual input and isolating foot and ankle proprioception.

Muscle Length/Joint ROM Impairments
- Based on length, ROM tests, and accessory joint assessments
- Limited physiological and accessory motion of involved and surrounding foot and ankle joints
- With degenerative changes, repeated passive ROM to end-range should decrease pain or improve symptoms

MMT, Manual muscle testing; *OA*, osteoarthritis; *ORIF*, open reduction internal fixation; *ROM*, range of motion.

Source of Signs and Symptoms

Joint/Bone Symptoms

- Joint clearing tests (end-range joint motion with overpressure) will be painful

Associated Signs or Contributing Factors

- Palpation: Tenderness at the site of fracture/surgery
- The foot is generally sore

Muscle Strength/Performance Impairments

- Based on MMT and/or functional performance
  - Weakness in all foot and ankle musculature, particularly the gastrocnemius

Balance/Proprioception

- Inability to maintain single-leg stance on the involved side with the control and for the duration that is performed on the uninvolved side; performance worsens with eyes closed

Differential Diagnosis

Movement Diagnosis

- Tissue impairment

Potential Diagnosis Requiring Referral Suggested by Signs and Symptoms

- Unstable fracture
- DJD
- Sympathetically maintained pain

Treatment

Inflammation and Pain Control

- Ice (may be contraindicated if patient is hypersensitive or with OA or RA)
- Heat is often helpful in decreasing feelings of joint stiffness and pain
- Compression garment

Walking and/or Running

- The presence of OA and/or RA often requires the individual to discontinue weight-bearing, high impact, and high repetition activities (walking or running for fitness). The patient often needs to be guided into lower impact activities, such as stationary bicycling, water aerobics, or use of a StairMaster/elliptical, or activities, such as rowing, that involve aerobic fitness through the upper extremities. Weight loss can also significantly impact pain with weight-bearing activities and should be discussed if appropriate for the patient.
- Walking with a limp can result in injury to other areas of the body (knee, hip, back, or uninvolved foot). All efforts to correct the gait pattern should be employed, including work on weight shifting, a gradual increase in weight-bearing tolerance, and addressing the strength and motion impairments contributing to the gait pattern. Use of assistive devices may be temporarily or permanently indicated for patients.

Muscle Performance

- Weakness of the plantarflexors (gastrocnemius, posterior tibialis muscles)
  - Thera-Band resistance exercise into plantar flexion and plantar flexion inversion
  - Heel raises
  - Eccentric training
  - Bilateral and single-leg hopping
  - Cutting, sprinting, and sport-specific activities
- Weakness of the anterior tibialis muscle
  - Thera-Band resistance exercise into dorsiflexion and/or inversion
- Weakness of the fibular (peroneal) muscles
  - Thera-Band resistance exercise into plantarflexion and/or eversion
- Weakness of the intrinsic muscles of the foot
  - Towel crunches: Towel is placed on the floor, using toes to grab towel, then pull it under the foot. Weight can be added to the towel to increase resistance. The arch should lift; do not allow the patient to only use the flexor digitorum longus.

After the tissue injury has been protected from excessive stresses and the inflammation has subsided, the involved muscle and tendon should undergo a progressive strengthening program and a progressive return to activity. In general, exercise or activity is permissible if pain remains at 2/10 on a 0 to 10 scale. The strengthening exercise should be completed at a minimum of 70% maximum voluntary contraction for 10 repetitions, 3 sets, 3 to 5 times/week.

Decreased Range of Motion

- Decreased dorsiflexion: Short gastrocnemius/soleus muscle/calcaneal tendon
  - Wall stretch: The knee is extended for gastrocnemius muscle shortness and flexed for soleus length deficits. The patient should be instructed to keep the foot facing forward or in line with the femur and tibia. The heel should be kept on the ground during the stretch. The patient should prevent subtalar joint pronation through active correction and by wearing good footwear. The stretch should be held for 30 seconds, completed 2 to 3 times/session, and done regularly throughout the day (5 to 8 times/day).
  - Heel-hang stretch: The knee can be extended or flexed as described for the wall stretch. The patient should prevent subtalar joint pronation through active patient correction and/or wearing good footwear.
  - Long sitting towel-assisted dorsiflexion: The patient should prevent subtalar joint pronation through active correction and by modifying the direction of force through the towel.
  - A night splint to maintain dorsiflexion position is often helpful.
  - Stretches should be held for 30 seconds, 2 to 3 repetitions, completed regularly throughout the day (5 to 8 times/day), and done 5 to 7 days/week.
- Talocrural joint limitation
  - Mobilize the talocrural joint using a posterior glide of the talus on the ankle mortise.
  - Mobilize the talocrural joint using a distraction technique.
  - May need to include a heel lift in the shoe until length changes are apparent.
- Decreased plantar flexion: Short dorsiflexor muscles
  - Hands and knees rocking back.
  - Sustained active ROM (AROM) and PROM.
- Decreased inversion/eversion: Subtalar joint limitation
  - Mobilize the subtalar joint using lateral and medial glides.
- Decreased intertarsal mobility
  - Mobilize specific intertarsal joints primarily using anterior and posterior glides.
- Decreased MTP and interphalangeal flexion and extension
  - Mobilize MTP and IP joint primarily using anterior (for extension) and posterior (for flexion) glides.

General ROM Activities

- Stationary bike.
- Baps board or wobble in sitting when weight-bearing tolerance is limited, progressing to standing activities when weight-bearing tolerance increases.

Activity

- Progress weight bearing gradually, reducing dependence on and type of assistive device.

- Address cardiovascular fitness with use of low impact activities (stationary bike, swimming, rowing, or Stair-Master/elliptical training).
- If appropriate for the patient's goals, progress to dynamic activities such as jumping, hopping, shuttle run, cutting, and so on.
- Running progression rules:
  - Start with straight plane jogging and jumping on a smooth flat surface.
  - Work on distance tolerance first.
  - Increase speed as tolerated.
  - Add varied terrain, hills, and cutting (these can include figure 8s).
  - Finally, add cuts and turns that are unexpected. For example, have the patient run straight forward and call cut right. He or she is expected to change directions immediately. Mix the calls, including cut left, 180 degrees turn, 360 degrees turn, and bend down.

External Tissue Support
Footwear
- Appropriate size, width, and depth to accommodate edematous foot.
- A last that looks like the foot. May be curved, straight, or in between (midlast), depending on the shape of the individual's foot.
- Footwear should include the standard shoe components to provide the necessary support and cushion. This includes a firm heel counter, the appropriate amount of arch support, and cushion, which is indicated only as needed for shock absorption.
- For individuals with OA or RA or those who have had fusion of joints in their foot, a steel shank in the sole of the shoe will make the sole of the shoe rigid and a rocker at the toe break will allow the patient to more easily roll over the foot without needing as much talocrural dorsiflexion or MTP dorsiflexion.

Orthoses
- For individuals with OA or RA, a total contact insert made of accommodative material is often indicated. Deformities of the foot should be considered in the design and materials chosen for the orthosis.
- A heel lift may be necessary to manage the loss of dorsiflexion ROM.

- Temporary orthoses with additional arch support are often indicated to manage foot pain that is often related to the new onset of a pronation impairment that results from the limited foot and ankle mobility.

Scar
- Firm and raised
  - TopiGel sheeting (chemical reaction)
  - Pressure
- Immobile
  - Gradual application of stress to scar helps the scar remodel in such a way that it allows gliding between structures.
  - AROM and PROM
- Immobile or adhered scar
  - Massage: Use circular motions and friction, minimum 5 to 6 times/day, 5 minutes each time. Using Dycem or wearing a latex glove on the uninvolved hand may help increase friction.

Hypersensitivity
- Desensitization exercises
  - Progress from light touch to more firm touch.
  - Progress from soft texture to a rough texture.
  - Add additional sensation such as vibration and tapping as tolerated.
  - Emphasize weight-bearing and ROM exercises.
  - Activity and exercise is better tolerated if heat has been applied (hot pack or exercise in warm whirlpool or pool).

Balance and Proprioception
- Stand on the involved leg with eyes open.
- Stand on the involved leg with eyes closed.
- Stand on the involved leg on foam or uneven surface with eyes open.
- Stand on the involved leg on foam or uneven surface with eyes closed.
- Stand on one leg and do the following:
  - Kick and stop a ball.
  - Throw and catch a ball.
  - Reach with hand.
- Do similar activities on a mini-trampoline or other challenging surface.

Foot and Ankle Impairment

A key criterion for placement into the foot and ankle impairment classification is the need to protect tissue. Usually, the tissue involved is stressed by a surgical procedure or trauma and may cause significant pain at rest and during movement. The patient is unable to tolerate a typical movement system examination. The limitation in movement is not primarily related to a chronic pain condition. Tissue healing and normal movement are expected. These are general guidelines and not intended to stand alone. Consult the physician's protocol for specific precautions and progressions. The physical therapist must be familiar with the tissues that were affected in the surgical procedure.

Symptoms and History
- Patient has history of surgery or acute injury.
- Knowledge of specific surgical approach or injury is mandatory.
- Patient may report severe pain.

Physiological Factors
Factors that affect the physical stress of tissue and/or thresholds of tissue adaptation and injury[1] specific to the foot are as follows.

Tissue Factors
- Bone
  - Fractures of the base of the fifth metatarsal have a high probability of nonunion secondary to the pull of the fibularis brevis. Additionally, stress fractures of the anterior lateral tibial diaphysis, medial malleolus, talus, navicular, and sesamoids are high-risk areas that often fail to heal, re-fracture, and/or need operative intervention.[2]
- Cartilage
- Muscle
  - Common to lose dorsiflexion ROM with immobilization.
  - Common to experience atrophy of gastrocnemius/soleus muscle with immobilization.
- Tendon
  - Calcaneal tendon rupture: Gastrocnemius/soleus muscle contraction contraindicated; may have dorsiflexion ROM restrictions.
  - Posterior tibial tendon injury or insufficiency: If severe, may result in significant deformity of the arch (flattening); may require long periods of immobilization or surgery. Contraction of the posterior tibial muscle would be contraindicated after surgery.
- Ligament
  - Lateral ankle sprain: Often accompanied by an avulsion fracture of the lateral malleolus.
  - Syndesmotic ankle sprain ("high ankle sprain"): Associated with greater discomfort during weight-bearing function and longer healing time and may require immobilization.[3]
- Skin
  - Edema has the potential to limit mobility and compromise the space occupied by nerves and arteries; often encountered under the extensor retinaculum and the flexor retinaculum; note location and measure extent of edema; assess whether it is brawny or pitting.
  - Scar: Note location, appearance, mobility, sensitivity, and if incision appears healed (approximately 10 days).
  - Color: Note location and size of discoloration, including bruising and other important changes in color (red, white, blue, or black).
  - Temperature: Note location of warmth.
- Nerve
  - Deep fibular (peroneal) nerve can be compromised as it runs beneath the extensor retinaculum.
  - Tibial nerve can be compressed as it runs beneath the flexor retinaculum.
  - Interdigital nerve.

Types of Surgeries (Indications)
- Stabilization (fracture, avascular necrosis [AVN], osteosarcoma)
  - ORIF
  - External fixation
  - Fusion
  - Bone graft
- Osteotomy (malalignment or osteosarcoma)
  - Calcaneal
  - Metatarsal
  - Phalangeal
- Arthroplasty (DJD, arthritis, joint destruction)
- Compartment decompression (crush injury, overuse with loss of arterial blood flow)
- Debridement (tear, arthritis, or infection)
  - Capsule
  - Cartilage
  - Wound
- Repair (tear, graft, or cell injections—open or arthroscopic)
  - Ligament
  - Cartilage
  - Tendon
- Soft tissue release (short tissue or spastic muscle)
  - Gastrocnemius/soleus muscle/calcaneal tendon
  - Plantar fascia
- Excision
  - Neuromas
  - Tumors
  - Bone

Medications
- Consider side effects and effects of medications on tissue, exam, and intervention
  - Nonsteroidal antiinflammatory drugs (NSAIDs)

- Muscle relaxants
- Analgesics
- Steroids

Medical Complications
- DVT
- Pulmonary embolus
- Fibular (peroneal) nerve neurapraxia
- Neurovascular compromise
- Compartment syndrome
- Infection
- Nonunion and malunion

Movement and Alignment Factors
- Variations
  - Anthropomorphics
  - Structural impairments
  - Scar adhesions
- Standing alignment
  - May demonstrate protective stance or rotational impairments

Underlying Movement Impairment Syndromes
- Pronation
- Supination
- Insufficient dorsiflexion
- Hypomobility

Extrinsic Factors
- Assistive devices to unload extremity
- Orthotic devices or braces

Psychosocial Factors
- Response to pain and/or anxiety

Treatment for Foot and Ankle Impairment

Emphasis of treatment is to restore ROM of the ankle and strength of the lower extremity without adding excessive stresses to the injured tissues and within the precautions outlined by the physician. Underlying movement impairments should be addressed during rehabilitation and functional activities to ensure optimal stresses to the healing tissues.

Impairments

Pain

Be sure to clarify the location, quality, and intensity of the pain.

Stage 1

Surgical: Within the first 2 weeks of the postoperative period, some pain will be associated with exercises. Gradually over the next few weeks, pain associated with the exercise should lessen. Pain can be used as a guide to rehabilitation. Sharp, stabbing pain should be avoided. Mild aching is expected after exercises but should be tolerable for the patient. This postexercise discomfort should decrease within 1 to 2 hours of the rehabilitation. A sudden increase in symptoms or symptoms that last longer than 2 hours after exercise may indicate that the rehabilitation program is too aggressive. Coordinating the use of analgesics with exercise sessions is important.

Acute Injury: Despite discomfort, tests may need to be performed to rule out serious injury. Modalities and taping/bracing may be helpful to decrease pain. The patient may also require the use of an assistive device, walker, or crutches in the early phases of healing.

Stage 2 to 3

Surgical/Acute Injury: Pain associated with the specific tissue that was involved in the surgery should be decreased by weeks 4 to 6. As the activity level of the patient is progressed, the patient may report increased pain or discomfort with new activities such as returning to daily activities and fitness. Pain or discomfort location should be monitored closely. Muscle soreness is expected, similar to the response of muscle to overload stimulus (e.g., weight training). General muscle soreness should be allowed to resolve, usually 1 to 2 days before repeating the bout of activity. Pain described as stabbing should always be avoided.

Edema

Stage 1

Surgical/Acute Injury: Edema is quite common in the foot and ankle s/p surgery or injury. The patient should be educated in use of edema-controlling techniques, such as the following:

- Ice[4]
- Elevation
- Compression: Ace wraps, compression stockings

Patient should be encouraged to keep extremity elevated as much as possible particularly in the early phases (1 to 3 weeks). Application of ice after exercise is recommended. Other methods to control edema in the foot and ankle include electrical stimulation or compression pumps.

Measurement of edema should be taken at each visit. A sudden increase in edema may indicate that the rehabilitation program is too aggressive or the patient possibly has an infection.

Stage 2 to 3

Surgical/Acute Injury: Time until swelling is resolved is variable among patients and surgical procedures. As the patient increases the time spent on their feet in regular daily activities or more weight-bearing exercises, the patient may experience a slight increase in edema. This is to be expected; however, the patient should be encouraged to continue to use techniques stated previously to manage the edema.

Appearance

Stage 1

Surgical: Infections should be suspected if the area around the incision or the involved joint is red, hot, and/or swollen. An increase in drainage from the incision, particularly if it has a foul odor or is no longer a clear color, is also indication of an infection. Red streaks following the lymphatic system can also appear with infection. The physician should be consulted immediately if infection is suspected. It is common to observe bruising after surgery. This should be monitored continuously for any changes; an increase in bruising during the rehabilitation phases may indicate infection. Stitches are typically removed in 7 to 14 days.

Stage 2 to 3

Surgical: Incisions should be well healed. Bruising may still be present for as long as 3 to 4 weeks; however, it should be diminishing. Signs of increased bruising are a red flag and should be immediately referred to the physician.

ROM

Stage 1

Surgical/Acute Injury: To prevent contracture, ROM exercises should begin as soon as possible as allowed by the precautions. In the early phases of rehabilitation, the patient should perform ROM exercises at least three times per day and all exercises should be performed within pain tolerance. All uninvolved lower extremity joints should be exercised to prevent the development of restricted ROM at those joints. The typical exercise progression begins with gentle PROM, assisted AROM, or AROM. The choice between PROM, assisted AROM, and AROM is based in part on the tissue injured or repaired. If resistance is allowed, proprioceptive neuromuscular facilitation (PNF) techniques, such as contract-relax or hold-relax, can assist in achieving greater ROM. During Stage 1, resistance should be very gentle and can be progressed to a submaximum level as the patient tolerates. When performing ROM exercises of the ankle in the patient with a fracture, attention to hand placement during the exercises can minimize the stresses placed on the healing fracture site. Decreasing pain and edema and improving ROM are typical signs that it is safe to progress the exercises. Refer to specific protocols for guidelines regarding progression of the exercises.

The patient may have ROM precautions per the physician. A common example is tendon transfer with no ROM of the ankle.

Mobilizations to the following specific joints may be indicated (see the next section):

- Talocrural joint
- Midtarsal joints
- Tarsometatarsal joints
- Metatarsophalangeal and interphalangeal joints

Stage 2 to 3

Surgical/Acute Injury: Precautions are typically lifted by the time the patient reaches this stage. ROM should be approaching normal. Exercises may need to be progressed using passive force. Patient should be instructed that a stretching discomfort is expected; however, sharp pain should be avoided. Mobilizations may be indicated in later stages of rehabilitation to improve ROM. Consult with the physician before initiating joint mobilization after surgery of the knee.

Decreased Dorsiflexion

- Short gastrocnemius/soleus muscle/calcaneal tendon
  - Wall stretch: The knee is extended for gastrocnemius muscle shortness and flexed for soleus muscle length deficits. The patient should be instructed to keep their foot facing forward or in line with the femur and tibia. The heel should be kept on the ground during the stretch. The patient should prevent subtalar joint pronation through active correction and by wearing good footwear. The stretch should be held for 30 seconds, completed 2 to 3 times/session, and done regularly throughout the day (5 to 8 times/day).
  - Heel hang stretch: The knee can be extended or flexed as described for the wall stretch. The patient should prevent subtalar joint pronation through active correction and by wearing good footwear.
  - Long sitting towel-assisted dorsiflexion: The patient should prevent subtalar joint pronation through active correction and by modifying the direction of force through the towel.
  - A night splint to maintain dorsiflexion position is often helpful.
  - Stretches should be held for 30 seconds, 2 to 3 repetitions, completed regularly throughout the day (5 to 8 times/day), and done 5 to 7 days/week.
- Talocrural joint limitation
  - Mobilize the talocrural joint using a posterior glide of the talus on the ankle mortise.

- Mobilize the talocrural joint using a distraction technique.
- May need to include a heel lift in the shoe until length changes are apparent.

Decreased Plantar Flexion

- Short dorsiflexor muscles
  - Hands and knees rocking back
  - Sustained AROM/PROM
- Talocrural joint limitation
  - Mobilize the talocrural joint using an anterior glide of the talus on the ankle mortise.
  - Mobilize the talocrural joint using a distraction technique.

Decreased Inversion/Eversion

- Subtalar joint limitation
  - Mobilize the subtalar joint using lateral and medial glides.

Decreased Intertarsal Mobility

- Mobilize specific intertarsal joints, primarily using anterior and posterior glides.

Decreased Metatarsophalangeal and Interphalangeal Flexion and Extension

- Mobilize MTP and interphalangeal joints, primarily using anterior (for extension) and posterior (for flexion) glides.

General Range-of-Motion Activities

- Stationary bike.
- Baps board or wobble in sitting when weight-bearing tolerance is limited, progressing to standing activities when weight-bearing tolerance increases.

Muscle Performance

Stage 1

Surgical/Acute Injury: Strengthening often begins after the initial phase of healing (4 weeks). The emphasis should be placed on proper movement patterns in preparation for strengthening activities. After 4 weeks, strengthening may be gradually incorporated. Progression to resistive exercise is based on the patient's ability to perform ROM with a good movement pattern and without increase in pain. Weights, Thera-Band, or isokinetic equipment may be used. Specific exercise protocols provided by physicians and physical therapists should be evaluated to ensure that all exercises are appropriate for the individual's situation. Gastrocnemius/soleus muscles are most commonly affected with surgery or injury to the ankle; however, others may be involved. Electrical stimulation or biofeedback may be used to improve strengthening (see the "Medications, Modalities, and Additional Interventions" section). The patient may have strengthening precautions per the physician.

Stage 2 to 3

Surgical/Acute Injury: After the tissue injury has been protected from excessive stresses and the inflammation has subsided, the involved muscle and tendon should undergo a progressive strengthening program and a progressive return to activity. At this stage, precautions are typically lifted. Strength activities can be progressed as tolerated by the patient. In general, exercise or activity is permissible if pain remains at 2/10 on a 0 to 10 scale. The strengthening exercise should be completed at a minimum of 70% maximum voluntary contraction for 10 repetitions, 3 sets, 3 to 5 times/week.

- Plantarflexors (gastrocnemius, posterior tibialis muscles)
  - Thera-Band resistance exercise into plantarflexion and plantarflexion inversion.
  - Heel raises: This exercise can be started with both feet on the ground with greater weight on the uninvolved side. As strength improves, the patient is instructed to increase weight on the involved extremity with the goal of completing the heel raise with all of the individual's weight on the involved side (single heel raise). The exercise should be performed with good control during the concentric and eccentric portions of the exercise.
  - Bilateral and single-leg hops.
- Anterior tibialis muscle
  - Thera-Band resistance exercise into dorsiflexion inversion: Have the patient curl the toes down if the extensor digitorum and extensor hallucis are dominant.
- Fibular (peroneal) muscles
  - Thera-Band resistance exercise into plantarflexion eversion.
- Intrinsic muscles of the foot
  - Towel crunches: Towel placed on the floor, use the toes to grab the towel, pulling it under the foot. Weight can be added to the towel to increase resistance. The arch should lift; do not allow the patient to only use the flexor digitorum longus.

Proprioception and Balance[5-12]
Stage 1
Surgical/Acute Injury: Activities to improve proprioception of the lower extremity should be incorporated as soon as possible. Begin early in treatment, using activities such as weight shifting, progressive increases in weight-bearing function on the involved lower extremity, and then eventually unilateral stance. As the patient improves, the eyes should be closed to increase the challenge for the lower extremity. As the patient can take full weight on the involved lower extremity, activities are progressed to use of a balance board and closed chained activities such as wall sits and lunges.

Stage 2 to 3
Surgical/Acute Injury: In this stage, precautions are typically lifted. Activities should be progressed to prepare patient to return to daily activities, fitness routines, and work or sporting activities. As the patient progresses, proprioception can be challenged by asking the patient to stand on unstable surfaces (pillows, trampoline, or BOSU ball), perturbations can be applied through having the patient catch a ball being thrown to him or her while standing on one leg. Sliding board activities have been shown to be beneficial to patients after surgery.[13] The prescription regarding frequency and duration of proprioceptive exercise training remains unclear, but research in this area supports a measurable and sustainable change in balance measures with a maximum of 10 weeks of training, 3 to 5 days/week, for 10 to 15 minutes.[6-12]

Cardiovascular and Muscular Endurance
Stage 1
Surgical/Acute Injury: Stationary bicycle riding can be started early in the rehabilitation if the patient's weight-bearing precautions allow. If weight-bearing precautions prohibit riding with the involved extremity, unilateral cycling can be performed with the uninvolved extremity. The involved extremity is supported on a stationary surface, while the patient pedals with the uninvolved extremity. The individual should start with low resistance stationary cycling and as strength improves, resistance should be increased. Water walking and swimming are good substitutes for full weight-bearing activities. For swimming, if kicking against the resistance is contraindicated, the patient may participate in swim drills that mainly challenge the upper extremities for conditioning.

Stage 2 to 3
Surgical/Acute Injury: The patient may be progressed to activities such as water walking, to walking on a treadmill, to an elliptical machine, to a Nordic ski machine, to a StairMaster, and then running and hopping when appropriate. The patient should be given specific instructions in gradual progression of these activities. See the "Work, School, and Higher-Level Activities" section for progression of running.

Patient Education
Stage 1 to 3
Surgical/Acute Injury: Educate the patient in specific medical precautions when indicated.

- Instruct the patient in proper method to don and doff brace if indicated.
- Educate the patient in timeline to return to activity, often driven by physician's guidelines.
- Educate the patient in maintaining precautions during various functional activities (e.g., ambulation, stairs, and transfers).
- Educate the patient in appropriate wound care and monitoring.

Scar and Sensitivity
Stage 1 to 3
Surgical: The gradual application of stress to scars, incisions, or port holes helps the scar remodel. Exercise, massage, compression, silicone gel sheets, and vibration are used in the management of scar. A hypersensitive scar requires desensitization. A dry incision that has been closed and reopens as the result of the stresses applied

with scar massage indicates that the scar massage is too aggressive. Refer to specific guidelines for management of scar for more treatment suggestions. Scars may require desensitization exercises as follows:

- Progress from light touch to more firm touch.
- Progress from soft texture to a rough texture.
- Add additional sensation such as vibration and tapping as tolerated.
- Emphasize weight-bearing and ROM exercises.
- Activity and exercise is better tolerated if heat has been applied (hot pack or exercise in warm whirlpool or pool).

Changes in Status
Stage 1 to 3
Surgical/Acute Injury: Consider carefully reports of increased pain or edema or significant change in ROM, especially in combination. The patient should be questioned regarding precipitating events (e.g., time of onset, activity, and so on). If the integrity of the surgery is in doubt, contact the physician promptly. If the patient has fever and erythema spreading from the incision, the physician should be contacted because of the possibility of infection.

Functional Mobility
Basic Mobility
Stage 1
Surgical/Acute Injury: The patient should be instructed in mobility while following medical precautions.

Sit to Stand: The patient should be instructed in the proper use of assistive device if a device is indicated and performance maintains prescribed weight-bearing precautions.

Ambulation: The patient may have weight-bearing precautions. The patient should be instructed in the proper use of an assistive device and proper gait pattern. Emphasis should be placed on normalizing the patient's gait pattern. If the patient is given partial or toe-touch weight-bearing restrictions, the patient should be instructed in using a heel-to-toe pattern while restricting the amount of weight that is accepted by the lower extremity. The patient should not place his weight on the ball of his foot only.

Stairs: The patient should be instructed in the proper stair ambulation with use of an assistive device (if indicated). In the early phases of healing (s/p surgery or acute injury), the patient should be instructed to use a step-to cadence, lead with the involved lower extremity when descending stairs, and lead with the uninvolved lower extremity when ascending stairs.

Stage 2 and 3
Surgical/Acute Injury:

All Mobility: As weight-bearing precautions are lifted, the patient should be instructed to gradually reduce the level or type of assistive device required. Progression

away from the device depends on the ability of the patient to achieve a normal gait pattern. If the patient demonstrates a significant gait deviation secondary to pain or weakness, the patient should continue to use the device. This may prevent the adaptation of movement impairment and development of pain problems in the future. A progression may be as follows: walker to crutches to one crutch to cane to no assistive device.

Stairs: As the patient progresses through the healing stages and can accept more weight on the involved leg, he or she should be instructed in normal stair ambulation for ascending and descending.

Work, School, and Higher-Level Activities
Stage 1
Surgical/Acute Injury: The patient may be off work or school in the immediate postoperative period or after acute injury. When the patient is cleared to return to work/school, he or she should be instructed in gradual resumption of activities. Emphasis should also be placed on edema control, particularly elevation and compression.

Stage 2 and 3
Surgical/Acute Injury: The patient should be prepared to return to their previous activities. Suggestions for improving proprioception and balance are provided in a previous section. In preparation for the return to sports, sport-specific activities should be added. The initial phases of these activities will include straight plane activities at a slow pace and then gradually increase the level of difficulty. The following sections are examples of activity progression:

Agility Exercises: Emphasis is placed on proper form.

- Hopping timed: Within each level, begin with short bouts of hopping and longer rests between (15 seconds on, 30 seconds off), then increase on time and decrease off time (30 seconds on, 15 seconds off).
- Hopping bilateral lower extremities with support of the upper extremities to decrease the amount of stress through the knee.
- Hopping bilateral lower extremities without support.
- Hopping bilateral lower extremities in different directions: Side-to-side, back and forth, box, V, and zigzag hopping.
- Progress to same activities with unilateral lower extremities.
- Jumping from short surface (2 inches). Emphasis should be placed on landing on both feet evenly, knees flexed, and with neutral knees over toes (avoid excessive valgus or femoral medial rotation). The patient should also think about landing softly to help absorb the landing.[5,14]
- Jump forward, backward, and off to each side.
- Progress by increasing the height of the surface.
- Jumping up on to surface: Begin with shorter surface and increase height when appropriate.
- Other plyometrics: Ladder drills.

Running: Early in the phases of running, the emphasis is placed on achieving an ideal gait pattern; speed or distance should not be emphasized. Assess gait pattern and instruct as appropriate. Cues are often needed to achieve a heel-toe gait pattern. The patient should run on even and soft surfaces initially. It is expected that the patient may experience some generalized discomfort or swelling with the initiation of running. If this generalized pain and swelling persists longer than 48 hours, then the running must be decreased. If the patient describes a stabbing pain or a pain that is consistent with tissue injury, running should be stopped and the patient reevaluated.

- Patient should be able to walk 30 minutes without an increase in pain or swelling to begin.
- Run 1: Walk 4 minutes, run 1 minute, repeat 4 times for 20 minutes.
- Rest day.
- Run 2: Walk 3 minutes, run 2 minutes, repeat 4 times for 20 minutes.
- Rest day.
- Run 3: Walk 2 minutes, run 3 minutes, repeat 4 times for 20 minutes.
- Continue to progress running appropriately. This example will not be appropriate for all patients and must be adjusted as needed.

Once the patient can run 1 mile without increasing pain or swelling, begin with other running drills such as the following:

- Figure 8 running, beginning with a large "8," then decreasing the size of the "8" gradually.
- Zigzag running with soft cuts, hard cuts, cut and spin: Care should be taken to evaluate how the patient chooses to cut. Often (particularly in non-contact injuries), you will note that the patient has adopted in inefficient cutting pattern such as planting the left foot when trying to cut to the left.

Drills: Once the patient can complete cutting drills without pain or swelling and demonstrates good control of the lower extremity, variations can be added such as the following:

- Drills with sport-specific equipment (e.g., basketball, hockey stick, soccer ball)
- Partner drills

Special notes: If plyometrics and strengthening are to be performed during the same visit, plyometrics should be performed before the strengthening activities.[5]

Functional testing: Consider functional tests before the patient's return to sport. There are many functional tests available. The validity of these tests is controversial; however, each test can offer some insight to how the patient may perform in their specific sport. It is recommended that a battery of tests be used to assess the aspects of balance, coordination, agility, and strength. Common test items for the ankle/foot include the following:

- Single-leg hop for distance[15]
- Triple-leg hop for distance[15]
- 6-Meter hop for time[15,16]
- Crossover hop for distance[15]
- 6-Meter shuttle run[17,18]
- Vertical jump[19,20]
- Lateral step[21]

Sleeping
Stage 1 to 3
Surgical/Acute Injury: Sleeping is often disrupted in the immediate postoperative period or after acute injury. The lower extremity should be slightly elevated (foot higher than the knee and knee higher than the hip) to minimize edema.

Support
Stage 1
Surgical: A brace may be used to protect the surgical site, depending on the procedure or type of fracture. A brace should fit comfortably. The patient should be educated in the timeline for wearing the brace. Refer to specific protocol or consult with physician if the wearing time is not clear.

Stage 2 to 3
Surgical: The recommendations concerning the need for bracing long term are varied. Communication among the team (patient, physician, and physical therapist) is necessary. Functional bracing is recommended if the patient wishes to return to high level sporting activities and demonstrates either laxity in the joint and/or performs poorly on functional tests.

Medications, Modalities, and Additional Interventions
Medications
Surgical: During the acute stage, physical therapy treatments should be timed with analgesics, typically 30 minutes after administration of oral medication. If medication is given intravenously, therapy often can occur immediately after administration. Communication with nurses and physicians is critical to provide optimal pain relief for the patient.

Acute Injury: The patient's medications should be reviewed to ensure that the patient is taking the medications appropriately.

Modalities: Thermal
Surgical/Acute Injury: Instruct the patient in proper home use of thermal modalities to decrease pain. Ice has been shown to be beneficial, particularly in the immediate postoperative phases.[22]

Electrical Stimulation
Stage 1 to 3
Surgical/Acute Injury: Electrical stimulation can be used for three purposes: Pain relief, edema control, and strengthening. Interferential current has been shown to be helpful in decreasing pain and edema.[23-25] Sensory level transcutaneous electrical stimulation (TENS) can assist in decreasing pain.

Currently, there is no definitive answer for the use of electrical stimulation for gastrocnemius/soleus muscle strengthening. It was once believed that electrical stimulation did not provide a distinct advantage over high-intensity exercise training.[26,27] However, more recent studies support the use of stimulation to improve motor recruitment and strength.[27-30] When strengthening the gastrocnemius/soleus muscles, portable units may not provide adequate stimulation and wall units are preferred; however, recent advances have produced more efficient portable units.

Be sure to check for contraindications. Avoid areas where metal is in close approximation of the skin.

Aquatic Therapy

Surgical/Acute Injury: Aquatic therapy to decrease weight bearing during ambulation may be helpful in the rehabilitation of patients after fracture or surgical procedures. Often, this medium is not available but should be considered if the patient's progress is slowed secondary to pain or the patient has difficulty maintaining weight-bearing precautions. Incisions must be healed before aquatic therapy is initiated.

Discharge Planning: Equipment

Stage 1

Surgical: Equipment that may be needed depends on the patient's abilities, precautions, and home environment.

- Assistive device: Walker, crutches, or cane
- Reacher
- Tub bench and hand-held shower

Discharge Planning: Therapy

Assess the need for physical therapy after discharge from an acute stay at a skilled nursing or rehabilitation facility, or if the patient has been discharged from a home health program or outpatient physical therapy.

After the acute phase of recovery, the patient should be reassessed to determine whether a movement impairment diagnosis exists. The patient should be given documentation for consistency of care. Documentation should include the following:

- Physician protocol, including precautions and progression of activities
- Progress of patient during physical therapist's care
- Expected outcomes

Proximal Tibiofibular Glide Syndrome

The principal movement impairment in proximal tibiofibular glide syndrome is posterior or superior motion of the fibula on the tibia during active hamstring contraction (especially during running). The principal positional impairment is the fibula located anterior, posterior, superior, or inferior to the normal position on the tibia after trauma, particularly an ankle sprain.

Symptoms and History

- Pain in posterolateral or lateral aspect of tibiofibular joint often associated with running or a history of lateral ankle sprains
- Numbness in the lateral/anterolateral knee and/or leg

Common Referring Diagnoses

- Knee pain
- Hamstring tendinopathy
- Fibular (lateral) collateral ligament sprain
- Posterolateral corner injury
- Entrapment of superficial fibular nerve

Key Tests and Signs for Movement Impairment

Alignment Analysis

- Palpation of the fibula location on tibia, relative to uninvolved side reveals malalignment (anterior, posterior, and/or superior).
  - A glide in the direction of the positional or movement impairment increases pain.
  - A glide in the opposite direction of the positional or movement impairment decreases symptoms.

Movement Impairment Analysis
Sitting

- Resisted hamstring contraction increases pain at the tibiofibular joint.
  - Manual stabilization of tibiofibular joint during hamstring contraction decreases pain.

Muscle Length/Joint ROM Impairments

- Positioning of limb at end-range of hamstrings muscle length (single-leg raise position of sitting knee extension) increases symptoms.

Source of Signs and Symptoms

Proximal Tibiofibular Joint Symptoms

- Palpation reveals local tenderness at the joint

Common Fibular (Peroneal) Nerve Symptoms

- Positive Tinel's test

Associated Signs or Contributing Factors

Muscle Length/Joint ROM Impairments

- Based on length or ROM tests

Talocrural Dorsiflexion

- Limited if dorsiflexion <10 degrees with knee extended
  - Gastrocnemius muscle short if dorsiflexion ≥10 degrees with knee flexed
  - Soleus muscle short if dorsiflexion ≤10 degrees with knee flexed and normal accessory talocrural motion
  - Talocrural joint limitation if dorsiflexion ≤10 degrees, regardless of knee position and limited accessory talocrural joint motion (cannot rule out soleus muscle length limitation in this case)

Hamstring Muscle Length

- Knee extension limited >20 degrees from full extension

Differential Diagnosis

Movement Diagnosis

- Hip extension with knee extension
- Hip extension with medial rotation
- Tibiofemoral rotation
- Knee extension

Potential Diagnosis Requiring Referral Suggested by Signs and Symptoms

Musculoskeletal

- L3-L5 radiculopathy
- Meniscal injury
- Fibular (lateral) collateral ligament sprain
- Posterolateral corner injury
- Fracture

Neurological

- Fibular nerve compression palsy

Treatment
Inflammation and Pain Control
- Ice
- Iontophoresis
- Electrical stimulation

Walking and/or Running
- Walking and running cues focus on using proximal hip extensors and lateral rotator (gluteus maximus, gluteus medius, and intrinsic hip lateral rotators) to assist with controlling hip motion and decreasing use of lateral hamstrings.

Muscle Performance
- Gluteus maximus
  - Prone hip extension with the knee flexed.
  - Positioning: Patient's that have short hip flexors will require a pillow under the pelvis. Patient must be able to control the tibial positioning during prone knee flexion to begin this exercise.
  - Lunges, squats.
- Intrinsic hip lateral rotators and posterior gluteus medius (if indicated)
  - Prone hip lateral rotation isometrics (prone foot pushes)
  - Prone hip abduction
  - Sidelying hip abduction with lateral rotation (level 1, 2, or 3)

Monitor that patient feels the contraction in the "seat" region; the therapist must palpate to be sure that the patient is recruiting the correct muscles. Common cues for improve performance of the hip lateral rotators include the following:
  - Positioning: The pelvis may be rotated posteriorly too far. Ask the patient to roll the pelvis anteriorly.
  - Positioning: Place a pillow between the knees.
  - Spin the thigh around an axis longitudinally through the femur.
  - Weight shifting with gluteal squeeze on the stance lower extremity; progress to standing on one leg with correct alignment; progress to resisted activities of the opposite leg while standing on the affected leg.
  - Lunges: Resisted; using Thera-Band around proximal thigh, the therapist pulls in the direction of medial rotation and adduction.

After the tissue injury has been protected from excessive stresses and the inflammation has subsided, the involved muscle and tendon should undergo a progressive strengthening program and a progressive return to activity. In general, exercise or activity is permissible if pain remains at 2/10 on a 0 to 10 scale. The strengthening exercise should be completed at a minimum of 70% maximum voluntary contraction for 10 repetitions, 3 sets, 3 to 5 times/week.

Decreased Dorsiflexion
- Short gastrocnemius/soleus muscle/calcaneal tendon
  - Wall stretch: The knee is extended for gastrocnemius muscle shortness and flexed for soleus muscle length deficits. The patient should be instructed to keep their foot facing forward or in line with the femur and tibia. The heel should be kept on the ground during the stretch. The patient should prevent subtalar joint pronation through active patient correction and by wearing good footwear. The stretch should be held for 30 seconds, completed 2 to 3 times/session, and done regularly throughout the day (5 to 8 times/day).
  - Heel hang stretch: The knee can be extended or flexed as described for the wall stretch. The patient should prevent subtalar joint pronation through active correction and by wearing good footwear.
  - Long sitting towel-assisted dorsiflexion. The patient should prevent subtalar joint pronation through active correction and by modifying the direction of force through the towel.
  - A night splint to maintain dorsiflexion position is often helpful.
  - Stretches should be held for 30 seconds, 2 to 3 repetitions, completed regularly throughout the day (5 to 8 times/day), and done 5 to 7 days/week.
- Talocrural joint limitation
  - Mobilize the talocrural joint using a posterior glide of the talus on the ankle mortise.
  - Mobilize the talocrural joint using a distraction technique.
  - May need to include a heel lift in the shoe until length changes are apparent.

Decreased Hamstring Muscle Length
- Hamstrings
  - Active sitting knee extension with dorsiflexion with hip in neutral rotation.

Positional Fault
- Mobilization/manipulation of the fibula on the tibia as indicated by evaluation findings.
  - The choice of which grade of movement to choose depends on how much shortening has occurred to the associated joint structures. Chronic conditions typically have shortening of the tissues surrounding the joint. Thus chronic conditions usually respond to prolonged stretching (creep) of the tissues gained with grade IV oscillations, primarily ending with grade III oscillations to ease the joint gently out of the grade IV stretching that was just performed.
- Acute conditions are not likely to have shortening of surrounding tissues and often are too painful to be mobilized back and forth. Rather, a high-velocity movement is much less painful and corrects the fault.

External Tissue Support
Orthoses/Taping
- Potential to develop a taping strategy to attempt to immobilize or limit motion between the proximal tibia and fibula

REFERENCES

1. Mueller MJ, Maluf KS: Tissue adaptations to physical stress: a proposed "Physical Stress Theory" to guide physical therapist practice, education and research, *Phys Ther* 82(4):383-403, 2002.
2. Kaeding CC, Yu JR, Wright R, et al: Management and return to play of stress fractures, *Clin J Sport Med* 15(6):442-447, 2005.
3. Boytim MJ, Fischer DA, Neumann L: Syndesmotic ankle sprains, *Am J Sports Med* 19(3):294-298, 1991.
4. Lessard L, Scudds R, Amendola A, et al: The efficacy of cryotherapy following arthroscopic knee surgery, *J Orthop Sports Phys Ther* 26(1):14-22, 1997.
5. Hewett TE, Paterno MV, Myer GD: Strategies for enhancing proprioception and neuromuscular control of the knee, *Clin Orthop* 1(402):76-94, 2002.
6. Tropp H, Askling C, Gillquist J: Prevention of ankle sprains, *Am J Sports Med* 13(4):259-262, 1985.
7. Bernier JN, Perrin DH: Effect of coordination training on proprioception of the functionally unstable ankle, *J Orthop Sports Phys Ther* 27(4):264-275, 1998.
8. Wester JU, Jespersen SM, Nielsen KD, et al: Wobble board training after partial sprains of the lateral ligaments of the ankle: a prospective randomized study, *J Orthop Sports Phys Ther* 23(5):332-336, 1996.
9. Rozzi SL, Lephart SM, Sterner R, et al: Balance training for persons with functionally unstable ankles, *J Orthop Sports Phys Ther* 29(8):478-486, 1999.
10. Eils E, Rosenbaum D: A multi-station proprioceptive exercise program in patients with ankle instability, *Med Sci Sports Exerc* 33(12):1991-1998, 2001.
11. Osborne MD, Chou LS, Laskowski ER, et al: The effect of ankle disk training on muscle reaction time in subjects with a history of ankle sprain, *Am J Sports Med* 29(5):627-632, 2001.
12. Matsusaka N, Yokoyama S, Tsurusaki T, et al: Effect of ankle disk training combined with tactile stimulation to the leg and foot on functional instability of the ankle, *Am J Sports Med* 29(1):25-30, 2001.
13. Blanpied P, Carroll R, Douglas T, et al: Effectiveness of lateral slide exercise in an anterior cruciate ligament reconstruction rehabilitation home exercise program, *Phys Ther* 30(10):609-611, 2000.
14. Hewett TE, Lindenfeld TN, Riccobene JV, et al: The effect of neuromuscular training on the incidence of knee injury in female athletes. A prospective study, *Am J Sports Med* 27(6):699-706, 1999.
15. Ross MD, Langford B, Whelan PJ: Test-retest reliability of 4 single-leg horizontal hop tests, *J Strength Cond Res* 16(4):617-622, 2002.
16. Bolgla LA, Keskula DR: Reliability of lower extremity functional performance tests, *J Orthop Sports Phys Ther* 26(3):138-142, 1997.
17. Demeritt KM, Shultz SJ, Docherty CL, et al: Chronic ankle instability does not affect lower extremity functional performance, *J Athl Train* 37(4):507-511, 2002.
18. Nadler SF, Malanga GA, Feinberg JH, et al: Functional performance deficits in athletes with previous lower extremity injury, *Clin J Sport Med* 12(2):73-78, 2002.
19. Petschnig R, Baron R, Albrecht M: The relationship between isokinetic quadriceps strength test and hop tests for distance and one-legged vertical jump test following anterior cruciate ligament reconstruction, *J Orthop Sports Phys Ther* 28(1):23-31, 1998.
20. Blackburn JR, Morrissey MC: The relationship between open and closed kinetic chain strength of the lower limb and jumping performance, *J Orthop Sports Phys Ther* 27(6):430-435, 1998.
21. Ross M: Test-retest reliability of the lateral step-up test in young adult healthy subjects, *J Orthop Sports Phys Ther* 25(2):128-132, 1997.
22. Lessard L, Scudds R, Amendola A, et al: The efficacy of cryotherapy following arthroscopic knee surgery, *J Orthop Sports Phys Ther* 26(1):14-22, 1997.
23. Christie AD, Willoughby GL: The effect of interferential therapy on swelling following open reduction and internal fixation of ankle fractures, *Physiother Theory Pract* 6:3-7, 1990.
24. Johnson MI, Wilson H: The analgesic effects of different swing patterns of interferential currents on cold-induced pain, *Physiotherapy* 83:461-467, 1997.
25. Young SL, Woodbury MG, Fryday-Field K: Efficacy of interferential current stimulation alone for pain reduction in patients with osteoarthritis of the knee: a randomized placebo control clinical trial, *Phys Ther* 71(Suppl):252, 1991.
26. Lieber RL, Silva PD, Daniel DM: Equal effectiveness of electrical and volitional strength training for quadriceps femoris muscles after anterior cruciate ligament surgery, *J Orthop Res* 14(1):131-138, 1996.
27. Van Swearingen J: Electrical stimulation for improving muscle performance. In Nelson RM, Hayes KW, Currier DP, eds: *Clinical electrotherapy*, Stamford, CT, 1999, Appleton & Lange.
28. Delitto A, Rose SJ, Lehman RC, et al: Electrical stimulation versus voluntary exercise in strengthening the thigh musculature after anterior cruciate ligament surgery, *Phys Ther* 68:660-663, 1988.
29. Stevens JE, Mizner RL, Snyder-Mackler L: Neuromuscular electrical stimulation for quadriceps muscle strengthening after bilateral total knee arthroplasty: a case series, *J Orthop Sports Phys Ther* 34(1):21-29, 2004.
30. Fitzgerald GK, Piva SR, Irrgang JJ: A modified neuromuscular electrical stimulation protocol for quadriceps strength training following anterior cruciate ligament reconstruction, *J Orthop Sports Phys Ther* 33(9):492-501, 2003.

Index

Page numbers followed by *f* indicate figures; *t*, tables; *b*, boxes.

Gluteus maximus muscle
  and Kext syndrome treatment, 423
  and Khext syndrome treatment,
      426-427
  and pronation syndrome performance,
      455
  and proximal tibiofibular glide
      syndrome, 508
  and TFHypo syndrome treatment, 417
  and TFR syndrome treatment, 411
Gluteus medius muscle
  and Khext syndrome treatment, 426
Gluteus medius muscle, posterior, 366
  pronation syndrome performance and,
      455
  TFHypo syndrome treatment and,
      417
  TFR syndrome treatment and, 411
Golfer's elbow. *See* Wrist flexion with
      forearm pronation syndrome
Gout, 449
Grasping, thenar muscles and, 201
Gravity
  cycling and, 12
  muscular adaptations and, 53
  muscular recruitment pattern and, 6
  wrist flexion and, 175
Grip dynamometer
  wrist extension with forearm pronation
      syndrome and, 301
Grip, cylindrical
  ED joint stabilization and, 199
  flexion movements and, 199
  FPL activity and, 202
  hypothenar muscles and, 202
  lumbricals and, 200
Gripping objects
  and active finger extension, 198
  and finger flexion syndrome, 226-227
  and finger flexion syndrome with
      rotation, 229
  and first web space stretching, 260
  and hand/wrist functional activities,
      195, 196f
  and hypothenar muscles, 202
  and insufficient flexion in finger/
      thumb syndrome, 203
  and insufficient thumb palmar
      abduction/opposition syndrome,
      218
  and intrinsic plus type grip, 195, 196f
  and radial tunnel syndrome treatment,
      340
  and wrist muscles, 197
Gripping, end-range power, 200

H

Hamstring contraction, resisted, 478
Hamstring muscle
  and imprecise movement, 28-29
  and improved extensibility exercise,
      412
  and Khext syndrome treatment, 427
  and knee flexors, 363, 368f
  and length assessment, 15-16, 16f-17f
  and proximal tibiofibular glide
      syndrome, 478, 508
  and short muscle, 15

Hamstring muscle (*Continued*)
  and stiffness/flexibility, 15-23, 16f-17f
  and stretching exercises, 397
  and TFHypo syndrome treatment,
      385, 397f, 418
  and TFR syndrome treatment, 410
Hand. *See also* Hand and wrist movement
      systems; Movement system
      syndromes
  dysfunction of, 165
    physical therapist guide and, 202
  key treatment elements of, 167
  movement system syndrome of
    finger flexion syndrome of, 226-227
    finger flexion syndrome without
        rotation, 229-231
    finger flexion syndrome with
        rotation of, 227-229
    insufficient finger/thumb extension
        syndrome of, 216
    insufficient finger/thumb flexion
        syndrome of, 203-216
    insufficient thumb palmar
        abduction/opposition syndrome
        of, 216-220
    introduction to, 202-232
    source or regional impairment of
        hand and, 231-232, 270-271,
        270t-271t
    thumb carpometacarpal accessory
        hypermobility syndrome of,
        220-226
  numbness/tingling in, 305
  source/regional impairment of,
      231-232, 232b-233b, 270-271,
      270t-271t
  therapy for, 165-166
  treatment guidelines for, 272
  weights for, 20-21
Hand and wrist functional activities
  computer use and, 193-195, 194f-195f
  gripping objects and, 195, 196f
  lifting and, 195
  manual therapy and, 197f
  playing an instrument and, 195-196
  reading and, 195, 196f-197f
  sleeping and, 195, 196f
  writing and, 193, 193f-194f
Hand and wrist movement system
      syndrome
  alignment of, 168-176
    impaired alignment of, 170-176
    normal standing alignment of,
        169-170
  conclusion for, 232
  examination and key tests for, 168
    objective examination and, 168
    subjective examination and, 168
  functional activities of, 192-202
    subjective examination of, 192-196
  introduction to, 165-167, 166b
  movement system diagnosis for wrist
      and, 232
  muscular actions of, 197
    extrinsic muscles of fingers and,
        198-200
    extrinsic muscles of thumb and,
        201-202

Hand and wrist movement system
      syndrome (*Continued*)
  hypothenar muscles and, 202
  intrinsic muscles of fingers and,
      200-201
  muscles of the wrist and, 197-198
  thenar muscles and, 201
  normal motions of, 176-192
    finger motions of, 176-184
    thumb motions of, 184
    wrist motions of, 176
  ROM assessment for, 184-192
  syndromes of the hand and, 202-232
  treatment guidelines for, 232b-233b
Hand and wrist muscular action
  finger extrinsic muscles and, 198-200
    finger extensors and, 198-199
    finger flexors and, 199-200
  finger intrinsic muscles and, 200-201
  hypothenor muscles and, 202
  muscles of the wrist and, 197-198
  thenar muscles and, 201
  thumb extrinsic muscles and, 201-202
Hand impairment
  treatment guidelines for, 272
    activity limitations/participation
        restrictions and, 274-275
      general guidelines for, 274
      specific suggestions for, 274-275
    body functions/structures and,
        272-274, 275t
      appearance and, 272
      cardiovascular/muscular
          endurance and, 273-274
      change in status and, 274
      coordination and, 273
      edema and, 272
      pain and, 272
      patient education and, 274
      ROM and, 273
      scar and, 272
      strength and, 273
    medications/modalities for, 275-276
      electrical stimulation and, 275
      paraffin/hot pack and, 275
      whirlpool treatment and, 275
    moderators of, 272
Headache, cervicogenic, 54
Headache, chronic tension, 53
Headache, suboccipital, 58
Healing, physical stress and, 36
Health care, trends in, 32
Hearing, cervical alignment and, 53
Heat
  and elbow hypomobility syndrome,
      304
    treatment for, 324
  and hypomobility syndrome, 496-497
  and tissue extensibility, 43
Heat, moist
  for insufficient finger/thumb extension
      syndrome
    caused by extensor tendon adhesion,
        252
    caused by flexor tendon adhesions/
        shortness, 252
  for insufficient finger/thumb flexion
      syndrome, 244